Anesthesia for
CARDIAC SURGERY

second edition

James A. DiNardo, MD, FAAP
Associate Professor of Clinical Anesthesiology
Director, Cardiothoracic Anesthesiology
University of Arizona Health Sciences Center
Tucson, Arizona

Appleton & Lange
Stamford, Connecticut

Notice: The authors and the publisher of this volume have taken care to make certain that the doses of drugs and schedules of treatment are correct and compatible with the standards generally accepted at the time of publication. Nevertheless, as new information becomes available, changes in treatment and in the use of drugs become necessary. The reader is advised to carefully consult the instruction and information material included in the package insert of each drug or therapeutic agent before administration. This advice is especially important when using, administering, or recommending new or infrequently used drugs. The authors and publisher disclaim all responsibility for any liability, loss, injury, or damage incurred as a consequence, directly or indirectly, of the use and application of any of the contents of this volume.

Prentice Hall International (UK) Limited, *London*
Prentice Hall of Australia Pty. Limited, *Sydney*
Prentice Hall Canada, Inc., *Toronto*
Prentice Hall Hispanoamericana, S.A., *Mexico*
Prentice Hall of India Private Limited, *New Delhi*
Prentice Hall of Japan, Inc., *Tokyo*
Simon & Schuster Asia Pte. Ltd., *Singapore*
Editora Prentice Hall do Brasil Ltda., *Rio de Janeiro*
Prentice Hall, *Upper Saddle River, New Jersey*

Library of Congress Cataloging-in-Publication Data

DiNardo, James A.
    Anesthesia for cardiac surgery / James A. DiNardo. — 2nd ed.
      p. cm.
    Includes bibliographical references and index.
    ISBN 0-8385-0253-9 (case : alk. paper)
    1. Anesthesia in cardiology. 2. Heart—Surgery. I. Title.
    [DNLM: 1. Heart Surgery. 2. Anesthesia.   WG 169 D583a 1998]
RD87.3.H43D5   1998
617.9′67412—dc21
DNLM/DLC
for Library of Congress   97-8137
                                 CIP

ISBN 0-8385-0253-9

9 780838 502532
90000

Acquisitions Editor: Michael P. Medina
Production Service: York Production Services
Cover Design: Libby Schmitz

PRINTED IN THE UNITED STATES OF AMERICA

Contents

iii

Contributors

Brian J. Cammarata, MD
Instructor, Clinical Anesthesiology
Department of Anesthesiology
University of Arizona Health Sciences Center
Tucson, Arizona

James A. DiNardo, MD, FAAP
Associate Professor of Clinical Anesthesiology
Director, Cardiothoracic Anesthesiology
University of Arizona Health Sciences Center
Tucson, Arizona

Bradley J. Hindman, MD
Associate Professor, Vice-Chairman for Research
Department of Anesthesia
University of Iowa, College of Medicine
Iowa City, Iowa

Introduction

Anesthesia for cardiac surgery requires that the anesthesiologist possess much of the knowledge conventionally within the domain of the cardiologist and cardiac surgeon. This book is written with the goal of providing the background information and approach necessary for the sophisticated, informed evaluation and management of patients undergoing cardiac surgery. The impetus for writing this book came from the desire to provide textual material for anesthesia residents, fellows, and attending anesthesiologists that integrated an overall conceptual framework for the anesthetic management of cardiac surgical patients with the specific anesthetic considerations each condition presented. This book is an attempt to provide the more experienced reader with timely reviews of the current literature, together with conceptual structures and detailed management recommendations for those individuals who do not care for cardiac surgical patients on a daily basis. The hope is that many will find this book useful: not only anesthesia residents and cardiac anesthesia fellows, but also attending anesthesiologists, intensivists, surgeons, perfusionists, and nurses. Readers are strongly encouraged to evaluate the suggestions herein in light of their own experience, recognizing that practices vary among surgeons, cardiologists, and institutions, as well as among anesthesiologists. I have endeavored to be as accurate and complete as possible, and take full responsibility for any errors and omissions.

Where appropriate, chapters are organized to review the relevant physiology; to outline the specific goals toward which the anesthetic plan is oriented; and to describe a specific anesthetic plan, from preoperative preparations, through induction and maintenance of anesthesia, and ending with postbypass management.

Chapter 1 describes the preoperative evaluation of the "rest of the patient," detailing specific management suggestions for associated, noncardiac illnesses that may be present. It is placed as the first chapter to emphasize the uniqueness of each patient and the necessity of integrating all of the clinical information available to tailor the most effective anesthetic possible.

Chapter 2 describes in detail the data available from a cardiac catheterization and how the data are obtained. Interpretation of these data for both acquired and congenital lesions is discussed. The application of these interpreted data to the anesthetic plan is discussed in the chapter on that lesion.

Chapter 3 provides an overview of the monitoring techniques commonly used during cardiac surgery. A detailed discussion of the advantages, limitations, and pitfalls in interpretation of pulmonary artery pressure measurements is presented. The uses and limitations of right ventricular ejection fraction, continuous cardiac output, and mixed venous oxygenation saturation pulmonary artery catheters also are discussed. Thromboelastography is reviewed and guidelines to its interpretation are presented.

An extensive section on transesophageal echocardiography (TEE) in both children and adults is presented. The chapter provides a comprehensive review of the TEE views obtainable with single-plane, biplane, and multiplane probes. In addition, practical guidelines to the use of continuous wave, pulsed wave, and color flow Doppler imaging are included. Emphasis is placed on obtaining the appropriate TEE views to answer specific questions. The TEE observations and measurements that should be made during a comprehensive examination are outlined in detail. In addition, the TEE findings encountered in various pathologic states are presented, along with the interpretation of these findings. Relevant TEE findings also are discussed in the other chapters on specific lesions and procedures.

Chapter 4 unites a discussion of the physiology of coronary perfusion and the pathophysiology of coronary stenoses with detailed recommendations for the management of patients presenting for coronary revascularization both electively and emergently. The prevalence, diagnosis, treatment, and consequences of myocardial ischemia are covered in detail. The modifications of anesthetic technique necessary to provide "fast-track" care are reviewed as well.

Chapter 5 provides a conceptual framework in which to evaluate any valvular lesion. This framework is then used to identify the pathophysiological processes that guide anesthetic management decisions in the pre- and postcardiopulmonary bypass periods.

Chapter 6 provides a conceptual framework in which to evaluate any congenital heart lesion. This includes construction of the "box heart," an exercise that provides a visual image of each congenital lesion based on preoperative catheterization and echocardiographic data consolidated with physiologic principles. The pre- and postcardiopulmonary bypass management of a number of simple and complex congenital cardiac lesions is presented in the context of the conceptual framework. The implications of the various palliative and corrective surgical options available for each lesion are discussed as well.

Chapter 7 provides a comprehensive overview of the disease states that lead to consideration for heart, heart–lung, and lung transplantation. Both orthotopic and heterotopic heart transplantations are discussed. Similarly, double-lung, bilateral single-lung, and single-lung transplantations are covered. The pre- and postcardiopulmonary bypass management of these patients for each of these procedures is covered in detail. The anesthetic management of patients with heart, heart–lung, or lung transplants for subsequent surgical procedures also is covered.

Chapter 8 covers the physiology of the normal and diseased pericardium, followed by a review of the disease states that alter pericardial function. The integration of pericardial and extracardiac manifestations of each disease state provides a practical approach to management of these patients.

Chapter 9 provides an organized approach to management of patients with lesions of the thoracic aorta for both emergent and elective surgical repair. In addition, the management of cardiopulmonary bypass and other circulatory support methods used in conjunction with repair of thoracic aortic lesions is discussed in detail.

Chapter 10 provides a thorough overview of the components of the cardiopulmonary bypass circuit as it applies to both children and adults. Routine initiation, maintenance, and termination of cardiopulmonary bypass is discussed, along with management of problems encountered during cardiopulmonary bypass. Current areas of controversy, including acid–base management, normothermic cardiopulmonary bypass, and hypothermic circulatory arrest, are reviewed. Management of coagulation abnormalities after cardiopulmonary bypass is covered in detail with specific emphasis on the renewed interest in antifibrinolytic agents, including aprotinin.

Chapter 11 is an overview of the currently available mechanical circulatory assist devices ranging from the intra-aortic balloon pump to the total artifical heart. The function and appropriate applications of each device is covered. Guidelines for management of patients needing a device and patients with a device in place are provided.

Chapter 12 reviews, in depth, the theory and practical application of myocardial preservation techniques during cardiac surgery.

Chapter 13 provides a state-of-the-art review of the effects of the various aspects of cardiac surgery and cardiopulmonary bypass on the central nervous system. Specific recommendations based on currently available information are given.

This work is an extension of the tremendous satisfaction that comes from working with enthusiastic, inquisitive residents, dedicated faculty, and caring, proficient cardiac surgeons. I am grateful to my wife, Mary Ann, for her infinite patience and unflagging support throughout this project and to Michael Medina at Appleton & Lange for his guidance, understanding, and support.

James A. DiNardo, MD, FAAP

Preoperative Assessment

James A. DiNardo

It goes without saying that for all patients undergoing cardiac surgery, a comprehensive evaluation of the cardiovascular system is required. However, these patients may have coexisting diseases that have contributed to the development of cardiac dysfunction. Furthermore, organ dysfunction may develop as the result of cardiac dysfunction. It is therefore important for cardiac surgical patients to undergo a comprehensive, multisystem preoperative evaluation. Many patients will have undergone a comprehensive screening before being seen by the anesthesiologist. Others will require additional tests after preoperative evaluation by the anesthesiologist. The cardiac anesthesiologist must be capable of conducting a comprehensive preoperative evaluation and should be familiar with the methodology, limitations, and accuracy of the tests used most commonly in evaluation of cardiac surgical patients.

■ ENDOCRINE EVALUATION

A careful evaluation for endocrine abnormalities should be sought in the history and physical examination. Diabetes mellitus and hypothyroidism deserve special consideration.

Diabetes Mellitus (DM)

Diabetes mellitus (DM) is a risk factor for development of coronary artery disease; therefore, perioperative management of DM is a common problem facing those who anesthetize patients for cardiac surgery. Recall that patients with insulin-dependent diabetes have reduced or absent insulin production due to destruction of pancreatic beta cells. Patients with non-insulin-dependent diabetes have normal or supranormal production of insulin but suffer from insulin resistance. This resistance may be due to a reduction in insulin receptors, a defect in the second messenger once insulin binds to receptors, or both. Patients with non-insulin-dependent diabetes may be managed with diet, oral hypoglycemic agents (agents that increase pancreatic insulin production), or exogenous insulin. Patients with insulin-dependent diabetes, on the other hand, must receive exogenous insulin.

Cardiopulmonary bypass (CPB) is associated with changes in glucose and insulin homeostasis in both diabetic and nondiabetic patients. During normothermic CPB, elevations in glucagon, cortisol, growth hormone, and catecholamine levels produce hyperglycemia through increased hepatic glucose production, reduced peripheral use of glucose, and reduced insulin production.[1,2] During hypothermic CPB, hepatic glucose production is reduced and insulin production remains low, such that blood glucose levels remain relatively constant.[1] Rewarming on CPB also is associated with increases in glucagon, cortisol, growth hormone, and catecholamine levels and is accompanied by enhanced hepatic production of glucose, enhanced insulin production, and insulin resistance.[1,3] The transfusion of blood preserved with acid-citrate-dextrose, the use of glucose solutions in the CPB prime, and the use of beta-adrenergic agents for inotropic support, further increase exogenous insulin requirements.[1,3,4] For nondiabetic patients, these hormonally mediated changes usually result in mild hyperglycemia.[2,4] For diabetic patients, these changes may produce significant hyperglycemia and ketoacidosis.[2]

Because of the varying insulin requirements during cardiac surgery and the unreliable absorption of subcutaneously administered insulin in patients undergoing large changes in body temperature and peripheral perfusion, insulin is best delivered intravenously for patients undergoing cardiac surgery. Perioperative management of blood glucose levels during cardiac surgical procedures has been accomplished with the use of both open[3] and closed-loop[3,5] insulin infusions in adults. Closed-loop systems require a system capable of measuring blood glucose levels and making appropriate adjustments in the insulin infusion rate. Open-loop systems require a method of determining blood glucose levels that the operator uses to adjust the insulin infusion rate. A comparison of open and closed-loop systems demonstrated both to be satisfactory in controlling intraoperative blood glucose levels in adults undergoing cardiac surgery.[3]

An open-loop system can be used with a minimum of equipment to manage patients with insulin-dependent diabetes and patients with non-insulin-dependent diabetes who take insulin. The goal of therapy should be maintenance of normoglycemia during the pre-CPB, CPB, and post-CPB periods. On the morning of surgery, the usual insulin dose is withheld. On arrival in the operating room, the patient's blood glucose is measured with a Dextrostix and glucometer. This technology allows accurate determination of blood glucose in just a few minutes. A continuous infusion of exogenous glucose at a rate of 1.0 mg/kg/min (approximately 1.2 mL/kg/h of 5% dextrose) is then started and maintained throughout the operative procedure. A continuous regular insulin infusion also is started and is used to maintain blood glucose between 100 and 200 mg/dL during the operative procedure. Determinations of blood glucose are made every 15 to 30 minutes with the Dextrostix and glucometer and the insulin infusion is adjusted accordingly. Generally, the following guidelines are useful:

Blood glucose (mg/dL)	Insulin infusion rate (units/kg/h)
200–250	0.015
250–300	0.03
300–350	0.045
350–400	0.06

It must be emphasized that the alterations in glucose homeostasis and the insulin resistance that accompany hypothermic CPB may necessitate insulin infusion rates in excess of 0.15 units/kg/h.[3,5]

Patients taking oral hypoglycemic agents should discontinue them at least 12 hours before surgery. For patients managed with these agents and patients managed with diet, blood glucose determinations should be made every 30 to 60 minutes during the operative procedure. They rarely require insulin infusions to maintain glucose homeostasis.

Hypothyroidism

Hypothroidism is characterized by a reduction in the basal metabolic rate. Patients with hypothyroidism have reductions in cardiac output that are appropriate for this reduction in metabolic rate. Cardiac output may be reduced by up to 40% due to reductions in both heart rate and stroke volume.[6] In addition, both hypoxic and hypercapnic ventilatory drive are blunted by hypothyroidism.[6] Furthermore, hypothyroidism may be associated with blunting of baroreceptor reflexes, reduced drug metabolism and renal excretion, reduced bowel motility, hypothermia, hyponatremia from syndrome of inappropriate antidiuretic hormone (SIADH), and adrenal insufficiency.[7,8] To further complicate matters, antianginal drugs such as nitrates and propranolol may be poorly tolerated by the depressed cardiovascular system. Propranolol-induced reduction in metabolic rate was believed to be a factor in the unusually low ventilatory and anesthetic drug requirements of a hypothyroid patient undergoing coronary revascularization.[9]

Despite these problems, thyroid replacement for cardiac surgical patients, particularly those with ischemic heart disease, is not always desirable. For hypothyroid patients requiring coronary revascularization, thyroid hormone replacement may precipitate myocardial ischemia, myocardial infarction, or adrenal insufficiency.[7,10,11] On the other hand, coronary revascularization has been managed successfully for hypothyroid patients with thyroid replacement withheld until the postoperative period.[10-13] A review of 66 clinically or biochemically mild to moderate hypothyroid patients undergoing cardiac surgery revealed minimal perioperative morbidity and mortality.[7] Among the complications observed were delayed emergence from anesthesia, persistent hypotension, tissue friability and bleeding, and adrenal insufficiency requiring exogenous steroids. The review concluded that preoperative thyroid hormone replacement does not seem to improve surgical outcome as long as serum thyroxine is less than 7 µg/dL at the time of surgery.[7] It may be difficult or impossible to safely achieve levels higher than 7 µg/dL in patients with coronary artery disease and myocardial ischemia. However, some degree of careful thyroid replacement probably is warranted for severely hypothyroid patients who have been scheduled for cardiac surgery.[8]

■ RESPIRATORY EVALUATION

A history of pulmonary disease should be sought. Emphasis should be placed on determining the extent and length of cigarette use, any history of asthma, the existence of recurrent pulmonary infections, and the presence of dyspnea. Physical examination should focus on the detection of wheezes, flattened diaphrams, air trapping, consolidations, and clubbing of the nails. Chest radiographs of all cardiac surgical patients should be taken. Pulmonary function tests (PFTs) should be ordered for all adults and older children with valvular heart disease in whom pulmonary vascular congestion exists, and in all other such patients with a history and physical examination consistent with pulmonary dysfunction. Spirometry will allow assessment of all lung volumes and capacities except residual volume and total lung capacity, which require measurement of the functional residual capacity. Spirometric measurement of expiratory flow rates allows measurement of the forced expiratory volume in 1 second (FEV_1), the forced vital capacity (FVC), and the forced midexpiratory flow (FEF 25–75%). Arterial blood gases should be obtained for patients in whom CO_2 retention is suspected and for those with severe pulmonary dysfunction as determined by history, physical examination, PFTs, and cardiac catheterization. The conditions covered in the next sections deserve special consideration.

Congenital Heart Disease

Lesions that produce excessive pulmonary blood flow (large ventricular septal defect, truncus arteriosus, dextrotransposition of the great arteries, and patent ductus arteriosus) are associated with pulmonary dysfunction (*see* Chapter 6). Occasionally, compression of large airways may occur secondary to enlargement of the pulmonary arteries. More commonly, these lesions produce pulmonary vascular changes that affect pulmonary function. The pulmonary vascular smooth muscle hypertrophy that accompanies increased pulmonary blood flow[14,15] produces peripheral airway obstruction and reduced expiratory flow rates characteristic of obstructive lung disease.[16,17] In addition, smooth muscle hypertrophy in respiratory bronchioles and alveolar ducts in patients with increased pulmonary blood flow also may contribute to this obstructive pathology.[17] These changes predispose the patient to atelectasis and pneumonia. Children with Down's syndrome seem to have a more extensive degree of pulmonary vascular and parenchymal lung disease than other children with similar heart lesions.[18] This predisposes patients with Down's syndrome to greater postoperative respiratory morbidity and mortality.[19,20]

Patients with lesions that reduce pulmonary blood flow (pulmonary atresia or stenosis, tetralogy of Fallot) also have characteristic pulmonary function changes. These patients have normal lung compliance as compared with the decreased compliance seen in patients with increased pulmonary blood flow. However, the large dead space to tidal volume ratio in these patients greatly reduces ventilatory efficiency, and large tidal volumes are required to maintain a normal alveolar ventilation.[21] Finally, 3 to 6% of patients with tetralogy of Fallot will have an absent pulmonary valve and aneurysmal dilatation of the pulmonary arteries. This aneurysmal dilatation produces bronchial compression and respiratory distress at birth.[22]

Acquired Heart Disease

The presence of clinically and PFT-diagnosed pulmonary dysfunction has important implications in assessing operative morbidity and mortality in adults undergoing cardiac surgical procedures. In one investigation, pulmonary dysfunction was defined as productive cough, wheeze, or dyspnea plus $FEV_1 < 2.0$ L or $FEV_1/FVC < 65\%$, plus either vital capacity (VC) < 3.0 L or maximum voluntary ventilation (MVV) < 80 L/min.[23] For patients undergoing valvular surgery, the presence of pulmonary dysfunction was associated with a 2.5-fold increase in perioperative mortality and a 2.5-fold increase in postoperative respiratory complications.[23] For patients undergoing coronary revascularization, the presence of pulmonary dysfunction was not associated with an increase in morbidity or mortality.[23] The presence of pulmonary dysfunction in patients with valvular heart disease may be due to the changes in lung parenchyma that parallel the development of pulmonary hypertension. Thus, the presence of pulmonary dysfunction in these patients may be indicative of severe myocardial dysfunction, which carries a high perioperative mortality rate. On the other hand, the presence of pulmonary dysfunction in patients with coronary artery disease is less likely to be secondary to myocardial dysfunction and more likely to be secondary to other causes, such as cigarette smoking.

Cigarette Smoking

Chronic cigarette use has several physiologic effects that complicate a patient's anesthetic management. Cigarette smoking may accelerate the development of atherosclerosis[24] and, in combination with preexisting stenoses, may be responsible for acute reductions in coronary blood flow by inducing increases in blood viscosity, platelet aggregation, and coronary vascular resistance.[25,26] Nicotine, through activation of the sympathetic nervous system, increases myocardial oxygen consumption by increasing heart rate and blood pressure.[24,25,27] Furthermore, the increased carboxyhemoglobin levels that accompany chronic cigarette use reduce systemic and myocardial oxygen delivery.[27] This is particularly detrimental to the patient with coronary artery disease due to the high extraction of oxygen that normally occurs in the myocardium. It has been shown that the threshold for exercise-induced angina is reduced by carboxyhemoglobin levels as low as 4.5%.[28] Short-term abstinence (12 to 48 hours) is sufficient to reduce carboxyhemoglobin and nicotine levels and improve the work capacity of the myocardium.[27]

Numerous studies have demonstrated that an increased incidence of postoperative respiratory morbidity exists in patients who smoke. The mechanisms at work seem to be a smoking-induced increase in mucus secretion, impairment of tracheobronchial clearance, and small airway narrowing.[27] For patients undergoing coronary revascularization, abstinence from smoking for 2 months or more reduced the incidence of postoperative respiratory complications to nearly that seen in nonsmokers (11%).[29] On the other hand, abstinence for less than 2 months was ineffective in reducing the incidence of postoperative respiratory complications.[29] Similar studies of patients undergoing other surgical procedures have confirmed the necessity of a 4- to 6-week abstinence period.[27]

Bronchospasm

Patients with asthma may present for cardiac surgery. In addition, patients with chronic obstructive pulmonary disease (COPD) and patients with pulmonary parenchymal disease secondary to valvular heart disease may have a bronchospastic component to their pulmonary dysfunction. Treatment of bronchospasm in the cardiac surgical patient is complicated by the fact that many bronchodilator drugs have cardiovascular side effects and that many cardiac drugs may worsen bronchospasm.

The major drugs used to treat bronchospasm are sympathomimetic agents, xanthines, and corticosteroids.

Sympathomimetic Agents.   Bronchodilation is mediated through beta-2-agonist-induced increases in intracellular cyclic adenosine monophosphate (AMP). Undesirable cardiovascular side effects of bronchodilator drugs, such as tachycardia and dysrhythmias, are mediated primarily through beta-1 agonism, although intense vasodilation via beta-2 agonism may initiate a reflex tachycardia. Nonetheless, cardiac side effects can be minimized by using beta-2-selective agonists. Terbutaline, albuterol, bitolterol, pirbuterol, and calmeterol are the beta-2-selective agents currently available.[30] Terbutaline can be administered subcutaneously, in a nebulized solution, or via a metered-dose inhaler (200 µg/puff). Albuterol can be administered orally, as a nebulized solution, or via a metered-dose inhaler (90 µg/puff). Bitolterol is available via a metered-dose inhaler (370 µg/puff). Pirbuterol is available as a metered-dose inhaler (200 µg/puff). Salmeterol is available as a metered-dose inhaler (25 µg/puff).

Bronchospasm may be exacerbated by beta-blocking agents and therefore must be used cautiously for patients who have a history of bronchospasm. Ideally, when intravenous beta-blocker therapy is indicated for these patients, a beta-1-selective agent such as metoprolol or esmolol is preferable to a nonselective agent such as propranolol.

Xanthines.   Xanthines promote bronchodilation by increasing intracellular levels of cyclic AMP through inhibition of phosphodiesterase. Theophylline is the prototypical parenteral xanthine used to treat bronchospasm. Aminopylline is a preparation of theophylline and the salt ethylenediamine, which is 20 times more soluble than theophylline and thus suitable for intravenous use.[31] Aminophylline contains approximately 80% theophylline by weight. Generally, a serum theophylline level of 10 to 20 mg/L is considered to be therapeutic. The incidence and severity of jitteriness, headache, nausea, vomiting, and cardiovascular side effects increase progressively at higher serum levels. Levels higher than 20 mg/L are considered to be toxic, although this may vary from patient to patient. For patients taking oral theophylline preparations, conversion to an infusion of aminophylline may be necessary in the perioperative period. If the theophylline level is subtherapeutic, a loading dose of aminophylline may be necessary. Each 1.25 mg/kg of aminophylline results in a 2-mg/L increase in the serum theophylline level. Infusion rates of aminophylline to maintain a steady serum theophylline concentration vary with age and other factors that affect metabolism:

- Children younger than 9 years of age: 1.0 mg/kg/h
- Children older than 9 years of age and for healthy adult smokers: 0.8 mg/kg/h
- Healthy adult nonsmokers: 0.5 mg/kg/h
- Elderly patients: 0.3 mg/kg/h
- Patients with congestive heart or liver failure: 0.1–0.2 mg/kg/h

These can only be taken as guidelines. It is essential that serum levels be monitored if aminophylline is to be used safely.

Theophylline has well-documented effects on the cardiovascular system. It increases cardiac output both by increasing stroke volume and heart rate.[31] In addition, theophylline is dysrhythmogenic, with this effect particularly prominent at higher serum concentrations.[31] Verapamil has been shown to be effective in terminating multifocal and unifocal atrial tachycardia associated with theophylline, whereas lidocaine is useful in treating ventricular ectopy.[32,33]

Corticosteroids. Corticosteroids are reserved for patients in whom bronchospasm cannot be controlled with bronchodilators alone. Prednisone, on an alternate-day basis, is the most commonly used oral preparation, whereas beclomethasone dipropionate, flunisolide, and triamcinolone acetonide are available via metered-dose inhalers used daily.[30] Generally, suppression of the hypothalamic-pituitary-adrenal axis does not occur with inhaled corticosteroids, although it has been reported in children.[30] On the other hand, systemic corticosteroid replacement may be necessary to prevent adrenal crisis during surgery for patients receiving high-dose alternate-day prednisone therapy.

For patients in whom bronchospasm is well controlled preoperatively, it is essential to continue therapy during the perioperative period. Beta-2-agonist metered-dose inhaler or nebulizer therapy can be continued until arrival in the operating room and can be restarted as soon as the patient is awake. Intraoperatively and postoperatively, metered-dose inhalation therapy can be delivered via the endotracheal tube with the aid of a T-piece designed for this purpose. Theophylline therapy can be converted to aminophylline therapy until the patient's gastrointestinal tract is functioning normally. Likewise, intravenous hydrocortisone therapy may be used in place of oral prednisone.

For patients not on bronchodilator therapy who present for surgery with bronchospasm, a trial of bronchodilators with measurement of PFTs before and after therapy is warranted.[34] An increase in the FEV_1 of 15% or more after inhalation of a nebulized bronchodilator suggests a reversible component of bronchospasm.[34] For these patients, continued bronchodilator therapy is indicated. Therapy for the cardiac surgical patient should be initiated with a beta-2-selective metered-dose inhaler or nebulized solution. The addition of theophylline preparations and corticosteroids should be reserved for patients who do not have a satisfactory response to beta-adrenergic therapy alone.

■ HEMATOLOGIC EVALUATION

For all patients scheduled for cardiac surgical procedures, a careful bleeding history should be taken, with emphasis on abnormal bleeding occurring after surgical procedures, dental extractions, and trauma. Signs of easy bruising should be sought on physical examination. All patients should undergo laboratory screening for the presence of abnormalities in hemostasis. A platelet count, bleeding time (BT), partial thromboplastin time (PTT), and prothrombin time (PT) should be obtained. Any abnormalities should be worked up before surgery so that post-CPB hemostasis is not complicated by unknown or unsuspected abnormalities.

PT and PTT Elevations

Elevations in PTT and PT should be investigated regarding factor deficiencies, factor inhibitors, and the presence of anticoagulants such as warfarin and heparin. It is important that documentation of a normal PTT and PT existing before warfarin or heparin administration is made so that other causes of an elevated PTT and PT are not overlooked. Deficiencies of factors VIII, IX, and XI are most commonly encountered.[35] These deficiencies and their management are summarized in the following sections.

Factor VIII Deficiency (Hemophilia A). The half-life of factor VIII in plasma is 8 to 12 hours; normal persons have approximately 1 unit of factor VIII activity per 1 mL of plasma (100% activity). Patients with severe hemophilia A will have as little as 1% factor VIII activity, whereas mildly affected patients will have up to 50% activity. Patients present with an elevated PTT and varying degrees of clinical bleeding. Diagnosis is made by factor assay. Safe conduct of cardiac surgery requires 50 to 100% factor VIII activity during the operative procedure, with maintenance of activity levels in the 30 to 50% range for 7 days postoperatively.[35,36] Calculation of the required factor VIII transfusion requirement can be based on the fact that infusion of 1.0 unit of factor VIII per kg of body weight will increase the patient's factor VIII activity level by 2%.[36] This relationship is expressed by the following equation:

$$\text{Units of factor VIII required} =$$
$$[(\text{desired factor VIII level} - \text{current factor VIII level})$$
$$/2 \times \text{weight in kg}]$$

Thus, a patient weighing 50 kg with a factor VIII level of 10% will require 2250 units of factor VIII to obtain an activity level of 100%. The 12-hour half-life of factor VIII requires that factor VIII be reinfused every 12 hours during the perioperative period. Factor VIII may be provided with cryoprecipitate, which contains 100 units of factor VIII per bag (10 to 20 mL). Factor VIII also may be provided by factor VIII concentrates that contain 1000 units of factor VIII in 30 to 100 mL.

Factor IX Deficiency (Hemophilia B). The half-life of factor IX in plasma is 24 hours; normal persons have approximately 1 unit of factor IX activity per 1 mL of plasma (100% activity). Factor IX deficiency is clinically indistinguishable from factor VIII deficiency. Diagnosis is made by factor assay. Safe conduct of cardiac surgery requires 60% factor IX activity during the operative procedure, with maintenance of activity levels in the 30 to 50% range for 7 days postoperatively.[35,36] Calculation of the required factor IX transfusion requirement can be based on the fact that infusion of 1.0 unit of factor IX per kg of body weight will increase the patient's factor IX activity level by 1%.[36] This relationship is expressed in the following equation:

$$\text{Units of factor IX required} =$$
$$(\text{desired factor IX level} - \text{current factor IX level})$$
$$\times \text{ weight in kg}$$

Thus, a patient weighing 50 kg with a factor IX level of 10% will require 2500 units of factor IX to obtain an activity level of 60%. The 24-hour half-life of factor IX requires that factor IX be reinfused only every 24 hours during the perioperative period. Fresh frozen plasma (FFP) contains 0.8 unit of all of the procoagulants per mL and generally is used to replace factor IX. A 250-mL bag of FFP will provide 200 units of factor IX. For patients in whom factor IX replacement with FFP will require infusion of prohibitively large volumes, factor IX concentrates are used.

Factor XI Deficiency (Rosenthal's Syndrome).

The half-life of factor XI in plasma is 60 to 80 hours; normal persons have approximately 1 unit of factor XI activity per 1 mL of plasma (100% activity). Factor XI deficiency is most common among patients of Jewish descent and is associated with a prolonged PTT. Many of these patients have no symptoms or have a history of bleeding only with surgery or major trauma. Diagnosis is made by factor assay. FFP generally is used to replace factor XI. It is recommended that 10 to 20 mL of FFP/kg/d be used during the preoperative and postoperative periods to manage this deficiency.[37]

Platelet Dysfunction

Traditionally, the BT has been used as a method of assessing platelet function and predicting blood loss. Recent review of the use of BT suggests that for coronary artery bypass surgery patients with a negative history of bleeding and no recent nonsteroidal anti-inflammatory drugs (NSAIDs) or aspirin intake, BT is not a reliable predictor of perioperative or postoperative bleeding.[38] For patients with a recent history of aspirin ingestion, a prolonged BT can be used to identify the 15 to 20% of patients who are aspirin hyperresponders and, thus, prone to aspirin-induced increased blood loss.[39]

Platelet dysfunction can result from a variety of causes, which are summarized below.

Thrombocytopenia.

Thrombocytopenia may occur for a variety of reasons, but thrombocytopenia secondary to preoperative heparin therapy deserves particular attention. Patients may receive heparin preoperatively as part of the therapeutic regimen for unstable angina, in place of warfarin for chronic atrial fibrillation, or for anticoagulation during use of the intra-aortic balloon pump. Heparin-induced thrombocytopenia and thrombosis occur due to the presence of a heparin-dependent platelet-aggregating antibody.[40,41] The condition can be terminated by withdrawal of heparin therapy. Ideally, heparin therapy should not be restarted until in-vitro platelet aggregation in response to heparin no longer occurs.[41] Unfortunately, heparin-induced thrombocytopenia may reoccur up to 12 months after the initial episode.[41] Patients with heparin-induced thrombocytopenia requiring CPB before the antibody can be cleared present a management problem. These patients have successfully received heparin for CPB after pretreatment with drugs that inhibit heparin-induced platelet aggregation, such as aspirin and dipyridamole.[39,40] The use of iloprost and prostaglandin E_1 (PGE_1) has been advocated to prevent heparin-induced platelet aggregation.[42,43] Iloprost [an analog of prostaglandin I_2 (PGI_2)] and PGE_1 inhibit platelet aggregation by increasing intracellular levels of cyclic AMP. Although aspirin produces irreversible inhibition of platelet aggregation, the effects of PGI_2 and PGE_1 are quickly terminated when the drug is withdrawn. In addition, iloprost is effective in the subset of patients with heparin-induced thrombocytopenia that is not mediated via the thromboxane pathway, in which aspirin is ineffective.[42]

Qualitative Platelet Defects.

These defects may exist for a variety of reasons. Platelet dysfunction may result from aspirin or nonsteroidal anti-inflammatory drug (NSAID) ingestion. In the case of NSAIDs, platelet function is normalized when these drugs are cleared from the blood. Despite normalization of the BT in 2 to 3 days, aspirin platelet dysfunction continues for up to 7 days after ingestion due to acetylation of platelet cyclooxygenase.

Preoperative aspirin ingestion is common in patients undergoing coronary artery bypass surgery because it is beneficial for patients with stable angina, unstable angina, and evolving myocardial infarction.[44] In addition, preoperative aspirin ingestion improves short-term coronary artery graft patency.[45] Preoperative aspirin ingestion has been implicated in increasing blood loss and transfusion requirements in cardiac surgical patients.[39] Recent data suggest that measures can be taken to attenuate the effects of aspirin. The use of autotransfused blood, intraoperative hemoconcentration, and stricter transfusion criteria can reduce transfusion requirements despite increased mediastinal drainage, whereas the use of antifibrinolytic agents, strict heparin and protamine dosing, and meticulous surgical technique may reduce bleeding even in reoperative patients taking aspirin.[45a,45b] Nonetheless aspirin induced platelet dysfunction does play a role in exacerbating post-CPB platelet dysfunction (*see* Chapter 10). Qualitative defects have been observed in children with congenital heart disease,[46,47] uremic patients, and patients taking a wide variety of drugs, including propranolol, calcium channel blockers, dipyridamole, and antibiotics.[48]

Von Willebrand's Disease (VWD).   Von Willebrand's disease (VWD) is caused by a deficient or defective plasma von Willebrand factor (VWF). VWF is a large glycoprotein responsible for mediating platelet adherence to vessel walls. Several types of VWD exist:[49]

- Type 1: the most common variant. Transmission is via an autosomal dominant pattern. Most patients are heterozygous and have a history of mild to moderate mucosal bleeding or marked bleeding associated with surgery and trauma. These patients usually have depressed levels of factor VIII procoagulant activity (VIII:C) and VWF. Ristocetin-induced platelet aggregation is depressed and the PTT usually is normal or slightly elevated.
- Type 2a: patients have depressed ristocetin-induced platelet aggregation, and immunoelectrophoresis reveals a decrease or absence of large VWF multimers.
- Type 2b: patients exhibit enhanced ristocetin-induced platelet aggregation and enhanced binding of large multimers to platelets. These patients also may exhibit chronic thrombocytopenia.
- Type 3: the rare homozygous or doubly heterozygous version of type 1 disease. These patients have severe bleeding, very low or nondetectable levels of VIII:C and VWF, and a prolonged PTT.

Preoperative preparation of the patient with VWD who has been scheduled for cardiac surgery is geared toward maintainance of a VIII:C level of approximately 70% and normalization of the BT.[35,49] Cryoprecipitate provides VWF as well as VIII:C; each bag of cryoprecipitate contains 100 units of VIII:C and of VWF. Before surgery, three bags of cryoprecipitate for each 10 kg of body weight should be infused for patients with severe VWD.[49] For patients with milder disease, 1.5 to two bags for each 10 kg of body weight are recommended.[49] After infusion of cryoprecipitate in patients with VWD, the half-life of VWF is 12 hours, whereas that of VIII:C is more than 24 hours. Therefore, it may be necessary to

continue cryoprecipitate infusion every 12 hours for several days after cardiac surgery.

For some patients with VWD, 1-deamino-8-D-arginevasopression (DDAVP) has been shown to increase VWF and shorten the BT by causing release of VWF from endothelial cells. The response to DDAVP in VWD is variable. Patients with severe type 1 disease and patients with type 3 disease have a limited response due to low tissue levels of VWF. Patients with type 2b disease should not receive VWF because thrombocytopenia is likely to result. When DDAVP is used, 0.03 µg/kg is infused intravenously over 15 minutes and the half-life of its activity is 8 hours.[49]

Congenital Heart Disease

Coagulopathies in children with congenital heart disease have been well described.[46,47,50] The etiology of these coagulopathies seems to be multifactorial.[51] Quantitative and qualitative platelet dysfunction plays a role in patients with both cyanotic and acyanotic lesions.[46,50] In acyanotic patients, an acquired deficiency of the large VWF multimers has been demonstrated.[52] In cyanotic patients, hypofibrinogenemia, low-grade disseminated intravascular coagulation (DIC), deficiencies in factors V and VIII, and deficiencies in the vitamin-K-dependent factors (II, VII, IX, X) have all been implicated.[43,46,47,50,52] Furthermore, in patients who are cyanotic and polycythemic, the plasma volume and quantity of coagulation factors are reduced, and this may contribute to the development of a coagulopathy.[47] In some instances, erythrophoresis with whole blood removed and replaced with fresh frozen plasma[46] or isotonic saline[53] may be justified. Finally, factors synthesized in the liver may be reduced in both cyanotic and acyanotic patients in whom severe right heart failure results in passive hepatic congestion and secondary parenchymal disease.[47]

The volume and factor contents of commonly used plasma and platelet products are summarized in Table 1-1.

TABLE 1-1. PLASMA AND PLATELET PRODUCTS

Product	Volume	Factors
Cryoprecipitate	10–20 mL/bag	100 units factor VIII:C
		100 units factor vWF
		60 units factor XIII
		250 mg fibrinogen
FFP	250 mL/bag	200 units of all procoagulants
		550 mg fibrinogen
Platelets	10–25 mL/single donor unit	5.5×10^{10} platelets/unit
	50–70 mL/multiple donor unit	

FFP = fresh frozen plasma; vWF = von Willebrand's factor.

■ RENAL/METABOLIC EVALUATION

Renal function and electrolyte balance should be evaluated before cardiac surgical procedures.

Renal Dysfunction

Patients presenting for cardiac surgery may possess varying degrees of renal dysfunction ranging from mild elevations in creatinine to dependence on dialysis. In addition, patients with renal transplants also may present for surgery. For all of these patients, optimization of renal function before the operative procedure is imperative. The dialysis-dependent patient will require dialysis preoperatively. If the patient is too hemodynamically unstable to tolerate preoperative dialysis, it can be managed intraoperatively, as discussed in Chapter 10. Dialysis will correct or improve the abnormalities in potassium, phosphate, sodium, chloride, and magnesium. In addition, the platelet dysfunction that accompanies uremia will be improved. DDAVP administration also has been shown to improve uremia-induced platelet dysfunction[54] and should be considered if clinically significant postdialysis platelet dysfunction exists (*see* Chapter 10). Dialysis will not favorably affect the anemia, renovascular hypertension, or immune-system compromise associated with chronic renal failure.

For nondialysis-dependent patients, preoperative hydration is necessary to prevent prerenal azotemia from complicating the underlying renal dysfunction. This is particularly important after procedures such as cardiac catheterization and arteriography, which use intravascular contrast agents. All patients seem to suffer a fall in creatinine clearance after contrast arteriography[55]; however, for patients with preexisting azotemia, this reduction is much more likely to result in the clinical manifestations of worsened renal function.[56] Hydration before and after angiographic procedures may ameliorate contrast-induced renal dysfunction.[56]

Patients with renal transplants have successfully undergone cardiac surgical procedures.[57] The extrarenal component of renal blood flow autoregulation will be absent in the denervated kidney. Therefore, preoperative hydration and maintenance of systemic perfusion pressure are particularly important to maintain renal perfusion. In addition, these patients must be treated meticulously with regard to sterile technique due to their immune-compromised status.

Hypokalemia

Theoretically, hypokalemia predisposes the development of ventricular dysrythymias by increasing the rate of phase 4 depolarization and by promoting unidirection atrioventricular (AV) nodal block. Reductions in potassium below 2.5 mEq/L predispose ventricular dys-

rhythmias and cardiovascular collapse. Serum potassium levels below 3.5 mEq/L predispose ventricular fibrillation in the setting of acute myocardial infarction[58] and the potentiation of digitalis toxicity by hypokalemia is well documented. Finally, acute reductions in potassium seem to be more likely to induce ventricular tachydysrhythmias than chronic hypokalemia.[59]

Hypokalemia defined as a serum potassium less than 3.5 mEq/L is not an uncommon finding in the preoperative evaluation of the cardiac surgical patient. The most common etiology is chronic diuretic therapy, but more acute causes such as nasogastric suction and vigorous in-hospital diuretic therapy must be considered. In a patient population with a low incidence of cardiac disease and digitalis use not undergoing cardiac surgical procedures, the incidence of atrial and ventricular dysrhythmias during anesthesia in chronically hypokalemic patients (2.6 to 3.4 mEq/L) has been shown to be no greater than that found in normokalemic patients (3.5 to 5.0 mEq/L).[60] Likewise, the incidence of atrial and ventricular dysrhythmias during anesthesia for cardiac surgery was similar in normokalemic, hypokalemic (3.1 to 3.5 mEq/L), and severely hypokalemic (<3.0 mEq/L) patients.[61] Although the incidence of dysrhythmias was greatest in patients taking digoxin and in patients with congestive heart failure, the increased incidence in this subset was not related to the presence of hypokalemia.[61] Thus, on the basis of the currently available information, routine potassium repletion does not seem to be warranted in all cardiac surgical patients with chronic hypokalemia. It may be prudent to maintain serum potassium higher than 3.5 mEq/L for cardiac surgical patients taking digitalis, those at high risk for myocardial ischemia, and those who have suffered acute reductions in serum potassium.

■ CARDIOVASCULAR EVALUATION

A comprehensive cardiovascular evaluation must be obtained before cardiac surgical procedures. The tests chosen to obtain this evaluation may vary from institution to institution and certainly will vary with the lesion being evaluated. The following description is intended to clarify the strength and limitations of the various tests that will need to be interpreted by the consulting anesthesiologist.

Electrocardiogram (ECG)

A preoperative electrocardiogram (ECG) should be obtained in all cardiac surgical patients. The ECG should be examined for evidence of left and right ventricular hypertrophy, atrial enlargement, conduction defects (both AV nodal and bundle branch block), premature atrial and ventricular activity, and drug effects. In addition, the ECG should be examined for findings consistent with the working preoperative diagnosis. The next sections describe ECG findings and associated lesions.

Left Atrial Enlargement (LAE). In adults, left atrial enlargement (LAE) may be found in association with mitral stenosis, aortic stenosis, systemic hypertension, and mitral regurgitation. In mitral stenosis, LAE occurs secondary to the increased impedance to atrial emptying across the stenotic mitral valve. In aortic stenosis and systemic hypertension, an elevated left-ventricular end-diastolic pressure results in left atrial hypertrophy. In mitral regurgitation, LAE occurs as a result of the large volumes of blood regurgitated in the left atrium during systole.

Right Atrial Enlargement (RAE). Right atrial enlargement (RAE) may be present in infants and children with right ventricular hypertrophy, as occurs with stenotic pulmonary lesions. RAE also may be observed in patients with tricuspid stenosis, tricuspid atresia, or Ebstein's abnormality. RAE also may be present in patients with right ventricular hypertrophy and pulmonary hypertension secondary to chronic lung disease.

Left Ventricular Hypertrophy (LVH). In adults, left ventricular hypertrophy (LVH) commonly occurs in left ventricular pressure overload lesions such as aortic stenosis and severe systemic hypertension. In children, LVH may be present with coarctation of the aorta and congenital aortic stenosis.

Right Ventricular Hypertrophy (RVH). Right ventricular hypertrophy (RVH) is a common finding in patients with congenital heart disease and may be seen in pulmonic stenosis, tetralogy of Fallot, and transposition of the great arteries. In adults, RVH may accompany the pulmonary hypertension induced by chronic lung disease.

It must be emphasized that a normal ECG does not preclude the presence of significant cardiac disease in the adult, infant, or child. The ECG is normal in 25 to 50% of adults with chronic stable angina.[62] Likewise, the ECG may be normal in children with left ventricular pressure overload (aortic stenosis) and volume overload (patent ductus arteriosus or ventricular septal defect) lesions.[63]

Chest Radiograph

In addition to providing information on pulmonary status, the posterior-anterior and lateral chest radiograph may prove useful in assessment of the cardiovascular system. Obviously, radiographic evidence of pulmonary vascular congestion suggests poor systolic function. For patients with valvular heart disease, a normal chest radiograph is more useful than an abnormal radiograph in assessing ventricular function. The presence of a cardiothoracic ratio less than 50% is a sensitive indicator of an ejection fraction greater than 50% and of a cardiac index greater than 2.5 L/min/m².[64] On the other hand, a cardiothoracic ratio greater than 50% is not a specific indicator and thus may be associated with both normal and abnormal ventricular function.[64] For patients with coronary artery disease, an abnormal chest radiograph is more useful than a normal radiograph in assessing ventricular function. Cardiomegaly is a sensitive indicator of a reduced ejection fraction, whereas a normal-sized heart may be associated with both normal and reduced ejection fractions.[65]

As with the ECG, efforts should be made to correlate radiographic findings with the working preoperative diagnosis. Left atrial enlargement is expected in mitral stenosis and regurgitation. As these diseases progress, enlargement of the pulmonary artery and right ventricle can be expected. Left ventricular enlargement would be expected from the eccentric hypertrophy that results from mitral and aortic regurgitation but usually is not observed in patients with concentric hypertrophy from aortic stenosis until severe ventricular dysfunction occurs. In infants and children with increased pulmonary blood flow (as with a large ventricular septal or atrial septal defect), the pulmonary artery and pulmonary vasculature in general will be prominent. In contrast, patients with reduced pulmonary blood flow (as with tetralogy of Fallot or pulmonary atresia) may manifest a small pulmonary artery and diminished vascularity. In addition, some congenital lesions are associated with classic radiographic cardiac silhouettes: the boot-shaped heart of tetralogy of Fallot, the "figure 8" heart of total anomalous pulmonary venous return, and the "egg-on-its-side"-shaped heart seen in D-transposition of the great arteries.

Stress Testing

Patients presenting for cardiac surgery may have undergone stress testing to establish the diagnosis of coronary artery disease (CAD), to assess the severity of known CAD, to establish the viability of regions of myocardium, and to evaluate antianginal therapy. Stress testing may use exercise or pharmacological agents. Pharmacological agents are useful for patients with physical disabilities that preclude effective exercise. It also is useful for patients who cannot reach an optimal exercise heart rate because they are taking beta or calcium channel blockers.

Pharmacological Stress Testing. Pharmacologic stress testing uses dipyridamole, adenosine, and dobutamine. Dipyridamole, adenosine, and dobutamine stress testing can be performed in conjunction with myocardial perfusion scintigraphy or echocardiography (as follows).

Adenosine and dipyridamole are both potent coronary vasodilators that increase myocardial blood flow 3- to 5-fold, independent of myocardial work. Adenosine is a direct vascular smooth muscle relaxant via A_2 receptors, whereas dipyridamole increases adenosine levels by inhibiting adenosine deaminase. Dobutamine increases myocardial work through increases in heart rate and contractility via $beta_1$ receptors. This, in turn, produces proportional increases in myocardial blood flow. In this sense, dobutamine stress testing is similar to exercise stress testing.

The hyperemic response to adenosine and dipyridamole produces increased myocardial blood flow in regions supplied by normal coronary arteries. In regions of myocardium supplied by steal prone anatomy (*see* Chapter 4) or diseased coronary arteries, myocardial blood flow increases will be attenuated or may actually decrease below resting levels. This is the result of baseline coronary vasodilation in areas of myocardium supplied by diseased vessels. This response expends coronary vasodilator reserve and attenuates the response to a vasodilatory stimulus.

Dipyridamole is infused at 0.56 to 0.84 mg/kg for 4 minutes, followed by injection of the radiopharmaceutical for myocardial perfusion scintigraphy 3 minutes later. If infusion produces headache, flushing, gastrointestinal (GI) distress, ectopy, angina, or ECG evidence of ischemia, the effect can be terminated with aminophylline 75 to 150 mg intravenously. Adenosine is infused at 140 µg/kg/min for 6 minutes with injection of the radiopharmaceutical for myocardial perfusion scintigraphy 3 minutes later. Side effects are similar to dipyridamole and usually can be terminated without aminophylline by stopping the infusion due to the very short half-life (40 seconds) of adenosine. Dobutamine is infused initially at 5 µg/kg/min for 3 minutes and then is increased to 10 µg/kg/min for 3 minutes. The dose is increased by 5 µg/kg/min every 3 minutes until a maximum of 40 µg/kg/min is reached or until significant increases in heart rate and blood pressure occur. Injection of the radiopharmaceutical for myocardial perfusion scintigraphy takes place 1 minute after the desired dose is reached, and the infusion is continued for 1 to 2 minutes after injection. Side effects of dobutamine (headache, flushing, GI distress, ectopy, angina, or ECG evidence of ischemia) can be terminated by discontinuing the infusion due to the short half-life (2 minutes) of the drug. If necessary, esmolol can be used.

Exercise Stress Testing. Exercise stress testing uses exercise-induced increases in myocardial oxygen consumption to detect limitations in the ability of the coronary arterial system to deliver appropriately increased blood flow. Exercise induces increases in cardiac output primarily through increases in heart rate.

Despite vasodilation in skeletal muscle, exercise typically induces an increase in arterial blood pressure as well. As a result, exercise is accompanied by increases in the major determinants of myocardial oxygen consumption: heart rate, wall tension, and contractility. Exercise increases coronary blood flow through vasodilation. The ability of the coronary circulation to increase blood flow to match exercise-induced increases in demand is compromised in the distribution of stenosed coronary arteries because vasodilatory reserve is exhausted in these beds.

All exercise tests involve inducing progressive increases in metabolic rate and oxygen consumption (VO_2). Isometric exercise may be used to increase the work load, but more commonly, dynamic exercise using either a treadmill or a bicycle is used. VO_2max is the maximal amount of oxygen a person can use while performing dynamic exercise. VO_2max is influenced by age, gender, exercise habits, and cardiovascular status. Exercise protocols are compared by comparing metabolic equivalents (METs). One MET is equal to a VO_2 of 3.5 ml O_2/kg/min and represents resting oxygen uptake. Different exercise protocols are compared by comparing the number of METs consumed at various stages.

The Bruce treadmill protocol is probably the most widely used. This protocol uses seven 3-minute stages. Each progressive stage involves an increase in both the grade and the speed of the treadmill. During stage 1, the treadmill speed is 1.7 miles per hour on a 10% grade (5 METs); during stage 5, the treadmill speed is 5 miles per hour on a 18% grade (16 METs). In the modified protocol, two warm-up stages on a level grade precede stage 1. The test is continued until the appearance of patient exhaustion, attainment of the target heart rate (90% of age predicted maximal heart rate) without evidence of ischemia, or until the appearance of ischemia as described below.

When exercise-induced increases in myocardial oxygen demand outstrip supply, myocardial ischemia results. For exercise testing to be a sensitive and specific indicator of myocardial ischemia, it must be capable of the detecting the various manifestations of ischemia. Exercise stress testing can be performed in conjunction with traditional ECG analysis, myocardial perfusion scintigraphy, or echocardiography. The details of stress myocardial perfusion scintigraphy, stress radionuclide angiography, and stress echocardiography are discussed in their respective sections below.

The following factors must be considered in interpretation of an ECG exercise stress test:[66]

- Angina—ischemia may present as the patient's typical angina pattern; however, angina is not a universal manifestation of ischemia in all patients. Ischemic pain induced by exercise is strongly predictive of CAD.

- VO$_2$max—if patients with CAD reach 13 METs, their prognosis is good regardless of other factors; patients with an exercise capacity of less than 5 METs have a poor prognosis.
- Dysrhythmias—for patients with CAD, ventricular dysrhythmias may be precipitated or aggravated by exercise testing. The appearance of reproducible sustained (>30 seconds) or symptomatic ventricular tachycardia (VT) is predictive of multivessel disease and adverse prognosis.
- ST segment changes—the 12-lead ECG is monitored before, during, and after exercise. ST segment depression is the most common manifestation of exercise-induced myocardial ischemia. The standard criteria for an abnormal response is horizontal or downsloping (>1 mm) depression 80 msec after the J point. Downsloping segments carry a worse prognosis than horizontal segments. The amount of ST segment depression (>2 mm), the time of appearance (starting with <6 METs), the duration of depression (persisting >5 minutes into recovery), and the number of ECG leads involved (>5 leads) are all predictive of multivessel CAD and adverse prognosis.
- Blood pressure changes—failure to increase systolic arterial blood pressure to greater than 120 mm Hg or a sustained decrease in systolic blood pressure with progressive exercise is indicative of a failure of cardiac output to increase as vasodilation in exercising muscle occurs. This finding suggests ischemic impairment of a large portion of the left ventricle such as that seen with severe multivessel or left main CAD.

Comparison of Stress Test Methods. The sensitivity of detection of CAD with exercise myocardial perfusion scintigraphy and exercise echocardiography is superior to that of exercise ECG testing (80 to 85% versus 65 to 70%).[67] The superiority of these two modalities over ECG testing in detecting CAD is greatest for patients with single vessel coronary artery disease.[67,68] The sensitivity and specificity of exercise ECG testing for patients with a normal resting ECG who are not taking digoxin and who have left main or three-vessel disease are almost as good as exercise myocardial perfusion scintigraphy and exercise echocardiography. The sensitivity and specificity for detection of CAD with stress (both exercise and pharmacologic) myocardial perfusion scintigraphy and echocardiography seem to be similar, with a trend toward greater sensitivity with myocardial perfusion scintigraphy, particularly for patients with single-vessel disease.[69]

Additional limitations of exercise ECG testing are the inability to accurately localize and assess the extent of ischemia. Furthermore, no direct information regarding left ventricle function is available. Stress myocardial perfusion scintigraphy, radionuclide angiography, and echocardiography provide this information. On the other hand, these methods are more expensive and technically demanding than exercise ECG testing.

Myocardial Perfusion Scintigraphy

Myocardial perfusion scintigraphy is a modality that allows blood flow to myocardium and myocardial viability to be assessed. Myocardial perfusion scintigraphy is performed most commonly in conjunction with stress testing. Stress testing can be accomplished with exercise or pharmacologically with dipyridamole, adenosine, or dobutamine. With this technology, it is possible to determine which regions of myocardium are perfused normally, which are ischemic, which are stunned or hibernating, and which are infarcted. The technique is based on the use of radiophamaceuticals that accumulate in myocardium proportional to regional blood flow.[70] Single-positron emission computed tomography (SPECT) or planar imaging is used to image the regional myocardial perfusion in multiple views and at various measurement intervals.

The radiopharmaceuticals currently in use are thallium-201 and technetium-99m methoxyisobutyl isonitrile (SestaMIBI).[71] Thallium has biologic properties similar to potassium and thus is transported across the myocardial cell membrane by the sodium–potassium ATPase pump proportional to regional myocardial blood flow. SestaMIBI is not dependent on ATP to enter myocardial cells because it is highly lipophilic but its distribution in myocardial is proportional to blood flow.

Thallium. Thallium-201 is injected at the peak level of a multistage exercise or pharmacological stress test. Scintillation imaging begins 6 to 8 minutes after injection (early views) and is repeated again 2.5 to 4 hours after injection (delayed or redistribution views). Identical views must be used so the early and delayed images can be compared. Thallium has the ability to redistribute after injection. During stress, myocardial blood flow and thallium-201 uptake will increase in areas of the myocardium supplied by normal coronary arteries. Subsequently, thallium redistributes to other tissues, thus clearing from myocardium slowly. Areas of myocardium supplied by diseased arteries are prone to ischemia during stress and have a reduced ability to increase myocardial blood flow and thallium-201 uptake. These areas will demonstrate a perfusion defect when compared with normal regions in the early views. In the delayed views, late accumulation or flat washout of thallium-201 from the ischemic areas compared with the nonischemic areas results in equalization of thallium-201 activity in the two areas. These *reversible perfusion* defects are typical of areas of myocardium that suffer transient, stress-induced ischemia. *Nonreversible perfusion defects* are present in both the early stress and delayed redistribution images. These defects are believed to represent areas of nonviable myocardium or scar. *Reverse redistribution* is the phenomenon in which early images are normal or show a defect and the delayed images show a defect or a more severe defect. This is seen frequently in patients who have recently undergone thrombolytic therapy or angioplasty and may result from higher-than-normal blood flow to the residual viable myocardium in the partially infarcted zone.

Recently, it has been demonstrated that modified thallium scintigraphy protocols are useful in detecting areas of viable, hibernating myocardium in areas previously believed to be nonviable. Hibernating myocardium exhibits persistent ischemic dysfunction secondary to a chronic reduction in coronary blood flow. Hibernating myocardium has been shown to exhibit functional improvement after surgical revascularization or angioplasty and restoration of coronary blood flow. Stunned myocardium has undergone a period of hypoperfusion with subsequent reperfusion. As a result, these regions exhibit transient postischemic dysfunction in the setting of normal coronary blood flow. Stunned myocardium is detected by identifying regions of dysfunctional myocardium in which no perfusion defect exists.

Some regions of myocardium that do not exhibit redistribution at 2.5 to 4 hours exhibit redistribution in late images at 18 to 24 hours.[72] This late redistribution represents areas of viable, hibernating myocardium. Another approach to detecting hibernating myocardium is reinjection of thallium at rest after acquisition of the 2.5 to 4-hour stress images. Persistent defects that show enhanced uptake after reinjection represent areas of viable myocardium. Finally, serial rest thallium imaging has proved useful in detecting viable, hibernating myocardium. Images are obtained at rest after injection of thallium and then are repeated 3 hours later. Regions of myocardium that exhibit rest redistribution represent areas of viable myocardium.

Increased lung uptake of thallium is related to exercise-induced LV dysfunction and suggests multivessel CAD. Because increased lung uptake of thallium is due to an elevated left atrial pressure (LAP), other factors besides extensive coronary artery disease and exercise-induced left ventricular (LV) dysfunction (such as mitral stenosis, mitral regurgitation, and nonischemic cardiomyopathy) must be considered when few or no myocardial perfusion defects are detected. Transcient LV dilation after exercise or pharmacologic stress also suggests severe myocardial ischemia.

SestaMIBI. SestaMIBI, unlike thallium, does not redistribute.[70] As a result, the distribution of myocardial blood flow at the time of injection remains fixed over the course of several hours. This necessitates two separate injections: one at rest and one at peak stress.[71] The two studies must be performed so that the myocardial activity from the first study decays enough not to interfere with the activity from the second study. A small dose is administered at rest with imaging approximately 45 to 60 minutes later. Several hours later, a larger dose is administered at peak stress, with imaging 15 to 30 minutes later. Reversible and fixed defects are detected by comparing the rest and stress images. As with thallium, late imaging after SestaMIBI stress imaging may be helpful in detecting viable, hibernating myocardium.[72]

SestaMIBI allows high-count-density images to be recorded, providing better resolution than thallium. In addition, use of SestaMIBI allows performance of first-pass radionuclide angiography (see below) to be performed in conjunction with myocardial perfusion scintigraphy. Use of stimultaneous radionuclide angiography and perfusion scintigraphy has proved useful in enhanced detection of viable myocardium.[72] Viable myocardium will exhibit perserved regional perfusion in conjunction with preserved regional wall motion.

Radionuclide Angiography

Two types of cardiac radionuclide imaging exist: first-pass radionuclide angiography (FPRNA)[73] and equilibrium radionuclide angiography (ERNA), also known as radionuclide ventriculography or gated blood pool imaging.[74] ERNA is also known as multiple-gated acquisition (MUGA) or multiple-gated equilibrium scintigraphy (MGES).

FPRNA involves injection of a radionuclide bolus (normally technetium-99m) into the central circulation via the external jugular or antecubital vein. Subsequent imaging with a scintillation camera in a fixed position provides a temporal pictorial presentation of the cardiac chambers as the radiolabeled bolus makes its way through the heart. First-pass studies may be gated or ungated. Gated studies involve synchronization of the presented images with the patient's ECG such that systole and diastole are identified. Ungated studies simply present a series of images over time.

ERNA involves use of technetium-99m-labeled red cells, which are allowed to distribute uniformly in the blood volume.[74] Radiolabeling of red cells is accomplished by initially injecting the patient with stannous pyrophosphate, which creates an stannous-hemoglobin complex over the course of 30 minutes. Subsequent injection of a technetium-99m bolus results in binding of technetium-99m to the stannous-hemoglobin complex, thus labeling the red cells. Because the binding of technetium-99m to the patient's red cells takes 5 minutes, a first-pass study can be performed immediately after the technetium-99m injection and before the start of the equilibrium study.

After equilibrium of the labeled red cells in the cardiac blood pool, gated imaging with a scintillation camera is performed. A computer divides the cardiac cycle into a predetermined number of frames (16 to 64).[74] Each frame represents a specific time interval relative to the ECG R wave. Data collected from each time interval over the course of several hundred cardiac cycles are then added together with the other images from the same time interval. The result is a sequence of 16 to 64 images, each representing a specific phase of the cardiac cycle. The images can be displayed in an endless loop format or individually. The procedure can then be repeated with the camera in a different position.

Below is a summary of the relative advantages and disadvantages of first-pass and equilibration studies. Both types of studies currently are used for adults, infants, and children.[73,74]

- With both FPRNA and ERNA studies, the number of radioactive counts during end systole and end diastole can be used to determine stroke volume, ejection fraction, and cardiac output.
- Both types of study allow reliable quantification of LV volume using count-proportional methods that do not require assumptions to be made about LV geometry.
- Although both studies allow determination of right ventricular (RV) and LV ejection fractions, determination of RV ejection fraction is more accurate with a first-pass study because the right atrium overlaps the right ventricle in equilibrium studies.
- First-pass studies allow detection and quantification of both right-to-left and left-to-right intracardiac shunts, whereas shunt detection is not possible with equilibration studies.
- First-pass studies also allow sequential analysis of right atrial (RA), RV, left atrial (LA), and LV size, whereas equilibration studies do not. Abnormalities in the progression of the radioactive tracer through the heart and great vessels is helpful in the diagnosis of congenital abnormalities.
- Equilibration studies provide better analysis of regional wall motion abnormalities than first-pass studies due to higher resolution.
- Both types of studies can be used for exercise studies. First-pass studies can be performed rapidly but do not allow assessment of ventricular wall motion at different exercise levels, nor do they allow assessment of wall motion from different angles.
- Mitral or aortic reguritation is detectable with both first-pass and equilibration studies by analysis of the stroke volume ratio. Normally, the LV-to-RV stroke volume ratio is slightly greater than 1. In the presence of aortic or mitral regurgitation, this ratio will increase. This method tends to overestimate regurgitant fraction and is not reliable for detection of minor degrees of regurgitation.

Echocardiography

Echocardiography has revolutionized the noninvasive structural and functional assessment of acquired and congenital heart disease. The technical details of echocardiography are discussed in detail in Chapter 3. Routine use of two-dimensional imaging, color flow Doppler, continuous wave Doppler, pulsed wave Doppler, and M-mode imaging allows the following:

- Assessment of cardiac anatomy—delineation of the most complex congenital heart lesions is feasible. In many instances, information acquired from a comprehensive echocardiographic examination is all that is necessary to undertake a surgical repair.
- Assessment of ventricular function—comprehensive assessment of RV and LV diastolic and systolic function is feasible.
- Assessment of valvular abnormalities—assessment of the functional status of all four cardiac valves is possible. In addition, quantification of valvular stenosis and insufficiency is accurate and reliable. Assessment of prosthetic valves also is feasible.
- Characterization of cardiomyopathics—hypertrophic, dilated, and restrictive cardiomyopathies can be identified.
- Assessment of the pericardium—pericardial effusions, cardiac tamponade, and constrictive pericarditis can be identified reliably.
- Assessment of cardiac and extracardiac masses—vegetations, foreign bodies, thrombi, and metastatic and primary cardiac tumors can be identified.
- Contrast echocardiography—use of contrast solutions containing microbubbles that act as scatterers of ultrasound allows assessment of myocardial perfusion, enhancement of intracardiac shunts, enhancement of Doppler signals, and improved assessment of regional and global LV function. Assessment of myocardial perfusion requires aortic injection of the contrast media, whereas the other applications can be accomplished with intravenous injection. Contrast agents are being developed that will allow myocardial perfusion contrast echocardiography to be accomplished using intravenous agent injection.

• Stress echocardiography—stress echocardiography is based on the concept that exercise or pharmacologically induced wall motion abnormalities develop early in the course of ischemia. Stress-induced wall motion abnormalities occur soon after perfusion defects are detected by radionuclide imaging because, in the ischemic cascade, hypoperfusion precedes wall motion abnormalities. Comparison of resting and stress images allows resting abnormalities to be distinguished from stress-induced abnormalities. Resting abnormalities indicate prior infarction or hibernating/stunned myocardium, whereas stress-induced abnormalities are specific for ischemia. Furthermore, dobutamine stress echocardiography may be useful in determining myocardial viability. Regions that are hypokinetic, akinetic, or dyskinetic at rest and improve with dobutamine administration probably contain areas of stunned or hibernating myocardium. Such areas demonstrate functional improvement after myocardial vascularization or angioplasty.

Cardiac Catheterization

Cardiac catheterization remains the gold standard for evaluation of acquired and congenital heart disease. Cardiac catheterization is covered in detail in Chapter 2.

■ REFERENCES

1. Kuntschen FR, Galletti PM, Hahn C: Glucose-insulin interactions during cardiopulmonary bypass. Hypothermia versus normothermia. *J Thorac Cardiovasc Surg* 1985; **91**:451-459.

2. Kuntschen FR, Galletti PM, Hahn C, et al: Alterations of insulin and glucose metabolism during cardiopulmonary bypass under normothermia. *J Thorac Cardiovasc Surg* 1985; **89**:97-106.

3. Elliott MJ, Gill GV, Home PH, et al: A comparison of two regimens for the management of diabetes during open heart surgery. *Anesthesiology* 1984; **60**:364-368.

4. McKnight CK, Elliott M, Pearson DT, et al: Continuous monitoring of blood glucose concentration during open-heart surgery. *Br J Anaesth* 1985; **57**:595-601.

5. Watson BG, Elliott MJ, Pay DA, Williamson M: Diabetes mellitus and open heart surgery. *Anaesthesia* 1986; **41**:250-257.

6. Murkin JM: Anesthesia and hypothyroidism: A review of thyroxine physiology, pharmacology, and anesthesic implications. *Anesth Analg* 1982; **61**:371-383.

7. Becker C: Hypothyroidism and atherosclerotic heart disease: Pathogenesis, medical management, and the role of coronary artery bypass surgery. *Endocrinol Rev* 1985; **6**:432-440.

8. Ladenson PW, Levin AA, Ridgway EC, Daniels GH: Complications of surgery in hypothyroid patients. *Am J Med* 1984; **77**:261-266.

9. Gyermek L, Henderson G: Low ventilatory and anesthetic drug requirements during myocardial revascularization in a hypothyroid patient. *J Cardiothorac Anesth* 1988; **2**:70-73.

10. Hay ID, Duick DS, Vlietstra RE, et al: Thyroxin therapy in hypothyroid patients undergoing coronary revascularization. A retrospective analysis. *Ann Intern Med* 1981; **95**:456-457.

11. Paine TD, Rogers WJ, Baxley WA, Russell RO: Coronary arterial surgery in patients with incapacitating angina pectoris and myxedema. *Am J Cardiol* 1977; **40**:226-231.

12. Myerowitz PD, Kamienski RW, Swanson DK, et al: Diagnosis and management of the hypothyroid patient with chest pain. *J Thorac Cardiovasc Surg* 1983; **86**:57-60.

13. Finlayson DC, Kaplan JA: Myxoedema and open heart surgery: Anaesthesia and intensive care unit experience. *Can Anaesth Soc J* 1982; **29**:543-549.

14. Rabinovitch M, Haworth SG, Castaneda AR, et al: Lung biopsy in congenital heart disease: A morphometric approach to pulmonary vascular disease. *Circulation* 1978; **58**:1107-1122.

15. Hoffman JIE, Rudolph AM, Heymann MA: Pulmonary vascular disease with congenital heart lesions: Pathologic features and causes. *Circulation* 1981; **64**:873-877.

16. Hordof AJ, Mellins RB, Gersony WM, Steeg CN: Reversibility of chronic obstructive lung disease in infants following repair of ventricular septal defect. *J Pediatr* 1977; **90**:187-191.

17. Motoyama EK, Tanaka T, Fricker EJ: Peripheral airway obstruction in children with congenital heart disease and pulmonary hypertension. *Am Rev Respir Dis* 1986; **133**:A10.

18. Yamaki S, Horiuchi T, Sekino Y: Quantitative analysis of pulmonary vascular disease in simple cardiac anomalies with the Down syndrome. *Am J Cardiol* 1983; **51**:1502-1506.

19. Morray JP, MacGillivray R, Duker G: Increased perioperative risk following repair of congenital heart disease in Down's syndrome. *Anesthesiology* 1986; **65**:221-224.

20. Yamaki S, Horiuchi T, Takahashi T: Pulmonary changes in congenital heart disease with Down's syndrome: Their significance as a cause of postoperative respiratory failure. *Thorax* 1985; **40**: 380-386.

21. Lindahl SGE, Olsson A-K: Congenital heart malformations and ventilatory efficiency in children. Effects of lung perfusion during halothane anaesthesia and spontaneous breathing. *Br J Anaesth* 1987; **59**:410-418.

22. Rabinovitch M, Grady S, David I: Compression of intrapulmonary branching pulmonary arteries associated with absent pulmonary valves. *Am J Cardiol* 1982; **50**:804-813.

23. Warner MA, Tinker JH, Frye RL, et al: Risk of cardiac operations in patients with concommitant pulmonary dysfunction. *Anesthesiology* 1982; **57**:A57.

24. Klein LW: Cigarette smoking, atherosclerosis and the coronary hemodynamic response: A unifying hypothesis. *J Am Coll Cardiol* 1984; **4**:972-974.

25. Nicod P, Rehr P, Winniford MD: Acute systemic and coronary hemodynamic and serologic responses to cigarette smoking in long term smokers with atherosclerotic coronary artery disease. *J Am Coll Cardiol* 1984; **4**:964-971.

26. Conti CR, Mehta JL: Acute myocardial ischemia: Role of atherosclerosis, thrombosis, platelet activation, coronary vasospasm, and altered arachidonic acid metabolism. *Circulation* 1987; **75**(suppl 5):84-95.

27. Pearce AC, Jones RM: Smoking and anesthesia: Preoperative abstinence and perioperative morbidity. *Anesthesiology* 1984; **61**: 576-584.

28. Anderson EW, Andelman RJ, Strauch JM, et al: Effect of low carbon monoxide exposure on onset and duration of angina pectoris. *Ann Intern Med* 1973; **79**:4650.

29. Warner MA, Divertie MB, Tinker JH: Preoperative cessation smoking and pulmonary complications in coronary artery bypass patients. *Anesthesiology* 1984; **60**:380-383.

30. *Drug Facts and Comparisons.* Philadelphia, JB Lippincott, 1994, pp 173-178.

31. Stirt JA, Sullivan SF: Aminophylline. *Anesth Analg* 1981; **60**: 587-602.

32. Marchlinski FE, Miller JM: Atrial arrhythmias exacerbated by theophylline. Response to verapamil and evidence for triggered activity in man. *Chest* 1985; **88**:931-934.

33. Greenberg A, Piraino BH, Kroboth PD, Weiss J: Severe theophylline toxicity. Role of conservative measures, antiarrhythmic agents, and charcoal hemoperfusion. *Am J Med* 1984; **76**: 854-860.

34. Kingston HGG, Hirshman CA: Perioperative management of the patient with asthma. *Anesth Analg* 1984; **63**:844-855.

35. Vander Woude JC, Milam JD, Walker WE, et al: Cardiovascular surgery in patients with congenital plasma coagulopathies. *Ann Thorac Surg* 1988; **46**:283-288.

36. Levine PH: Clinical manifestations and therapy of hemophilias A and B, in Colman RW, Hirsh J, Marder VJ, Salzman EW (eds): *Hemostasis and Thrombis: Basic Principles and Clinical Practice.* 2nd ed. Philadelphia, Lippincott, 1987, pp 97-111.

37. Schmaier AH, Silverberg M, Kaplan AP, Colman RW: Contact activation and its abnormalities, in Colman RW, Hirsh J, Marder VJ, Salzman EW (eds): *Hemostasis and Thrombis: Basic Principles and Clinical Practice.* 2nd ed. Philadelphia, Lippincott, 1987, pp 18-38.

38. De Caterina R, Lanza M, Manca G, et al: Bleeding time and bleeding: An analysis of the bleeding time test with parameters of surgical bleeding. *Blood* 1994; **84**:3363-3370.

39. Ferraris VA, Ferraris SP: Preoperative aspirin ingestion increases operative blood loss after coronary artery bypass grafting (updated in 1995). *Ann Thorac Surg* 1995; **59**:1036-1037.

40. Palmer Smith J, Walls JT, Muscato MS, et al: Extracorporeal circulation in a patient with heparin-induced thrombocytopenia. *Anesthesiology* 1985; **62**:363-365.

41. Makhoul RG, McCann RL, Austin EH, et al: Management of patients with heparin-associated thrombocytopenia and thrombosis requiring cardiac surgery. *Ann Thorac Surg* 1987; **43**:617-621.

42. Kappa JR, Horn MK, Fischer CA: Efficacy of iloprost (ZK36374) versus aspirin in preventing heparin-induced platelet activation during open heart surgery. *J Thorac Cardiovasc Surg* 1987; **94**:405-413.

43. Shorten G, Commule ME, Johnson RG: Management of cardiopulmonary bypass in a patient with heparin-induced thrombocytopenia using prostaglandin E$_1$ and aspirin. *J Cardiothorac Vasc Anesth* 1994; **8**:556-558.

44. Willard JE, Lange RA, Hillis LD: The use of aspirin in ischemic heart disease. *N Engl J Med* 1992; **327**:175-181.

45. Sethi GK, Copeland JC, Goldman S: Implications of preoperative administration of aspirin in patients undergoing coronary artery bypass surgery. *J Am Coll Cardiol* 1990; **15**:15-20.

45a. Tuman KJ, McCarthy RJ, O'Connor CJ, et al: Aspirin does not increase allogenic blood transfusion in reoperative coronary artery surgery. *Anesth Analg* 1996; **83**:1178-1184.

45b. Reich DL, Patel GC, Vela-Cantos F, et al: Aspirin does not increase homologous blood requirements in elective coronary bypass surgery. *Anesth Analg* 1994; **79**:4-8.

46. Maurer HM: Hematologic effects of cardiac disease. *Pediatr Clin North Am* 1972; **19**:1083-1093.

47. Milam JD, Austin SF, Nihill MR, et al: Use of sufficient hemodilution to prevent coagulopathies following surgical correction of cyanotic heart disease. *J Thorac Cardiovasc Surg* 1985; **89**: 623-629.

48. Hindman BJ, Koka BV: Usefulness of the post-aspirin bleeding time. *Anesthesiology* 1986; **64**:368-370.

49. Coller BS: von Willebrand disease, in Colman RW, Hirsh J, Marder VJ, Salzman EW (eds): *Hemostasis and Thrombis: Basic Principles and Clinical Practice.* 2nd ed. Philadelphia, Lippincott, 1987, pp 60-96.

50. Komp DM, Sparrow AW: Polycythemia in cyanotic heart disease—A study of altered coagulation. *J Pediatr* 1970; **76**:231-236.

51. Colon-Otero G, Gilchrist GS, Holcomb GR, et al: Preoperative evaluation of hemostasis in patients with congenital heart disease. *Mayo Clin Proc* 1987; **62**:379-385.

52. Gill JC, Wilson AD, Endres-Brooks J, Montgomery RR: Loss of the largest von Willebrand factor multimers from the plasma of patients with congenital cardiac defects. *Blood* 1986; **67**:758-761.

53. Perloff JK, Rosove MH, Child JS, Wright GB: Adults with cyanotic congenital heart disease: Hematologic management. *Ann Intern Med* 1988; **109**:406-413.

54. Mannucci PM, Remuzzi G, Pusineri F: Deamino-8-arginine vasopressin shortens the bleeding time in uremia. *N Engl J Med* 1983; **308**:8-12.

55. Mason RA, Arbeit LA, Giron F: Renal dysfunction after arteriography. *JAMA* 1985; **253**:1001-1004.

56. D'Elia JA, Gleason RE, Alday M, et al: Nephrotoxicity from angiographic contrast material. A prospective study. *Am J Med* 1982; **72**:719-725.

57. Bolman RM, Anderson RW, Molina JE: Cardiac operations in patients with functioning renal allografts. *J Thorac Cardiovasc Surg* 1984; **88**:537-543.

58. Nordrehaug JE, Van Der Lippe G: Hypokalemia and ventricular fibrillation in acute myocardial infarction. *Br Heart J* 1983; **50**:525-529.

59. McGovern B: Hypokalemia and cardiac arrhythmias. *Anesthesiology* 1985; **63**:127-129.

60. Vitez TS, Soper LE, Wong WC, Soper P: Chronic hypokalemia and intraoperative dysrhythmias. *Anesthesiology* 1985; **63**:130-133.

61. Hirsch IA, Tomlinson DL, Slogoff S, Keats AS: The overstated risk of preoperative hypokalemia. *Anesth Analg* 1988; **67**:131-136.

62. Gorlin R: Evaluation of the patient with coronary heart disease, in Gorlin R (ed): *Coronary Artery Disease.* Philadelphia, Saunders, 1976, pp 177-178.

63. Marriott HJL: The heart in childhood and congenital lesions, in Marriott HJL (ed): *Practical Electrocardiography.* Baltimore, Williams & Wilkins, 1980, pp 274-275.

64. Mangano DT, Hedgcock MW, Wisneski J: Non-invasive prediction of ventricular dysfunction: Valvular heart disease. *Anesthesiology* 1985; **63**:A65.

65. Mangano DT: Preoperative assessment, in Kaplan JA (ed): *Cardiac Anesthesia.* 2nd ed. Orlando, Grune & Stratton, 1987, pp 341-392.

66. Chaitman B: Exercise stress testing, in Braunwald E (ed): *Heart Disease, A Textbook of Cardiovascular Medicine.* 4th ed. Philadelphia, WB Saunders, 1992, pp 161-179.

67. Mayo Clinic Cardiovascular Working Group on Stress Testing: Cardiovascular stress testing: A description of the various types of stress tests and indications for their use. *Mayo Clin Proc* 1996; **71**:43-52.

68. Ryan T: Stress echocardiography, in Skorton DJ (ed): *Marcus Cardiac Imaging.* 2nd ed. Philadelphia, WB Saunders, 1996, pp 503-522.

69. Brown KA: Prognostic value of cardiac imaging in patients with known or suspected coronary artery disease: Comparison of myocardial perfusion imaging, stress echocardiography, and positron emission tomography. *Am J Cardiol* 1995; **75**:35D-41D.

70. Dahlberg ST, Leppo JA: Single-positron emitting tracers for imaging myocardial perfusion and cell membrane integrity, in Skorton DJ (ed): *Marcus Cardiac Imaging.* 2nd ed. Philadelphia, WB Saunders, 1996, pp 963-971.

71. Maddahi J: Myocardial perfusion imaging for the detection and evaluation of coronary artery disease, in Skorton DJ (ed): *Marcus Cardiac Imaging.* 2nd ed. Philadelphia, WB Saunders, 1996, pp 971-995.

72. Beller GA: Myocardial imaging for the assessment of myocardial viability, in Skorton DJ (ed): *Marcus Cardiac Imaging*. 2nd ed. Philadelphia, WB Saunders, 1996, pp 971–995.

73. Port S: First-pass radionuclide angiography, in Skorton DJ (ed): *Marcus Cardiac Imaging*. 2nd ed. Philadelphia, WB Saunders, 1996, pp 923–941.

74. Gibbons RJ, Miller TD: Equilibrium radionuclide angiography, in Skorton DJ (ed): *Marcus Cardiac Imaging*. 2nd ed. Philadelphia, WB Saunders, 1996, pp 941–963.

2

Interpreting Cardiac Catheterization Data

James A. DiNardo

The ability to interpret cardiac catheterization data is essential to the cardiac anesthesiologist. Properly interpreted catheterization data provide information about the extent and distribution of coronary stenosis, the type and extent of valvular lesions, the location and quantitation of intracardiac shunts and congenital lesions, and an assessment of systolic and diastolic function. This information is important both as part of a complete preoperative evaluation and as a predictor of postoperative functional status.

The following procedures are part of a routine cardiac catheterization at our institution. It is expected that there will be variation from institution to institution.

Right Heart Catheterization. A fluid-filled catheter capable of making high-fidelity systolic, diastolic, and mean pressure measurements in the right atrium, right ventricle, pulmonary artery, and pulmonary capillary wedge position is passed antegrade via a basilic, cephalic, or femoral vein under fluoroscopic guidance. In addition, the catheter may have the capability of making thermodilution cardiac output measurements. Angiography is performed by recording several cardiac cycles on cine film while radiographic contrast material is injected into the right heart chambers.

For infants and children, the femoral vein is the usual access site; however, right heart catheterization via the umbilical vein may be possible in the first few days after birth. Catheterization of the right ventricle and

pulmonary arteries may be difficult via the umbilical route because umbilical vein catheters tend to pass directly into the left atrium via the foramen ovale. Right atrial, right ventricular, and pulmonary angiography may be performed on infants and children to delineate congenital lesions.

Left Heart Catheterization. A fluid-filled catheter capable of making high-fidelity systolic, diastolic, and mean pressure measurements and capable of allowing angiographic dye injection is used. The catheter may be passed retrograde via the brachial or femoral artery to the aortic root under fluoroscopic guidance where pressures are recorded. For infants and children, the atrial septum usually can be crossed via a patent foramen ovale or an atrial septal defect, and left heart catheterization can be performed antegrade via the right atrium. If this approach is unsuccessful, retrograde catheterization via the femoral artery is performed. The course of the umbilical artery is tortuous and it generally is not useful except for pressure monitoring and angiography of the descending aorta.

Pressures in the aorta, left ventricle, and left atrium are recorded. Aortography may be performed by recording on cine film the injection of radiographic contrast material into the aortic root. This will allow detection of aortic regurgitation, congenital aortic arch abnormalities such as coarctation or aortic arch interruption, and acquired aortic lesions such as aortic dissection. Left atrial

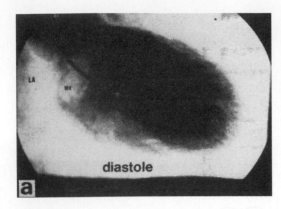
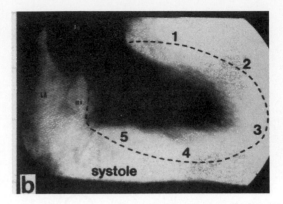

FIGURE 2–1. Left ventriculogram in right anterior oblique (RAO) projection. Ao = aorta, LA = left atrium, mv = mitral valve. End-diastolic image is seen on the left (a) while end-systolic image is seen on the right (b). For purposes of comparison, end diastole is represented by dotted outline on end-systolic image. Numbers 1 to 5 refer to five segments analyzed for wall motion in RAO projection (see Fig. 2–13). *(From: Jamieson SW, Shumway NE: Rob and Smith's Operative Surgery: Cardiac Surgery. 4th ed. London, Butterworths, 1995, p 6. Reprinted by permission.)*

and ventricular angiography allows detection of congenital anomalies. For adults, left ventriculography is performed by recording several cardiac cycles on cine film as radiographic contrast material is injected into the midleft ventricle. The left ventriculogram allows detection of mitral regurgitation as well as comparison of both regional and global wall motion in systole and diastole (*see* Fig. 2–1). The left ventriculogram also allows calculation of left ventricular end-diastolic volume (LVEDV) and left ventricular end-systolic volume (LVESV). The innermost margin of the left ventricular silhouette in systole and diastole is traced out by hand. Computer-assisted planimetry calculates left ventricular volumes from these two-dimensional pictures based on the assumption that ventricular shape is approximated by an ellipsoid.[1] Angiographic stroke volume (SV) is then defined as LVEDV − LVESV. Ejection fraction (EF) is defined as (LVEDV − LVESV)/LVEDV, which is SV/LVEDV.

Coronary Angiography. Cine recordings of radiographic contrast material selectively injected into the coronary ostia are made. Special catheters are used for the selective cannulization of the ostia and are advanced under fluoroscopic guidance via the same artery used for left heart catheterization (*see* Figs. 2–2 and 2–3).

Cardiac Output Determination. Two methods are used that compliment each other: the thermodilution determination and the Fick determination. Both methods measure forward cardiac outputs. Forward cardiac output and total cardiac output are equal only if there are no regurgitant lesions or shunt fractions.

Themodilution cardiac output is a modification of the indicator dilution method, in which flow is determined from the following relationship:

$$\frac{\text{Known amount of indicator injected}}{\text{Measured concentration of indicator}} \times \text{time}$$

In the thermodilution method, cold water is the indicator. A predetermined volume of injectate of known temperature is injected into the right atrium, where the temperature of the blood also is known. The subsequent change in temperature over time is measured by a ther-

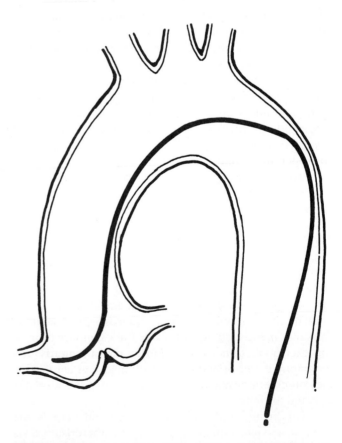

FIGURE 2–2. Left anterior oblique (LAO) projection of aorta illustrating use of Judkins technique to catheterize the right coronary ostia retrograde via femoral artery.

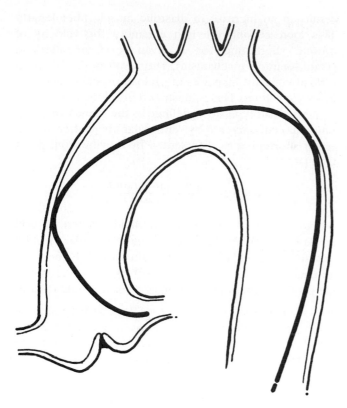

FIGURE 2–3. Left anterior oblique (LAO) projection of aorta illustrating use of Judkins technique to catheterize the left coronary ostia retrograde via femoral artery.

mistor in the pulmonary artery. This method measures pulmonary blood flow, which is equal to forward right heart output. It is not accurate at low cardiac outputs, in tricuspid regurgitation, or where an intracardiac left-to-right shunt exists. Thermodilution cardiac outputs are discussed in detail in Chapter 3.

The Fick determination is based on the relationship of O_2 uptake/AV O_2 difference. O_2 uptake or consumption can be determined from calculations made on a 3-minute expired air sample collected in a Douglas bag. More commonly, an estimate of O_2 consumption is obtained from tables that relate O_2 consumption to body surface area or to heart rate and age. AV O_2 difference is calculated from the difference between the arterial and mixed venous O_2 contents:

$$\text{Content} = (\% \ O_2 \text{ saturation of arterial or}$$
$$\text{mixed venous blood} \times \text{hemoglobin concentration}$$
$$\times (1.36) + (0.003 \times O_2 \text{ partial pressure}$$
$$\text{of arterial or mixed venous blood})$$

This method measures systemic blood flow, which equals forward left heart output. It also can be used to measure pulmonary blood flow or forward right heart output, when O_2 uptake is divided by pulmonary arterial content subtracted from pulmonary venous content.

The method is more accurate at low cardiac outputs, where the arterial to venous O_2 difference is great. It also is accurate in the presence of intracardiac shunts when the mixed venous O_2 content and pulmonary venous O_2 content are properly determined. This will be discussed further in the section on intracardiac shunts.

Resistances.   Systemic and pulmonary vascular resistances are made using hemodynamic and cardiac output data as follows:

- Systemic vascular resistance (SVR)
- Pulmonary vascular resistance (PVR)
- Transpulmonary gradient (TPG)
- Mean arterial blood pressure (MAP)
- Mean pulmonary artery pressure (mPAP)
- Pulmonary capillary wedge pressure (PCWP)
- Central venous pressure (CVP)
- Cardiac output (C.O.)

$$SVR = \frac{(MAP - CVP)\ 80}{C.O.} \qquad nl = 700–1600 \text{ dynes sec cm}^{-5}$$

$$SVR = \frac{(MAP - CVP)}{C.O.} \qquad nl = 9–20 \text{ Woods units}$$

$$PVR = \frac{(mPAP - PCWP)\ 80}{C.O.} \qquad nl = 20–130 \text{ dynes sec cm}^{-5}$$

$$PVR = \frac{(mPAP - PCWP)}{C.O.} \qquad nl = 0.25–1.6 \text{ Woods units}$$

$$TPG = mPAP - PCWP \qquad nl = 5–10 \text{ mm Hg}$$

The use of these parameters in evaluation of patients is discussed in detail in Chapters 4-9.

Saturation Data.   The percent saturation of blood in the low superior vena cava, the main pulmonary artery, and the aorta are obtained to screen for intracardiac shunts. If an intracardiac shunt is suspected, multiple samples from locations in the great vessels and cardiac chambers are necessary to localize the shunt and determine its magnitude and direction.

Assessment of Valve Lesions.   Analysis of the pressure data from right and left heart catheterization, in combination with analysis of ventriculography and aortography data, will delineate the extent and nature of valvular lesions.

Assessment of Pulmonary Vascular Anatomy. For infants and children with congenital heart disease, special procedures may be necessary to assess the pulmonary vasculature and the extent of pulmonary vascular disease.

To fully understand catheter data, it is necessary to be familiar with ventricular pressure–volume loops. A normal left ventricular pressure–volume loop is illustrated in Figure 2-4. Curve AB represents the diastolic

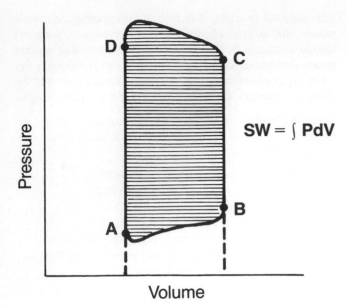

$$SW = \int PdV$$

FIGURE 2–4. Schematic representation of ventricular pressure–volume loop. Cross-hatched area represents stroke work or total external mechanical work. Curve AB = diastolic filling, BC = isovolumic contraction, CD = systolic ejection, DA = isovolumic relaxation.

pressure–volume relationship. Ventricular filling begins when left atrial pressure (LAP) exceeds left ventricular pressure at point A and the mitral valve opens. Point B represents left ventricular end-diastolic pressure (LVEDP) and left ventricular end-diastolic volume (LVEDV). Point B also represents the onset of isovolumic contraction at which left ventricular (LV) pressure exceeds LAP and the mitral valve closes. Changes in diastolic function can be represented by changes in the position and shape of the curve AB and will be discussed later.

Curve BC represents isovolumic contraction. Left ventricular pressure increases while left ventricular volume remains constant. At point C, left ventricular pressure exceeds aortic diastolic pressure and the aortic valve opens.

Curve CD represents the ejection phase of ventricular contraction. At point D, aortic pressure exceeds left ventricular pressure and the aortic valve closes. Point D represents the left ventricular end-systolic pressure (LVESP) and the left ventricular end-systolic volume (LVESV).

Curve DA represents isovolumic relaxation — that is, a constant left ventricular volume in the face of a decreasing left ventricular pressure.

The area encompassed by ABCD represents the stroke work (SW), which is external mechanical work.[2]

Preload is defined as an increase in end-diastolic fiber length or volume and is represented by a point B farther to the left on the curve AB. Augmented preload

results in an increase in diastolic muscle fiber length. This increased fiber length enhances the velocity of muscle shortening for a given level of afterload (Frank–Starling mechanism). The result is that with afterload constant increases in preload produce increases in stroke volume. This is illustrated in Figure 2–5.

Afterload typically is defined as the stress (force per unit area) encountered by ventricular fibers after the onset of shortening as represented by moving from point C to D.

$$Stress = \frac{pressure \times radius}{2\,h}$$

where h is wall thickness. Afterload defined as wall stress is constantly changing during ventricular ejection because ventricular pressure, radius, and thickness are all changing as ejection progresses. Because the ventricle produces pulsatile ejection of a viscous fluid (blood)

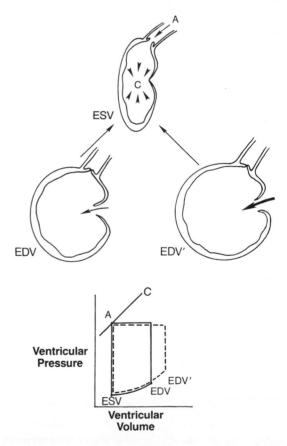

FIGURE 2–5. Top. Long-axis cross section of left ventricle illustrating the effect of increasing preload or end-diastolic volume (EDV) with afterload (A) and contractility (C) constant. Increasing preload from EDV to EDV′ increases stroke volume by Frank–Starling mechanism. Note that end-systolic volume is not changed and stroke volume is enhanced solely by increase in preload. **Bottom.** Ventricular pressure–volume loop illustrating effect of increased preload (EDV′) with afterload (A) and contractility (C) constant. Again note that stroke volume is increased (from EDV–ESV to EDV′–ESV) and ESV is unchanged.

into a viscoelastic reservoir (the arterial system), it is worth considering the characteristics of the arterial system and of the blood, both of which constitute impedance to ventricular ejection.[3] Pulsatile and nonpulsatile flow must be considered because both exist in the intact arterial system. The nonpulsatile component of afterload is measured as peripheral vascular resistance. This is a familiar concept and is defined as:

$$\frac{\text{Mean arterial pressure} - \text{central venous pressure}}{\text{cardiac output}}$$

Blood viscosity and the caliber of the arterioles are the major determinants of peripheral vascular resistance. The pulsatile component of afterload is measured as frequency-dependent aortic input impedance, which is determined by the elastic properties of the proximal aorta and by the reflection of pulse waves from the peripheral arterial tree.[3]

Contractility is defined as the state of cardiac performance independent of preload and afterload. In the pressure–volume loop scheme, end-systolic fiber length or LVESV (point D) is independent of preload and is uniquely determined by the contractile state and the afterload.[4] A linear end-systolic pressure-volume relationship is obtained by connecting LVESV's obtained at different levels of afterload. The slope and position of this line uniquely defines the contractile state of the ventricle. For a given contractile state, an increase in afterload results in a larger LVESV, represented by moving upward and to the right on the line, whereas a decrease in afterload results in a smaller LVESV, represented by moving downward and to the left on the line (*see* Fig. 2–6). Increased contractility is represented by a linear end-systolic pressure–volume relationship that is steeper and shifted upward to the left. An increase in contractility with preload and afterload fixed obviously augments

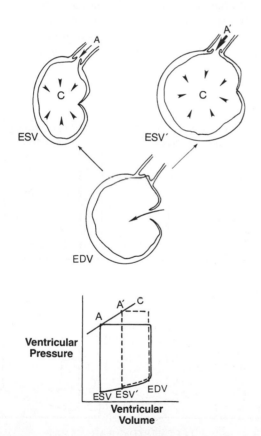

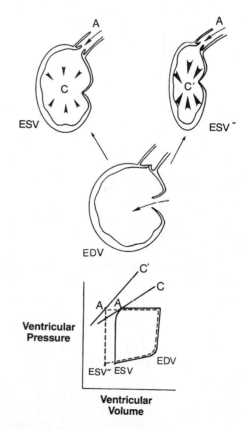

FIGURE 2–6. Top. Long-axis cross section of left ventricle illustrating effect of increasing afterload (A) with preload (EDV) and contractility (C) constant. Increasing afterload from A to A' results in increase in end-systolic volume (ESV) from ESV to ESV'. With EDV constant this results in reduction in stroke volume. **Bottom.** Ventricular pressure–volume loop illustrating effect of increased afterload (A') with preload (EDV) and contractility (C) constant. Increased afterload is represented by point (A') further to right on line C, which describes contractility. Increased afterload results in increase in end-systolic volume (from ESV to ESV'), which causes reduction in stroke volume (from EDV–ESV to EDV–ESV').

FIGURE 2–7. Top. Long-axis cross section of left ventricle illustrating effect of increasing contractility (C) with preload (EDV) and afterload (A) constant. Increasing contractility from C to C' results in decrease in end-systolic volume from ESV' to ESV''. With EDV constant, this results in increase in stroke volume. **Bottom.** Ventricular pressure–volume loop illustrating effect of increased contractility (C) with preload (EDV) and afterload (A) constant. Increased contractility is represented by line (C') shifted to left of line C and with steeper slope than line C. Increased contractility results in decrease in end-systolic volume (from ESV to ESV''), which causes an increase in stroke volume (from EDV–ESV to EDV–ESV'').

stroke volume because of the marked decrease in LVESV with LVEDV (preload) constant (see Fig. 2-7). Decreased contractility is represented by a linear end-systolic pressure–volume relationship that has a less positive slope and that is shifted downward to the right. With preload and afterload fixed, stroke volume is diminished when contractility decreases (see Fig. 2-7).

Figure 2-8 serves to unify these concepts. Loop 1 represents the control situation. Loop 2 represents an abrupt increase in afterload with contractility constant. The result is an increased LVESV and an unchanged LVEDV. The result is a reduction in stroke volume. In subsequent beats (loop 3) of a normal heart, LVEDV is increased such that the original stroke volume is now maintained at the new increased afterload. The ability of the ventricle to maintain stroke volume in the face of increased afterload by increasing preload is defined as preload reserve.[4] Preload reserve is exhausted when the sarcomeres are stretched to their maximum diastolic length. When this occurs, there will be no further augmentation of the velocity of shortening by increasing diastolic fiber length and the ventricle behaves as if preload is fixed. For a given level of contractility, after preload reserve is ex-

hausted, additional increases in afterload will be accompanied by parallel decreases in stroke volume (loop 4). This is defined as a state of afterload mismatch.[4] Therefore, afterload mismatch is the inability of the ventricle at a given level of contractility to maintain stroke volume in the face of an increased wall stress.

■ DIASTOLIC FUNCTION

Normal diastolic function is dependent on normal ventricular diastolic compliance, distensibility, and relaxation. Both extrinsic and intrinsic factors affect ventricular diastolic function.[5] It is necessary to differentiate between compliance, distensibility, and relaxation, and this is best accomplished by examining diastolic pressure–volume diagrams (see Fig. 2-9). It is possible for any or all of these abnormalities to exist in a given patient.

Compliance. Compliance is defined as the ratio of a volume change to the corresponding pressure change or as the slope of the pressure–volume relationship ($\Delta V/\Delta P$). Stiffness is the inverse of compliance ($\Delta P/\Delta V$). Decreased compliance or increased stiffness is thus de-

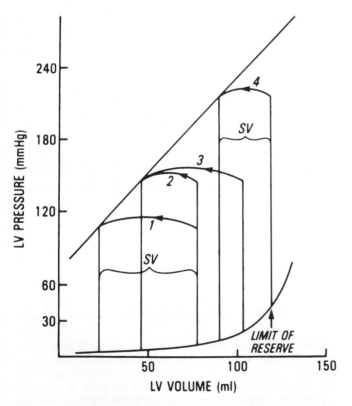

FIGURE 2–8. Ventricular pressure–volume loops illustrating compensation of intact ventricle for progressive increases in afterload with contractility fixed. Stroke volume can be maintained in face of progressive afterload increases until preload reserve is exhausted. *(From: Hurst JW: The Heart. 6th ed. New York: McGraw-Hill, 1986, p 813.)*

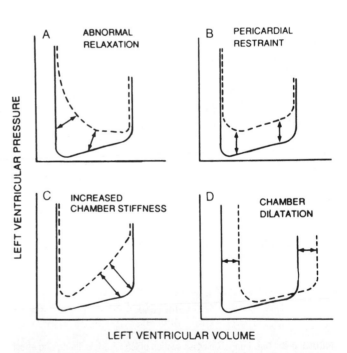

FIGURE 2–9. Series of diastolic pressure–volume curves. The solid curve in each example represents a normal diastolic pressure–volume relationship, whereas the dotted curve represents the altered diastolic pressure–volume relationship. **A.** The diastolic pressure–volume relationship when ventricular relaxation is impaired. **B.** The diastolic pressure–volume relationship when distensibility is reduced as with pericardial restraint. **C.** The diastolic pressure–volume relationship when ventricular chamber stiffness is increased or ventricular chamber compliance is reduced. **D.** The effect of chamber dilatation on a normal diastolic pressure–volume relationship.

fined as an increase in the steepness of the pressure-volume plot (*see* Fig. 2-9C). Strictly speaking, diastolic compliance is determined by the intrinsic pressure-volume relationship of completely relaxed myocytes. There are two causes of poor diastolic compliance:

1. Increased chamber stiffness — as occurs in aortic stenosis or sytemic hypertension. In these cases, there is an increase in the amount of myocardial tissue due to concentric hypertrophy. Diastolic compliance of the ventricle as a whole is diminished despite that fact that the compliance of the individual muscle units is normal.
2. Increased muscle stiffness — as occurs in restrictive cardiomyopathies due to amyoidosis and hemochromatosis. In these cases, the compliance of the individual muscle units is diminished due to an infiltrative process.

Normally, the diastolic pressure-volume relationship does not exhibit constant compliance; there is high compliance at low volumes with a progressive decrease in compliance at higher volumes. As a result, reduced diastolic compliance is not limited to ventricles with altered pressure-volume slopes. A ventricle forced to make use of preload reserve to maintain stroke volume may function on the steep portion of an otherwise normal compliance curve (*see* Fig. 2-9D).

Distensibility.   Decreased ventricular distensibility is defined as an increased diastolic pressure at a given volume. This would be represented in a diastolic pressure-volume diagram by a parallel upward shift of the entire pressure-volume relation (*see* Fig. 2-9B).

Reduced distensibility can occur from intrinsic and extrinsic causes:

1. Intrinisic — It has been demonstrated clearly that pacing-induced ischemia in humans with coronary artery disease (CAD) is responsible for diminished diastolic distensibility.[6-10] Although impaired relaxation certainly plays a role in diastolic dysfunction with ischemia, the pressure-volume relation in ischemia more closely resembles the pattern seen with pericardial restraint (*see* Fig. 2-9B). This diminished diastolic distensibility often precedes systolic dysfunction.[11] In addition, pacing-induced ischemia elicits diminished diastolic distensibility in humans with aortic stenosis without CAD.[12] Differences in the diastolic behavior of ischemic and nonischemic segments of the same ventricle subjected to pacing-induced ischemia have been demonstrated.[13] An upward shift (diminished distensibility) in the pressure-length relationship is observed in ischemic segments. For a given diastolic volume, this results in an increase in diastolic pressure, which causes the nonischemic segments to move to a steeper (less compliant) portion of their original pressure-length relationship.
2. Extrinsic — Reduced distensibility may be caused by extrinsic limitations to ventricular expansion in diastole. Diminished distensibility occurs due to ventricular interdependence via an intact ventricular septum and the restraining effect of the pericardium (*see* Fig. 2-9B). For example, distension of the right ventricle with a leftward septal shift will result in diminished distensibility of the left ventricle. In addition, reduced distensibility may occur due to the presence of a diseased or fluid-filled pericardium (*see* Chapter 7).

Relaxation.   Ventricular relaxation is an energy-consumptive process. ATP is required for calcium sequestration back into the sarcoplasmic reticulum and for detachment of actin-myocin crossbridges. When isovolumic relaxation is delayed, early diastolic filling is impeded. When relaxation is incomplete, filling is impeded throughout diastole (*see* Fig. 2-9a). Relaxation is impaired in myocardial ischemia and in hypertrophic and congestive cardiomyopathies.

Normally, the right ventricular end-diastolic pressure (RVEDP) is 1 to 2 mm Hg greater than the mean right atrial pressure (RAP), and the left ventricular end-diastolic pressure (LVEDP) is 2 to 3 mm Hg greater than the mean pulmonary capillary wedge pressure (PCWP) or left atrial pressure (LAP).[14] These small differences in pressure are due to the volume added to the ventricle by atrial systole. When LV compliance is poor, the A wave produced by atrial systole will be large and the additional volume provided by the atrial kick in end diastole will result in a large increase in LVEDP. For these patients, the peak A-wave pressure in the LAP or PCWP trace is a better measure of LVEDP than the mean LAP or PCWP because the mean LAP or PCWP pressure will underestimate LVEDP.[15,16] Even large A waves only slightly elevate mean LAP because their duration is short. Thus, well-timed atrial contraction results in a large elevation of LVEDV with only a small elevation of mean LAP and limited pulmonary congestion.[15,17] For patients who chronically function on a steep portion of the compliance curve, a large A wave, left atrial enlargement on electrocardiogram (ECG) and an S_4 on physical examination are expected findings.

ANALYSIS OF DIASTOLIC PRESSURE-VOLUME CURVES

Ideally, we would like to be able to examine the diastolic pressure-volume curve over its entire range and under baseline and stress conditions. Unfortunately, this

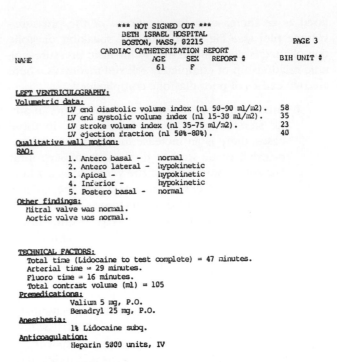

BETH ISRAEL HOSPITAL
BOSTON, MASS, 02215
CARDIAC CATHETERIZATION REPORT   PAGE 2
NAME   AGE   SEX   REPORT #   BIH UNIT #
                              61   F

                                    BODY SURFACE AREA: 1.85 m2
                                    HEMOGLOBIN: 13.4 gms %

HEMODYNAMICS

		NORMALS	
**PRESSURES			
RIGHT ATRIUM {a/v/m}	2-10/2-10/0-8	9/7/6	
RIGHT VENTRICLE {s/ed}	15-30/0-8	34/7	
PULMONARY ARTERY {s/d/m}	15-30/4-12/9-16	34/16/23	
PULMONARY WEDGE {a/v/m}	3-15/3-15/1-10	13/10/9	
LEFT VENTRICLE {s/ed}	100-140/3-12	138/13	
AORTA {s/d/m}	110-140/60-90/70-105	138/66/97	
**CARDIAC OUTPUT			
HEART RATE {beats/min}	60-100	82	
RHYTHM	NSR	NSR	
O2 CONS. IND {ml/min/m2}	110-150	121	
A-V O2 DIFFERENCE {ml/ltr}	30-50	49	
CARD. OP/IND FICK {l/mn/m2}	2.5-4.2	4.6/2.5	
**RESISTANCES			
SYSTEMIC VASC. RESISTANCE	770-1500	1583	
PULMONARY VASC. RESISTANCE	20-120	243	
**% SATURATION DATA (NL)			
SVC LOW		65	
PA MAIN		65,65	
AO		91,93	
**ARTERIAL BLOOD GAS			
INSPIRED O2 CONCENTR'N		0.21	
pO2		63	
pCO2		39	
pH		7.46	

(OVER)

FIGURE 2–10. Reproduction of portion of cardiac catheterization report from 61-year-old woman with severe three-vessel coronary artery disease and systolic dysfunction. Right and left ventricular pressure measurements. Fick CO determination, and derived hemodynamic variables are reported.

BETH ISRAEL HOSPITAL
BOSTON, MASS, 02215
CARDIAC CATHETERIZATION REPORT   PAGE 3
NAME   AGE   SEX   REPORT #   BIH UNIT #
                              61   F

LEFT VENTRICULOGRAPHY:
Volumetric data:
        LV end diastolic volume index (nl 50-90 ml/m2).   58
        LV end systolic volume index (nl 15-30 ml/m2).   35
        LV stroke volume index (nl 35-75 ml/m2).   23
        LV ejection fraction (nl 50%-80%).   40
Qualitative wall motion:
RAO:
        1. Antero basal -   normal
        2. Antero lateral -   hypokinetic
        3. Apical -   hypokinetic
        4. Inferior -   hypokinetic
        5. Postero basal -   normal
Other findings:
   Mitral valve was normal.
   Aortic valve was normal.

TECHNICAL FACTORS:
   Total time (Lidocaine to test complete) = 47 minutes.
   Arterial time = 29 minutes.
   Fluoro time = 16 minutes.
   Total contrast volume (ml) = 105
Premedications:
        Valium 5 mg, P.O.
        Benadryl 25 mg, P.O.
Anesthesia:
        1% Lidocaine subq.
Anticoagulation:
        Heparin 5000 units, IV

FIGURE 2–11. Reproduction of portion of catheterization report from the patient described in Figure 2–10. Section reports information obtained from left ventriculography: Left ventricular end-diastolic volume index (LVEDVI), left ventricular end-systolic volume index (LVESVI), stroke volume index (SVI), and ejection fraction (EF) are reported. In addition, qualitative descriptions of left ventricular wall motion in five wall segments seen in right anterior oblique (RAO) projection are reported.

information is not routinely available to us from cardiac catheterization data. At our institution, we are provided with the A-wave, V-wave, and mean pressures of the RAP and PCWP tracing, the RVEDP and LVEDP, and the left ventricular end-systolic and end-diastolic volume indices (LVESVI and LVEDVI). The LVESVI and the LVEDVI are simply the LVESV and LVEDV obtained by planimetry of left ventricular end-systolic and end-diastolic angiograms divided by the Dubois determination of the patient's body surface area. Pressure and volume data from a representative catheterization report are reproduced in Figures 2–10 and 2–11.

One point on the LV diastolic pressure–volume curve is obtained if the pressure and volume measurements are made under identical conditions of preload, heart rate, and ischemia. Thus, we must use incomplete information to draw inferences on overall diastolic performance. For patients in sinus rhythm without pericardial disease, the flow diagram in Figure 2–12 is useful.

Clinically, a dilated heart would be expected in patients who are dependent on a large LVEDV to maintain an adequate forward SV. Patients with chronic volume overload valvular lesions such as mitral regurgitation and aortic insufficiency are good examples. Here, a large LVEDV is needed because only a portion of the total SV

becomes forward SV. Early in the disease, these patients operate on the flat portion of a diastolic pressure–volume curve and have enormous preload reserve. As the disease progresses and systolic function deteriorates, larger LVEDVs are needed to maintain SV. Eventually, these patients operate on the steep portion of the diastolic pressure–volume relationship and are unable to augment preload without large increases in diastolic pressure and subsequent pulmonary congestion. Unfortunately, in patients with mitral regurgitation this analysis of diastolic function is complicated by the presence of regurgitant V waves in the LAP or PCWP trace during ventricular systole. The electronically determined mean LAP or PCWP will be increased in direct porportion to the height and duration of the regurgitant V wave. This will cause the mean LAP or PCWP to overestimate LVEDP. An estimate of the LVEDP can be obtained by examining a calibrated PCWP or LAP paper trace and determining the A-wave amplitude. For patients without an atrial systole, the best estimate of LVEDP will be the PCWP or LAP at end diastole (*see* Chapter 3).

A heart with a normal LVEDV and diminished ventricular compliance is seen most commonly in patients with left ventricular pressure overload valve lesions such as aortic stenosis and, to a lesser degree, in patients with

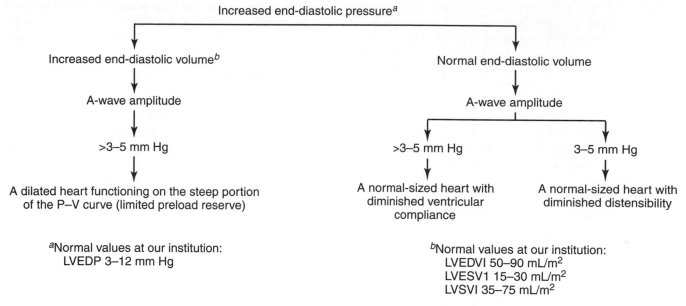

FIGURE 2–12. Flow diagram that uses diastolic pressure and volume data to delineate diastolic function.

systemic hypertension. For these patients, the LVEDV necessary to maintain an adequate SV is maintained at the expense of a high LVEDP because compliance is poor. The volume contributed by atrial systole represents a larger proportion of the LVEDV than it does in ventricles with normal compliance because the early diastolic filling is compromised by low compliance and is compensated for by a well-timed forceful atrial systole.[18] Loss of atrial systole for these patients is disastrous because LVEDV can then be maintained only by large elevations of mean LAP with consequent pulmonary congestion.

A ventricle with abnormal LVEDV and diminished distensibility is characteristic of patients with severe coronary artery disease in whom the energy requirements necessary to guarantee complete ventricular relaxation at rest are not met. Such diastolic dysfunction precedes the development of systolic dysfunction.[11]

■ SYSTOLIC FUNCTION

Systolic function is not synonymous with contractility. Normal systolic function is the ability of the ventricle to perform external work (generate a stroke volume) under varying conditions of preload, afterload, and contractility. Any assessment of systolic function must take the contribution of these three factors into account.

Ejection Fraction

Defined as (LVEDV − LVESV)/LVEDV, the EF is an ejection-phase index and the most commonly used assessment of global systolic function. The LVEDV and the LVESV are obtained from planimetry of LV end-diastolic and end-systolic angiograms (*see* Fig. 2-1). The normal value is 50 to 80%. Determination of EF is dependent on variations in preload, afterload, and contractility (*see* Figs. 2-5 through 2-7). It is obvious that increases or decreases in preload have relatively small influences on EF, because both the numerator (stroke volume) and the denominator (LVEDV) are increasing or decreasing simultaneously. An increase in LVEDVI from 75 to 90 mL/m² with LVESVI constant at 25 mL/m², as would occur with afterload and contractility constant, would result in an increase in EF from 66 to 72%. Thus, a 20% increase in preload results in a 9% increase in EF.

An increase in afterload with preload and contractility constant will diminish EF. An increase in afterload will result in an increased LVESV with LVEDV constant; thus, stroke volume and EF will fall. Likewise, a decrease in afterload will increase EF. How much effect an increase in afterload has on EF will depend on the slope of the linear pressure–volume relationship. The more positive the slope, the less the incremental increase in LVESV for a given increase in afterload. Thus, ventricles with depressed contractile function (more negative slope) have greater reductions in EF for a given increase in afterload. An increase in contractility augments EF because with preload and afterload constant there is a marked decrease in the LVESV.

EF is not a very sensitive index of coronary artery disease because areas of regional myocardial dysfunction secondary to ischemia may exist without depression of global systolic function. EF is diminished in all patients with three-vessel disease but is diminished in patients with one- and two-vessel coronary disease only in the presence of a previous myocardial infarction.[19] Nonetheless, EF reliably separates patients with normal LV function from those with LV dysfunction and is reliable in following changes in systolic function in individual patients.[20,21] An EF lower than 40% in the absence of acute afterload elevations represents depressed systolic function and corresponds clinically with New York Heart Association class 3 symptoms. An EF lower than 25% represents severe depression of LV systolic function and corresponds to New York Heart Association class 4 symptoms.

EF may overestimate systolic function in mitral regurgitation because of the unique systolic loading conditions in this lesion. The left ventricle is presented with two outflow tracts in systole: the aortic valve and the incompetent mitral valve. The mitral valve provides a low-impedance outflow tract and the aortic valve provides a normal-impedance outflow tract. EF may remain near normal in the face of depressed systolic function due to this low mean afterload state.[4] With mitral valve replacement and the elimination of the low-impedance outflow tract, the ventricle is presented with more normal systolic loading conditions. EF may actually decrease substantially postoperatively in such patients because depressed systolic function is now unmasked.[4,22,23]

Stroke Work

Another ejection-phase index of systolic function is stroke work (SW) or external LV work, represented by the area ABCD in Figure 2–4. When the shape of the LV pressure–volume loop is normal, as is true in the absence of pressure or volume overload conditions, left ventricular stroke work (LVSW) is a good measure of systolic function. Chronic volume and pressure overload conditions alter the shape of the pressure–volume loop and the calculated LVSW is increased above the normal value of 60 to 120 gram–meters/beat. LVSW is defined as:

$$(\text{Mean LV systolic pressure} - \text{mean LV diastolic pressure}) \times SV \times 0.0136$$

When aortic and mitral regurgitation are absent, this can be simplified to:

$$(\text{Mean arterial pressure} - \text{mean pulmonary capillary wedge pressure}) \times SV \times 0.0136$$

because mean arterial pressure approximates mean LV systolic pressure and mean pulmonary capillary wedge pressure closely approximates mean LV diastolic pressure. In direct contrast to EF, alterations in afterload have little effect on calculated SW.[24] SV declines or increases in proportion to the afterload elevation or reduction such that the area of the loop remains unchanged. SW, unlike EF, is very sensitive to changes in preload.[24] The area of the loop is increased or decreased by increases or decreases in preload.

Left Ventricular End-Systolic Pressure–Volume Relationships

Attempts to assess myocardial contractility independent of pressure and volume loading conditions have led to the use of LV end-systolic pressure–volume relationships. As previously discussed, the line determined by the relationship of LV end-systolic pressure to volume uniquely defines contractility independent of loading conditions. Grossman et al. plotted LVESP versus LVESV at two levels of afterload and were able to clearly separate patients with normal, intermediate, and depressed contractility.[25] This method requires the ability to simultaneously record LVESV and LVESP and is not in routine clinical use.

Left Ventriculography

Qualitative analysis of regional wall motion by left ventriculography is another index of systolic function. Ventriculography is performed by making cine recordings as contrast material is injected directly into the midleft ventricle. Left ventriculography is performed in the right anterior oblique (RAO) projection or in the right and left anterior oblique (LAO) projections. The ventricle is divided into segments (see Fig. 2–13) and visual analysis of regional wall motion is made by comparison of end-diastolic and end-systolic cineangiograms (see Fig. 2–1). At our institution, five segments are analyzed in the RAO projection: anterobasal, anterolateral, apical, diaphragmatic (inferior), and posterobasal. Five segments also may be analyzed in the LAO projection: basal septal, apical septal, apical inferior, posterolateral, and superior lateral. These areas are graded qualitatively for dyssynergy. Normal areas exhibit concentric inward movement in systole. Hypokinetic areas exhibit reduced concentric inward motion in systole. Akinetic areas exhibit no motion with systole. Dyskinetic areas exhibit a paradoxical outward bulging with systole. Aneurysmal areas exhibit frank aneurysm formation.

Areas of hypokinesis generally are composed of ischemic myocardium, whereas akinetic areas are composed of ischemic myocardium and fibrous scar.[26] Improvements in wall motion have been demonstrated in hypokinetic and akinetic areas when ischemic tissue has been "salvaged" by revascularization or by pharmacologic interventions to improve perfusion such as nitrate therapy.[26,27] The presence of collaterals, the absence of surface ECG Q waves, and the presence of an associated proximal coronary stenosis less than 90% improve the likelihood that medical or surgical intervention will improve the dyssynergy in a given area.[28] Dyskinetic and

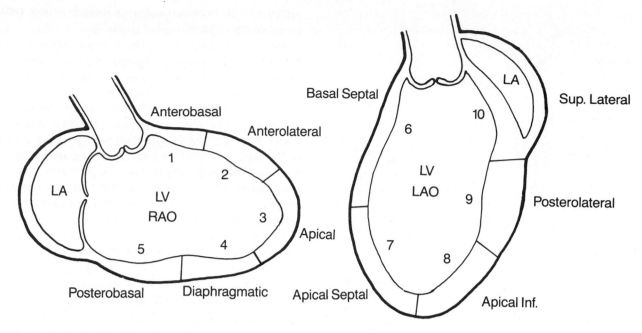

FIGURE 2–13. Schematic delineation of five wall segments seen in RAO and LAO projections during left ventriculography. Following is summary of coronary arterial supply to these regions (LMCA = left main coronary artery, LAD = left anterior descending artery, CIRC = circumflex artery, RCA = right coronary artery, PDA = posterior descending artery):

1. Anterobasal — LMCA; proximal LAD; 1st diagonal
2. Anterolateral — LMCA; proximal or mid-LAD; 1st diagonal
3. Apical — LMCA; proximal, mid, or distal LAD; 2nd diagonal
4. Diaphramatic (inferior) — proximal, mid, or distal RCA; PDA
5. Posterobasal — proximal, mid, or distal RCA; PDA
6. Basal septal — LMCA; proximal or mid-LAD, 1st septal
7. Apical septal — LMCA; proximal, mid, or distal LAD
8. Apical inferior — proximal, mid, or distal RCA
9. Posterolateral — LMCA; proximal or distal CIRC marginals
10. Superior lateral — LMCA; proximal CIRC marginals

aneurysmal areas, respectively, represent regions with little or no viable myocardium and rarely show improvement in wall motion with surgical or pharmacologic intervention.[26,27]

Regional dyssynergy is a more sensitive indicator of coronary artery disease than is a reduction in a global ejection-phase index of systolic function like EF. This is because global systolic function can be maintained in the presence of regional dyssynergy by compensatory increases in wall shortening in areas of normal wall motion as long as large areas of myocardium are not dyssynergic.

■ CORONARY ANGIOGRAPHY

Coronary angiography is a diagnostic procedure intended to delineate the normal and pathologic features of the coronary circulation. Normally, angiography is performed in the 60° LAO projection and the 30° RAO projection with caudal or cranial angulated views if necessary.[29] There are several categories of information to be interpreted.

Coronary Anatomy

To know what areas of myocardium are at risk with a particular stenotic or vasospastic lesion, it is necessary to know the regional blood supply pattern. The right and left coronary anatomy is illustrated in Figures 2–14 and 2–15. Most patients (85%) have a right dominant system of coronary circulation. Here, the right coronary artery extends to the crux cordis in the atrioventricular groove and gives rise to the posterior descending branch, left atrial branch, atrioventricular (AV) nodal branch, and one or more posterior left ventricular branches. In a left-dominant system (8%), these branches are supplied by the left circumflex artery and the right coronary artery supplies only the right atria and ventricle. In 7% of patients, the system is balanced, with the right coronary artery supplying the posterior descending, left atria, and

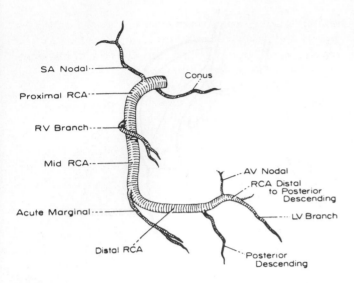

FIGURE 2–14. Anatomy of right coronary artery. *(From: Hurst JW: The Heart. 5th ed. New York, McGraw-Hill, 1981, p 1872.)*

AV nodal branches, whereas the left circumflex artery supplies the posterior left ventricular branches.

There is variation in the blood supply to various regions of myocardium, but some generalizations can be made. This information is summarized in Figure 2–13. Normally, the anterobasal region is supplied by a proximal branch of the left circumflex artery. The anterolateral region is supplied by contributions from both the diagional branch of the left anterior descending (LAD)

artery and the obtuse marginal branch of the left circumflex. The apical region is supplied by the terminal portion of the LAD artery. The inferior region is a combination of the posterior lateral and diaphragmatic regions, which are best seen in an LAO projection. The posterior lateral region is supplied by the posterior lateral branch of the left circumflex artery. The diaphragmatic region is supplied by the posterior descending artery, which, as previously discussed, is either a branch of the right coronary or left circumflex artery. The posterobasal region is supplied by the proximal right coronary artery. The anterior two-thirds of the ventricular septum is supplied by the septal branches of the LAD artery, and the posterior one-third is supplied by branches of the right coronary and posterior descending arteries. The SA node is supplied by a branch of the right coronary artery in 55% of patients and by a branch of the left circumflex artery in the other 45%.

The bulk of the right ventricle is located in the diaphragmatic and posterobasal regions supplied by the right coronary artery in a right dominant system. Obviously, small portions of the right ventricle also are included in the apical and septal areas. It is for this reason that involvement of the LAD results in compromise of perfusion to the anterior right ventricular wall near the ventricular septum and to the right ventricular apex. Conversely, involvement of the right coronary artery in a right dominant system results in compromise of perfusion to the portions of the left ventricle located in the diaphragmatic and posterobasal regions. How severely the posterior portion of the left ventricle will be com-

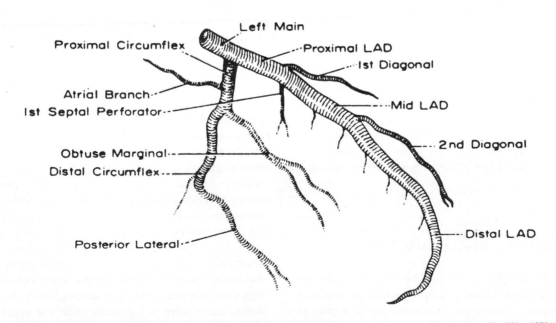

FIGURE 2–15. Anatomy of left coronary artery (right oblique). *(From: Hurst JW: The Heart. 5th ed. New York, McGraw-Hill, 1981, p 1873.)*

promised in this setting will depend on how much of this region is also supplied by the distal branches of the circumflex artery.

Anatomic Coronary Lesions

Coronary atherosclerotic stenotic lesions are quantitated visually from moving cineangiograms in several projections. Coronary arteriography from a representative catheterization report is reproduced in Figure 2–16. Stenotic areas of artery are compared with adjacent normal areas and the percent reduction in lumen diameter caused by the stenosis is quantified. Thus, in standard parlance, a 90% lesion refers to a stenosis that causes a 90% reduction in lumen diameter. It is generally acknowledged that resting coronary blood flow does not decrease until there is an 85% reduction in lumen diameter.[30,31] This corresponds to a greater than 90% reduc-

tion in lumen cross-sectional area. By contrast, a 50% diameter reduction corresponds to a 75% reduction in cross-sectional area. Maximal coronary flow in response to a stimulus for vasodilation is blunted when there is a 30 to 45% reduction in lumen diameter and is absent when lumen diameter is reduced 88 to 93%.[31] It has been demonstrated that interobserver variability exists in the grading of stenotic lesions.[32] In addition, coronary angiography typically underestimates the severity of stenotic lesions[33] and may not accurately predict the physiologic significance of a particular lesion.[34] Nonetheless, at present, it is the gold standard.

Coronary Spasm

True coronary spasm is diagnosed at the time of coronary angiography with an ergonovine provocation test. The test is considered positive if focal spasm occurs in the presence of clinical symptoms or ECG changes (*see* Chapter 4).

Coronary Thrombus Formation

A thrombus superimposed on an obstructive coronary lesion has been implicated in the pathogenesis of unstable angina and is the direct cause of acute transmural myocardial infarction in most patients.[35] Currently, protocols designed to intervene in the early stages of myocardial infarction incorporate thrombolytic therapy, percutaneous transluminal coronary angioplasty, or both (*see* Chapter 8).

Coronary Collaterals

An extensive network of coronary collaterals is normally present at birth. However, these collaterals are not demonstrable by angiography in normal hearts due to their small diameter. It is only when the collateral channels enlarge secondary to regional myocardial oxygen deprivation that they are visible angiographically. The development of collateral pathways in patients with comparable degrees of coronary insufficiency is variable in both extent and time course. The presence of collaterals has been identified as a determinant of reversible dyssynergy,[28] and left ventricular function in the region of an occluded coronary artery is better maintained in the presence of collaterals than in their absence.[36]

Interpretation of Coronary Angiography Data

To properly interpret the coronary angiograms it is necessary to integrate data from the angiograms with data from the right and left heart catheterizations and from the left ventriculograms. Several questions should be answered:

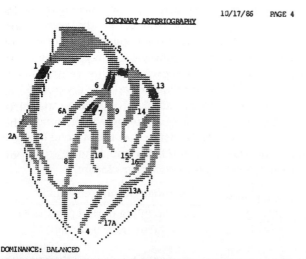

CORONARY ARTERIOGRAPHY   10/17/86   PAGE 4

DOMINANCE: BALANCED

ARTERIAL SEGMENT	MORPHOLOGY	% STENOSIS	COLLAT FROM
RIGHT CORONARY			
1) PROXIMAL RCA	DISCRETE	100	
2) MID RCA	NORMAL		
2A) ACUTE MARGINAL	NORMAL		
3) DISTAL RCA	NORMAL		
4) R-PDA	NORMAL		
4A) R-POST-LAT	NORMAL		
4B) R-LV	NORMAL		
LEFT CORONARY			
5) LEFT MAIN	NORMAL		
6) PROXIMAL LAD	TUBULAR	70	
6A) SEPTAL-1	NORMAL		
7) MID-LAD	DISCRETE	50	
8) DISTAL LAD	NORMAL		
9) DIAGONAL-1	NORMAL		
10) DIAGONAL-2	NORMAL		
12) PROXIMAL CX	DISCRETE	85	
13) MID CX	DISCRETE	90	
13A) DISTAL CX	NORMAL		
14) OBTUSE MARGINAL-1	NORMAL		
17) LEFT PDA	NORMAL		

FIGURE 2–16. Reproduction of portion of catheterization report from patient described in Figure 2–10. This section reports information obtained from coronary angiography. Morphology of stenoses, percent reduction in lumen diameter, and sources of collateralization are reported. A pictorial representation of coronary arterial anatomy also is given.

1. What is the status of systolic function? Global function in the absence of mitral regurgitation is best evaluated with EF. Regional function is assessed by analysis of the ventriculogram. Patients with an EF greater than 55% would be expected to have limited areas of dyssynergy and no history of a prior myocardial infarct. Patients with a history of prior myocardial infarction or three-vessel coronary disease would be expected to have a reduced EF and more extensive areas of dyssynergy. Ejection fractions in the range of 40% are common in this subset of patients.[19] Patients with three-vessel disease and a history of myocardial infarction have ejection fractions in the range of 35%.[19] More extensive areas of dyssynergy would be expected. Patients with an EF lower than 25% have poor ventricular function and will have large areas of akinesis and dyskinesis.

2. What is the status of diastolic function? It is necessary to determine whether coronary insufficiency is responsible for diminished ventricular distensibility as discussed in the section on diastolic function. An elevated LVEDP is characteristic of diastolic dysfunction; although this also may exist in concert with systolic dysfunction, an elevated LVEDP is not synonymous with systolic dysfunction.

3. What regions of myocardium are jeopardized? Significant stenotic lesions jeopardize the myocardium in specific regions as discussed previously. A region is at high risk of developing ischemic dysfunction if it is poorly collaterized and distal to a proximal, severe stenosis. It also is necessary to determine whether the regional myocardium distal to a stenosis is viable. If the area of myocardium is dyskinetic or aneurysmal with evidence of surface Q waves, pharmacologic and surgical efforts to salvage the area will not be fruitful. If the area seems to be viable and salvageable, then efforts must be made to optimize blood flow to the area until revascularization can occur.

4. What are the consequences of deteriorating function in a given region? Deteriorating function in a given region may cause major management problems. Continued compromise of flow to the AV node may cause progressive heart block with subsequent hemodynamic compromise. A patient with depressed global systolic function whose hypokinetic anterior lateral wall becomes akinetic may develop cardiogenic shock. The anesthesiologist should have a myocardial map in his or her mind and should be prepared to look for deterioration in regions of high risk.

■ EVALUATION OF VALVULAR LESIONS

The impressive technological advances in Doppler echocardiography[37] and nuclear cardiac[38] imaging now allow noninvasive assessment of valvular pathology. Evaluation via cardiac catheterization, however, remains the gold standard.

Stenotic Lesions

The analysis of stenotic valve lesions is based on obtaining a valve orifice area from flow and pressure-gradient data. The Gorlins[39] used the basic hydraulic formula: area = flow/velocity. They then combined this with an equation that relates velocity to mean pressure gradient: velocity = k × √mean pressure gradient, where k is a specific constant for either the aortic or mitral valve. For the mitral valve, then, the equation is: valve area = flow/37.7 × √mean pressure gradient. For the aortic valve, the equation is: valve area = flow/44.5 × √mean pressure gradient. Obviously, flow occurs across the mitral valve only in diastole and across the aortic valve only in systole. Therefore, cardiac output cannot be substituted for flow in the equations. The time per heartbeat during which blood flows across the mitral valve is defined as the diastolic filling period. The diastolic filling period is measured from mitral valve opening to end diastole. The time per heartbeat during which blood flows across the aortic valve is defined as the systolic ejection period. The systolic ejection period is measured from aortic valve opening to aortic valve closure.

$$\text{Mitral valve flow (cm}^3\text{/sec)} = \frac{\text{Cardiac output (cm}^3\text{/min)}}{\text{diastolic filling period (sec/beat)} \times \text{heart rate (beat/min)}}$$

$$\text{Mitral valve area (cm}^2\text{)} = \frac{\text{mitral valve flow (cm}^3\text{/sec)}}{37.7 \times \sqrt{\text{mean pressure gradient}} \text{ (cm/sec)}}$$

$$\text{Aortic valve flow (cm}^3\text{/sec)} = \frac{\text{cardiac output (cm}^3\text{/min)}}{\text{systolic ejection period (sec/beat)} \times \text{heart rate (beat/min)}}$$

$$\text{Aortic valve area (cm}^2\text{)} = \frac{\text{aortic valve flow (cm}^3\text{/sec)}}{44.5 \times \sqrt{\text{mean pressure gradient}} \text{ (cm/sec)}}$$

The mean pressure gradient for mitral stenosis is obtained by using planimetry to determine the area between simultaneous tracings of the left atrial or wedge pressure and the left ventricular pressure during the diastolic filling period and then dividing this area by the length of the diastolic filling period. Figure 2–17 illus-

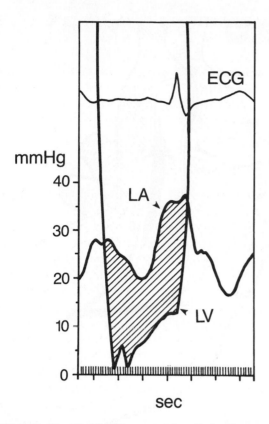

FIGURE 2–17. One diastolic filling period in patient with severe mitral stenosis. Simultaneous tracings of electrocardiogram (ECG), left atrial pressure, and left ventricular pressure are shown. Pressure gradient across mitral valve is cross-hatched and seen to vary during diastolic filling period. Length of diastolic filling period can be seen in seconds.

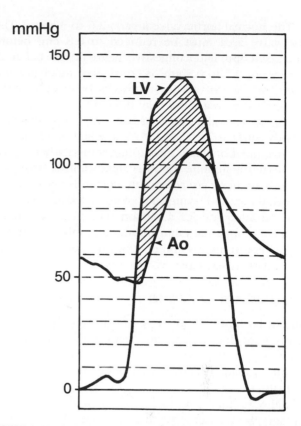

FIGURE 2–18. One systolic ejection period in patient with severe aortic stenosis. Simultaneous recordings of proximal aortic pressure and left ventricular pressure are recorded. Pressure gradient across the aortic valve is cross-hatched and seen to vary during systolic ejection period. Time scale for length of systolic ejection period not shown.

trates this area during one diastolic filling period. Normally, the pressure gradients for several beats are determined and the average is taken. For aortic stenosis, analogous measurements are made using planimetry to determine the area between simultaneous tracings of the proximal aortic pressure and the left ventricular pressure during the systolic ejection period. Figure 2–18 illustrates this area during one ejection period. Again, the gradients for several beats are determined and averaged.

It is essential that proper assessment of flow be used for lesions in which stenosis and regurgitation coexist. A thermodilution or Fick cardiac output determination is an assessment of forward flow across a valve orifice. If regurgitation exists, total flow across the valve orifice will be forward flow plus regurgitant flow. If forward flow instead of total flow is used, the valve area for a given gradient will be underestimated; the degree of stenosis will be exaggerated. Total flow is best obtained from angiographic determination of cardiac output. Left ventriculography is used to determine stroke volume (as described previously) and stroke volume is multiplied by heart rate.

It is important when evaluating stenotic lesions that the pressure gradient alone is not evaluated. At low flows (low cardiac output), it is possible for a valve to be critically stenotic with a small transvalvular pressure gradient. Several other relationships should be kept in mind. The mean pressure gradient is directly related to the square of flow. Thus, if cardiac output doubles, the mean pressure gradient will increase by a factor of four. The mean pressure gradient is inversely related to the square of the valve area. Thus, if valve area is reduced by one-half, the mean pressure gradient will increase by a factor of four.

The normal mitral valve area in an adult is 4 to 6 cm^2. The mitral valve area must be reduced to 2.6 cm^2 before symptoms occur, and a valve area of 1.5 to 2.5 cm^2 is considered mild mitral stenosis, with symptoms occurring during exercise.[40] A valve area of 1.1 to 1.5 cm^2 is considered moderate mitral stenosis, with an elevated left atrial pressure necessary to maintain a diminished cardiac output.[40] A valve area of 1.0 cm^2 is considered severe mitral stenosis, with a left atrial pressure of 25 mm Hg necessary to maintain minimal cardiac output.[40]

The normal aortic valve area is 2.6 to 3.5 cm². The aortic valve area must be reduced to 0.8 cm² before angina, syncope, and congestive heart failure occur. A valve area of 0.5 to 0.8 cm² is considered moderate aortic stenosis. Severe aortic stenosis is believed to exist when the valve area is less than 0.5 cm².

For adults, valve areas usually are not normalized for body surface area (BSA). As a result, extremes of body size must be taken into consideration when deciding whether a stenotic lesion is significant. A large person with higher cardiac output demands may have a large gradient and symptoms with a valve area that would be adequate for a person with smaller cardiac output requirements. Valve areas commonly are normalized for BSA in infants and children because large variations in patient size exist.

Regurgitant Lesions

Quantification of regurgitant lesions is more difficult and less accurate than for stenotic lesions. Two approaches are available at the time of cardiac catheterization. One method is qualitative; the other is quantitative. Qualitative analysis is based on assessing the amount of contrast material regurgitated into the left atrium during left ventriculography for mitral regurgitation (*see* Fig. 2–19) or into the left ventricle during aortography for aortic regurgitation (*see* Fig. 2–20). The degree of regurgitation is graded 1+ to 4+. In 1+ aortic regurgitation, a small amount of contrast enters the left ventricle during diastole but clears with each systole. In 1+ mitral regurgitation, a small amount of contrast enters the left atrium during systole but clears in diastole. In 4+ aortic regurgitation, the left ventricle is filled with contrast after the first diastole and it remains opacified for several systoles. In 4+ mitral regurgitation, the left atrium is filled with contrast after the first systole and becomes progressively opacified with each beat. In addition, contrast is seen refluxing into the pulmonary veins. Similar qualitative analysis is used to grade tricuspid regurgitation as well.

The quantitative method of assessing regurgitation is based on calculation of the regurgitant fraction.

$$\text{Regurgitant fraction} = \frac{\text{regurgitant stroke volume}}{\text{total stroke volume}}$$

$$\frac{\text{Regurgitant}}{\text{stroke volume}} = \frac{\text{total stroke volume} - \text{forward}}{\text{stroke volume}}$$

Angiographic or total stroke volume is determined from left ventriculography as described previously and forward stroke volume is determined by the Fick method. A regurgitant fraction lower than 30% indicates mild mitral regurgitation, 30 to 60% indicates moderate mitral regurgitation, and higher than 60% indicates severe mitral regurgitation.[41] A regurgitant fraction of 10 to 40%

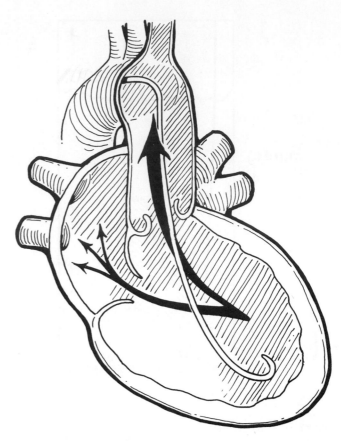

FIGURE 2–19. Long-axis cross-sectional view of left atrium, left ventricle, and aorta in severe mitral regurgitation. Injection of contrast material into left ventricle demonstrates regurgitation of contrast into left atrium and pulmonary veins.

indicates mild aortic regurgitation, 40 to 60% indicates moderate aortic regurgitation, and more than 60% severe aortic regurgitation.[41]

It is important to note that the height and duration of V waves are not a direct assessment of the degree of mitral regurgitation. It has been demonstrated that afterload reduction with sodium nitroprusside abolished the V wave in a patient with severe mitral regurgitation while the regurgitant fraction was reduced from 80 to 64%.[42,43] Thus, severe mitral regurgitation can exist in the absence of a significant V wave. It has been stated that, for an individual patient, the height of the V wave correlates with the degree of regurgitation under conditions of changing afterload.[44] Such conclusions must be drawn carefully, because there are several factors that affect the height and duration of V waves:

1. The degree of mechanical mitral valve impairment. Mechanical impairment occurs with a ruptured papillary muscle, a torn prosthetic valve leaflet, or a perivalvular leak.
2. The degree of functional mitral valve impairment. Functional impairment occurs with papil-

6. The length of ventricular systole. A decrease in the length of ventricular systole will reduce the time available for regurgitant flow to take place. However, forward stroke volume may be compromised as well.

Analysis of the V wave in tricuspid regurgitation is hampered by similar considerations. Nonetheless, with severe tricuspid regurgitation, the right atrial pressure trace takes on the shape of the right ventricular pressure trace.

■ EVALUATION OF CARDIAC SHUNTS

O_2 saturation measurements in multiple cardiac chambers and the great vessels are used to localize and quantify cardiac shunts. Additionally, angiography during cardiac catheterization may be used to locate cardiac shunts. The most common sources of shunting are atrial and ventricular septal defects, a patent ductus arteriosus, and surgical shunts from the aorta to the pulmonary arterial system (Blalock–Tausig shunt, Waterston shunt, Potts shunt).

Shunt Location

The mainstay of shunt location is detection of an O_2 saturation step-up in the right heart in the case of a left-to-right shunt or a step-down in the left heart in the case of a right-to-left shunt. A step-up is defined as an increase in the saturation of blood in a particular location that exceeds the normal variability in that location, whereas a step-down is a greater-than-expected decrease in saturation for a given location. Grossman has summarized the criteria for a step-up based on sample locations.[48] To localize a step-up in the right heart, blood samples for saturation analysis are drawn from 14 locations: low and high superior vena cava; low and high inferior vena cava; multiple right atrial and ventricular sites; right, left, and main pulmonary artery; left ventricle; and aorta.[48] If a step-up occurs at the level of the right atrium, it is likely that an atrial septal defect exists with a left-to-right shunt.

Similar logic is used to locate right-to-left shunts. An O_2 saturation step-down is sought by sampling multiple locations in the left heart.

Shunt Quantification

Shunt quantification is based on comparison of systemic and pulmonary blood flows. Systemic (Q_s) and pulmonary (Q_p) blood flows are calculated by the Fick method previously described.

$$Q_p = O_2 \text{ uptake}/(\text{P}v_{O_2} \text{ content} - \text{PA}_{O_2} \text{ content})$$

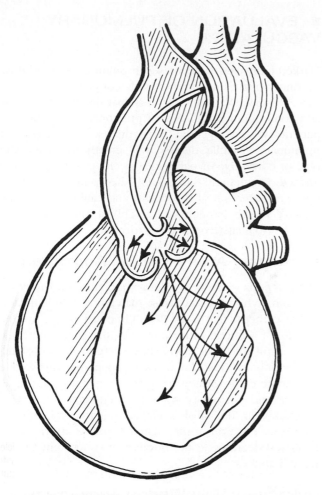

FIGURE 2–20. Long-axis cross-sectional view of left ventricle, right ventricle, and aorta in severe aortic regurgitation. Injection of contrast material into proximal aorta demonstrates regurgitation of contrast into left ventricle.

lary muscle ischemia or ventricular dilation with deformation of the valvular annulus.[45,46]

3. The compliance characteristics of the left atrium and pulmonary veins. For a given regurgitant volume, a dilated, compliant left atrium will exhibit a smaller V wave than a small, noncompliant left atrium.[47]

4. The relative impedance to ejection through the aortic valve versus that through the incompetent mitral valve. An increase in the impedance to aortic ejection will favor increased outflow through the lower impedance of the incompetent mitral valve. With all other variables constant, this will increase the magnitude of the V wave.

5. The inotropic state of the left ventricle. An increase in left ventricular contractility will tend to decrease left ventricular dimensions, decrease the size of the valvular annulus, and thus decrease the amount of regurgitant flow.[45,46]

PVO_2 content is pulmonary venous O_2 content, which in the absence of a right-to-left shunt is equal to systemic arterial O_2 content. If a right-to-left shunt exists, PVO_2 saturation must be measured directly or assumed to be 95 to 98%. PaO_2 content is pulmonary artery O_2 content.

$$Q_s = O_2 \text{ uptake (SAO}_2 \text{ content} - MVO_2 \text{ content)}$$

SAO_2 is systemic arterial O_2 content. MVO_2 content is mixed venous O_2 content. True mixed venous blood is a mixture of desaturated blood from the inferior vena cava, superior vena cava, and coronary sinus. Normally, it is assumed that MVO_2 saturation is the same as PAO_2 saturation. In the presence of an intracardiac left-to-right shunt, PAO_2 saturation will overestimate true MVO_2 saturation because pulmonary arterial blood will be a mixture of mixed venous blood and oxygenated blood from the left heart. In this setting, true mixed venous saturation must be determined from samples taken from the superior and inferior vena cavae. Flamm et al.[49] developed an empiric formula for patients at rest that states:

$$\begin{array}{l} MVO_2 \\ \text{saturation} \end{array} = \begin{array}{l} (3/4 \times \text{superior vena cava } O_2 \\ \text{saturation}) + (1/4 \times \text{inferior} \\ \text{vena cava } O_2 \text{ saturation}) \end{array}$$

This formula may be used to determine MVO_2 in the catheterization laboratory when left-to-right shunts exist. Alternatively, the superior vena cava O_2 saturation may be used as an estimate of the MVO_2 saturation.

After Q_s and Q_p have been calculated, shunts can be quantitated. For a left-to-right shunt, the magnitude of the shunt is $Q_p - Q_s$. For a right-to-left shunt, the magnitude of the shunt is $Q_s - Q_p$. The ratio Q_p/Q_s also is a useful calculation. It can be calculated from saturation data alone because the O_2 uptake terms cancel out.

$$Q_p/Q_s = (SAO_2 = MVO_2)/(PVO_2 - PAO_2)$$

A Q_p/Q_s ratio greater than 2.0 constitutes a large shunt, whereas one less than 1.5 constitutes a small shunt. Obviously, a ratio less than 1.0 indicates a right-to-left shunt. For example, for a left-to-right shunt at the atrial level Q_p might be 8 L/min and Q_s 4 L/min. This would constitute a shunt of 4 L/min and a Q_p/Q_s of 2:1.

For bidirectional shunts, it is necessary to calculate effective pulmonary blood flow ($Q_p$eff) and effective systemic blood flow ($Q_s$eff). $Q_p$eff is the amount of desaturated systemic venous blood that traverses the pulmonary capillaries to be oxygenated. $Q_s$eff is the amount of oxygenated pulmonary venous blood that traverses the systemic capillaries to deliver oxygen. $Q_p$eff is always equal to $Q_s$eff.

$$Q_p\text{eff} = O_2 \text{ uptake}/(PVO_2 \text{ content} - MVO_2 \text{ content})$$

The left-to-right shunt is defined as $Q_p - Q_p$eff while the right-to-left shunt is defined as $Q_s - Q_p$eff. The net shunt is the difference between these two calculated shunts.

EVALUATION OF PULMONARY VASCULATURE

Marked increases or decreases in pulmonary blood flow routinely occur in patients with congenital heart disease. Obstructive pulmonary vascular disease may occur as a consequence of increased pulmonary blood flow in patients with congenital heart disease. The extent of pulmonary vascular disease will greatly influence the type of corrective or palliative operative procedure performed. For patients with diminished pulmonary blood flow, an evaluation of the extent and caliber of the pulmonary vessels is necessary to choose the proper corrective or palliative operative procedure.

Pulmonary Artery Wedge Angiogram

The pulmonary artery wedge angiogram is recorded on cine film while radiocontrast material is hand-injected into a catheter that is in the pulmonary artery wedge position.[50] Generally, the artery to the posterior basal segment of the right lower lobe is studied. As obstructive pulmonary vascular disease progresses, the wedge angiogram demonstrates progressive increases in the diameter and tortuosity of the pulmonary arteries, a diminution in the blush seen as capillaries fill, and the abrupt termination of the dilated, tortuous arteries with a marked decrease in the number of supernumerary arterial branches.

Pulmonary Vein Wedge Angiogram

In many congenital cardiac lesions with reduced pulmonary blood flow, the pulmonary vasculature may be well visualized with injection of contrast into collaterals that arise off the aorta. For patients with pulmonary atresia, pulmonary blood flow is markedly diminished and the pulmonary arteries may not be well visualized with contrast injections into collateral vessels. In this instance, the pulmonary vein wedge angiogram may be used to delineate the pulmonary vasculature. Retrograde filling of the parenchymal pulmonary vessels can be seen on cine recordings when contrast is hand-injected into a catheter wedged in a pulmonary vein. When pulmonary blood flow is severely diminished, retrograde filling of even the main pulmonary artery can occur.

REFERENCES

1. Dodge HT, Sandler H, Ballew DW, Lord JD Jr: The use of biplane angiocardiography for the measurement of left ventricular volume in man. *Am Heart J* 1960; **60:**762–776.
2. Suga H, Yamada O, Goto Y: Energetics of ventricular contraction as traced in the pressure–volume diagram. *Federation Proc* 1984; **43:**2411-2413.

3. Suga H, Sagawa K: Instantaneous pressure-volume relationships and their ratio in the excised, supported canine left ventricle. *Circ Res* 1974; **35**:117-126.

4. Ross J: Cardiac function and myocardial contractility: A perspective. *J Am Coll Cardiol* 1983; **1**:52-62.

5. Grossman W, McLaurin LP: Diastolic properties of the left ventricle. *Ann Intern Med* 1976; **84**:316-326.

6. McLaurin LP, Rolet EL, Grossman W: Impaired left ventricular relaxation during pacing induced ischemia. *Am J Cardiol* 1973; **32**:751-757.

7. Barry WH, Brooker JZ, Alderman EL, Harrison DC: Changes in diastolic stiffness and tone of the left ventricle during angina pectoris. *Circulation* 1974; **49**:255-263.

8. Mann JT, Brodie RR, Grossman W, McLaurin LP: Effect of angina on left ventricular pressure-volume relationships. *Circulation* 1977; **55**:761-766.

9. Grossman W, Mann JT: Evidence for impaired left ventricular relaxation during acute ischemia in man. *Eur J Cardiol* 1978; **7**:239-249.

10. Bourdillion PD, Lorell BH, Mirsky I, et al: Increased regional myocardial stiffness of the left ventricle during pacing-induced angina in man. *Circulation* 1983; **67**:316-323.

11. Aroesty JM, McKay RG, Heller GV, et al: Simultaneous assessment of left ventricular systolic and diastolic dysfunction during pacing-induced ischemia. *Circulation* 1983; **5**:889-900.

12. Fifer MA, Bourdillon PD, Lorell BH: Altered left ventricular diastolic properties during pacing-induced angina in patients with aortic stenosis. *Circulation* 1986; **74**:675-683.

13. Sasayama S, Nonogi H, Miyazaki S, et al: Changes in diastolic properties of the regional myocardium during pacing-induced ischemia in human subjects. *J Am Coll Cardiol* 1985; **5**:599-606.

14. Braunwald E, Frahm CJ: Studies on Starling's law of the heart. IV. Observations on the hemodynamic functions of the left atrium in man. *Circulation* 1961; **24**:633-642.

15. Rahimtoola SH: Left ventricular end-diastolic and filling pressure in assessment of ventricular function. *Chest* 1973; **63**:858-860.

16. Forsberg SH: Relationship between the pressures in the pulmonary artery, left atrium and left ventricle with special reference to the events at end diastole. *Br Heart J* 1971; **33**:494-499.

17. Rahimtoola SH, Ehsani A, Sinn MZ, et al: Left atrial transport function in myocardial infarction: Importance of the booster pump function. *Am J Med* 1979; **59**:686-694.

18. Hanrath P, Mathey DG, Siegert R, Bleifeld W: Left ventricular relaxation and filling pattern in different forms of left ventricular hypertrophy: An echocardiographic study. *Am J Cardiol* 1980; **45**:15-23.

19. Moraski RE, Russell RO, McKamy S, Rackley CE: Left ventricular function in patients with and without myocardial infarction and one, two or three vessel coronary artery disease. *Am J Cardiol* 1975; **35**:1-10.

20. Peterson KL, Sklovan D, Ludbrook P, et al: Comparison of isovolumic and ejection phase indices of myocardial performance in man. *Circulation* 1974; **49**:1088-1101.

21. Kreulen T, Bove AA, McDonough MT, et al: The evaluation of left ventricular function in man: A comparison of methods. *Circulation* 1975; **51**:677-700.

22. Ross J: Left ventricular function and the timing of surgical treatment in valvular heart disease. *Ann Intern Med* 1981; **94**:498-504.

23. Ross J: Afterload mismatch in aortic and mitral valve disease: Implications for surgical therapy. *J Am Coll Cardiol* 1985; **5**:811-826.

24. Kass DA, Maughan WL, Guo ZM, et al: Comparative influence of load versus inotropic states on indexes of ventricular contractility: Experimental and theoretic analysis based on pressure-volume relationships. *Circulation* 1987; **76**:1422-1436.

25. Grossman W, Braunwald E, Mann T, et al: Contractile state of the left ventricle in man as evaluated from endsystolic pressure-volume relations. *Circulation* 1977; **56**:845-852.

26. Bodenheimer MM, Banka VS, Hermann GA, et al: Reversible asynergy. Histopathologic and electrographic correlations in patients with coronary artery disease. *Circulation* 1976; **53**:792-796.

27. Helfant RH, Bodenheimer MM, Banka VS: Asynergy in coronary heart disease. Evolving clinical and pathophysiologic concepts. *Ann Intern Med* 1977; **87**:475-482.

28. Banka VS, Bodenheimer MM, Helfant RH: Determinants of reversible asynergy. Effect of pathologic Q waves, coronary collaterals, and anatomic location. *Circulation* 1974; **50**:714-719.

29. Aldridge HE: Special projections. A generation of coronary arteriography. *Cleveland Clin Quart* 1979; **47**:145-146.

30. Gould KL, Liscomb K: Effects of coronary stenosis on coronary flow reserve and resistance. *Am J Cardiol* 1974; **34**:48-55.

31. Gould KL, Liscomb K, Hamilton GW: Physiologic basis for assessing critical coronary stenosis. Instantaneous flow response and regional distribution during coronary hyperemia as measures of coronary flow reserve. *Am J Cardiol* 1974; **33**:87-94.

32. Zir LM, Miller SW, Dinsmore RE, et al: Interobserver variability in coronary angiography. *Circulation* 1976; **54**:627-632.

33. Arnett EN, Isner JM, Redwood DR, et al: Coronary artery narrowing in coronary heart disease: Comparison of cineangiographic and necropsy findings. *Ann Intern Med* 1979; **91**:350-356.

34. White CW, Wright CB, Doty DB, et al: Does visual interpretation of the coronary arteriogram predict the physiologic importance of a coronary stenosis? *N Engl J Med* 1984; **310**:819-824.

35. DeWood MA, Spores J, Notske R: Prevalence of total coronary occlusion during the early hours of transmural M.I. *N Engl J Med* 1980; **303**:897-902.

36. Levin DC: Pathways and functional significance of the coronary collateral circulation. *Circulation* 1974; **50**:831-837.

37. Stevenson JG: Doppler echocardiography: Technique and cardiovascular applications, in Come PC (ed): *Diagnostic Cardiology: Noninvasive Imaging Techniques.* Philadelphia, Lippincott, 1985, pp 539-574.

38. Kiess MC, Boucher CA, Strauss HW: Nuclear imaging: The assessment of cardiac performance, in Come PC (ed): *Diagnostic Cardiology: Noninvasive Imaging Techniques.* Philadelphia, Lippincott, 1985, pp 85-123.

39. Gorlin R, Gorlin SG: Hydraulic formula for calculation of the area of the stenotic valve, other cardiac valves and central circulatory shunts. *Am Heart J* 1951; **41**:1-29.

40. Rapaport E: Natural history of aortic and mitral valve disease. *Am J Cardiol* 1975; **35**:221-242.

41. Tyrell MG, Ellison RC, Hugenholtz PC: Correlation of the degree of left ventricle volume overload with clinical course in aortic and mitral regurgitation. *Br Heart J* 1970; **32**:683-690.

42. Harshaw CW, Munro AB, McLaurin LP, Grossman W: Reduced systemic vascular resistance as therapy for severe mitral regurgitation of valvular origin. *Ann Intern Med* 1975; **83**:312-316.

43. Grossman W, Harshaw CW, Munro AB, et al: Lowered aortic impedance as therapy for severe mitral regurgitation. *JAMA* 1974; **230**:1011-1013.

44. Chatterjee K, Parmley WW: The role of vasodilator therapy in heart failure. *Prog Cardiovasc Dis* 1977; **19**:301-325.

45. Yoran C, Yellin EL, Becker RM, et al: Dynamic aspects of acute mitral regurgitation: Effects of ventricular volume, pressure and contractility on the effective regurgitant orifice area. *Circulation* 1979; **60**:170-176.

46. Borgenhagen DM, Serur JR, Gorlin R, et al: The effects of left ventricular load and contractility on mitral regurgitant orifice size and flow in the dog. *Circulation* 1976; **56**:106-113.

47. Roberts WC, Perloff JK: Mitral valvular disease: A clinicopathologic survey of the conditions causing the mitral valve to function abnormally. *Ann Intern Med* 1972; **77**:939-975.

48. Grossman W: Shunt detection and measurement, in Grossman W (ed): *Cardiac Catheterization and Angiography.* 4th ed. Philadelphia, Lea & Febiger, 1991, pp 166–181.

49. Flamm MD, Cohn KE, Hancock EW: Measurement of systemic cardiac output at rest and exercise in patients with atrial septal defect. *Am J Cardiol* 1969; **23:**258–265.

50. Nihill MR, McNamara DG: Magnification pulmonary wedge angiography in the evaluation of children with congenital heart disease and pulmonary hypertension. *Circulation* 1978; **58:**1094–1106.

3

Monitoring

James A. DiNardo

Basic monitoring of cardiopulmonary function is essential to the safe conduct of any anesthetic. For patients undergoing cardiac surgery, extensive monitoring of cardiac, pulmonary, and cerebral function will allow measurement of the physiologic variables necessary to make sound clinical decisions. The extent of monitoring required for a given case should be made on a patient-by-patient basis and the anesthesiologist should be familiar with the advantages, limitations, and risks of the available monitoring systems. This chapter will provide an overview of the monitoring systems used most commonly in the management of cardiac surgical patients.

■ END-TIDAL CO$_2$ MONITORING

End-tidal CO$_2$ (ETco$_2$) monitoring uses infrared absorption analysis to determine the end-tidal partial pressure of CO$_2$ in expired respiratory gases. Two types of capnometers exist. In-line devices determine the CO$_2$ content of the gas that passes through a cuvette placed at the proximal end of the endotracheal tube. Aspiration devices aspirate small samples of gas from the proximal or distal end of the endotracheal tube and deliver the samples to the monitor to be analyzed for CO$_2$ content. Both types determine the partial pressure of CO$_2$ throughout the respiratory cycle; ETco$_2$ is the highest partial pressure of CO$_2$ obtained.

Ideally, ETco$_2$ will slightly underestimate arterial CO$_2$ due to dilution of the expired alveolar gas sample, which contains CO$_2$, with gas from the physiologic dead space (alveolar dead space plus anatomic dead space), which does not contain CO$_2$. Unfortunately physiologic deadspace may not remain constant during the course of an operative procedure; furthermore, changes in physiologic deadspace are not predictable from commonly obtained clinical parameters. Therefore, unheralded changes in the arterial-to-ETco$_2$ difference may occur during surgery, making ETco$_2$ unreliable approximation of arterial partial pressure of CO$_2$ (Pco$_2$). In fact, the arterial-to-ETco$_2$ difference has been demonstrated to vary during cardiac surgical and other operative procedures in adults.[1-3] For infants and small children, the analysis of ETco$_2$ is further complicated by dilution of the ETco$_2$ sample with fresh gas flow. Contributing to this problem are the low ratio of tidal volume to equipment deadspace in these patients; the necessary use of rapid ventilatory rates and high fresh gas flows; the use of partial rebreathing circuits such as the Mapleson D circuit, which allow fresh gas to flow past the sampling site in expiration; and the high sampling rates of some aspiration-type analyzers.[4-6] When a continuous-flow, time-cycled ventilator and a partial rebreathing circuit are used for infants and children weighing less than 12 kg, aspiration sampling at the distal end of the endotracheal tube provides better approximation of arterial Pco$_2$ than aspiration sampling at the proximal end of the endotracheal tube.[7] This is largely due to sampling of end-tidal gas before its dilution with fresh gas flow. Aspiration sampling of ET_{CO_2} at the proximal end of the endotracheal tube provides a good approximation of arterial P_{CO_2} when a Siemens-Elema "Servo" 900C nonrebreathing circuit is used in children weighing less than 8 kg.[6]

■ PULSE OXIMETRY

Pulse oximeters are intended to provide continuous determination of heart rate and continuous estimation of arterial oxygen saturation. Pulse oximeters function by placing any pulsating vascular bed between a light source and a detector.[8] The pulsations cause a change in the light path length, which allows identification and light absorption analysis of the arterial pulse. The light source consists of two wavelengths of light: 660 nm and 925 nm. The 660-nm wavelength approaches the maximal difference between light absorption by oxyhemoglobin (low light absorption) and reduced hemoglobin (high light absorption).[9] The 925-nm wavelength functionally mimics the isobestic point (810 nm) at which the absorption coefficients of oxyhemoglobin and reduced hemoglobin are equal.[9] The ratio of light absorption at 660 nm and at the reference point of 925 nm is used by a microprocessor to determine the arterial oxygen saturation based on information obtained over 5 to 7 heartbeats.

Pulse oximeters have been demonstrated to provide accurate determination of arterial oxygen saturation from 55 to 100% for infants, children, and adults.[8,10-13] In addition, pulse oximetry has been used intraoperatively to guide tightening of pulmonary artery bands in infants with large ventricular septal defects. Arterial desaturation was seen to precede hypotension and bradycardia by 2 to 3 minutes in cases in which the pulmonary band was too tight.[14]

There may be problems with pulse oximetry. Peripheral vasoconstriction from drugs, hypothermia, peripheral vascular disease, and hypotension will all reduce arterial pulsations and compromise the ability of the monitor to calculate arterial saturation.[8] Overhead fluorescent lights and the infrared heat lamps used to heat infants and children may give falsely high saturation values due to detection of ambient light by the oximeter.[15-17] Covering the oximeter with opaque material such as a surgical drape and applying an appropriately sized sensor to the patient will prevent this problem. Finally, after prolonged application of an oximeter, burning and tanning of the skin under the phototransmitter side of the oximeter probe have been reported in pediatric patients.[18]

Problems may arise because currently available pulse oximeters use only two wavelengths of light and calculate saturation based on the premise that only two species of hemoglobin (oxy- and deoxy-) exist. Substances that absorb light at or near 660 nm may mimic deoxyhemoglobin. Falsely low saturation readings will occur when a pulse oximeter is placed on a fingernail polished with colors such as blue, green, black, and purple, which have high absorption for light at or near 660 nm.[19,20] Obviously, nail polish should be removed when a pulse oximeter is to be placed on a finger. Intravenous injection of the dyes methylene blue, indigo carmine, and indocyanine green may result in falsely low oxygen saturation readings by mimicking reduced hemoglobin.[21,22] The absorption characteristics of methemoglobin are such that as the concentration of methemoglobin increases, the pulse oximeteric estimation of arterial saturation will approach 85%, regardless of the real arterial saturation.[23] Because carboxyhemoglobin and oxyhemoglobin have essentially identical absorption coefficients for light with a wavelength of 660 nm, the pulse oximeter will overestimate arterial saturation in the presence of carboxyhemoglobin.[24]

■ TRANSESOPHAGEAL ECHOCARDIOGRAPHY

Transesophageal echocardiography (TEE) is an intraoperative diagnostic and monitoring modality that has wide use among cardiovascular anesthesiologists. Because the esophagus lies in direct proximity to the heart and great vessels, imaging can be obtained without interference from the ribs and lungs as occurs with standard transthoracic echocardiography. Furthermore, TEE allows intraoperative use without disrupting the surgical procedure. Its use is not limited to the operating room, however. It is a valuable tool in the intensive care unit (ICU) and in the evaluation of trauma patients. Every cardiovascular anesthesiologist should at least be familiar with the basic advantages and limitations of TEE.

Basics of Ultrasound

A brief review of the principles of ultrasound is necessary. Ultrasound is sound above 20,000 cycles/sec (Hertz). This is the upper limit of the audible range in humans. In current echocardiographic equipment, pizoelectric crystals form the transducers that generate and receive ultrasound. A high frequency electrical current is applied to the crystal, which causes it to vibrate and generate sound waves. As the generated sound waves pass through inhomogenous human tissue, they are either absorbed, reflected, refrated, or scattered. When there is a big difference between the density and impedance through which the ultrasound wave must travel and when the structures are perpendicular to the ultrasound wave, they are more likely to be reflected. Reflected ultrasound waves are the basis of an echocardiographic image.

The frequency of the ultrasound waves produced by the pizoelectric crystals is important. Recall that wavelength equals velocity divided by frequency: $1 = V/F$. Because ultrasound travels at 1540 m/sec through soft tissue, there is a constant relationship between frequency and wavelength. As the frequency of the vibrations of the pizoelectric crystals increases, the length of the waves produced decreases. A smaller wavelength signal allows better image resolution but is prone to greater signal attentuation with increasing distance from the transducer.

When the pizoelectric crystal receives a reflected sound wave, it vibrates and generates an electrical signal. Because the wavelength, the frequency, and the speed of the transmitted and reflected waves are known, the time it takes for the signal to be transmitted and reflected back can be used to determine the depth of the reflecting object. With proper amplification and processing, these signals can be displayed as a real-time display of reflected wave activity.

Doppler echocardiography is based on the Doppler principle, which states that when a wave of a given frequency strikes a moving target it will be reflected and the reflected wave will show a frequency shift proportional to the velocity of the target, which is parallel to the path of the emitted wave. If the target is moving toward the emitted wave, the frequency of the reflected wave will be higher. If the target is moving away from the emitted wave, the frequency of the reflected wave will be lower. Red blood cells act as excellent reflectors and move throughout the heart. Measuring the red blood cell flow velocity in the heart is the application of Doppler technology in echocardiography. The Doppler principle, when used to calculate the velocity of red blood cells, can be summarized in the following equation:

$$v = (cf_d)/2f_o \cos \theta$$

where v = velocity of red cells
c = speed of sound in tissue (1540 m/sec)
f_d = shifted or Doppler frequency
f_o = transmitted frequency
θ = the angle of incidence between the transmitted wave and the velocity vector being interrogated.

Recall that $\cos 90°$ and $\cos 270° = 0$ and $\cos 0° = 1$ and $\cos 180° = -1$; therefore, detection of velocity is most accurate when the transmitted beam and the velocity vector are parallel ($\cos 0°$ and $180°$) and detection of velocity is impossible when the transmitted beam and the velocity vector are perpendicular ($\cos 90°$ and $270°$). In practice, aligning the Doppler beam and the velocity vector within 20° produces acceptable results (6% underestimation of velocity). By convention, flow away from the transducer ($\cos 180°$) has a negative value and flow toward the transducer has a positive value ($\cos 0°$).

M-Mode Echocardiography

M-mode echocardiography is the simplest echocardiographic imaging technique (*see* color plate Figure 1). Ultrasonic waves of known frequency and wavelength are transmitted in a single beam path. This provides an "ice pick" view of the portion of the heart through which the beam passes. M mode is used in conjunction with two-dimensional imaging and the cursor line is used to direct the beam path through the desired area. The reflected waves are displayed in real time as a time-motion study. Distance of the returning waves from the transducer is displayed in the vertical axis from the top down, amplitude of the returning waves is displayed as shades of brightness, and time is displaced on the horizontal axis. Thus, blood-filled chambers with little or no reflected wave activity are black, whereas valve tissue and myocardium with high wave reflectivity are gray or white.

Ultrasound waves through a single beam path can be transmitted and received back in 0.001 seconds. As a result, the display is a real-time repetitive display of cardiac activity along this single beam line at 1000 frames/sec. This means that M mode provides very high resolution images of moving cardiac structures. It also means that M mode is useful in making measurements of cardiac dimensions at specific stages of the cardiac cycle as the relationship of the displayed image to the ECG is also displayed.

Two-dimensional Echocardiography

Two-dimensional imaging is the display of reflected images obtained for transmission of waves not along a single beam line but across a multiple beam line constituting a sector. This sector usually is 60 to 90° wide (*see* Fig. 3–1). This sector scan is accomplished most frequently by use of a phased-array technology. This is a process whereby a set of pizoelectric crystals are electronically activated in certain sequences to create what amounts to scanning a single beam through a defined sector. This results in a sector sweep that contains approximately 100 single scan lines. Obviously, obtaining 100 scan lines is more time consuming than obtaining 1 scan line, as in M mode.

Two-dimensional images are presented in real time with the sector scan updated 30 to 60 times/sec as opposed to the 1000 times/sec of M mode. As with M mode, distance of the reflected wave from the transducer is displayed from the top of the scan down and the displayed brightness of the reflected wave is proportional to its amplitude.

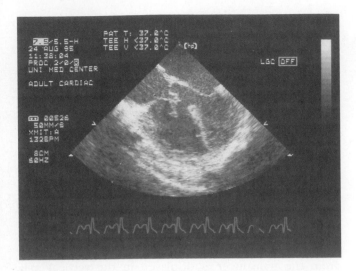

FIGURE 3–1. A real-time two-dimensional echocardiographic image of a patient with a large perimembranous ventricular septal defect (VSD). The image was frozen at a point that corresponded with the QRS of the ECG (see boxed out QRS complex at the right side of the continuous ECG trace) and photographed.

Pulsed-wave Doppler

Pulsed-wave (PW) Doppler makes use of the same transducer used for two-dimensional imaging to intermittently transmit and then receive reflected ultrasonic signals to be analyzed for frequency shifts. In practice, the transmitter emits a signal, waits a period of time (t), and then opens back up to receive reflected signals. This arrangement allows the position of the reflected signal to be localized because the distance of the reflecting object from the transducer is defined by:

$$d = c\,t/2$$

where d = distance of the reflecting object from the transducer

c = 1540 m/sec

t = time between emission and reception of signal

In practice, the PW Doppler cursor and sample volume are positioned on an updated two-dimensional image. After the Doppler cursor and sample volume are positioned, only reflected signals from that position are analyzed. The sample volume also can be selected (usually from 2 to 6 mm). This allows the interrogated area to be expanded or contracted. Data are displayed as a spectra, which is a real-time presentation of velocity over time (*see* color plate Figure 2).

This arrangement also introduces some limitations. The Nyquist criterion states that for the frequency shift induced by the reflecting object (and hence its velocity) to be detected reliably, the reflected wave must be sampled at a frequency at least twice its own frequency. The sampling frequency of pulsed wave Doppler is called the pulse repetition frequency (PRF). Thus, the maximal detected velocity for a given PRF is PFR/2. This is called the Nyquist limit. Thus, the mamimum velocity that can be detected is limited. An additional problem is that the PRF must decrease as the distance of the sampling site from the transducer increases. This must occur because it takes longer for the emitted wave to reach the increased depth and for the reflected wave to return.

When the Nyquist limit is exceeded, aliasing or wraparound occurs. The signal literally wraps around to the velocity scale in the other direction. It then becomes difficult or impossible to determine red cell velocity or direction. The trade-off is unambiguous distance information but ambiguous velocity and direction information. There are two strategies to deal with aliaising during pulsed wave Doppler interrogation. The first is to increase the available scale to the maximum. This simple maneuver is often overlooked. The second is to shift the baseline. When the baseline is maximally shifted, the velocity in one direction, which can be viewed without wraparound, is doubled over that which can be seen with the baseline in the middle. If wraparound still occurs, then continuous-wave Doppler must be used to determine peak velocity and direction.

PW Doppler is useful for measuring low velocities at very specific locations such as mitral and tricuspid inflow or pulmonary and hepatic veins.

Continuous-wave Doppler

Continuous-wave (CW) Doppler uses one transducer to continuously emit signals and a separate transducer to continuously receive reflected signals. These transducers are not the same ones used to obtain two-dimensional images. This arrangement allows very high velocities to be measured reliably because there is no lag between emission and reception of signals. In other words, the PRF is extremely high. Because reflected signals returning from all points along the Doppler beam are analyzed, the location of returning signals is ambiguous. In addition, lower velocity signals are buried in the higher velocity signals. The trade-off is unambiguous peak velocity and direction information but ambiguous distance information.

In practice, the CW Doppler cursor is positioned on an updated two-dimensional image just like PW except that there is no sample volume (*see* color plate Figure 3). Data are displayed as a spectra, which is a real-time presentation of velocity over time (*see* color plate Figure 3). CW Doppler is useful for measuring high velocities such as those seen with aortic stenosis or with intracardiac shunts. With the baseline shifted, velocities up to 600 to 800 cm/sec can be measured.

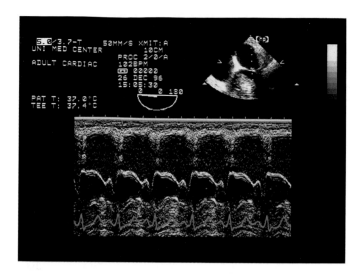

FIGURE 1. M-mode display through a portion of the anterior mitral valve leaflet. The M-mode cursor has been positioned using the two-dimensional image in the right corner. The M-mode display is 1000 frames/sec and in the course of one screen sweep, four cardiac cycles have been captured. Cardiac motion along this single beam line has been captured and, as a result, a high-resolution repetitive image of anterior mitral valve motion through this line has been captured.

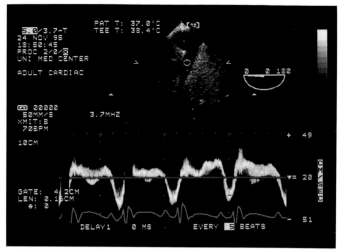

FIGURE 2. PW Doppler spectra from a hepatic vein. The Doppler cursor and sample volume (the circle open at the sides) are positioned in the hepatic vein using a two-dimensional image. The Doppler spectra over four cardiac cycles is displaced below the two-dimensional image. Velocity is on the vertical axis and time on the horizontal axis. The horizontal line through the center of the spectra is the zero baseline. The 20 to the right of baseline means that each gradation of the velocity scale is 20 cm/sec. Peak velocities of 49 cm/sec are detectable toward the transducer (above the baseline) and peak velocities of –51 cm/sec are detectable away from the transducer (below the baseline). There is prominent flow reversal (into the hepatic veins) associated with atrial systole.

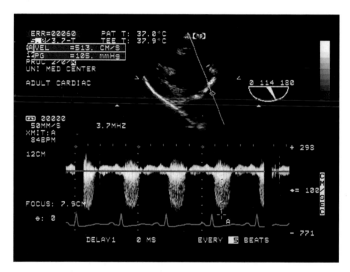

FIGURE 3. CW Doppler spectra across a stenotic aortic valve. The Doppler cursor is placed across the valve in the two-dimensional image. The position of the diamond is for reference only as the velocities along the entire length of the cursor line are measured. The Doppler spectra over four cardiac cycles are displaced below the two-dimensional image. Velocity is on the vertical axis and time is shown on the horizontal axis. The horizontal line through the center of the spectra is the zero baseline. The 100 to the right of baseline means that each gradation of the velocity scale is 100 cm/sec. Peak velocities of 298 cm/sec are detectable toward the transducer (above the baseline) and peak velocities of –771 cm/sec are detectable away from the transducer (below the baseline). The baseline has been shifted upward to allow greater velocities away from the transducer to be detected.

Point A was chosen by the operator as the peak instantaneous velocity (VEL). The machine software determines VEL to be 513 cm/sec. This corresponds to a peak instantaneous gradient (PG) of $4(5.13)^2$ or 105 mm Hg. This information is displayed in the upper left corner.

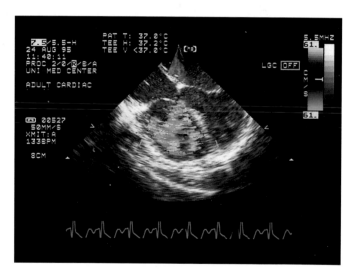

FIGURE 4. Simultaneous two-dimensional image and CF Doppler image of the same large perimembranous VSD shown in Figure 3–2. The image was frozen at a point just before the QRS of the ECG (see boxed out portion of the ECG just before the QRS complex at the right side of the continuous ECG trace) and photographed. The color map is located in the upper right corner, with the peak velocities detectable being 61 cm/sec both toward and away from the transducer. The color red indicates flow toward the transducer (toward the top of the image) and blue represents flow away from the transducer (toward the bottom of the image).

The flow pattern is abnormal because there should not be flow in this location in a normal heart. The direction and spatial extent of this abnormal flow is seen clearly. The presence of the color mosaic (multiple colors in proximity) indicates aliasing. Thus, there are velocities in excess of 61 cm/sec but no reliable information about peak velocity is available from this CF Doppler presentation. Peak velocity data could be obtained with a CW Doppler spectra.

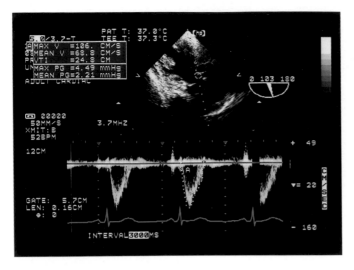

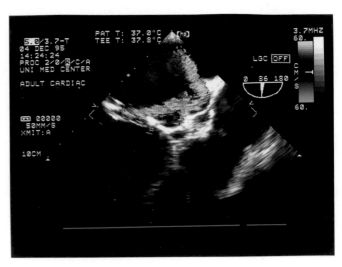

FIGURE 5. PW Doppler spectra from the LVOT of a normal patient. A representative Doppler spectra is frozen on the screen and traced by hand using a trackball. This area is marked by the dotted trace. The machine software uses the trace to determine VTI, mean velocity, and max velocity. From these data, the peak instantaneous gradient (MAX PG) and the mean gradient (MEAN PG) are determined using machine software.

FIGURE 6. Color-flow (CF) Doppler and two-dimensional echocardiographic image in a patient with 4+ MR. The regurgitation jet is constrained and exhibits the Coanda effect (hugging the atrial wall). The jet is deceiving because it is not large relative to the left atrial (LA) size. This patient had systolic velocity reversal in the pulmonary veins and the jet is seen to enter the LA appendage.

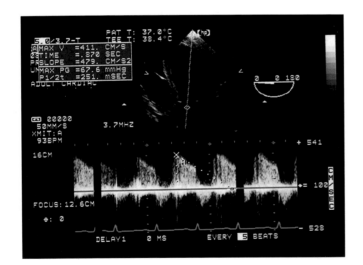

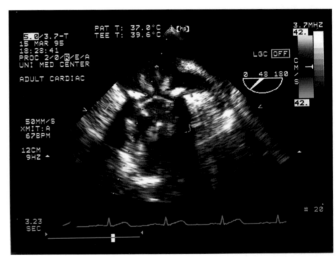

FIGURE 7. Continuous-wave (CW) Doppler spectra from a patient with severe aortic regurgitation. Notice how in this deep transgastric view the Doppler beam is parallel to the left ventricular outflow tract (LVOT), aortic valve, and proximal ascending aorta. Calculations are in the upper left corner. The pressure half-time (PHT) here is 251 msec as calculated by the machine software using a deceleration time (DT) line extended to the zero baseline from the peak velocity.

FIGURE 8. Color-flow (CF) Doppler and two-dimensional echocardiographic image of a normally functioning bileaflet mechanical valve (Carbomedics) in the mitral position. The regurgitant jets are small, low velocity, and centrally located. Both leaflets are in the closed position.

Color-flow Doppler

Color-flow (CF) Doppler is a modification of pulsed-waved Doppler called multigated PW Doppler. Blood-flow velocity is sampled at many locations along many lines in a sector. The sample volumes are called packets. The average velocity and direction for the spectra in a sample volume are determined and assigned a predetermined color. Generally, 8 to 16 samples per frame are used to determine the average. The set of velocities that are averaged in a sample volume for a single frame is called a packet or packet size. Velocity toward the transducer is presented as one color and velocity away as another. A popular presentation is BART (blue away, red toward). In this scheme, velocities toward the transducer are red and those away are blue. As velocity increases, the intensity of color increases as well. The CF Doppler image is presented in real time as a sector displayed over a real-time two-dimensional image (see color plate Figure 4).

CF Doppler has some of the same limitations as PW Doppler. There is no position ambiguity, but the peak velocity that can be presented is limited and decreases with the distance from the transducer. Aliasing or wrap-around occurs and is presented as a color mosaic (see color plate Figure 4). Because the color image is presented over the real-time two-dimensional image, the direction of the aliased signal can be determined easily. This is an obvious advantage when compared with viewing an aliased PW Doppler signal. Because valuable spectral data are lost by the averaging process, CF Doppler is useful for detection of abnormal flows and the direction and spatial extent of these flows. Reliable determination of peak velocities requires PW or CW Doppler spectral analysis.

Doppler Spectra Measurements

As discussed previously, Doppler spectra represent velocity data over time. Velocities toward the transducer are presented above the zero velocity line or baseline and are assigned + values. Velocities away from the transducer are presented below the zero line or baseline and are assigned − values. Accurate Doppler measurements are dependent on the Doppler beam being parallel (or within 20° of parallel) to the interrogated flow. Several important Doppler spectra measurements are discussed:

Pressure Gradients. A velocity measurement (m/sec or cm/sec) can be converted to a pressure gradient (mm Hg) using a modification of the Bernoulli equation $4V^2$ where V = velocity in m/sec. Peak instantaneous pressure gradients are determined by identifying the peak velocity (Max V) of the desired Doppler spectra and using the equation $4V^2$. In practice, machine software will calculate the peak pressure gradient using

a peak velocity identified by the operator. An example of a peak instantaneous pressure gradient is shown in color plate Figure 3. Peak instantaneous gradients are always greater than the peak-to-peak gradients determined at catheterization.

Mean pressure gradient determinations are more complicated and are discussed below.

Velocity–time Integral. Velocity–time integral (VTI) is determined by tracing (planimetry) the entire Doppler spectra over the desired portion of the cardiac cycle (systole or diastole). Machine software integrates the area under the traced spectra to determine VTI in cm. This is illustrated in color plate Figure 5. VTI can be used to determine the following.

Mean gradient — the mean velocity (cm/sec) is determined by machine software by dividing the VTI (cm) by the duration of flow (sec). Mean velocity cannot be used to calculate the mean gradient because the mean gradient is actually the average of multiple instantaneous gradients within the VTI trace. Machine software determines, totals, and averages these individual pressure gradients to determine the mean gradient.

Stroke volume and cardiac output — VTI can be used to determine stroke volume (cm^3) by multiplying the VTI (cm) obtained at a given location by the area of the location (cm^2). Cardiac output is then stroke volume × heart rate (HR). In theory, this can be done in the main pulmonary artery, in the right ventricular outflow tract (RVOT), at the mitral valve annulus, in the left ventricular outflow tract (LVOT), or at the level of the aortic valve. The feasibility depends on two factors:

- obtaining a Doppler spectra from the desired area with the Doppler beam within 20° of parallel to blood flow.
- obtaining an accurate measure of the area from which the Doppler sample was obtained. Diameter (D) can be converted to area using the equation:

$$\text{Area} = 3.14\,(D/2)^2 \text{ or } 0.785\,(D)^2$$

Alternatively, a direct measurement of area can be obtained using planimetry.

Continuity equation — the continuity equation makes use of the VTI to calculate valve areas. The continuity equation makes use of the fact that flows immediately upstream and downstream of a stenotic valve must be equal. This is true even if the valve in question is regurgitant. Thus,

$$(A_1) \times (\text{VTI}_1) = (A_2) \times (\text{VTI}_2)$$

where:
A_1 = area of region 1
A_2 = area of region 2
VTI_1 = VTI from area 1
VTI_2 = VTI from area

The concept can be extended to state that the flows across all valves in the heart must be equal, but this is true only in the absence of regurgitant lesions or shunts. Thus, in theory, the continuity equation could be used to determine aortic valve area using mitral valve or pulmonary artery flows or vice versa.

Deceleration Time, Acceleration Time, Pressure Half-Time. Deceleration Time (DT) — this is the time it takes (msec) for the peak velocity of a Doppler spectra to fall to the zero baseline. In instances in which the zero baseline is not reached, the natural slope of the Doppler spectra is extended to the baseline (*see* Fig. 3-2).

Acceleration Time (AT) — this is the time it takes (msec) for the Doppler spectra to reach peak velocity from the zero baseline.

Pressure Half-Time (PHT) — this is the time it takes (msec) for the peak velocity gradient of a Doppler spectra to decrease by one-half (*see* Fig. 3-2). In other words, it is the time it takes for the peak velocity to decline to the peak velocity divided by $\sqrt{2}$. In addition, the PHT (msec) is always $0.29 \times DT$. The PHT is important because it can be used to calculate mitral valve area (MVA) over a wide range of values using the formula:

$$MVA = 220/PHT$$

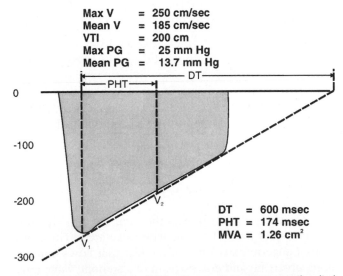

FIGURE 3–2. Schematic of a CW Doppler spectra across a stenotic mitral valve. The VTI is the shaded area inside the spectra. The values calculated from VTI are shown in the upper left hand corner. The deceleration time is obtained by extending the slope of the spectra to the zero baseline. The pressure half-time (PHT) can be determined by calculating V_2 and measuring the time between V_1 and V_2. In reality machine software will determine PHT and use it to determine mitral valve area. The values calculated from DT are shown in the lower right hand corner. DT = deceleration time, MVA = mitral valve area, VTI = velocity–time integral.

TEE Probes

TEE probes consist of an echocardiographic transducer or combination of transducers fitted to the distal, flexible end of a gastroscope. The transducer consists of an array of pizoelectric crystals. Most current adult TEE transducers have a 64-crystal element, whereas pediatric probes have a 48-crystal element. Adult TEE transducers generally operate at 5 mHz, whereas pediatric probes operate at 7.5 mHz. Some adult TEE probes possess frequency agility or the ability to function at 3.7 mHz and 5 mHz, whereas some pediatric probes can function at 7.5 mHz and 5.5 mHz. The higher frequency transducers can be used without significant signal attenuation because of the proximity of the transducer to the heart. In addition to two-dimensional imaging, current TEE probes also possess M-mode, PW Doppler, CW Doppler, and CF Doppler capabilities.

Hand controls allow flexion of the transducer both side to side and anterior and posterior. These controls allow 70° of lateral mobility in each direction (right and left) and 90° of anteflexion and retroflexion (*see* Figs. 3-3 and 3-4). Presently, there are single-plane, biplane, and multiplane adult TEE probes available. Both single-plane and biplane pediatric probes are available. These pediatric probes can be used for neonates and infants as small as 2 to 3 kg. With care, adult probes can be used for children as small as 15 to 20 kg.

Single-plane probes have a single transducer that transmits and receives ultrasonic signals in the transverse or 0° plane, which is also called the horizontal plane. Biplane probes have two transducers mounted one above the other. One transducer transmits and receives ultrasonic signals in the transverse or 0° plane and the other transmits and receives ultrasonic signals in the longitudinal or 90° plane. The longitudinal plane is also called the sagittal plane. Changing planes requires switching from one transducer to the other. Because the transducers are at different levels, subtle (1 to 1.5 cm) advancement or withdrawal of the probe is necessary after transducers are switched to ensure imaging at the same anatomic level. Multiplane probes have the ability to transmit and receive ultrasonic signals in any plane from 0 to 180°. These probes use either mechanical rotation or phased-array activation (varying sequential activation of the pizoelectric crystals in the transducer) of a single transducer to accomplish this. Activation of multiplane capability is obtained with a switch on the handle of the probe (Fig. 3-3).

Insertion of the TEE Probe

Insertion of the TEE probe in the anesthetized adult or pediatric patient with an endotracheal tube in place is relatively easy if a few simple steps are taken. The patient should have an orogastric tube placed and the

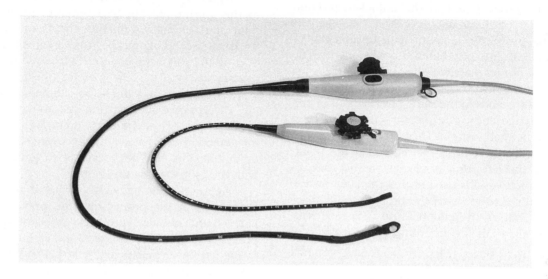

FIGURE 3–3. Photograph of a multiplane adult probe and a biplane pediatric probe. The inner knobs control anteflexion and retroflexion, the outer knobs control left and right flexion. On the handle of the adult probe, the two buttons that control the image plane can be seen.

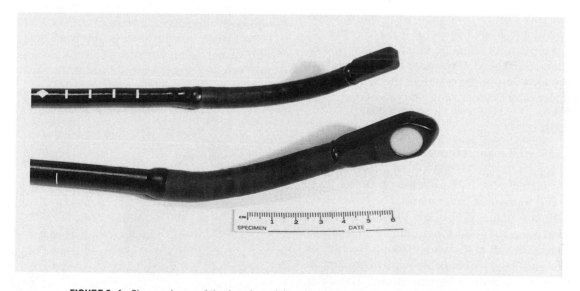

FIGURE 3–4. Close-up image of the tips of an adult multiplane probe and a pediatric biplane TEE probe.

stomach should be emptied as well as possible. Even a small volume of fluid in the stomach can interfere with imaging from the transgastric position. The orogastric tube should be removed before probe insertion. The presence of a tube in the esophagus also will interfere with imaging. The endotracheal tube should be well secured. The TEE probe is left in the unlocked position and is lubricated with ultrasonic gel. A bite block is placed on the probe for patients with any teeth. For edentulous patients, the bite block is not necessary. The bite block need not be placed in the patient's mouth until after the probe is inserted.

The operator stands in the same position as if to perform direct laryngoscopy. The patient's head and neck should be in a neutral position. There should be no positioning rolls under the patient's shoulders at this point. The thumb of the left hand is placed on the patient's tongue and the left hand is used to pull the jaw upward. The right hand is used to insert the probe into the pharynx to the left side of the endotracheal (ET) tube with the probe transducer facing anteriorly. The remainder of the probe can be looped around the operator's neck and shoulder, held by an assistant, or rested on the head of the bed near the patient. The probe is advanced with steady gentle pressure. The unlocked probe will follow the natural curve of the pharynx. At the pharnygeal-esophageal junction (10 cm from the lips in neonates, 20 cm from the lips in adults), some mild resistance will characteristically be met. This can be overcome with gentle, steady pressure. If a lot of resistance is met, it is possible that the probe is in the piraform sinus or vallecula. It should be withdrawn and readvanced. If resistance is met and there is any doubt regarding probe position, the probe should be placed under direct vision using a laryngoscope.

TEE Views

The basic TEE views are summarized in Figures 3-5 through 3-15.

Views available with a single-plane probe are those obtained in the transverse or 0° plane. The basic views available with a biplane probe are those obtained in both the transverse (0°) and longitudinal (90°) planes. Multiplane views are all of the views from 0° to 180°. In fact, most of the views obtainable with a multiplane probe are obtainable with a biplane probe. The difference is that use of a biplane probe requires significantly more probe manipulation than a multiplane probe. The following is useful when using a biplane probe:

- Angles 0–45°: flex the transverse probe to the patient's left
- Angles 45–90°: flex the longitudinal probe to the patient's right
- Angles 90–135°: flex the longitudinal probe to the patient's left

- Angles 135–180°: flex the transverse probe to the patient's right

In this text, rotation to the right always means to the patient's right (clockwise) and rotation to the left always means to the patient's left (counterclockwise).

Figure 3-5 shows views from the upper esophagus. At this level, there can be interference from air in the right and left main stem bronchi. Good views of the proximal ascending aorta can be obtained. The view at 0° is useful for Doppler interrogation of the main pulmonary artery. For some patients, the pulmonic valve and a small portion of the RVOT can be seen as well.

CF Doppler interrogation just above this level but at a level just below the aortic arch (Fig. 3-20) is useful for detection of a patent ductus arteriosus (PDA). Gentle anteflexion may be necessary to get good contact with the esophagus at this level.

Figure 3-6 shows views obtained with slight advancement of the probe from the previous level (see Fig. 3-10). This level provides excellent views of the pulmonary veins and allows Doppler interrogation. At 0° the left lower pulmonary vein (LLPV) is lateral to and seen at a slightly deeper level (10 to 50 mm) than the left upper pulmonary vein (LUPV). The LLPV usually is seen in conjunction with the descending aorta. At 0°, the right lower pulmonary vein is posterior to and at a slightly deeper level (10 to 50 mm) than the right upper pulmonary vein (RUPV). The RUPV is seen in conjunction with the superior vena cava (SVC). The LUPV and LLPV usually can be seen in the same image at 100 to 110°. A persistent left superior vena cava would appear as a vascular structure (circular in the sulcus between the left atrial appendage and the LUPV).

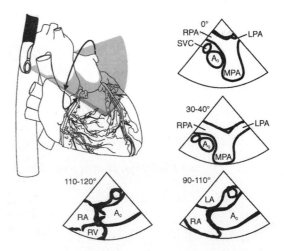

FIGURE 3–5. TEE views at the base of the heart. See text for description. LA = left atrium, RA = right atrium, Ao = aorta, MPA = main pulmonary artery, LPA = left pulmonary artery, RPA = right pulmonary artery, SVC = superior vena cava.

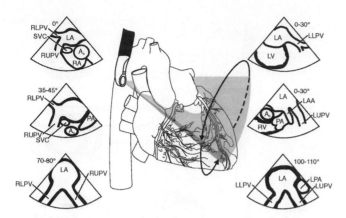

FIGURE 3–6. TEE views of the pulmonary veins at the base of the heart. See text for description. LA = left atrium, RA = right atrium, Ao = aorta, MPA = main pulmonary artery, LPA = left pulmonary artery, RPA = right pulmonary artery, SVC = superior vena cava, RUPV = right upper pulmonary vein, RLPV = right lower pulmonary vein, LLPV = left lower pulmonary vein, LUPV = left upper pulmonary vein, LAA = left atrial appendage.

Figure 3–7 shows views obtained at a slightly deeper level in the upper esophagus. Some of the most valuable views are obtained at this level. Both long- and short-axis views of the aortic valve are seen. In the short-axis views, the right coronary cusp is anterior, the noncoronary cusp is next to the right atrium, and the left coronary cusp is next to the left atrial appendage (LAA). In the long-axis views, two cusps are seen: the right coronary cusp is anterior and the noncoronary cusp is in continuity with the anterior mitral valve leaflet. A good long-axis view of the main pulmonary artery and two leaflets of the pulmonic valve are seen. Views of the tricuspid valve suitable for Doppler interrogation are seen as well.

Figure 3–8 shows views obtained at the midesophageal level. Varying amounts of retroflexion are needed to prevent foreshortening of the left ventricle (LV) and right ventricle (RV). The classic four-chamber view is seen at 0°. These views allow good alignment for Doppler interrogation of the mitral valve. The anterior mitral valve leaflet is seen in continuity with the interventricular septum at 0° and in continuity with the noncoronary cusp of the aortic valve at 130 to 150°. The LAA also is seen. Slight withdrawal and anteflexion will give a short-axis view of the aorta. The coronary arteries can be seen at this level. The left coronary artery often can be seen dividing into the left anterior descending (LAD) and circumflex branches in the area near the LAA. The right coronary artery is anterior and usually requires very slight probe advancement to be seen. Slight off angles (20 to 30°) often will allow better visualization.

Figure 3–9 shows views also obtained at the midesophageal level. The probe is rotated to the patient's right to obtain these views from the previous angles. These views provide excellent visualization of the intraatrial septum, which makes them useful for detection of a patent foramen ovale or atrial septal defect. Good visualization of the right atrium/superior vena cava and right atrium/inferior vena cava (IVC) junctions also is obtained.

Figure 3–10 shows views obtained at the gastroesophageal junction (36 to 38 cm from the teeth). Gentle anteflexion usually is needed to obtain these views. The coronary sinus (CS) is seen entering the right atrium. A large CS should alert one to the possibility of a persistent left superior vena cava or anomalous pulmonary venous return. The right atrium/inferior vena cava junction and eustachian valve are seen as is the right atrial appendage.

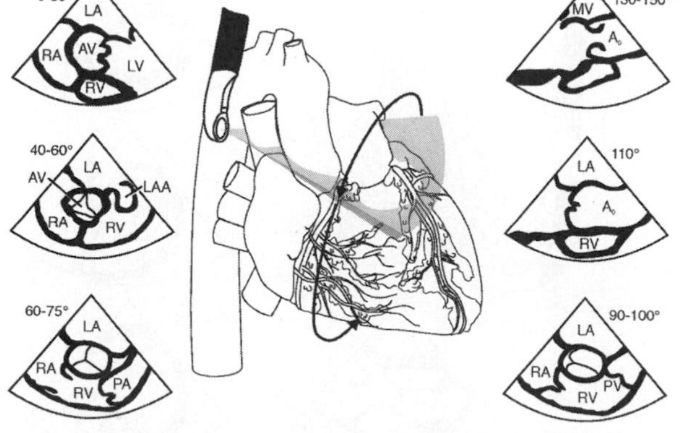

FIGURE 3–7. TEE views obtained from the upper esophagus. See text for description. LA = left atrium, LV = left ventricle, RA = right atrium, RV = right ventricle, Ao = aorta, PA = pulmonary artery, LA = left atrium, LV = left ventricle, RA = right atrium, RV = right ventricle, A_0 = aorta, PV = pulmonic valve, AV = aortic valve, MV = mitral valve.

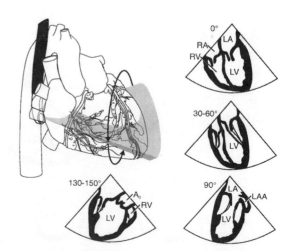

FIGURE 3–8. TEE views obtained from the mid esophagus. See text for description. LA = left atrium, LV = left ventricle, RA = right atrium, RV = right ventricle, A_0 = aorta, LA = left atrium, LV = left ventricle, RA = right atrium, RV = right ventricle, A_0 = aorta, LAA = left atrial appendage.

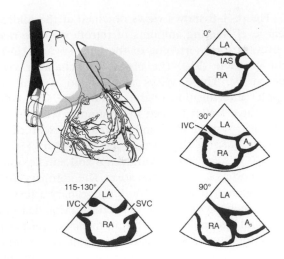

FIGURE 3–9. TEE views of the atria obtained from the midesophagus. See text for description. LA = left atrium, RA = right atrium, A_0 = aorta, IAS = interatria septum, IVC = inferior vena cava, SVC = superior vena cava.

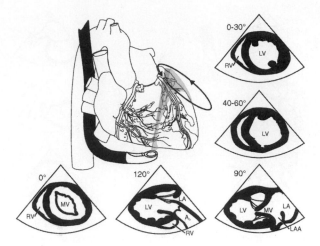

FIGURE 3–11. TEE views obtained from the transgastric position. See text for description. LA = left atrium, LV = left ventricle, RA = right atrium, RV = right ventricle, SVC = superior vena cava, LAA = left atrial appendage, MV = mitral valve, A_0 = aorta.

Figure 3-11 shows transgastric views of the left heart structures. Varying degrees of anteflexion are required to obtain these views. These provide the short-axis views of the LV and RV used in regional wall motion analysis. The anterior and posterior papillary muscles are seen. With manipulation, the view at or around 120° can provide views of the LVOT and aortic valve amenable to Doppler interrogation. A short-axis view of the mitral valve suitable for planimetry often is obtainable either by withdrawing the probe slightly or anteflexing it to a greater degree.

Figure 3-12 shows transgastric views of the right heart structures. Varying degrees of anteflexion are re-

quired to obtain these views. They are obtained by rightward rotation of the probe from the previous position. These views provide excellent visualization of the RVOT, which is very useful in the congenital heart disease patient. They also provide good visualization of wall motion in the RV inferior wall and free wall.

Figure 3-13 shows the deep transgastric views. These views are obtained by passing the probe in a neutral position all the way into the stomach. At this point, the probe is maximally flexed and withdrawn until contact is made and resistance is felt. Flexion of the probe to the left and rotation to the patient's right helps align the image so that the LVOT, aortic valve, and proximal

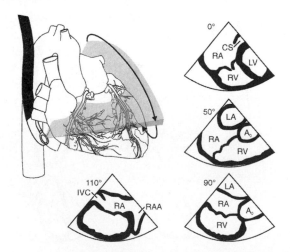

FIGURE 3–10. TEE views obtained at the gastroesophageal junction. See text for description. CS = coronary sinus, RAA = right atrial appendage, LA = left atrium, LV = left ventricle, RA = right atrium, RV = right ventricle, IVC = inferior vena cava, SVC = superior vena cava, A_0 = aorta.

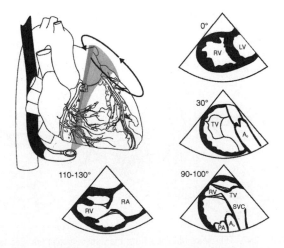

FIGURE 3–12. TEE views of the right ventricle obtained from the transgastric position. See text for description. SVC = superior vena cava, TV = tricuspid valve, LV = left ventricle, RA = right atrium, RV = right ventricle, A_0 = aorta, PA = pulmonary artery.

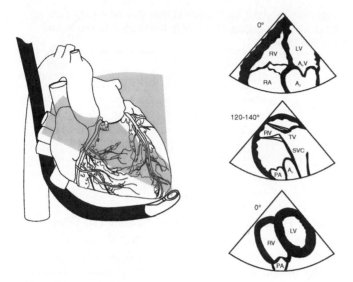

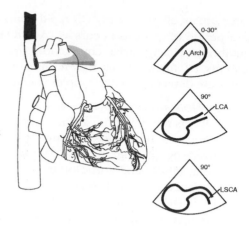

FIGURE 3–15. TEE views of the aortic arch. See text for description. LSCA = left subclavian artery, LCA = left carotid artery, A_0 = aorta.

FIGURE 3–13. TEE views obtained from the deep transgastric position. See text for description. SVC = superior vena cava, TV = tricuspid valve, LV = left ventricle, RA = right atrium, RV = right ventricle, A_0 = aorta, PA = pulmonary artery, A_0V = aortic valve.

ascending aorta are vertical. This location reliably provides views of the LVOT and aortic valve amenable to Doppler interrogation.

Figure 3–14 shows the probe set in the transverse plane and positioned as depicted in Figure 3–8. Next, the probe is rotated 90 to 100° to the patient's left and the descending thoracic aorta is visualized. Once it is located, it can be viewed from the arch (see below) to just below the diaphragm. Inability to see the descending aorta to the left should arouse suspicion that there is a right aortic arch. This can be localized by rotating the probe to the patient's right from the original position.

Figure 3–15 shows, with the descending thoracic aorta visualized, the probe being withdrawn, keeping the image of the aorta in the center of the screen. As the

arch is approached in the upper esophagus, the probe is rotated slightly to the patient's right. At this point, the inferior portion of the aortic arch is seen. At 90°, a short axis view of the arch is obtained. With slight further withdrawal and rotation to the patient's right, the left carotid artery can be seen. With rotation to the left, the left subclavian artery can be seen curving off inferiorly.

TEE Examination

There is no one way to conduct a comprehensive TEE examination. Each examiner has a particular protocol. What is important is that the examiner conduct the same examination on every patient in a consistent format. This is the only way to avoid missing what may turn out to be critical findings. The examiner should concentrate on known diseases, but not to the exclusion of a complete examination. This should include complete two-dimensional imaging with a comprehensive Doppler examination. When the TEE probe is not being used, it should be left in the unlocked position and the image should be frozen. Freezing the image will terminate ultrasound transmission. Some examiners advocate advancing the probe to the stomach when it is not being used to prevent undue pressure on the esophagus from the probe tip.

The analysis of specific enities that can be encountered in a complete examination are summarized below.

LV Diastolic Function

LV diastolic function can be characterized using an integrated approach, which involves analysis of both the mitral inflow pattern and the pulmonary venous blood-flow pattern.

Diastole commences with isovolumic relaxation. As ventricular relaxation continues, LV pressure falls. LA pressure (LAP) eventually exceeds LV pressure and the

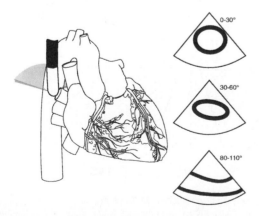

FIGURE 3–14. TEE views of the descending thoracic aorta. See text for description.

mitral valve opens, allowing early (E) rapid filling of the LV. Next, a period of diastasis occurs as LA and LV pressure equilibrate. Finally, atrial contraction (A) occurs and augments LV filling as diastole terminates. All of these events are detectable with Doppler spectra.

Isovolumic Relaxation Time.   Isovolumic relaxation time (IVRT) is the time from aortic valve closure to the commencement of flow across the mitral valve. IVRT can be detected by placing the CW Doppler cursor across the mitral inflow and aortic outflow tracts. This can be accomplished with the TEE view shown in Figure 3–8, 130 to 150°. The time from the aortic valve closure click to the commencement of mitral flow is the IVRT.

Mitral Inflow.   Mitral inflow can be assessed with the PW Doppler sample volume placed at the tips of the mitral leaflets. This generates an accurate Doppler spectra. The spectra will contain E and A velocities, which correspond to passive (E) and atrial (A) filling of the LV. A normal mitral inflow spectra is shown in Figure 3–16. Normal values for the parameters derived from the spectra are shown in Table 3–1.

Pulmonary Venous Flow.   Pulmonary venous flow is assessed by placing the PW sample volume 1.0 to 2.0 cm into the pulmonary vein from its junction at the left atrium. Typically, the LUPV or LLPV is used. A typical pulmonary vein spectra is shown in Figure 3–16. The systolic (S) velocity occurs as a result of LA filling

TABLE 3–1. NORMAL VALUES FOR MITRAL INFLOW PARAMETERS AS WELL AS THOSE ENCOUNTERED WITH IMPAIRED RELAXATION AND RESTRICTION

	Abnormal Relaxation	Normal	Restriction
DT	>240 msec	160–240 msec	<160 msec
E	↓	0.8–1.5 M/sec	↔↑
A	↑	0.75 M/sec	↓
E/A	E<A	E>A(>1.0)	E>>A
IVRT	↑	55–90 msec	<70 msec

during LV systole, whereas the diastolic (D) velocity occurs as the result of LA filling during LV diastole. There is flow reversal seen with atrial systole (AC). The D velocity usually mirrors the E velocity of mitral inflow. The S velocity often is seen to have an early (S_1) and late (S_2) velocity with $S_1 < S_2$. S_1 is the result of LA relaxation, whereas S_2 is the result of movement of the mitral annulus toward the LV apex during LV contraction.

Abnormalities of LV Diastolic Function.   The range of LV diastolic abnormalities is summarized in Figure 3–17. With impaired relaxation, the E velocity is reduced, the A velocity is increased, and the mitral DT and IVRT are increased. The pulmonary venous spectra mirror these changes with a reduction in the velocity and an increase in the DT of the diastolic component (D) of

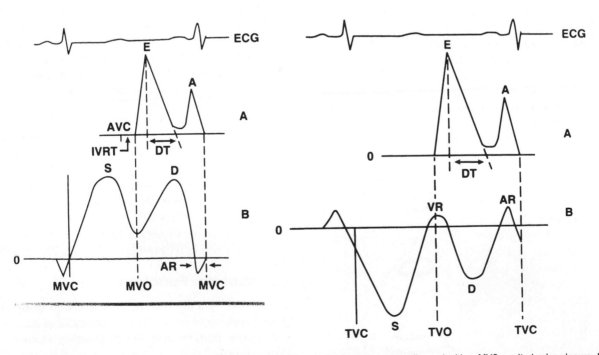

FIGURE 3–16. Left. Schematic of the normal relationship between mitral inflow and pulmonary venous flow velocities. MVC = mitral valve closure, MVO = mitral valve opening, AVC = aortic valve closure, AR = flow reversal after atrial contraction. Other abbreviations are as in the text. **Right.** Schematic of the normal relationship between tricuspid inflow and hepatic venous flow velocities. TVC = tricuspid valve closure, TVO = tricuspid valve opening, AR = flow reversal after atrial contraction, VR = flow reversal during late ventricular systole. Other abbreviations are as in the text.

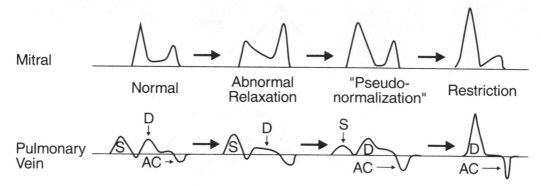

FIGURE 3–17. Schematic of the relationship between mitral inflow and pulmonary venous flow velocities in various types of LV diastolic dysfunction. See text for description.

pulmonary venous return. These changes all are a consequence of prolonged ventricular filling during early diastole. This pattern is very common in patients with coronary artery disease and in patients with left ventricular hypertrophy.

Pseudonormalization occurs due to an elevation in mean LAP. This normalizes the passive mitral filling, mitral DT, and IVRT by increasing the pressure gradient between the LA and LV and masking the impaired relaxation. This pattern is distinguished from the normal pattern by analysis of the pulmonary venous blood flow. The systolic component (S) of pulmonary venous return is reduced because of the elevated LAP. In addition, the flow reversal with atrial contraction is more prominent because of enhanced atrial contraction in the expanded atrium and reduced ventricular compliance.

The restrictive pattern is characterized by rapid mitral DT and IVRT. Restriction to ventricular filling results in rapid equilibration of LAP and LV pressure. The velocity of early filling (E) is high because of an elevated LAP. There is little contribution to LV filling from atrial contraction, and thus, atrial filling velocity (A) is low. The pulmonary veins exhibit marked reduction of the systolic component (S) of filling due the high LAP. The velocity of the diastolic component (D) is high as it corresponds to the early filling (E) velocity across the mitral valve. There is pronounced flow reversal with atrial contraction because of enhanced atrial contraction and minimal antegrade flow across the mitral valve with atrial systole. This restrictive pattern is common in patients with dilated cardiomyopathies and in patients with ventricular volume overload.

Unfortunately, the velocity patterns are load dependent, which can make application difficult. A normal pattern can be converted to an impaired relaxation pattern with hypovolemia or afterload increases. Similarly, an impaired relaxation pattern can be pseudonormalized with volume expansion. The intelligent use of these parameters requires integration of the entire hemodynamic and echocardiographic picture.

Preload and EF Assessment

Intraoperative changes in the shape and position of the left ventricular pressure-volume relationship make the traditional pressure measurements used to assess LV preload unreliable,[25-27] whereas hemodynamic assessment of LV ejection fraction is not possible. Both qualitative and quantitative assessment of LV end-diastolic area (EDA), end-systolic area (ESA), and fractional area change (FAC) are possible using TEE.

Quantitative assessment of EDA using TEE has been demonstrated consistently to provide accurate assessment of preload in adults and children.[27-33] Quantitative assessment of LV EDA is traditionally performed using the short-axis view of the LV at the level of the papillary muscles. EDA is determined one of two ways:

1. Computer planimetry — this method requires freezing the LV end-diastolic echocardiographic image and tracing the endocardial border using a trackball and the leading edge–leading edge technique (*see* Fig. 3-18). The computer then calculates EDA. Usually, the short-axis EDA for several cardiac cycles are obtained and averaged. This method also can be used to determine ESA using the frozen end-systolic echocardiographic image. ESA and EDA can be used for FAC, which is analogous to EF.

$$FAC = (EDA - ESA)/EDA$$

2. Automated border detection (ABD) — also called acoustic quantification (AQ), this method makes use of backscattered signals from the blood-tissue interface to outline the endocardiac borders in real time. When the data are gated to

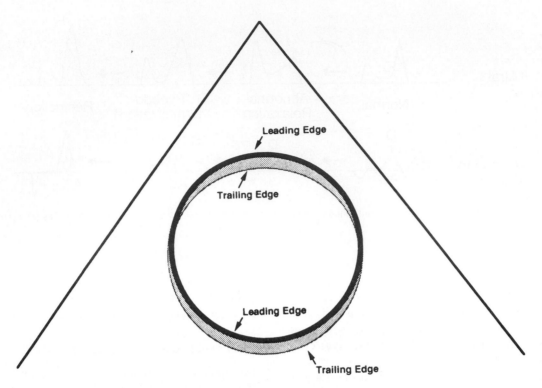

FIGURE 3–18. Schematic of the leading edge–leading edge technique for defining endocardial borders. The endocardial borders are thickest at the points at which they are perpendicular to the ultrasonic beam. The leading edge–leading edge technique provides the most accurate results.

the electrocardiogram (ECG), a beat-to-beat display of EDA, ESA, and FAC is provided. Only one manufacturer currently provides this technology (Hewlett-Packard).

Both methods can be performed online, but obviously, the first method is more time consuming and is not a continuous real-time assessment. ABD is a continuous real-time assessment but is cumbersome and, for 20 to 30% of patients, is unreliable because of poor image quality.[32,33] FAC obtained by both methods has been shown to correlate well with EF obtained by radionuclide angiography.[34,35]

Qualitative assessment of EDA, ESA, and FAC requires no special techniques except a trained eye. In practice, this is used by many anesthesiologists. It is quick and can be as continuous as desired. Several cautions are in order. The development of end-systolic cavity obliteration commonly is used as one of the visual signs of a reduced EDA. However, it has been demonstrated that although many of the episodes of end-systolic cavity obliteration are associated with reduced EDA, end-systolic cavity obliteration does not always indicate reduced EDA.[36] End-systolic cavity obliteration may be caused by increases in contractility or decreases in afterload. It also has been demonstrated that anesthesiologists can estimate FAC or ejection fraction area (EFA) to within 10% of offline values in 75% of cases

and that assessment of EDA as either low or normal corresponds well with offline assessment of EDA.[37]

Regional Wall Motion Analysis

As discussed in detail in Chapter 4, TEE analysis of regional wall motion abnormalities (RWMA) can be used to detect myocardial ischemic and has predictive value in regard to adverse clinical outcomes.

Traditionally, intraoperative assessment of RWMA has been accomplished using the short-axis view of the ventricles at the level of the papillary muscles (*see* Fig. 3–11). This view is chosen because it is easily and reproducibly obtained and because it contains regions of myocardium supplied by all three coronary arteries. Most data regarding intraoperative use of TEE to monitor for ischemia uses this view with analysis that has been performed offline. With the advent of biplane and multiplane probes, more comprehensive analysis is possible (*see* Fig. 3–19). In addition, analysis of RV wall motion, which has received little attention, is possible (*see* Fig. 3–19).

Wall motion is graded both on excursion and wall thickening. Excursion is defined as inward movement along an imaginary radius to the center of the ventricular cavity. Both assessments are necessary because it is possible for an infarcted segment of myocardium to be moved passively by surrounding areas of normal myocardium but the infarcted myocardium will not

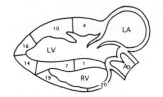 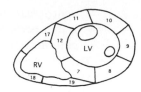

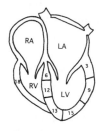 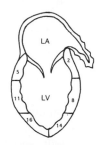

vere RWMA. Only recently, investigations have been performed to determine whether real-time assessment of ischemia is reliable and/or practical[37] and whether the information is useful in making clinical decisions.[38]

Mitral Stenosis

Two-dimensional Anatomy

- Reliable views are obtained as shown in Figures 3–8 (long axis) and 3–11 (short axis).
- A grading system originally described for use in balloon valvuloplasty is used commonly (*see* Table 3–3). A grade of higher than 8 out of 16 suggests that the patient is a candidate for a MV repair rather than replacement, but this decision is individualized.
- The left atrium will be enlarged and hypokinetic and may be filled with spontaneous contrast (swirling, smoke-like contrast). Spontaneous contrast is indicative of a low flow state and is predictive of subsequent development of LA thrombus. The LA should be examined carefully for thrombus, particularly in the LAA. If there is atrial fibrillation or flutter, the atrium will appear akinetic.

FIGURE 3–19. Schematic of the 20 LV and RV wall segments that can be visualized using a biplane or multiplane TEE probe. These views are presented in an inverted orientation from that most commonly used. 1 = basal anteroseptal wall, 2 = basal anterior wall, 3 = basal anterolateral wall, 4 = basal posterolateral wall, 5 = posterobasal wall, 6 = inferobasal septum, 7 = midanteroseptum, 8 = mid anterior wall, 9 = mid anterolateral wall, 10 = midposterolateral wall, 11 = mid inferior wall, 12 = midinferoseptum, 13 = apical septum, 14 = anteroapex, 15 = lateral apex, 16 = inferoapex, 17 = RV inferior wall, 18 = RV lateral wall, 19 = RV anterior wall, 20 = RVOT anterior wall. A₀ = aorta, LA = left atrium, LV = left ventricle, RA = right atrium, RV = right ventricle.

thicken. By concentrating on both excursion and thickening, it is possible to account for the translation (lateral motion of the entire heart) and rotation of the echocardiographic image during contraction. Wall motion is graded from 0 to 4 as shown in Table 3-2.

A new wall motion abnormality is defined as a change in two grades or more for a sustained period of time (minutes). As discussed in Chapter 4, recognition of new RWMA is more difficult than it sounds, particularly in the presence of preexisting RWMA. Furthermore, recognition of mild degrees of RWMA are more difficult than recognition of normal wall motion or se-

TABLE 3–2. GRADING SYSTEM USED TO ASSESS REGIONAL WALL MOTION

Grade	Systolic Wall Thickening	Systolic Excursion
Normal (0)	30–50%	>30%
Mild hypokinesis (1)	30–50%	10–30%
Severe hypokinesis (2)	<30%	<10%
Akinesis (3)	0%	0%
Dyskinesis (4)	0% or thinning	outward bulge

TABLE 3–3. 16-POINT GRADING SYSTEM USED TO ASSESS THE SEVERITY OF MITRAL STENOSIS

Mitral Valve Morphology
  Mobility
    Grade 1 Highly mobile valve with restriction of leaflet tips only
    Grade 2 Leaflet middle and base portions have normal mobility
    Grade 3 Valve continues to move forward in diastole, mainly from the base
    Grade 4 No or minimal forward movement of the leaflets in diastole
Leaflet thickening
    Grade 1 Leaflets slightly increased in thickness (3–4 mm)
    Grade 2 Midleaflets normal; marked thickening of margins only (5–8 mm)
    Grade 3 Thickening extending through the entire leaflet (5–8 mm)
    Grade 4 Marked thickening of all leaflet tissue (>8–10 mm)
Subvalvular thickening
    Grade 1 Minimal thickening just below the mitral leaflets
    Grade 2 Thickening of chordal structures extending up to one-third of the chordal length
    Grade 3 Thickening extending to the distal third of the chords
    Grade 4 Extensive thickening and shortening of all chordal structures, extending down to the papillary muscles
Calcification
    Grade 1 A single area of increased echo brightness
    Grade 2 Scattered areas of brightness confined to the leaflet margins
    Grade 3 Brightness extending into the midportion of the leaflets
    Grade 4 Extensive brightness throughout much of the leaflet tissue

A grade of 1 to 4 is assigned for each of the four categories: leaflet mobility, leaflet thickening, subvalvular thickening, and calcification.

TABLE 3–4. GRADING OF THE SEVERITY OF MITRAL STENOSIS USING DOPPLER-DERIVED INDICES

	Mild	Moderate	Severe
Mean gradient (mm Hg)	6	6–12	>12
PHT (msec)	100–150	150–200	>220
MVA (cm²)	1.5–2.0	1.0–1.5	<1.0

Doppler

- CF Doppler is used to determine the position of the mitral stenosis (MS) jet to guide optimal placement of the CW cursor.
- CW Doppler is used to determine the mean velocity and mean grade using the VTI. Because the mean gradient can underestimate the severity of MS with low cardiac outputs and overestimate the severity in the presence of mitral regurgitation, the valve area should be determined. MVA can be calculated using the PHT method. The summary of mean gradients, PHT, and MVA in MS (see Table 3-4) is useful.

This method will overestimate MVA (underestimate severity) in conditions in which LV pressure rises quickly in diastole, such as aortic insufficiency (AI) or reduced LV compliance. PHT is unreliable when there is merging of the E and A waves or an alteration in the E-wave decay pattern due to tachycardiac, atrioventricular (AV) block, or A flutter. In these instances, the continuity equation using the MV_{VTI} and the $LVOT_{VTI}$ and $LVOT_{area}$ can be used to calculate MVA assuming there is no MR. Details of the use of $LVOT_{VTI}$ and $LVOT_{area}$ are explained in the section on aortic stenosis.

Mitral Regurgitation

Two-dimensional Anatomy

- Reliable views are obtained as shown in Figures 3-8 (long axis) and 3-11 (short axis).
- The etiology of the mitral regurgitation (MR) can be identified reliably based on the mitral leaflet motion:[39]
  - flail or prolapsing anterior leaflet (A)
  - flail or prolapsing posterior leaflet (B)
  - bileaflet chordal elongation (C)
  - posterior medial papillary muscle dysfunction or infarction with disruption of support to both leaflets at the posteriomedial commisure (D_1)
  - anterior lateral medial papillary muscle dysfunction or infarction with disruption of support to both leaflets at the anterolateral commisure (D_2)
  - leaflet restriction (E)

- ventricular annular dilatation (F)
- leaflet perforation, may be associated with vegetations (G)
- The left atrium will be enlarged and hypokinetic. Spontaneous contrast (swirling, smoke-like contrast) is unlikely when MR is severe because statis of blood is less likely. If there is atrial fibrillation or flutter, the atrium will appear akinetic.
- The LV will exhibit eccentric hypertrophy, and the FAC or EFA will be normal or low normal, even in the presence of systolic function because of the favorable loading conditions in MR.

Doppler

- CF Doppler patterns are relatively specific for each type of mitral reguritation lesion and are summarized below[39]:
- Comprehensive semiquantitative evaluation of MR should be performed intraoperatively. CF Doppler analysis of the regurgitant jet is performed in combination with PW Doppler interrogation of the pulmonary veins. The area of the regurgitant jet relative to the area of the LA is a useful CF Doppler technique. This should be performed in as many planes as possible to gain a good understanding of the extent of the MR. It should be performed at the level of the mitral valve using a full 180° sweep with a multiplane probe or at multiple angles using a biplane probe (see Fig. 3–8).
  - Mild MR = jet/LA ratio < 0.25
  - Moderate MR = jet/LA ratio = 0.25–0.50
  - Severe MR = jet/LA rato > 0.50
- Pulmonary venous blood flow is used to differentiate moderately severe MR from severe MR. The appropriate views are shown in Figure 3-9. Moderately severe MR is accompanied by attentuation or absence of the systolic (S) velocity of pulmonary venous return. Severe MR is accompanied by frank reversal of velocity in the pulmonary veins during systole. Thus, MR can be graded as:

TABLE 3–5. TWO-DIMENSIONAL ECHO ANALYSIS OF LEAFLET MOTION

	Excessive	Normal	Restricted
CF Doppler jet direction			
Anterior	A		
Posterior	B	F	E
Central	C	F	E
Commissural posterolateral jet	D_1		
Commissural posteromedial jet	D_2		
Eccentric		G	

- I: mild
- II: moderate
- III: moderately severe
- IV: severe

- Regurgitant jets, which hug the atrial wall (Coanda effect), are considered constrained jets and will be 30 to 40% smaller than a free jet (such as a central jet) under the same conditions of regurgitation. Jets that exhibit the Coanda effect usually are associated with 3 to 4+ MR (*see* color plate Figure 6). When the MR jet width at the mitral leaflet is greater than 0.6 cm, MR usually is severe as well.
- Quantitative methods to classify MR exist, such as regurgitant fraction calculations and proximal isovelocity surface area (PISA),[40] but they generally are cumbersome and time consuming.
- Several cautions are in order. Technical factors such as CF Doppler gain and Nyquist limit will affect how much of the actual regurgitant jet will be detected. We generally turn the color gain up all the way, then reduce it until the "sparkling" disappears, and start with the velocity scale peak at 50 to 60 cm/sec. Both right and left pulmonary veins should be examined because eccentric jets may reverse flow in the pulmonary veins, on only one side of the atrium.
- Loading conditions can dramatically effect the amount of MR, and it has been demonstrated that the amount of MR detected in an anesthetized patient is less than that detected in the same patient while awake.[41] It may be necessary to use phenylephrine[42] to elevate afterload and attempt to duplicate preoperative conditions for patients in whom the intraoperative assessment of MR is significantly different from the preoperative assessment.

After MV Repair. The repair should be assessed for both regurgitation and stenosis and should not be "blessed" until the extent of regurgitant is evaluated under the conditions of afterload and contractility likely to be encountered in the awake state. The presence of 1 to 2+ MR after MV repair does not confer increased morbidity or mortality.[43] The valve should be evaluated for stenosis either directly by planimetry or indirectly with the PHT method. Systolic anterior motion (SAM) leading to LVOT obstruction has been described after MV repair[44] and should be evaluated.

For information on MV replacement, see discussion on valve replacement below.

Aortic Stenosis

Two-dimensional Anatomy

- A number of views of the aortic valve are available, but the short- and long-axis views of the aortic valve, as shown in Figure 3–12, are particularly useful.
- Leaflet mobility should be observed. A stenotic valve will have limited opening and heavy calcification may be present in the leaflets and commissures. A biscuspid aortic valve can be identified easily in a short-axis view (*see* Fig. 3–20).
- The LV will exhibit concentric hypertrophy.

Doppler. Determination of the severity of aortic stenosis is made on the basis of the peak and mean gradients and the calculated aortic valve area. Before introduction of the deep transgastric views (*see* Fig. 3–18), the views necessary to obtain parallel alignment of the Doppler beam with the LVOT, aortic valve, and proximal ascending aorta were not possible. The introduction of biplane and multiplane TEE probes has provided an additional alternative, as shown in Figure 3–16.

The mean gradient and peak instantaneous gradient are determined with the VTI obtained by using CW Doppler aligned parallel (or within 20°) to the LVOT, aortic valve, and proximal ascending aorta. The initially obtained gradient may not be the largest one. It is necessary to be aggressive about finding the cleanest Doppler spectra with the highest peak velocity. CF Doppler is helpful in placing the CW cursor in the center of eccentric jets. The more severe the stenosis, the harder it is to find the optimal CW Doppler spectra because the ejection jet tends to be small.

Determination of aortic valve area requires use of the continuity equation:

$$A_{AV} = (A_{LVOT}) \times (VTI_{LVOT})/VTI_{AV}$$

LVOT area is determined using the diameter method. The long-axis view of the aortic valve in Figure

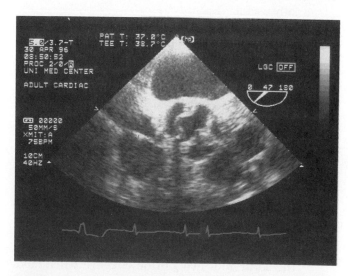

FIGURE 3–20. Two-dimensional echocardiographic short-axis image of a bicuspid aortic valve. Orientation is the same as shown in Figure 3–12.

3-7 can be used to measure the diameter at the point at which the aortic valve cusps abut the LVOT. VTI_{AV} is obtained with CW Doppler across the aortic valve in systole with the views used to obtain VTI. VTI_{LVOT} is obtained with PW Doppler in the LVOT just below the aortic valve leaflets in systole with the views used to obtain VTI.

The continuity equation, as described here, will be accurate in the presence of aortic regurgitation.

AS is classified as follows:

- mild AS = valve area > 1.0 cm²
- moderate AS = valve area 0.75–1.0 cm²
- severe AS = aortic valve area < 0.75 cm²
  peak velocity > 4.5 m/sec
  mean pressure gradient
  > 50 mm Hg

Remember that gradients will underestimate the severity of the stenosis when output is low and may overestimate it when output is high. If there is suspicion that the gradient is misleading, the aortic valve area should be calculated or the dimensionless index (DI) should be used.

$$DI = velocity_{VLOT}/velocity_{aortic\ valve}$$

A DI < 0.2 indicates severe aortic stenosis. Because the peak velocity in the LVOT and across the aortic valve will change proportionally, this index is independent of cardiac output.

Aortic Regurgitation

Two-dimensional Anatomy

- A number of views of the aortic valve are available, but the short- and long-axis views of the aortic valve, as shown in Figure 3–7, are particularly useful.
- Fluttering of the anterior mitral valve leaflet in diastole can be seen when the aortic regurgitation (AR) jet is directed along it.
- Enlargement of the ascending aorta and aortic root may cause poor coadaptation of the aortic leaflets and AR.
- Retrograde aortic dissection can cause mechanical deformation of the aortic valve annulus and AR. Visualization of the coronary ostia should be undertaken, because retrograde dissection can involve the ostia of one or both coronary arteries.
- AR may be associated with vegetations and leaflet perforation.
- The presence of AR may alter the manner in which cardioplegia is delivered as infusion into the aortic root may not be effective when moderate or severe AR is present.
- The LV will exhibit eccentric hypertrophy.

Doppler. CF Doppler imaging of the aortic valve in the long axis is used to measure the minimum width of the regurgitant jet (usually at the origin of the jet at the leaflets) relative to the width of the LVOT. AR is graded, based on this assessment, as follows:

Jet area/LVOT width

<0.25:	1+
0.25–0.46:	2+
0.47–0.64:	3+
>0.65:	4+

CF Doppler imaging of the aortic valve in the short axis at or just below the level of aortic valve leaflets is used to measure the regurgitant jet area relative to the circular LVOT area at this level. AR is graded, based on this assessment, as follows:

Jet area/LVOT area

<0.2:	1+
0.20–0.40:	2+
0.40–0.60:	3+
>0.60:	4+

CW is useful for quantifying AR by determining the PHT of the regurgitant spectra (*see* color plate Figure 7). A PHT < 300 msec is indicative of severe AR, whereas a PHT > 800 msec is associated with mild AR. This occurs because, in severe AR, there is more rapid equilibration between aortic and LV pressure in diastole and thus a more rapid decay in the velocity of the regurgitant spectra. In severe AR, the CW Doppler spectra will be dense, whereas in mild AR, it will be faint. CF Doppler will help guide positioning of the CW cursor.

PW Doppler of the mitral inflow will reveal a restrictive pattern in severe or acute AR. PW Doppler of the proximal descending thoracic aorta will reveal holodiastolic flow reversal in severe AR. It is impossible to align the Doppler beam parallel to the descending aorta, but it still may be possible to detect diastolic flow reversal.

RV Function

Global RV function can be assessed using the same techniques described for the LV to determine EDA, ESA, and FAC. This usually is performed in a short-axis view (Fig. 3–16), the four-chamber view (*see* Fig. 3–8), and the transgastric view (*see* Fig. 3–12). This allows all five wall segments of the RV to be analyzed: inferior wall, septal wall, lateral wall, anterior wall, and anterior wall of the RVOT (*see* Fig. 3–24). Use of the biplane and multiplane probes allows a long view of both the RV inflow and outflow tracts (*see* Fig. 3–12 and 3–13) and of the RV inferior wall and anterior wall of the RVOT. This view is valuable for assessing RV size and systolic function.

Valve Function. The same principles used to evaluate the aortic and mitral valves are used to evaluate the pulmonic and tricuspid valves. Figure 3–7 provides views of the tricuspid and pulmonic valves amenable to Doppler interrogation. The four-chamber view is also useful in assessment of TV function, and the pulmonary artery view shown in Figure 3–5 allows reliable Doppler interrogation.

The hepatic venous Doppler spectra provides information analogous to the pulmonary venous Doppler spectra. The hepatic venous blood flow pattern relative to the tricuspid inflow pattern is shown in Figure 3–16. The hepatic venous blood flow pattern typically exhibits a small amount of flow reversal at end systole. This is caused by descent of the tricuspid annulus valve toward the apex and enhanced flow to the RA.

Views of the hepatic veins are easily obtained by starting in the four-chamber view and rotating the probe to the patient's right to obtain a view of the RA. The probe is then advanced until the IVC is seen. Additional advancement and slight rightward rotation will bring the hepatic veins into view. Usually, a number of veins are visible. The PW sample volume can be placed in the hepatic vein, to which it lies parallel at a distance of 1.0 to 2.0 cm from the junction of the IVC.

Flow in the hepatic veins in tricuspid regurgitation (TR) will parallel those seen in MR, with 4+ TR causing reversal of the systolic component of hepatic venous return.

TEE After Valve Replacement

Discussion of all types of prosthetic valves is beyond the scope of this presentation. However, several important points deserve discussion. All mechanical valves have some small quantity of regurgitant flow built into their design to prevent thrombus formation. This regurgitant flow is characterized by low velocity, small area, and location within the annulus of the valve (*see* color plate Figure 8). If a leaflet is stuck in the open position, the amount of regurgitation present will be large. Tissue valves are not regurgitant unless they have degenerated. Perivalvular leaks generally have a high velocity and are located at the outer margin of the annulus or sewing ring.

Prosthetic valves should have transvalvular gradients that are physiologic for the particular position. If the gradient across a prosthetic valve is high, an aggressive examination to determine whether the leaflets are opening is warranted. A leaflet may be stuck closed because of impingement on surrounding tissue.

Deairing the Heart

All procedures in which the heart is opened have potential to introduce air into the systemic circulation (*see* Fig. 3–21.) In addition, closed procedures have the potential to introduce air as well because of the placement of vents to decompress the left side of the heart. TEE is

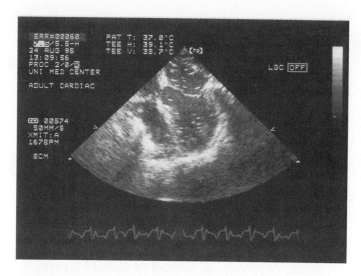

FIGURE 3–21. Two-dimensional echocardiographic image of retained intracardiac air in the left heart chambers.

valuable in detecting intracardiac air and guiding its evacuation before termination of cardiopulmonary bypass (CPB). Air is particularly likely to be retained in the LV apex, LA, right coronary sinus, and the pulmonary veins, particularly the right upper pulmonary vein.[45,46] Deairing procedures are discussed in Chapter 10.

Estimation of Intracardiac Pressures

Several methods exist to estimate intracardiac pressures, some of which are quite creative.

Peak Pressure Gradients. This method requires the presence of a regurgitant valve or a communication between cardiac chambers. It is based on the premise that the peak velocity of a regurgitant jet can be used to determine the pressure gradient between two cardiac chambers during either systole or diastole. Peak velocity is converted to the peak pressure gradient using $4V^2$.

For example, if there is a TR jet with a peak velocity of 3.0 m/sec, then a peak pressure gradient of 36 mm Hg exists between the RV and RA during systole because TR is a systolic event. If we measure the central venous pressure (CVP) to be 10 mm Hg (or assume that it is 10 mm Hg), then RV systolic pressure must be 36 + 10 = 46 mm Hg. If we know (or assume) that there is no RVOT obstruction, then PA systolic pressure is also 46 mm Hg.

A pulmonary regurgitation (PR) Doppler spectra can be used in the same way. The peak PR velocity (velocity at the beginning of diastole) is used to calculate the pressure difference between the pulmonary artery (PA) and the RV at the time of pulmonary valve closure in diastole which gives a good estimate of mean PA pressure (PAP).

Mean PAP = 4(peak PR velocity)^2 + RV end-diastolic pressure (EDP); RV EDP = CVP, which again is measured or assumed.

TABLE 3–6. SUMMARY OF PEAK VELOCITY DATA USED TO DETERMINE INTRACARDIAC PRESSURES

Measure	Measure or Assume	Calculate
Peak TR velocity	CVP	RV systolic pressure
		PA systolic pressure
Peak PR velocity	RVEDP = CVP	Mean PA pressure
End-diastolic PR velocity	RVEDP = CVP	PA end-diastolic pressure
Peak MR velocity	Systolic BP	LA pressure
End-diastolic AR velocity	Diastolic BP	LV end-diastolic pressure
ASD mean velocity	CVP	LA pressure
VSD systolic velocity	Systolic BP	RV systolic pressure

If the PR velocity at the end of diastole is used, PA EDP can be calculated.

PA EDP = 4(end-diastolic PR velocity)^2 + RV EDP; RV EDP = CVP, which again is measured or assumed.

The same arguments can be used with MR and AR velocities. This information is summarized in Table 3–6.

Movement of the Interatrial Septum. In general, the shape of the interatrial septum is determined by the interatrial pressure gradient. Normally, left atrial pressure (LAP) is greater than right atrial pressure (RAP) and the interatrial septum is bowed toward the LA. During the passive, expiratory phase of mechanical ventilation, there is a transient midsystolic reversal of inter-atrial septum position with bowing of the interatrial septum into the LA from the RA. This finding is highly predictive of a pulmonary capillary wedge pressure (PCWP) less than 15 mm Hg.[47] Conversely, absence of this finding is highly predictive of a PCWP greater than 15 mm Hg.

The observation of an interatrial septum continuously shifted to the left would predict elevated RAP.

Pulmonary and Hepatic Venous Blood Flow Velocities. Reductions in the systolic portion of the hepatic venous Doppler spectra relative to the diastolic portion are strongly correlated with increases in RAP. In fact, progressive decreases in the ratio

$$VTI_{systolic}/(VTI_{systolic} + VTI_{diastolic})$$

are associated with increasing RAP.[48] Similar observations have been made regarding pulmonary venous Doppler spectra and PCWP and LAP.[49] When LVEDP > 15 mm Hg the flow duration of pulmonary versus atrial flow reversal is more than 30 msec longer than the duration of the mitral A wave.

Thoracic Aorta

TEE is useful for examination of the ascending aorta, aortic arch, and descending thoracic aorta. The ascending aorta is seen well with the views shown in Figures 3–7 and 3–9. The aortic arch and descending aorta are seen in the views shown in Figures 3–14 and 3–15.

The primary limitation of the use of TEE in examining the thoracic aorta is that a blind spot in the distal ascending aorta and proximal aortic arch exists because of interposed interference from air in the trachea and/or left main stem bronchus. As much as 42% of the ascending aorta may not be visible in certain patients, even with the use of biplane TEE.[50] This area encompasses the region in which the aortic cannula, aortic cross-clamp, and proximal ends of the saphenous vein grafts are placed. Because of the higher incidence of stroke seen in patients with atheromata in the ascending[51] and descending aorta[52] who are undergoing cardiac surgery with CPB, there is concern about manipulation of the aortic if it contains atheroma. Presently, only epiaortic scanning (placement of a transducer directly on the aorta) can reliably visualize this area.

Atheromatous disease of the aorta is graded I to V as follows:

- I: normal
- II: extensive intimal thickening
- III: sessile atheroma protruding < 5 mm into the aorta
- IV: sessile atheroma protruding > 5 mm into the aorta
- V: mobile atheroma (*see* Fig. 3–22)

Obviously, observation of atheromata in the aorta should prompt attention to placement of the aortic cannula. Although TEE can rarely be used to visualize the site of aortic cannulation, it can be used to visualize the jet out of the aortic cannula. This is accomplished using CF Doppler in conjunction with a two-dimen-

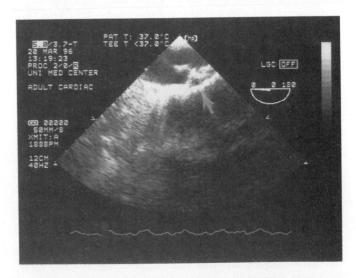

FIGURE 3–22. Two-dimensional image of the aortic arch. The proximal end is to the left and the distal end to the right. The arrow points to a mobile (grade V) aorta atheromata.

sional image of the aortic arch (*see* Fig. 3-15). The direction of the jet out of the aortic cannula is important because the jet can dislodge plaque. Misdirection of the cannula jet down the left subclavian artery or left carotid artery also can be detected using CF Doppler in conjunction with two-dimensional images of those vessels (*see* Fig. 3-15).

TEE also is used extensively to diagnosis aneurysm, dissection, and disruption of the ascending aorta, aortic arch, and descending aorta (*see* Chapter 9).

Ultrasound artifacts are found in 50 to 60% of patients and may result in misdiagnosis. There are two classes of artifacts: linear and mirror image.[53,54]

Linear artifacts occur in the ascending aorta and are the result of reflections from either the left atrium (LA) or right pulmonary artery (RPA). They can be distinguished from intimal flaps because they do not display rapid oscillatory motion, do not disrupt the CF Doppler flow pattern, are parallel to the posterior aortic wall, have movement (best seen with M mode) parallel to that of the posterior aortic wall, and are located twice as far from the posterior wall of the LA or RPA as from the posterior wall of the aorta.

Mirror image artifacts occur in the arch and descending aorta and give the appearance of a double-barreled aorta. They are caused by reflections from the lung-aorta interface. They can be distinguished from intimal flaps or false lumens by the double-barreled mirror image appearance and by the lack of interruption of the CF Doppler flow pattern.

Congenital Heart Disease

A comprehensive treatment of the use of TEE of the wide variety of congenital lesions the pediatric cardiac anesthesiologist is likely to encounter is beyond the scope of this chapter. An excellent comprehensive review is recommended.[55] However, by becoming familiar with some basic principles, the reader should be able to begin conducting a good quality examination in patients with congenital heart disease.

With a biplane probe, the views outlined in Figures 3-5 through 3-15 are available. These views allow comprehensive two-dimensional and Doppler examination of the heart, including the LVOT and RVOT. The LVOT and RVOT are not well oriented for performance of a Doppler examination with standard single-plane imaging. If only a single-plane probe is available, the deep transgastric position will allow visualization of the LVOT and RVOT and the ventriculoarterial connections. In some situations, deep transgastric imaging may provide superior delineation of antomy than biplane examination.[56] From a practical point of view, deep transgastric imaging with a biplane probe is difficult and much less satisfactory because the extra transducer element makes

the distance from the tip of the probe to the flexion point longer. This makes good tissue contact difficult, particularly in small infants.

The following issues should be addressed while performing an examination of a patient with congenital heart disease.

Atrial Identity and Location.   Identity of the atrial chamber by examining the appendage is helpful.

The right atrial appendage (RAA) is best seen in the transverse plane at the level demonstrated in Figure 3-7. Flexion of the probe will allow better visualization. The RAA has the following characteristics:

- a broad junction to the RA
- it is short and blunt (Snoopy's nose)

The LAA is seen in multiple views (*see* Figs. 3-6 and 3-7). It has the following characteristics:

- a narrow junction to the LA
- it is long, narrow, and crenulated (Snoopy's ear)
- The IVC almost always returns to the RA, the return patterns of the SVC and pulmonary veins are much less reliable.
- The RA will have a eustachian valve; the LA septal surface has the flap of the fossa ovalis.
- Atrial situs solitus = RA on the right side of the heart, LA on the left side of the heart.
- Atrial situs inversus = RA on the left side of the heart, LA on the right side of the heart.

Ventricular Size and Identity.   A chamber is considered a ventricle if it receives more than 50% of the ventricular inlet or fibrous ring of an AV valve. The AV valve need not be patent for the chamber to be considered a ventricle, as is the case with tricuspid or mitral atresia (*see* Chapter 6). Likewise, the chamber does not need to be large to be considered a ventricle, as is the case with hypoplastic left heart syndrome. The right and left ventricles have different morphologies:

- RV:
  - has the tricuspid valve (three leaflets) with one the leaflets having a chordal attachment to the septum; there are three papillary muscles that are located apically.
  - the septal leaflet of the tricuspid valve inserts slightly lower on the intraventricular septum than the anterior leaflet of the mitral valve.
  - the RV has a triangular shape and a trabeculated endocardial surface.
  - the RV has the moderator band, a band of tissue that stretches from lower intraventricular septum to the anterior RV wall and is best seen in the four-chamber view with retroflexion of the TEE probe

- LV:
  - has the mitral valve (two leaflets) with no chordal attachment to the septum; there are two papillary muscles that are located at the junction of the apical and middle two-thirds of the chamber.
  - has an ellipsoid shape and a smooth endocardial surface.

Great Vessel Orientation and Identity.   Normally, the great vessels are oriented at 45° to each other when they leave the heart with the pulmonary artery (PA) anterior to the aorta. When they are viewed echocardiographically, one vessel will be observed in the short axis and the other will have a sausage shape. This is seen in the transverse plane image in Figure 3-10. When the great vessels are transposed, they are oriented parallel to each other when they leave the heart. When they are viewed echocardiographically, both vessels will be observed in the same axis. The rule of thumb when viewing transposed vessels in the short axis is that the anterior vessel is invariably the aorta. When the vessels are aligned side to side, the determination is more difficult and usually requires finding the arch of the aorta or the branch pulmonary arteries to make the determination.

After the great vessels are identified, their relationship to the ventricles must be delineated. This requires creativity in finding the views that allow this to be seen. This is an instance in which deep transgastric views are useful, although biplane imaging also works well (*see* Fig. 3-23).

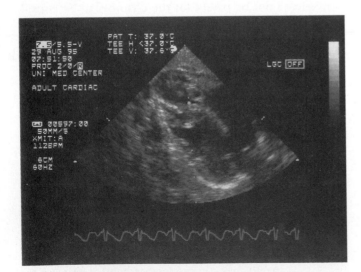

FIGURE 3–23. Transgastric biplane two-dimensional image (90° plane) of a patient with tetrology of Fallot. Apex of the heart is at the top of the image. The left ventricle (LV) is the chamber to the right, the right ventricle (RV) the chamber to the left. There is a large ventricular septal defect (VSD) with the aorta (at the bottom of the image) overriding the VSD.

Presence of Intracardiac Shunts and Obstructive Lesions.   CF Doppler is indispensable in identifying intracardiac shunts, including those not seen with two-dimensional imaging. CW Doppler is useful in determining velocities and gradients across restrictive communications or valves, whereas PW Doppler can be used to assess less restrictive orifices as well as hepatic and pulmonary venous blood flow. The RVOT must be examined carefully for both dynamic and fixed obstructive lesions. Two-dimensional echocardiography in combination with Doppler will clearly delineate dynamic obstructive lesions. The use of CW Doppler to determine intracardiac pressures as described previously is also valuable. Don't forget to look for a PDA.

Evaluation of the Surgical Repair.   A comprehensive preoperative intraoperative study is the foundation of repair assessment. This allows the operator to focus the examination on the repaired lesions. Specific lesions are discussed in detail in Chapter 6. Look for the common things:

- Patch leaks:
  - after ventricular septal defect (VSD) and atrial septal defect (ASD) repairs, detection of residual VSD leaks can be more difficult than it sounds, because the VSD patch produces areas of echo attenuation in the RV and RVOT that may mask leaks. The use of biplane imaging improves detection but does not completely resolve this problem.
- Regurgitant valves:
  - after valvuloplasty but also after transvalvular approaches to the lesion (such as approach to a VSD via the tricuspid valve)
- Stenotic anastomoses:
  - pulmonary vein anastomosis to LA in total anomalous pulmonary venous return (TAPVR)
  - SVC to PA in bidirectional cavopulmonary shunts and Fontan
- Residual outflow tract gradients:
  - after tetrology of Fallot repairs
  - after resection of subaortic membranes
- Residual gradients across ASD or VSD left open in the course of a staged repair (tricuspid atresia, double outlet RV, hypoplastic left heart syndrome)
- Ventricular function assessment:
  - after all repairs
  - particular attention paid to patients with (1) reimplanted coronary arteries such as vessel switch for transposition of the great vessels or Ross procedure (transplantation of the pulmonic valve to the aortic position and creation of an RV-to-PA conduit) and (2) patients

who may have had air in the coronary arteries during the deairing process
- Patency of aortopulmonary shunts:
  — CW Doppler will detect a high velocity signal with flow in systole and diastole. CF Doppler will help position the CW Doppler beam.
- Patency of cavopulmonary shunts
  — PW Doppler will reveal a phasic venous blood flow pattern that exhibits respiratory variation.

Saline-Contrast Echocardiography

Saline-contrast echocardiography is a technique that can be used to detect intracardiac shunting. The basis of the technique is opacification of the right heart chambers using agitated saline injected rapidly into a catheter. Microbubble formation occurs as the solution leaves the catheter orifice as dissolved gas escapes from solution. The presence of microbubbles in high concentrations opacifies the RA and RV. The amount of opacification with a properly performed procedure is impressive.

Saline-contrast studies are used most commonly in conjunction with a provocative maneuver to detect right-to-left flow patency of the foramen ovale. Agitated saline is produced by vigorously transferring 10 mL of saline with a small amount of air between two syringes connected by a stopcock. Alternatively, 8 mL of saline and 2 mL of the patient's blood can be used. The agitated mixture can be injected peripherally or centrally.

Detection of the right-to-left flow patency of the patent foramen ovale (PFO) is dependent on transiently increasing RAP above that of LAP. The easiest way to accomplish this is by applying a Valsalva maneuver during positive-pressure ventilation. This transiently impedes venous return to the right heart and subsequently to the left heart. Upon release of the Valsalva, the rapid increase in venous return to the right heart will precede the increase in return to the left heart and the result will be a transient elevation in RAP above that of LAP. The amount of inspiratory airway pressure necessary to make this effective can be judged by observing the interatrial septum with a biatrial TEE view (see Fig. 3-9) during and after release of the Valsalva maneuver. The interatrial septum must bow into the LA at some point for the test to be effective. The amount of inspiratory pressure necessary to accomplish this should be determined before injection of contrast.

The test is accomplished by injecting the saline contrast during the Valsalva maneuver. After opacification of the RA occurs, the Valsalva is released and the biatrial TEE view is observed for appearance of saline contrast in the LA. Appearance of three or more microbubbles in the LA within three cardiac cycles is indicative of a flow-patent PFO.

Intracardiac and Endovascular Catheters

TEE can be used in a wide variety of ways to image intracardiac and endovascular catheters and devices. A few of the most common and important are summarized here:

- IABP — (see Chapter 11) TEE views of the descending thoracic aorta can and should be used to document that the tip of the intra-aortic balloon pump (IABP) is below the level of the aortic arch and the takeoff of the left subclavian artery. In addition, inflation and deflation can be observed, which may aid in detection of a ruptured balloon.
- Coronary sinus cannula for cardioplegia — the CS is easily seen in most patients and is obliterated when the catheter is placed properly.
- Ventricular assist devices — (see Chapter 11) the inflow and outflow cannulae to the devices can be seen and should be checked to rule out obstruction (see Figs. 3-24 and 3-25).
- Venous cannulae for CPB — position in the IVC and SVC can be checked. In particular, the IVC cannula should not inpinge on any hepatic veins. Difficulty in placing an IVC cannula can be caused by a prominent eustachian valve — alert the surgeon.
- PA catheters — the position of a PA catheter can be documented by sequential views of the RA, RV, and PA. This may have some use if catheter placement is difficult.

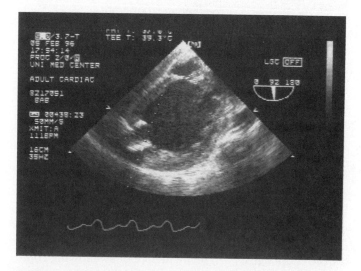

FIGURE 3–24. Proper, unobstructed placement of the inflow cannula of a Novacor left ventricular assist device in the apex of the left ventricle (LV).

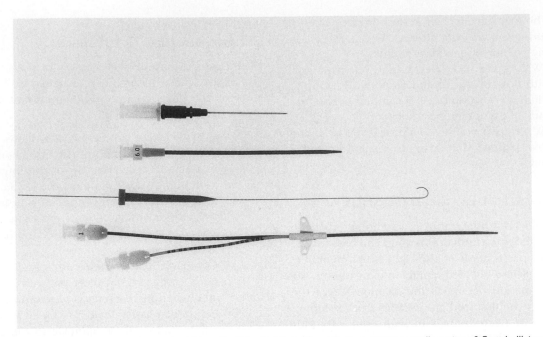

FIGURE 3–25. Central venous catheter system for use in children 10–40 kg. **Top to bottom:** 22-guage catheter–needle system; 6-French dilator, which is passed over guidewire before placement of central nervous catheter; 40-cm 0.018-inch-diameter J guide wire; and 5-French double-lumen central venous catheter. Double-lumen catheter has 20-gauge proximal lumen and 20-gauge distal lumen; 8 cm of catheter is available for placement in a central vein.

Contraindications and Complications

The relative and absolute contraindications to use of a TEE probe are summarized below:

- Relative:
  - Recent gastroesophageal operation
  - Esophageal varicies
  - Upper gastrointestinal bleed
  - Alantoaxial disease
  - Severe cervical arthritis
  - Unexplained dysphagia or odynophagia
- Absolute:
  - Esophageal obstruction (stricture, neoplasm)
  - Esophageal fistula, laceration, or perforation
  - Esophageal diverticulum
  - Cervical spine instability

A number of complications have been reported in association with use of TEE probes. Most complications in adults involve trauma to the upper gastrointestinal (GI) tract ranging from minor lacerations to perforation of the esophagus.[57-59] The incidence of swallowing complications after cardiac surgery in adults having undergone intraoperative TEE also may be higher.[60]

The complications reported in infants and children involve hemodynamic or respiratory compromise.[61-64] Vigilance is required when using TEE probes in a small child, even with the availability of pediatric probes. Airway obstruction may occur due to compression of the small trachea or bronchus between surrounding tissue and the rigid probe. Likewise, aortic or aotic arch vessel compression may occur.

Prophylactic antibiotic coverage for patients undergoing TEE examinations is debated because it carries a risk of inducing bacteremia like any other endoscopic procedure.[65] Most patients undergoing cardiac surgery receive prophylactic antibiotics of some kind, and many consider this sufficient prophylaxis for endocarditis, which further clouds the issue.

In general, use of the TEE probe with proper attention to detail is a safe and rewarding procedure.[66]

■ ARTERIAL ACCESS

Arterial access allows beat-to-beat monitoring of arterial blood pressure as well as the ability to obtain arterial blood samples for analysis of Po_2, Pco_2, pH, and bicarbonate. The preferred site of arterial cannulation is the radial, femoral, or umbilical artery.

Radial Artery

Radial artery cannulation can be accomplished in infants, children, and adults. We use a 22-gauge Teflon or polyurethane catheter for infants and children weighing less than 20 to 30 kg and a 20-gauge catheter for larger children and adults. The wrist is dorsiflexed over a roll of towel or gauze and secured on a short arm board. The thumb is taped back to reduce the mobility of the artery. Neither the dorsiflexion of the wrist nor the taping of the thumb should be so severe as to compromise the radial pulse. The course of the radial artery over an inch of length should be discerned. After appropriate sterile prepping, the area of proposed puncture is anesthetized with 1 to 2 mL of 1% lidocaine in the awake patient. The catheter–needle system should be flushed with a heparinized solution before puncture of the artery. The skin is nicked with a needle directly over the artery. The skin nick helps prevent deformation of the catheter tip, which is particularly likely with the 22-gauge catheter.

The catheter is introduced through the nick at an angle of 30° to the artery with the bevel of the needle directed upward. When blood flows freely out the end of the catheter, the angle between the catheter and the artery is reduced to 5° to 10°, the needle bevel is rotated 180° downward, and the catheter and needle are advanced approximately 1 to 2 mm. At this point, both the catheter and needle should be within the vessel lumen, as indicated by the presence of continued flow of blood out the needle, and the catheter can be advanced forward over the needle into the vessel. Rotating the bevel before advancement helps prevent impingement of the needle tip on the posterior wall of the artery. If there is no blood flow out the needle, it is likely that the posterior wall of the artery has been punctured. The needle and catheter are then intentionally advanced through the posterior wall. The needle is withdrawn partly from the catheter and the catheter is then withdrawn until its tip is located within the lumen of the artery and free flow of blood is noted. At this point, the catheter is readvanced into the artery using the needle as a stent. A 0.018-inch-diameter guide wire can be passed up a 22- or 20-gauge catheter into the artery and often will facilitate readvancement of the catheter.

The safety of radial arterial cannulation has been confirmed in large study populations of infants and children[67] as well as adults.[68] It is generally taught that an Allen's test to assess collateral circulation to the hand via the ulnar artery and palmar arch should be performed before cannulation of the radial artery. For patients without vascular disease of the arms and without previously cannulated arteries, the Allen's test does not seem to be useful in predicting complications from radial artery cannulation in adults[68] or in infants and children.[67,69]

Normally, the radial artery catheter is introduced into the wrist of the nondominant hand. In some instances, the radial artery catheter must be introduced preferentially into one radial artery or the other, as specified below.

- Blalock–Taussig shunts: For children undergoing these subclavian to pulmonary artery shunts, the radial artery contralateral to the subclavian artery being used must be cannulated. Likewise, for children with preexisting Blalock–Taussig shunts, accurate interarterial blood pressure will be obtained only in the contralateral arm.
- Coarctation repair: Arterial blood pressure is best monitored in the right radial artery for a variety of reasons — arterial blood pressure in the left arm may be lower than that in the right arm in the presence of a preductal coarctation, a left subclavian artery patch may be used to repair the coarctation, or left subclavian artery circulation may be compromised by placement of aortic cross-clamps during coarctation repair.
- Thoracic aortic surgery: Because left subclavian artery flow may be compromised by surgical procedures on the distal arch or descending aorta, blood pressure should be monitored in the right radial artery. For procedures involving the ascending aorta, the left radial artery is a better choice.
- Internal mammary artery grafting: Monitoring should be performed in the radial artery contralateral to the side on which the internal mammary artery is to be harvested (*see* Chapter 4).

Femoral Artery

The femoral artery can be cannulated in infants, children, and adults. We use a 22-gauge thin-wall needle to puncture the artery in infants and children weighing less than 30 kg. After free flow of blood is obtained, a straight wire is passed through the needle up into the artery. For infants, we then pass a 2-inch 20-gauge catheter into the artery over the wire. For children, we use a 3-inch 20-gauge catheter. For children weighing more than 30 kg, we use an 18-gauge thin-wall needle for arterial puncture and a 4-inch 18-gauge catheter. For larger children and adults, we use an 18-gauge thin-wall needle for arterial puncture and a 6-inch 16- or 18-gauge catheter.

Femoral artery catheters have been used with a low complication rate for infants and children[70] and adults.[71] Hesitation to use femoral artery catheters in children stems from concern that damage to the poorly encapsulated hip joint may occur directly or through sepsis or arterial occlusion. This does not seem to be a problem for infants and children when proper insertion techniques and catheter sizes are used. However, for infants younger than 1 month of age (neonates), the incidence of transient perfusion-related complications (loss of distal pulse, limb coolness) has been reported to be 25% when a 20-gauge catheter is used.[70] This is higher than the rate associated with radial or umbilical artery catheterization in this age group.

Umbilical Artery

The umbilical artery may be cannulated in the catheterization laboratory or in the intensive care unit in neonates being prepared for surgery. This site usually is cannulated with a 3.5- or 5-French catheter and can be used for arterial monitoring. The catheter tip should lie just above the aortic bifurcation but below L3, or alternatively, above the diaphram at the T7 to T8 level.

■ CENTRAL VENOUS ACCESS

Access to the central venous circulation may be desirable for cardiac surgical patients for a variety of reasons: drug infusion, monitoring of right heart pressures, or placement of a pulmonary artery catheter. The internal and external jugular veins are commonly used for central venous access in infants, children, and adults. We prefer the right internal or external jugular system because they offer fairly constant anatomy with a straight course to the right atrium and a low complication rate. Attempts at left internal jugular venous cannulation may lead to injury to the thoracic duct, and for patients with congenital heart disease, the left internal jugular may drain into a persistent left superior vena cava. For patients with communication between the right and left heart chambers, all peripheral and central venous lines must be kept clear of air bubbles to avoid potential systemic air embolization.

A wide variety of central venous catheters are available for use in adults, infants, and children via the internal or external jugular route. For adults and large children, 7- and 8-French double- and triple-lumen catheters are available. For infants and children weighing less than 4 kg, 4-French double-lumen catheters 5 cm in length are available. For children weighing more than 4 kg, 5-French double-lumen catheters 8 cm in length are used (Fig. 3–25).

Internal Jugular

Three general approaches to the internal jugular using anatomical landmarks have been described: central, anterior, and posterior. However, there are many variations on these general approaches.[72] The central approach involves localization of the internal jugular vein at the apex of the triangle formed by the two heads of the sternocleidomastoid muscle.[73] The apex lies lateral to the carotid pulse and generally is at the level of the cricoid cartilage (two to three finger-breadths above the clavicle in adults). This approach has been used successfully in infants and children and it is our preferred route for these patients.[74] The anterior approach involves localization of the vein at the lateral border of the medial head of the sternocleidomastoid at a point halfway between the clavicle and the mastoid.[75] The posterior approach involves localization of the vein under the lateral border of the medial head of the sternocleidomastoid at the level of the cricoid cartilage.[76]

Recently, it has been demonstrated using ultrasonography that the anatomic relationship of the internal jugular vein and carotid artery is not consistent. In 54% of adults[77] and 59%[78] of children, more than 75% of the right carotid artery (CA) is overlaid by the right internal jugular vein (IJ) when the head is rotated to the left. It also has been demonstrated that the amount of overlap can be reduced by rotating the head less than 40% from the neutral position.[79] When this information is combined with the knowledge that access to the internal jugular vein is obtained 50% of the time during needle advancement and 50% of the time during needle withdrawal,[80] it is easy to see how inadvertent carotid puncture might occur. Ultrasonic guidance has been demonstrated to increase the rate and decrease the complication rate of central venous catheter placement.[81-83]

The following is recommended for cannulation of the internal jugular vein:

1. The patient is positioned with the head turned as far to the left (for right IJ) or right (for left IJ) as is comfortable in the awake patient or until any resistance is met in the anesthetized patient. Supplemental O_2 is supplied to awake patients.
2. For adults and older children, the pillow is removed from beneath the head to produce a slightly extended neck position. For elderly patients with limited neck mobility, removal of the pillow may not be possible. For children, infants, and neonates, it may be necessary to place a small roll under the shoulders to prevent hyperflexion due to the larger head size.
3. The anatomic outline of the clavicle and of the two heads of the sternocleidomastoid muscle are outlined with a marking pen. In awake patients, lifting the head off the bed will help define these landmarks. An ultrasonic device (such as a Site Rite probe or the imaging probe from an echocardiography machine, 5.0 to 7.5 mHz) is placed on the neck using ultrasonic

gel. The relationship of the IJ and CA relative to each other and to the anatomic markings is noted. The depth of the vein below the skin surface also is determined. An illustrative ultrasonic image is shown in Figure 3–26. Head position should be altered to provide the least amount of overlap of the IJ and CA without compromising access to the neck. Ultrasonography will also allow one to determine whether the IJ is small or is compressed from hematoma from previous attempts. This may prompt a look at the contralateral IJ.

4. The neck is prepped and draped using sterile technique. The operator is gowned and gloved. For awake patients, local anesthesia in the form of a skin wheal is accomplished with 1% lidocaine in the area of the intended needle puncture. Deeper infiltration should be performed with caution because the vein is not very deep below the skin. The patient is placed in a 10° to 15° Trendelenberg position. This may increase the size of the IJ and does reduce the risk of air embolus. It is best to wait until the last minute to do this for patients with pulmonary venous congestion or poor ventricular failure because prolonged periods in the Trendelenberg position may exacerbate pulmonary venous congestion, resulting in patient discomfort with subsequent agitation and lack of cooperation.

5. A 25-gauge 5/8-inch needle on a tuberculin syringe is used to locate the center of the vein in all but the largest of adults. A 1-1/2-inch 22-gauge needle rarely is needed to localize the IJ. There is no need to keep a hand on the CA after the vein position has been localized with ultrasound. This maneuver only serves to compress the IJ.

6. After the vein is localized, the finder needle can be left in place or removed. The appropriate-sized thin-wall needle is inserted through the skin in the same orientation as the finder needle. The thin-wall needle is advanced. If the skin is depressed or dimpled inward, the vein is at least partially compressed. When dimpling occurs, the skin should be allowed to "rebound." This does not mean pulling the needle back out of the skin, it means relieving pressure to allow the skin to return to a neutral position. Some compression of the vein by the larger thin-wall needle is inevitable, but when the needle is advanced without compressing the skin, it is more likely that the vein will be entered on the way in and less likely that the vein will be transfixed and the carotid will be punctured. Often, when the skin is allowed to rebound, free flow of IJ blood is obtained without any further advancement of the needle.

7. When free flow of IJ blood is obtained, the thin-wall needle is fixed in place with the fingers of the left hand while the hypothenar eminence rests on the patient. A flexible J-wire is advanced into the thin wall needle and vein. If

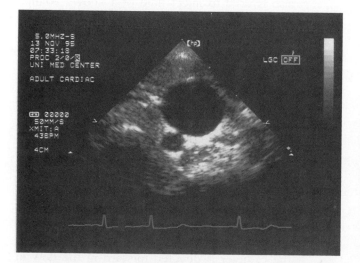
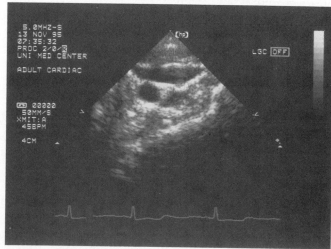

FIGURE 3–26. **Left.** Ultrasonic image of the internal jugular vein (IJ) and the carotid artery (CA) in an adult with an elevated central venous pressure (CVP). The very large IJ is seen to completely overlie the CA. **Right.** Only a small amount of pressure with the transducer is necessary to almost completely compress the IJ.

the wire goes a short distance out the end of the needle and resistance is met, advancement of the wire while spinning it with the right hand should be attempted. If resistance is still met, the wire can be left in place and the thin-wall needle can be removed. An appropriate-sized intravenous catheter is then placed over the wire and advanced into the vein. The guide wire is removed and a syringe is attached to the catheter. The syringe is aspirated and the catheter is withdrawn until free flow of blood is obtained. The catheter is then readvanced into the vein and the guide wire is reintroduced.

8. If there is any doubt that the thin-wall needle or catheter is in the IJ, the needle or catheter should be transduced. Color and blood flow rate, as an indication of arterial cannulation, are unreliable, particularly with the small needles used for children. Transduction can be achieved by attaching a piece of sterile tubing to a transducer or alternatively by using a piece of sterile tubing attached to the needle or catheter and observing the height of the column of blood.

9. When the guide wire is in place in the IJ (it is reassuring to see some ventricular ectopic activity (VEA) as the wire is advanced), a skin nick is made with a knife. The skin nick should be contiguous with the wire; that is, there should not be a skin bridge between the wire and the incision made with the knife. The dilator is passed over the wire. The dilator should only be passed once and only deep enough to pass through skin, soft tissue, platysma, and into the vein. The dilator is removed and gentle pressure is held over the dilated puncture site until the CVP catheter or pulmonary artery catheter introducer is placed.

10. For instances in which venous access is difficult or large transfusion requirements are anticipated, two catheters can be placed in the same IJ. In this "double-stick" technique, one guidewire is placed and then a second guidewire is placed through a second puncture site above or below the first one. The cannulation process is then the same as described previously. This technique is valuable and seems to offer no greater risk than single cannulation.[84]

11. Ultrasonic localization of the IJ is essential for patients who are aggressively anticoagulated when they present for surgery. These patients include heart and heart–lung transplant patients taking coumadin and patients on ventricular assist devices who may be taking coumadin, dipyridamole, aspirin, and other antiplatelet agents.

The most common complication of the internal jugular approach is carotid puncture (4%). Other potential complications of the internal jugular approach include pneumothorax, thoracic duct injury, brachial plexus injury, and air embolism.

External Jugular

The external jugular approach is complicated by the presence of a system of extrathoracic valves, which can make the placement of a guidewire and, subsquently, a catheter into the central circulation difficult. The advantage of this approach is that there is little or no risk of carotid puncture, pneumothorax, thoracic duct injury, or brachial plexus injury. For adults, the use of a guidewire with a flexible J-shaped tip increases the success rate of this approach to 75 to 95%, compared with 95% for the internal jugular route. For children, the success rate of this approach seems to be approximately 60%.[78] Clinically silent venous thrombosis in pediatric patients is high when the external jugular catheter does not reach the central circulation.

■ PULMONARY ARTERY CATHETERS

Pulmonary artery catheters are multilumen, multipurpose catheters available in a variety of sizes (5, 7, and 7.5 French). A typical pulmonary artery catheter (Fig. 3–27) contains the following components:

1. A proximal lumen that terminates in a port located 30 cm (7 and 7.5 French) or 15 cm (5 French) from the distal end of the catheter. When the catheter is positioned properly, this proximal port will be located in the right atrium. This lumen is used to transduce RAP and also is used to inject fluid of a known volume and temperature for determination of thermodilution cardiac outputs.

2. A distal lumen that terminates in a port located at the distal end of the catheter. This lumen is transduced as the catheter is advanced into position and, when the catheter is properly positioned, is used to transduce PAP and PCWP.

3. A balloon located 1 mm from the distal end of the catheter. This balloon is connected to the proximal end of the catheter by a lumen that runs the length of the catheter. The balloon can be filled with air with a syringe located at the proximal end. The 7- and 7.5-French catheters have a 1.5-mL balloon, and the 5-French catheter has a 1-mL balloon. When the balloon is inflated, the catheter is directed forward in the flow of blood. Balloon inflation is used whenever the catheter is advanced. When the catheter is posi-

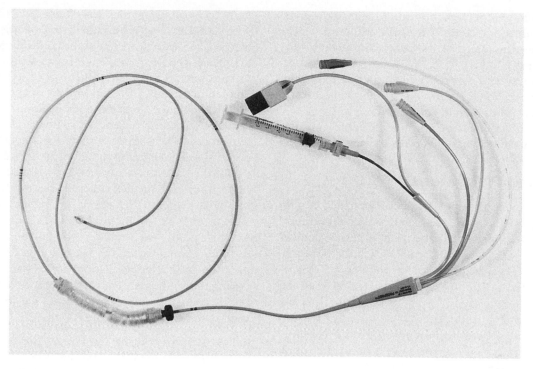

FIGURE 3–27. A 7.5-French pulmonary artery catheter. Sterile sheath is shown on catheter and balloon is partially inflated via syringe. Next to the syringe is a jack for connection to cardiac output computer. Connections for proximal, distal, and right ventricular ports are also visible. Right ventricular port can be used for drug infusion or placement of right ventricular bipolar endocardial pacing wire.

tioned properly, in the pulmonary artery, inflation of the balloon will result in the balloon occluding a branch of the pulmonary artery. The pressure tracing obtained from the distal port at this point will be a measure of the pulmonary artery wedge or occlusion pressure.

4. A thermistor is located at the distal end of the catheter just proximal to the distal port and the balloon. The thermistor is connected to one or more plugs at the proximal end of the catheter, which are used to interface the thermistor with a cardiac output computer.

5. The catheter is labeled in 10-cm increments from the distal end of the catheter.

More recently, 7.5 and 8.0-French pulmonary artery catheters have been manufactured with the following features:

- An additional lumen for drug infusion.
- An additional lumen for placement of a bipolar right ventricular endocardial pacing wire.
- Atrial and ventricular pacing electrodes for bipolar endocardial atrial, ventricular, and atrioventricular (AV) sequential pacing. These catheters contain three atrial electrodes and two ventricular electrodes. Two electrodes must be in contact with the endocardium for successful pacing. Considering the variations in patient size and the length of catheter necessary to properly position a pulmonary artery catheter (PAC), the presence of three atrial electrodes increases the likelihood that two electrodes will be in contact with the atrial endocardial surface. These catheters have been shown to be 80% effective in establishing atrial, ventricular, and AV sequential pacing.

- The addition of fiberoptic bundles, which allow continuous determination of mixed venous oxygen saturation by reflective spectrophotometry. Light of selected wavelengths is transmitted down a fiberoptic bundle, the tip of which is located in the pulmonary artery. This light is transmitted through blood flowing past the fiberoptic bundle and is reflected back to be transmitted down another fiberoptic bundle to be analyzed by a photodetector. The differential absorption of known wavelengths of light by oxyhemoglobin and deoxyhemoglobin is used by a computer to determine mixed venous oxygen saturation (*see* earlier section on Pulse Oximetry). Currently, two models of pulmonary artery catheter with this technology are available. The Baxter Edwards model uses two and the Abbott model three wavelengths of transmitted light.

The use of continuous mixed venous oxygen saturation measurements will be discussed in detail later.

- The ability to perform continuous cardiac output determinations using a thermal filament, which obviates the need for injectate (discussed in detail later).
- The ability to measure RV ejection fraction using a rapid-response thermistor pulmonary artery catheter (discussed in detail later).
- The ability to measure continuous cardiac output and continuous mixed venous oxygen saturation.

Access and Placement

Pulmonary artery catheters usually are introduced percutaneously into the right heart and pulmonary artery via an introducer placed in the right internal jugular vein. For adults and large children, 7, 7.5, and 8.0-French catheters are used and are placed through an 8.5 or 9.0-French introducer. The 5-French catheter is used in smaller children (weighing 15 to 40 kg) and is placed through a 6-French introducer.

The patient should be monitored with a continuous ECG display. A defibrillator should be in the room and in working order. The defibrillator should be capable of being synchronized with the ECG signal to allow cardioversion as well as defibrillation. Intravenous lidocaine should be available as well. The catheter must be placed under sterile conditions by the operator. The catheter is placed in a sterile sheath, and the proximal end of the catheter is handed off to an assistant, who uses the syringe to test balloon inflation. The fully inflated balloon should protrude out over the distal end of the catheter and inflate symmetrically. The assistant also should connect the proximal and distal lumens to their respective transducer/flush systems. The proximal lumen will be used to transduce the RAP while the distal lumen will be used to transduce the PAP and PCWP. The distal lumen trace must be visible on the monitor screen as the catheter is advanced.[82] Finally, the thermodilution cardiac output computer should be connected to the appropriate jack and the correction factor for the catheter being used should be programmed into the computer.

The catheter is held, loosely coiled, in the operator's hand with the tip pointed toward the patient's left (toward the right ventricle and pulmonary outflow tract). The catheter is placed into the introducer and advanced 20 cm for older children and adults and 10 cm for smaller children. At this point, the balloon is inflated and the catheter is advanced with a smooth motion. For adults and older children, a RAP trace will be seen on the distal lumen trace at approximately 20 to 30 cm. For smaller children, this will occur at approximately 10 to 15 cm. Smooth catheter advancement with the balloon inflated continues until the right ventricular trace is seen, followed by the PAP trace and finally the PCWP trace.

Catheter advancement stops when the PCWP trace is seen (see Fig. 3–29). For adults and older children, the PCWP trace will be seen at approximately 50 to 60 cm. In smaller children, the PCWP trace will be seen at approximately 25 to 35 cm. Deflation of the balloon at this time should result in reappearance of the PAP trace. If the PCWP trace remains after balloon deflation, the catheter should be pulled back. The catheter should not remain in the PCWP position for any longer than it takes to measure PCWP to avoid pulmonary infarction.[83]

If the catheter is advanced more than 10 to 15 cm (5 to 10 cm for smaller children) before the trace from the next expected chamber or vessel is noted, the catheter may be coiling in the right atrium or ventricle. At this point, the balloon should be deflated, the catheter should be drawn back, and readvance should be attempted after reinflation of the balloon. Catheter coiling may ultimately lead to catheter knotting.[84]

If coiling occurs, several things can be tried to advance the catheter out of the RA or RV:

1. Remove the catheter from the introducer and make certain that the balloon inflates properly.
2. Orient the curve of the catheter so that it is more anterior than medial as it enters the introducer. This may help direct it toward the TV orifice.
3. After multiple attempts, the catheter may soften. This can be remedied by flushing the distal port with 2 to 3 mL of iced saline or by gently torqueing the catheter as it is advanced.
4. For awake patients, taking a deep breath may enhance blood flow out the RA and RVOT. For anesthetized patients, release of a Valsalva maneuver may accomplish the same thing.
5. Occasionally putting the patient in the head-up position or rotating the bed left or right may help as well.

Most patients with congenital heart disease are not candidates for percutaneous placement of pulmonary artery catheters:

1. Some patients (less than approximately 15 kg) are too small for the 5-French catheters.
2. In some patients, percutaneous placement of a pulmonary artery catheter may be difficult or impossible. For example, the presence of a large atrial septal defect or a ventricular septal defect may make placement difficult without the use of fluroscopy. Similarly, the presence of tricuspid atresia, pulmonary atresia, or pulmonary stenosis make percutaneous placement impossible.
3. The pulmonary artery catheter may interfere with the surgical repair and may have to be removed intraoperatively.

If necessary, catheters can be placed directly into pediatric patients by the surgeon immediately before termination of cardiopulmonary bypass. A thermistor probe (2.5 French) or a thermistor probe combined with a distal lumen (4 French) may be placed directly into the pulmonary artery via the right ventricular outflow tract. When combined with a directly placed right atrial catheter (3.5 French), these will allow determination of thermodilution cardiac outputs. Because these catheters do not allow determination of PCWP, a left atrial pressure line may be placed by the surgeon as well. These lines may be placed directly into the left atrium or into the left atrium via the right superior pulmonary vein. Caution must be exercised with left atrial lines to avoid introduction of air into the systemic circulation.

Pressure Measurement

RAP and PCWP. The RAP is monitored directly through the proximal lumen, whereas LAP is not directly measured by the PAC. The PCWP will be an accurate assessment of LAP, except for instances in which there is pulmonary venous obstruction (rare) or in which the pulmonary alveolar pressure exceeds pulmonary venous pressure.[85] In these instances, PCWP will reflect pulmonary alveolar pressure (Palv). Pulmonary alveolar pressure will exceed pulmonary venous pressure (Pv) when the distal port lies in zone one (PAP < Palv > Pv) or zone two (PAP > Palv > Pv) of the lung. Fortunately, most catheters (93%) reside in zone three (PAP > Palv < Pv) portions of the right middle and lower lobes.[86]

The RAP trace usually is of higher quality than the PCWP trace because the LAP changes are damped as they are transmitted through the pulmonary vasculature to be detected by the distal port. The right and left atrial pressure traces normally contain A, C, and V waves as well as X and Y descents (see Fig. 3-28).

A WAVE. The A wave reflects the atrial pressure increase seen during atrial systole. Atrial systole occurs at ventricular end diastole and is commonly called the atrial kick (see Chapter 2). The peak of the right atrial A wave follows the peak of the P wave by 80 msec when simultaneous RAP and ECG traces are compared.[87] The peak of the left atrial A wave follows the peak of the P wave by 240 msec due to the later depolarization of the left atrium compared with the right atrium.[87] As discussed in Chapter 2, the peak A-wave pressure is the best estimate of ventricular end-diastolic pressure, particularly when ventricular compliance or distensibility is poor (see Fig. 3-29). Obviously, no A wave will be present when atrial systole is absent, as in atrial fibrillation or atrial flutter. For instances in which atrial systole is not synchronous with ventricular diastole, atrial contrac-

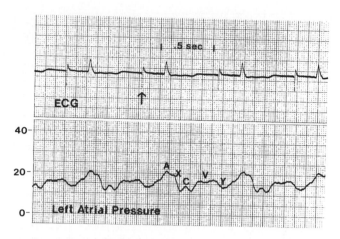

FIGURE 3–28. Left atrial pressure trace obtained from a patient undergoing atrial pacing. *Arrow* shows atrial pacer spike. Paper speed has been increased from 25 to 50 mm/sec to allow clear delineation of the A, C, and V waves as well as the X and Y descents.

tion may occur in the presence of a closed tricuspid or mitral valve during ventricular systole. This will result in production of a large A wave (cannon A wave) because the atrium cannot empty via the closed tricuspid or mitral valve. Cannon A waves may be seen during nodal rhythms with retrograde atrial depolarization (see Fig. 3-30), reentrant supraventricular tachycardia in which ventricular activation precedes atrial activation, and heart block with nonconducted atrial activity occurring during ventricular systole. Cannon A waves also may be seen in instances in which atrial and ventricular contraction are synchronous but in which atrial outflow is prevented by tricuspid or mitral atresia.

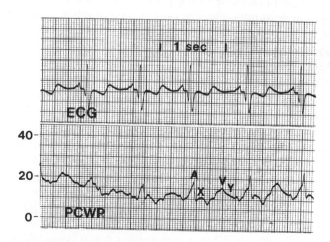

FIGURE 3–29. Pulmonary capillary wedge pressure (PCWP) trace from a patient with aortic stenosis and concentric left ventricular hypertrophy. Large A wave is clearly seen. C wave is not labeled but is clearly visible at bottom of X descent. Peak A-wave pressure at end expiration is approximately 18 mm Hg. The best estimate of left ventricular (LV) end-diastolic pressure (EDP) in this patient, therefore, is 18 mm Hg.

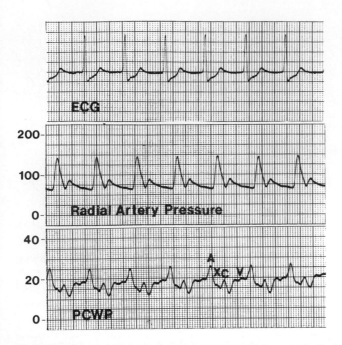

FIGURE 3–30. Pulmonary capillary wedge pressure (PCWP) trace obtained from a patient in nodal rhythm with retrograde atrial activation. Cannon A waves are clearly visible.

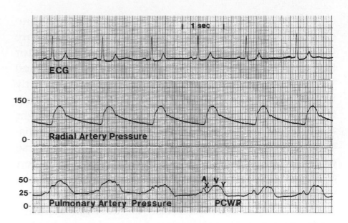

FIGURE 3–31. Pressure (PAP) and pulmonary capillary wedge pressure (PCWP) trace from a patient with mitral regurgitation. Presence of large V wave may make distinguishing pulmonary artery and PCWP traces difficult. However, it is clear that peak of PAP trace relative to electrocardiogram ECG and arterial pressure traces occurs much earlier than peak of V wave in PCWP trace. End-expiratory A-wave pressure of approximately 30 mm Hg is seen; this will be best estimate of LVEDP.

C WAVE. The C wave reflects movement of the tricuspid or mitral valve annulus into the atrium during the isovolumic phase of ventricular systole and is often not well seen (*see* Fig. 3–28). The C wave follows the A wave by a time interval equal to the P-R interval and is seen best when the P-R interval is prolonged.[87]

V WAVE. Normally, the V wave represents passive atrial filling while the tricuspid and mitral valves are closed during ventricular systole. The peak V-wave pressure will be determined by the compliance of the atrium and the volume of blood that enters the atrium during passive filling. In the right atrial trace, the V wave peaks near the end of the ECG T wave, whereas the left atrial V wave peaks after the T wave.

A large V wave may be produced by tricuspid or mitral regurgitation (*see* Figs. 3–31 and 3–32). In this setting, the V wave represents a combination of passive atrial filling and regurgitation of blood into the atrium via the incompetent valve during ventricular systole. Commonly, the height and duration of the V wave is used to quantitate tricuspid or mitral regurgitation. As discussed in detail in Chapter 2, such conclusions must be drawn carefully because the duration of systole, the extent of mitral or tricuspid valve impairment, atrial compliance, the systolic performance of the ventricle, and the impedance to ejection via the pulmonary artery or aorta all contribute to the height and duration of V waves.

It is important to note that other factors may be responsible for production of a large V wave. A large vol-ume of blood returning to the atrium and poor atrial compliance will both produce large V waves.[88] For example, in the presence of a ventricular septal defect with a two-to-one left-to-right shunt, left atrial venous return will be twice that of right atrial return. Likewise, in the presence of poor ventricular systolic performance, pre-load reserve may be exhausted to meet baseline cardiac

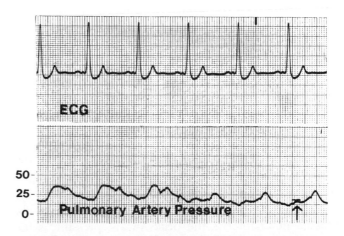

FIGURE 3–32. Pulmonary artery pressure (PAP) and pulmonary capillary wedge pressure (PCWP) trace from patient with mitral regurgitation. PCWP V wave is clearly seen. Arrow points to end-diastolic pressure in PCWP trace. End-diastolic PCWP is approximately 18 mm Hg; this is best estimate of left ventricular (LV) end-diastolic pressure (EDP). As in Figure 3–31, peak of PAP trace occurs earlier in electrocardiogram (ECG) cycle than peak of the PCWP V wave.

output demands. In both instances, the large preload requirements will result in atrial distension, with the atrium functioning on the steep portion of its compliance curve. This reduced atrial compliance will result in production of a large V wave during passive atrial filling.

Differentiating the PAP trace from the PCWP can be difficult in the presence of large V waves because of the morphologic similarity of the two traces. Failure to recognize the V wave of the PCWP can result in overadvancement of the PAC into a distal pulmonary artery, increasing the likelihood of a catheter-induced pulmonary artery perforation. Use of simultaneously obtained PAP and systemic artery pressure or ECG traces can be used to differentiate the two traces. It has been demonstrated that the peak of the pulmonary artery trace normally occurs approximately 130 msec after the upstroke of a simultaneously recorded systemic arterial trace, whereas the peak of the V wave occurs approximately 350 msec after the systemic arterial upstroke.[89] Similarly, the peak of the V wave will occur later in the ECG cycle than the peak of the pulmonary arterial pressure wave (*see* Figs. 3–31 and 3–32).

X AND Y DESCENTS. The X descent follows the A and C waves and reflects a combination of downward displacement of the tricuspid and mitral valve with the onset of ventricular systole and atrial relaxation following atrial systole. The Y descent follows the V wave and reflects rapid atrial emptying after opening of the tricuspid and mitral valves. Thus, the Y descent also reflects early diastolic filling of the ventricle (*see* Fig. 3–28).

In the presence of pericardial tamponade, the X descent usually will remain visible while the Y descent will be attenuated. In pericardial tamponade, diastolic filling of the heart chambers is impeded because the potential space available for expansion of the heart in the pericardium is largely eliminated when the pericardium is filled with fluid (*see* Chapter 8). For this reason, passive filling and expansion of the ventricle as reflected in the Y descent is attenuated. To the contrary, the X descent is preserved because it reflects a decrease in intrapericardial volume as atrial relaxation and ventricular systole begin.

For patients with constrictive pericarditis, early diastolic filling of the ventricle is not compromised as it is in pericardial tamponade (*see* Chapter 8). Constrictive pericarditis is characterized by impairment of ventricular filling in late diastole. Because early diastolic filling is not impaired and because atrial pressure is elevated, the Y descent is more prominent than normal in constrictive pericarditis. As in pericardial tamponade, the X descent remains prominent. This combination of prominent X and Y descents gives a characteristic shape to the atrial pressure curve, which is often referred to as the M or W sign.

Pulmonary Artery Pressure. A determination of systolic, mean, and diastolic PAP can be made with a PAC. In the presence of normal pulmonary vascular resistance, the diastolic PAP will overestimate the PCWP by 2 to 3 mm Hg. In the presence of increased pulmonary vascular resistance, the diastolic PAP will overestimate PCWP and cannot be used as a substitute measurement.

LIMITATIONS. There are major limitations to accurate measurement and interpretation of intracardiac and pulmonary artery pressures.

DETERMINATION OF MEAN PRESSURES. Monitor systems designate systolic, diastolic, and mean pressures as the average highest, lowest, and mean pressures obtained during a preset time interval or a series of such intervals. The electronically determined mean RAP and PCWP will be skewed upward by the presence of large V waves. This will cause mean RAP or PCWP to overestimate ventricular end-diastolic pressure. A device to provide calibrated paper printout of pressure traces is useful in analysis of pressure traces. These paper traces can be used for accurate determination of A- and V-wave pressures as well as systolic and diastolic PAP. The best estimate of ventricular end-diastolic pressure will be the peak A-wave pressure. For patients without an atrial systole, the best estimate of ventricular end-diastolic pressure will be the RAP or PCWP at end diastole. This can be determined by obtaining simultaneous ECG and RAP or PCWP paper traces. End-diastolic pressure in the RAP trace is determined at a point approximately 40 msec before the start of upstroke of the QRS complex. End-diastolic pressure in the PCWP trace is determined at the QRS ST segment junction (*see* Fig. 3–32).

CHANGES IN PLEURAL PRESSURE. Transmural pressure — the pressure acting to distend a heart chamber — is determined by the pressure–volume relationship of the chamber. Intracardiac pressures (such as RAP and PCWP) are equal to the transmural pressure plus the juxtacardiac pressure. Transmural and intracardiac pressure will be equal as long as juxtacardiac pressure is zero. Pleural pressure is a major determinant of juxtacardiac pressure. Pleural pressure will be negative during spontaneous inspiration and positive during controlled inspiration and forced exhalation. Large fluctuations in pleural pressure will cause intracardiac pressure to over- and underestimate transmural pressure and preload. Ideally, then, all intracardiac pressure determinations should be made at passive end expiration, when pleural pressure is close to zero (atmospheric pressure).

If positive end-expiratory pressure (PEEP) is added to the ventilatory circuit, the juxtacardiac pressure at end expiration may be greater than atmospheric pressure; this will cause intracardiac pressure to overestimate transmural pressure and preload. How much a given quantity of PEEP will elevate juxtacardiac pressure depends on the relationship of lung and thoracic compliance. Under normal circumstances, the juxtacardiac pressure is expected to rise by approximately one-half the value of the added PEEP.[90] Thus, if 10 cm H$_2$O of PEEP is added, the juxtacardiac pressure can be expected to increase by 5 cm H$_2$O. When lung compliance is high (emphysema) and thoracic compliance is low (obesity), a larger proportion of the added PEEP will be added to the juxtacardiac pressure.[85,90] A smaller proportion will be added in cases where lung compliance is poor (acute respiratory distress syndrome) and thoracic compliance is high (muscle relaxation).[85,90]

ASSUMPTIONS ABOUT VENTRICULAR PRELOAD BASED ON PRESSURE MEASUREMENTS.   Ventricular preload is defined as the ventricular end-diastolic volume. Unfortunately, methods of obtaining measurements of ventricular end-diastolic volume are not yet in common clinical use. In the absence of tricuspid or mitral stenosis, the A wave of the RAP and LAP (as measured by PCWP) traces are good estimates of the right and left ventricular end-diastolic pressures. If we assume that the ventricular pressure–volume relationship does not vary, then measurement of ventricular end-diastolic pressure is as good an assessment of preload as ventricular end-diastolic volume. Unfortunately, as discussed in Chapter 2, the shape of the ventricular pressure–volume relationship is not linear. Furthermore, changes in ventricular distensibility and compliance alter the relationship between ventricular pressure and volume. It is not surprising, then, that changes in PCWP and LAP have been shown to correlate poorly with changes in left ventricular end-diastolic volume in both the pre- and postcardiopulmonary bypass periods.

Thermodilution Cardiac Output Determination

Thermodilution (TD) cardiac output is a modification of the indicator dilution method in which flow is determined from the following relationship:

$$\frac{\text{known amount of indicator injected}}{\text{measured concentration of indicator}} \times \text{time}$$

In the bolus TD method, the indicator is a crystalloid injectate (usually 5% dextrose in water or isotonic saline) at a temperature lower than the blood temperature. Blood temperature is measured by a thermistor in the pulmonary artery. Crystalloid temperature is measured by separate injectate thermistor. A predetermined volume of crystalloid is injected into the right atrium. Adequate mixing of the crystalloid and blood occurs before passage into the pulmonary artery, and the change in blood temperature over time after injection of the crystalloid is measured by the thermistor in the pulmonary artery. Cardiac output in L/min can be calculated with the aid of a computer and the equation:

$$\text{Cardiac output} = \frac{V_I \times S_I \times C_I \times (T_B - T_I) \times 60}{S_B \times C_B \int_0^\infty \Delta T_B(t)\, dt}$$

where V_I is the volume of the injectate; S_I and S_B are the specific gravity of the indicator and the blood, respectively; C_I and C_B are the specific heat of the indicator and the blood, respectively; and T_I and T_B are the temperature of the indicator and the blood, respectively. $(S_I \times C_I)/(S_B \times C_B) = 1.08$ when isotonic saline or 5% dextrose is injected. $\Delta T_B(t)dt$ is the temperature–time curve measured by the pulmonary artery thermistor after indicator injection. $\int_0^\infty \Delta T_B(t)\, dt$ is the area under the temperature–time curve.

A computer extrapolates the exponential down slope of the temperature–time curve to the baseline and then determines the area under the curve (*see* Fig. 3–41). With all variables thus known or measured the computer solves the equation for cardiac output.

Two recent modifications of the bolus thermodilution technique deserve attention: continuous cardiac output (CCO) monitoring and RV ejection fraction (EF) catheters.

CCO — the currently available technique makes use of a thermal filament located between the 15- and 25-cm gradations on the PA catheter. No injectate is necessary. This filament infuses, on the average, 7.5 W of heat; the blood temperature always remains below 44°C. The thermal filament of one type of CCO catheter (Baxter-Edwards) transfers heat into the blood in a pseudorandom (varying frequencies) binary (on–off) sequence. The thermal filament of the other CCO catheter (Abbott) continuously transfers heat into the blood using a discrete-frequency binary (on–off) sequence. In both cases, the resulting temperature change is detected downstream in the pulmonary artery and cross-correlated with the input sequence to produce a thermodilution washout curve.[91] This requires use of a signal processing system with an enhanced signal-to-noise ratio because the thermal input is low relative to the background PA thermal activity. This is accomplished with a stochastic or spread spectral signal processing. The monitor displays the average cardiac output from the previous 3 to 7 minutes updated every 30 seconds. In the "stat" mode, a new, unaveraged cardiac output can be obtained every 45 to 54 seconds. In this mode, fast trend estimates of cardiac output can be obtained when a hemodynamically unstable thermal signal is present. These catheters also can be used to obtain standard bolus injectate cardiac outputs.

Clinical studies have demonstrated a close correlation between TDCO determinations made with the bolus and CCO techniques in a relatively stable ICU environment.[92,93] A major advantage of the CCO technique would be the ability to monitor acute changes in CO as they occur in real time. To date, the response time of the

CCO technique to acute changes in CO has not been impressive. Both laboratory and clinical studies indicate that the response time of a CCO catheter to acute changes in CO is long (on the order of 5 to 10 minutes).[94,95] In fact, the changes in CCO lag behind those seen with mixed venous saturation monitoring.[94]

RVEF catheter — these catheters are a modification of bolus injectate catheters. They incorporate:

- a rapid response thermistor, which has a reaction time of 50 msec compared with the 300 to 1000 msec response time of standard bolus injectate PA catheters.
- a multihole injectate port located 21 cm from the catheter tip to ensure complete mixing of the injectate in the RV.
- 2 ECG electrodes, which enable the computer to detect the R wave.

This arrangement allows beat-to-beat determination of PA temperature changes. The injectate mixes and equilibrates with RV blood within 2 beats. There is an exponential decrease in the amount of indicator ejected with each subsequent beat. PA concentrations of indicator for each beat are equal to the RV end-diastolic concentration of indicator for that beat. This produces a series of diastolic temperature plateaus that are identified by the computer. EF is calculated as follows from three diastolic plateaus using the equation:

$$EF = 1 - RF_{mean}$$
$$where: \quad RF_{mean} = (RF_1 + RF_2)/2$$

$$RF_1 = (T_2 - T_B)/(T_1 - T_B)$$
$$RF_2 = (T_3 - T_B)/(T_2 - T_B)$$

where:
T_1 = temperature at first diastolic plateau
T_2 = temperature at second diastolic plateau
T_3 = temperature at third diastolic plateau
T_B = blood temperature

Stroke volume (SV), RV end-diastolic volume (EDV) EDV, and RV end-systolic volume (ESV) are calculated as follows:

$$SV = CO/HR$$
$$RV\ EDV = SV/EF$$
$$RV\ ESV = RV\ EDV - SV$$

The normal RV EF = 0.4. Good correlations between PA catheter determined RV EF and radionuclide-determined RV EF have been reported.

Several points regarding TDCO techniques (bolus, RV EF, and CCO) are worth emphasizing:

1. TDCO is a measure of pulmonary blood flow, which in the absence of shunting (both intracardiac and systemic to pulmonary artery), is equal to forward right heart output.
2. Cardiac output is inversely proportional to the area under the pulmonary artery temperature–time curve (*see* Fig. 3–33).
3. There are large cyclical variations in the TD determination of cardiac output during the differ-

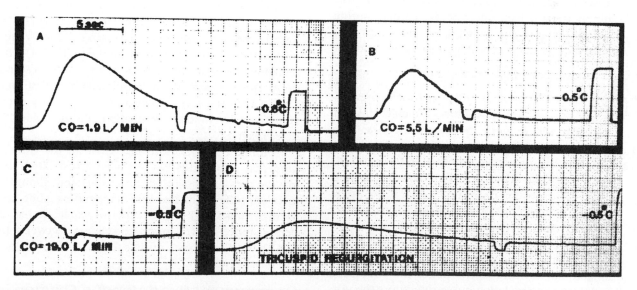

FIGURE 3–33. Examples of thermodilution cardiac output curves. The curves represent change in pulmonary artery temperature (*y* axis) over time (*x* axis). Curves **A, B,** and **C** demonstrate that the area under the temperature–time curve will decrease as cardiac output increases. Curves **A, B,** and **C** all demonstrate normal exponential downslope. This downslope is extrapolated to baseline by computer and the area under curve is determined. Curve **D** was obtained from patient with tricuspid regurgitation; curve is broad and of low amplitude, which results in inaccurate cardiac output determination by computer. (*From: Sharkey SW: Beyond the wedge: Clinical physiology and the Swan-Ganz catheter. Am J Med* 1987; **83:**1199. *Reprinted by permission.*)

ent phases of mechanical ventilation. This seems to be due to cyclic variations in pulmonary blood flow and temperature.[96] For this reason, bolus measurements obtained at random during the ventilatory cycle will exhibit a great deal of variability, whereas those obtained during the same phase of the ventilatory cycle will have the greatest reproducibility. It has been demonstrated that multiple cardiac output values obtained at end expiration or peak inspiration in ventilated patients have high reproducibility.[97,98] The highest measured TDCOs occur at peak inspiration, whereas the lowest occur at end expiration.[97-99] Triplicate TDCO determinations are commonly made at end expiration because end expiration is the easiest phase of respiration to detect clinically. This practice provides excellent reproducibility but tends to underestimate the average cardiac output over one full cycle of mechanical ventilation.[90,96]

4. The injectate volume can vary from 1 to 10 mL. For adults, use of 3- and 5-mL volumes results in more within-patient variation than a 10-mL volume.[100] Volumes of 1, 2, and 3 mL have been shown to produce reliable results in infants and small children.[101-103]

5. Injectate temperatures from 0°C to room temperature are used. The lower temperatures are obtained by placing the injectate in an ice bath. The accuracy and variability of TDCO in adults is similar with either 10 mL of room temperature or iced injectate.[100] Sinus bradycardia[104,105] and atrial fibrillation[106] have been reported in conjunction with iced injectate for cardiac output determination. The slowing of the sinus rate seems to be due to cooling of the sinus node.[107]

TDCOs are inaccurate in the presence of:

- Low cardiac outputs. Cardiac output is overestimated because low flow allows the cold injectate to warm and reduces the area under the thermodilution curve.
- Left-to-right intracardiac shunts (atrial septal defect, ventricular septal defect). Computer analysis of the temperature–time curve often is not possible due to recirculation of indicator (cold water) through the pulmonary vasculature, which results in interruption of the exponential downslope of the temperature–time curve with a prolonged, flat deflection. The larger the shunt, the earlier the recirculation curve interrupts the normal downslope. Manual planimetry has been used to determine the area under the two portions of these curves.[108] The ratio of the area under the terminal deflection of the curve to the

area under the entire curve has been shown to be an accurate estimate of the ratio of pulmonary to systemic blood flow.[108]

- Tricuspid regurgitation. Regurgitation of a fraction of the cold injectate results in delayed clearance of the indicator from the right heart. This causes the thermodilution curve to be broad and of low amplitude, which results in inaccurate assessment of forward cardiac output (*see* Fig. 3–41). Similar problems would be expected with CCO catheters.
- Rapid infusion of volume via peripheral intravenous catheters. Abrupt increases in the infusion rate of intravenous solutions within 20 seconds of a bolus TDCO determination have been shown to result in variations of up to 80% in TDCO.[109] The precise timing of the infusion rate increase relative to the TDCO measurement determines whether the output will be an over- or underestimate. It is recommended that volume infusions be terminated or held at a constant rate for at least 30 seconds before a TDCO determination.[109] Likewise, rapid infusions of cold intravenous solutions affect the accuracy of CCO catheters.[110]

The accuracy of bolus TDCO determinations in the period immediately following termination of CPB is questionable. Bolus TDCOs have been shown to underestimate true cardiac output by approximately 0.5 L/min in the first 10 minutes after termination of CPB due to a downward drift of the temperature baseline in the pulmonary artery.[110] Another source of bolus TDCO error in the first 30 minutes after termination of CPB is the presence of respiratory variations or thermal noise in the pulmonary artery blood temperature.[111] These thermal variations in pulmonary artery blood temperature may cause large variations in the bolus TDCO determinations made at the various points in the respiratory cycle. This problem can be minimized by measuring bolus TDCO at the same point in the respiratory cycle or eliminated by holding ventilation during bolus TDCO determination.

Similar considerations may exist for the CCO technique, but as yet, this has not been investigated. In theory, the data processing of the CCO system should minimize the effects of baseline temperature shift and of thermal noise and improve performance. It has been demonstrated that a poor correlation between bolus TDCO and CCO exists during the first 45 minutes after termination of CPB.[112]

Continuous Mixed Venous Oxygen Saturation (SvO₂) Monitoring

As described previously, SvO₂ monitoring is available as part of some PA catheters. The SvO₂ is measured in the main pulmonary artery by oximetry. The main pulmonary artery is chosen because this is the most reliable source of true mixed venous (SVC, IVC, and coronary sinus) blood. The SvO_2 is used to determine total tissue O_2 balance. It will not reflect regional O_2 imbalance.

Several definitions are in order:

- O_2 delivery (DO_2) = cardiac output (CO) × O_2 content
- Arterial O_2 content (CaO_2) = (Hgb × 13.8) (SaO_2)
- Mixed venous O_2 content (CvO_2) = (Hgb × 13.8) (SvO_2)
- O_2 consumption (VO_2) = the metabolic rate or the amount of O_2 consumed by the body. This is equal to the amount of O_2 delivered systemically (CO) (CaO_2) minus the amount of O_2 returned to the heart (CO) (CvO_2).

$$(CO)(CaO_2) - (CO)(CvO_2) =$$
$$[(Hgb \times 13.8)(SaO_2)(CO)] - [(Hgb \times 13.8)(SvO_2)$$
$$(CO)] = (Hgb \times 13.8)(CO) \times (SaO_2 - SvO_2)$$

This is simplified to:

$$SvO_2 = SaO_2 - [VO_2/(Hgb \times 13.8)(CO)]$$

Thus, mixed venous O_2 saturation as measured continuously by a mixed venous saturation PA catheter varies directly with CO, Hgb, and SaO_2 and varies inversely with VO_2. If SaO_2, Hgb, and VO_2 remain constant, then SvO_2 will directly reflect changes in CO. Under these circumstances, continuous measurement of SvO_2 is analogous to a continuous CO measurement. The response time of SvO_2 to acute changes in CO under conditions of constant SaO_2, Hgb, and VO_2 has been demonstrated to be more rapid than CCO measurements.[94]

A normal SvO_2 is 75%, which corresponds to a mixed venous PO_2 of 40 mm Hg. SvO_2 is a reflection of the adequacy of systemic O_2 delivery. A reduced SvO_2 indicates inadequate systemic O_2 delivery and increased peripheral O_2 extraction and should prompt an evaluation of SaO_2, Hgb, VO_2, and CO. Similarly, a "low" CO in the setting of a normal SvO_2 indicates that systemic O_2 delivery is adequate to meet present metabolic needs and that, in reality, the CO is not low. Although a high CO is reassuring, does not guarantee adequate systemic O_2 delivery under conditions of reduced Hgb and SaO_2 or increased VO_2. An SvO_2 measurement allows this determination to be made.

Hemodynamic Profiles

The information obtained from a PAC can be used in conjunction with arterial blood pressure monitoring to obtain a number of derived hemodynamic parameters. The most commonly used parameters, their derivation, and their units of measurement are given in Table 3–7.

TABLE 3–7. HEMODYNAMIC PARAMETERS, DERIVATION, AND MEASUREMENT

Formula	Units	Normal Value
$SV = \dfrac{CO}{HR} \times 1000$	mL/beat	60–90
$SI = \dfrac{SV}{BSA}$	mL/beat/m²	40–60
$LVSWI = \dfrac{1.36 \times (MAP - \overline{PCWP})}{100} \times SI$	$\dfrac{\text{gram-meters/m}^2}{\text{beat}}$	45–60
$RVSWI = \dfrac{1.36 \times (\overline{PAP} - \overline{CVP})}{100} \times SI$	$\dfrac{\text{gram-meters/m}^2}{\text{beat}}$	5–10
$SVR = \dfrac{MAP - \overline{CVP}}{CO} \times 80$	dynes-sec/cm⁵	900–1500
$PVR = \dfrac{\overline{PAP} - \overline{PCWP}}{CO} \times 80$	dynes-sec/cm⁵	50–150

BSA = body surface area; CO = cardiac output; $\overline{CVP}$ = mean central venous pressure; HR = heart rate; LVSWI = left ventricular stroke work index; MAP = mean systemic arterial pressure; PAP = mean pulmonary artery pressure; PCWP = mean pulmonary capillary wedge pressure; PVR = pulmonary vascular resistance; RVSWI = right ventricular stroke work index; SI = stroke index; SV = stroke volume; SVR = systemic vascular resistance.

For SVR and PVR, dynes-sec/cm⁵ can be converted to Wood Units by leaving out the correction factor of 80 in the calculations.

Complications

In general, PACs have been used without a high incidence of major complications.

Complications associated with obtaining central venous access were addressed in the section on that topic.

The incidence of catheter-induced transient premature ventricular contractions (PVCs) during advancement of PACs is approximately 65%,[113,114] whereas the incidence of persistent PVCs during catheter advancement seems to be approximately 3.0%.[114] These persistent PVCs generally resolve with an intravenous bolus of lidocaine (1.0 to 1.5 mg/kg). The prophylactic use of lidocaine does not seem to be warranted before placement of PACs as it does not reduce the incidence of these benign, transient catheter-induced PVCs.[113] The incidence of catheter-induced right bundle branch block is less than 0.05%.[114] Likewise, the risk of complete heart block in a patient with a preexisting left bundle branch block is extremely low.[114]

The incidence of pulmonary artery rupture, a potentially lethal complication, seems to be less than 0.07%.[114] The risk of pulmonary artery rupture seems to be increased by anticoagulation, pulmonary hypertension, distal catheter placement, and eccentric balloon inflation.[115-118] Pulmonary infarction occurs with low frequency (less than 0.07%)[114] and can be avoided by preventing the catheter from remaining in a continuous wedge position.[83] Placement of pulmonary catheters has resulted in direct tricuspid and pulmonary valvular damage[119,120] as well as tricuspid and pulmonary valvular endocarditis.[121]

■ ELECTROCARDIOGRAPHIC (ECG) MONITORING

The ECG is a standard monitor during cardiac surgical procedures for monitoring heart rate, rhythm, and ischemia. Normally, a five-electrode ECG system capable of monitoring seven leads (I, II, III, aVR, aVL, aVF, and V_5) is used.

Dysrhythmia Detection

Typically, lead II is used for dysrhythmia identification because the P-wave morphology is well seen. In some tachydysrhythmias (paroxysmal atrial tachycardia, nodal rhythm, ventricular tachycardia), the P wave may be difficult or impossible to see in any of the standard leads. In other tachydysrhythmias (atrial fibrillation, atrial flutter), the P wave is absent. In some cases of AV nodal block or AV dissociation, the relationship between the P waves and the QRS complex may be difficult to discern with standard ECG leads. In such instances, the bipolar esophageal or intra-atrial ECG may be very useful. Two electrodes are incorporated in either a 12-French esophageal stethoscope for pediatric patients[122] or an 18-French esophageal stethoscope for adults.[123,124] Alternatively, two of the three atrial electrodes from a pacing PAC can be used to obtain a bipolar intra-atrial ECG.[113] The two leads from these electrodes are connected to the right arm and left arm jacks of a standard three-lead ECG system. The third lead of the three-lead ECG is connected to the patient via a skin electrode and lead I is monitored. Because the esophageal and intra-atrial ECGs place electrodes so proximal to the atria, there is augmentation of atrial activity such that the P wave is often larger than the QRS complex. Use of the esophageal ECG has been shown to greatly improve the ability to identify intraoperative dysrhythmias both in adults[123] and in children.[122]

Ischemia Detection

The presence of ECG changes is useful in the detection of myocardial ischemia. Specifically, ischemia is heralded by the development of ST segment depressions with or without T-wave changes. These changes are related to alterations in the repolarization process. Progression to transmural ischemia and myocardial injury is associated with ST segment elevations. In the case of coronary spasm, ST segment elevations are likely to be the initial manifestation seen on ECG. For ECG monitoring to be effective in detecting ischemia, the appropriate leads must be monitored. Exercise treadmill testing has demonstrated that 89% of the significant ST segment depressions occurring during exercise can be detected in lead V_5.[125] The addition of leads II, aV$_F$, V_3, V_4, and V_6 to lead V_5 increases the sensitivity of ischemia detection to

100% during exercise testing.[125] Similarly, lead V_5 and the combination of leads V_5 and II have been shown to be effective in detecting intraoperative ischemic changes.[126-128] It has been demonstrated recently that the combination of leads V_5 and II has a sensitivity of 80% in detecting intraoperative ischemia, whereas the combination of V_4, V_5, and II has a sensitivity of 96%.[129]

Use of a five-electrode ECG system to simultaneously monitor leads II and V_5 has become popular as a method of detecting both ischemia and dysrhythmias. Because monitoring of the standard seven leads will not detect true posterior ischemia, use of an esophageal ECG lead has been suggested to monitor RV and posterior LV ischemia.[123,124] Despite appropriate lead selection, accurate detection of ischemic ECG changes by the anesthesiologist during the course of an operative procedure can be difficult:

- In most instances, the anesthesiologist observes one or two ECG traces on the oscilloscope during the case. Vigilance to other monitors and the numerous tasks that must be performed in the course of the operative procedure do not permit continuous visual monitoring of the ECG traces.
- The monitoring mode (0.5 to 40.0 Hz) filters out high and low frequency artifacts to attentuate the effects of extraneous interference from 60-cycle noise, electocautery, respiratory variation, and movement. Unfortunately, this mode makes analysis of subtle ST segment changes unreliable. The diagnostic mode (0.05 to 100.0 Hz) reflects the true extent of ST segment changes but is more prone to interference.

It is not surprising, then, that a large percentage of intraoperative ischemic ECG changes go undetected by the anesthesiologist even when lead V_5 is available for monitoring.[130,131] This has led to efforts to improve intraoperative analysis of ECG changes.

Automated ST segment software is currently available on many intraoperative monitoring systems. These ST segment analysis systems identify the QRS complex and then identify the isoelectric point in the P-R interval and a measurement point along the ST segment. The monitor analysis of the appropriate points for ST segment analysis are displayed. They can be subsequently altered by the operator. This is an important feature because computer analysis of the appropriate points for measurement may be rendered inaccurate by nontypical QRS patterns. In addition, this feature allows the operator to choose whether 60 msec or 80 msec after the J point is to be the analysis point. Most monitors can provide analysis of two leads simultaneously, some provide analysis of three. The monitors provide digital presentation of current ST segment data and graphical presentation of trended ST segment data. Alarms may be set for specific amounts of ST segment deviation. Extensive validation of these monitors is lacking, but a recent investigation demonstrated that two types of automated ST segment analysis (Hewlet Packard and Marquette) document most but not all of the episodes of ischemia seen with a printed eight-lead ECG.[132]

■ THROMBOELASTOGRAPHY

Thromboelastography (TEG) is a method of monitoring blood viscosity that can be used to evaluate various components of the coagulation system. Although the efficacy of using TEG analysis as the sole source of information on the coagulation system after CPB is debatable,[133-135] there is no doubt that TEG as part of the algorithm for treating post-CPB bleeding is valuable (*see* Chapter 10).

The TEG is a sensitive device that requires training and meticulous technique to use. The device usually contains two identical channels so that two blood samples can be run at once. Each channel consists of a disposable cylindrical plastic cup mounted in a base. The cup is filled with a 360 µl of blood sample from a pipette. The base is associated with a heated block that allows the blood sample to be warmed to and maintained at 37°C. A piston that is covered with a disposable plastic sheath is suspended in the blood sample by a wire. The base in which the cup is mounted rotates 4°45′ every 9 seconds in an alternating clockwise, counterclockwise pattern. There is a 1-second rest interval at the end of each rotation. Before the blood begins to coagulate, the oscillatory motion of the cup is not transferred to the piston. When coagulation begins, blood viscosity increases and progressively increasing increments of cup rotation are transferred to the piston. The torque on the piston is transferred to the suspending wire. These signals are amplified and transferred to an analog output such as a computer screen. With this presentation, the real-time development of the TEG pattern can be assessed. A TEG sample trace is shown in Figure 3–34. The symmetric nature of the trace is caused by the oscillary rotation of the cup and piston.

The TEG data are presented in a time-amplitude format with time on the hortizontal axis. The following data are derived and displayed:[136]

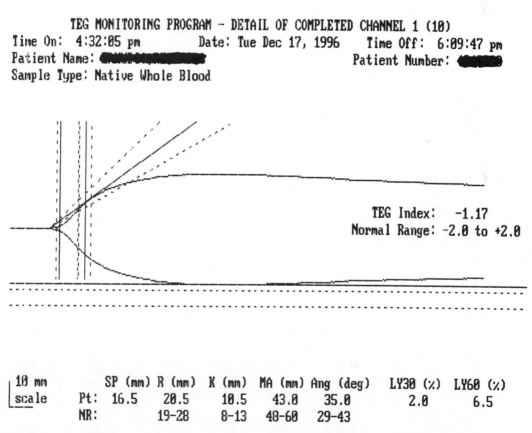

FIGURE 3–34 Thromboelastography (TEG) trace from a patient with normal initiation of coagulation, a low maximum amplitude (MA), and evidence of mild late clot lysis. LY30 = % clot lysis at 30 minutes after the MA, LY60 = % clot lysis at 60 minutes after the MA. Numeric values are given along the bottom of the trace. Pt = patient values, NR = normal range for the particular value. The normal ranges are indicated by the dotted lines on the TEG trace. The normal valve for LYS 60 < 15%. The patient values by the solid lines. Values here for *R* and *K* are given in mm; they are converted to minutes using 2.0 mm/min conversion. This patient had a normal fibrinogen level and platelet count after cardiopulmonary bypass. This TEG is indicative of a mild defect in platelet function which could be treated with administration of desmopressin acetate.

- R = reaction time; this is the time from the initiation of the test to the point of 2-mm divergence. The R value is similar to the whole blood clotting time. Prolongation of R is associated with clotting factor deficiencies or inhibitors and anticoagulants such as heparin. Thrombocytopenia may prolong R because platelets provide the phospholipid surface of coagulation reactions in the TEG.
- K = coagulation time; this is the time from R to the point of 20-mm divergence. This represents the rate of clot structure formation. K is increased by clotting factor deficiencies, thrombocytopenia, hypofibrinogenemia, and platelet dysfunction.
- $R + K$ = summation time.
- Ang = alpha angle; this the angle generated by the slope of the line tangent to the plot upstroke. This (like K) represents the rate of clot structure formation. The alpha angle is reduced by clotting factor deficiencies, thrombocytopenia, hypofibrinogenemia, and platelet dysfunction.

- MA = maximum amplitude; this the maximum amplitude reached by the plot. This is indicative of maximum clot strength and is primarily a function of platelet count and fibrinogen. MA also is reduced by severe factor deficiencies and heparin therapy.
- LY30 = percent decrease in MA at 30 minutes after MA is reached. This is a measure of early clot lysis.
- LYS 60 = percent decrease in MA at 60 minutes after MA is reached. This is a measure of late clot lysis. Normally, LYS 60 < 15%. LYS 60 can also be expressed as A_{60}: MA ratio, where A_{60} is the TEG amplitude at 60 minutes.
- TEG index = index created by weighted average of R, K, MA, and alpha angle. Useful as an overall index of coagulability.

It should be emphasized that the TEG is a test of whole blood coagulation. Each of the parameters determined by the TEG involves the interplay of several por-

TABLE 3–8. SUMMARY OF TEG DATA AND ASSOCIATED COAGULATION ABNORMALITIES

Normal R and K:	
MA < 40	Moderate functional platelet deficiency
MA = A_{60}	
MA < 40	Hypofibrinoginemia
R and K upper limit of normal	
MA < 40	Hyperfibrinolysis
MA >> A_{60}	
LYS30 and LYS60 close to 100%	
Prolonged R and K:	
MA normal	Factor deficiency
A_{60} normal	
R prolonged 3+	
K prolonged 1+	
MA = A_{60} (both may be reduced)	Anticoagulant therapy (heparin, coumadin)
R prolonged 3+	
K prolonged 3+	
30 > MA < 20	Severe functional platelet deficiency
MA = A_{60}	
MA < 50	Abnormal coagulation and fibrinolysis
A_{60} = 0	
LYS60 = 100%	
MA < 20	Near complete heparinization or severe functional platelet deficiency
MA = 0	Full heparinization or afibrinogenemia
Decreased R and K:	
R decreased 3+	Plasma-related hypercoagulability
K decreased 1+	
MA < 60	
R decreased 2+	Platelet-related hypercoagulability
K decreased 2+	
MA > 60	

tions of the complete coagulation system. As a result the correlation of individual TEG variables (*R, K,* MA) with standard coagulation test (PTT, PT, BT) is poor. The correlation of MA to platelet count and fibrinogen level is good.

The guidelines listed in Table 3-8 are useful in interpreting the TEG.[137]

A functional platelet deficiency can be the result of thrombocytopenia, defects in platelet function, or both. A platelet count and a fibrinogen level are useful in sorting the contribution of platelets and fibrinogen to the observed TEG pattern.

TEG would be valuable if it could be used to determine coagulation defects that have developed on CPB before termination of CPB. This would allow prompt treatment after CPB had been terminated and protamine had been administered. This has not been possible previously because heparin anticoagulation during CPB produces a flat TEG. Recently, the ability to add protamine or the enzyme heparinase to samples obtained on CPB has made determination of coagulation status on CPB possible.[138] We have found heparinase TEG on CPB a reliable way to predict dilutional factor and platelet deficiencies, particularly for small infants and neonates.

The use of aprotinin complicates TEG interpretation. Heparinase TEG on CPB in patients receiving aprotinin typically has a very prolonged *R.* This is presumably the result of the same factors that prolong ACT and PTT in patients receiving aprotinin (*see* Chapter 10).

Finally, TEG has also proved useful in titrating postoperative anticoagulation in patients on LVADs and with the total artificial heart.

■ REFERENCES

1. DiNardo JA, Satwicz PR: Nonlinear relationship of arterial to peak end tidal partial pressure of CO_2 during CABG surgery. *Anesth Analg* 1986; **65:**S41.
2. Fletcher R, Malmkvist G, Niklason L, Jonson B: Online measurement of gas-exchange during cardiac surgery. *Acta Anaesthesiol Scand* 1986; **30:**295-299.
3. Raemer DB, Francis D, Philip JM, Gabel RA: Variations in P_{CO_2} between arterial blood and peak expired gas during anesthesia. *Anesth Analg* 1983; **62:**1065-1069.
4. From RP, Scamman FL: Ventilatory frequency influences accuracy of end-tidal CO_2 measurements. Analysis of seven capnometers. *Anesth Analg* 1988; **67:**884-886.
5. McEvedy BAB, McLeod ME, Mulera M, et al: End-tidal, transcutaneous, and arterial P_{CO_2} measurements in critically ill neonates: A comparative study. *Anesthesiology* 1988; **69:**112-116.
6. Bagwell JM, Heavner JE, May WS, et al: End-tidal P_{CO_2} monitoring in infants and children ventilated with either a partial rebreathing or a nonrebreathing circuit. *Anesthesiology* 1987; **66:**405-410.
7. Bagwell JM, McLeod ME, Lerman J, Creighton RE: End-tidal P_{CO_2} measurements sampled at the distal and proximal ends of the endotracheal tube in infants and children. *Anesth Analg* 1987; **66:**959-964.
8. Yelderman M, New W: Evaluation of pulse oximetry. *Anesthesiology* 1983; **59:**349-352.
9. Kessler MR, Eide T, Humayun B, Poppers PJ: Spurious pulse oximeter desaturation with methylene blue injection. *Anesthesiology* 1986; **65:**435-436.
10. Mihm FG, Halperin BD: Noninvasive detection of profound arterial desaturations using a pulse oximetry device. *Anesthesiology* 1985; **62:**85-87.
11. Deckart R, Stewart DJ: Noninvasive arterial hemoglobin oxygen saturation versus transcutaneous oxygen tension monitoring in the preterm infant. *Crit Care Med* 1984; **12:**935-939.
12. Swedlow DB, Stern S: Continuous non-invasive oxygen saturation monitoring in children with a new pulse oximeter. *Crit Care Med* 1983; **11:**A228.
13. Deckart R, Steward DJ: Noninvasive arterial hemoglobin oxygen saturation versus transcutaneous oxygen tension monitoring in the preterm infant. *Crit Care Med* 1984; **12:**935-939.
14. Casthely PA, Redko V, Dluzneski J, et al: Pulse oximetry during pulmonary artery banding. *J Cardiothorac Anesth* 1987; **1:**297-299.
15. Brooks TD, Paulus DA, Winkle WE: Infrared heat lamps interfere with pulse oximeters. *Anesthesiology* 1984; **61:**630.
16. Eisele JH, Downs D: Ambient light affects pulse oximeters. *Anesthesiology* 1987; **67:**864-865.
17. Costarino AT, Davis DA, Keon TP: Falsely normal saturation reading with the pulse oximeter. *Anesthesiology* 1987; **67:**830-831.
18. Miyasaka K, Ohata J: Burn, erosion, and "sun" tan with the use of pulse oximeters in infants. *Anesthesiology* 1987; **67:**1008-1009.
19. Rubin AS: Nail polish color can affect pulse oximeter saturation. *Anesthesiology* 1988; **68:**825.
20. Cote CJ, Goldstein EA, Fuchsman WH, Hoaglin DC: The effect of nail polish on pulse oximetry. *Anesth Analg* 1988; **67:**683-686.
21. Scheller MS, Unger RJ, Kelner MJ: Effects of intravenously administered dyes on pulse oximetry readings. *Anesthesiology* 1986; **65:**550-552.
22. Eisenkraft JB: Pulse oximeter desaturation due to methemoglobinemia. *Anesthesiology* 1988; **68:**279-282.
23. Eisenkraft JB: Pulse oximeter desaturation due to methemoglobin. *Anesthesiology* 1988; **68:**279-282.
24. Barker SJ, Tremper KK: The effect of carbon monoxide inhalation on pulse oximetry and transcutaneous P_{O_2}. *Anesthesiology* 1987; **66:**677-679.
25. Hansen RM, Viquerat CE, Matthay MA, et al: Poor correlation between pulmonary arterial wedge pressure and left ventricular end-diastolic volume after coronary artery bypass graft surgery. *Anesthesiology* 1986; **64:**764-770.
26. Ellis RJ, Mangano DT, Van Dyke DC: Relationship of wedge pressure to end-diastolic volume in patients undergoing myocardial revascularization. *J Thorac Cardiovasc Surg* 1978; **78:**605-613.
27. Douglas PS, Edmunds H, Sutton M St J, et al: Unreliability of hemodynamic indexes of left ventricular size during cardiac surgery. *Ann Thorac Surg* 1987; **44:**31-34.
28. Thys DM, Hillel Z, Goldman ME, et al: A comparison of hemodynamic indices derived by invasive monitoring and two-dimensional echocardiography. *Anesthesiology* 1987, **67:**630-634.
29. Konstadt SN, Thys D, Mindich BP, et al: Validation of quantitative intraoperative transesophageal echocardiography. *Anesthesiology* 1986; **65:**418-421.
30. Cheung AT, Savino JS, Weiss SJ, et al: Echocardiographic and hemodynamic indexes of left ventricular preload in patients with normal and abnormal ventricular function. *Anesthesiology* 1994; **81:**376-387.
31. Reich DL, Konstadt SN, Nejat M, et al: Intraoperative transesophageal echocardiography for the detection of cardiac preload changes induced by transfusion and phlebotomy in pediatric patients. *Anesthesiology* 1993; **79:**10-15.

32. Perez J, Klein S, Prater D, et al: Automated, on-line quantification of left ventricular dimensions and function by echocardiography with backscatter imaging and lateral gain compensation. *Am J Cardiol* 1992; **70:**1200-1205.

33. Cahalan M, Ionescu P, Melton H, et al: Automated real-time analysis of intraoperative transesophageal echocardiography. *Anesthesiology* 1993; **78:**477-485.

34. Liu N, Darmon P-L, Saada M, et al: Comparison between radionuclide ejection fraction and fractional area changes derived from transesophageal echocardiography using automated border detection. *Anesthesiology* 1996; **85:**468-474.

35. Urbanowicz JH, Shaaban MJ, Cohen NH, et al: Comparison of transesophageal echocardiographic and scintigraphic estimates of left ventricular end-diastolic index and ejection fraction in patients following coronary artery bypass grafting. *Anesthesiology* 1990; **72:**607-612.

36. Leung JM, Levine EH: Left ventricular end-systolic cavity obliteration as an estimate of intraoperative hypovolemia. *Anesthesiology* 1994; **81:**1102-1109.

37. Berquist BD, Leung JM, Bellows WH: Transesophageal echocardiography in myocardial revascularization: I. Accuracy of intraoperative real-time interpetation. *Anesth Analg* 1996; **82:**1132-1138.

38. Berquist BD, Bellows WH, Leung JM: Transesophageal echocardiography in myocardial revascularization: II. Influence on intraoperative decision making. *Anesth Analg* 1996; **82:**1132-1138.

39. Stewart WJ, Currie PJ, Saledo EE, et al: Evaluation of mitral leaflet motion by echocardiography and jet direction by Doppler color flow mapping to determine the mechanism of mitral regurgitation. *J Am Coll Cardiol* 1992; **20:**1353-1361.

40. Simpson IA, Shiota T, Gharib M, et al: Current status of flow convergence for clinical applications: Is it a leaning tower of "PISA"? *J Am Coll Cardiol* 1996; **27:**504-509.

41. Bach DS, Deeb M, Bolling SF: Accuracy of intraoperative transesophageal echocardiography for estimating the severity of functional mitral regurgitation. *Am J Cardiol* 1995; **76:**508-512.

42. Czer LS, Maurer G, Bolger AF, et al: Intraoperative evaluation of mitral regurgitation by Doppler color-flow mapping. *Circulation* 1987; **76:**III-108-III-116.

43. Fix J, Isada L, Cosgrove D, et al: Do patients with less than "echo-perfect" results from mitral valve repair by intraoperative echocardiography have a different outcome? *Circulation* 1993; **88:**39-48.

44. Lee KS, Stewart WJ, Lever HM, et al: Mechanism of outflow tract obstruction causing failed mitral valve repair. Anterior displacement of leaflet coaptation. *Circulation* 1993; **88:**24-29.

45. Tingleff J, Joyce FS, Pettersson G: Intraoperative echocardiographic study of air embolism during cardiac operations. *Ann Thorac Surg* 1995; **60:**673-677.

46. Orihashi K, Matsuura Y, Hamanaka Y, et al: Retained intracardiac air in open heart operations examined by transesophageal echocardiography. *Ann Thorac Surg* 1993; **55:**467-471.

47. Kusumoto FM, Muhiudeen IA, Kuecherer HF, et al: Response of the interatrial septum to transatrial pressure gradients and its potential for predicting pulmonary capillary wedge pressure: An intraoperative study using transesophageal echocardiography in patients during mechanical ventilation. *J Am Coll Cardiol* 1993; **21:**721-728.

48. Nagueh SF, Kopelen HA, Zoghbi WA: Relation of mean right atrial pressure to echocardiographic and Doppler parameters of right atrial and right ventricular function. *Circulation* 1996; **93:**1160-1169.

49. Kuecherer H, Muhiudeen IA, Kusumoto FM, et al: Estimation of mean left atrial pressure from transesophageal pulsed Doppler echocardiography of pulmonary venous flow. *Circulation* 1990; **82:**1127-1139.

50. Konstadt SN, Reich DL, Quintana C, et al: The ascending aorta: How much does transesophageal echocardiography see? *Anesth Analg* 1994; **78:**240-244.

51. Katz ES, Tunik PA, Rusinek H, et al: Protruding aortic atheromas predict stroke in elderly patients undergoing cardiopulmonary bypass: Experience with intraoperative transesophageal echocardiography. *J Am Coll Cardiol* 1992; **20:**70-77.

52. Hartman GS, Yao F-S, Bruefach M, et al: Severity of aortic atheromatous disease diagnosed by transesophageal echocardiography predicts stroke and other outcomes associated with coronary artery disease: A prospective study. *Anesth Analg* 1996; **83:** 701-708.

53. Applbe AF, Walker PG, Yeoh JK, et al: Clinical significance and origin of artifacts in transesophageal echocardiography of the thoracic aorta. *J Am Coll Cardiol* 1993; **21:**754-760.

54. Evangelista A, Garcia-del-Castillo H, Gonzalez T, et al: Diagnosis of ascending aortic dissection by transesophageal echocardiography: Utility of M-mode in recognizing artifacts. *J Am Coll Cardiol* 1996; **27:**102-107.

55. Muhiudeen IA, Cahalan MK, Silverman NH: Intraoperative transesophageal echocardiography in patients with congenital heart disease. In Greeley WJ (ed): *Perioperative Management of the Patient with Congenital Heart Disease.* Baltimore, Williams & Wilkins, 1996, pp 43-65.

56. Muhiudeen IA, Silverman NH, Anderson RH: Transesophageal transgastric echocardiography in infants and children: The subcostal view equivalent. *J Am Soc Echocardiogr* 1995; **8:**231-244.

57. Savino JS, Hanson CW, Bigelow DC, et al: Oropharyngeal injury after transesophageal echocardiography. *J Cardiothorac Vasc Anesth* 1994; **8:**76-78.

58. Dewhurst WE, Stragand JJ, Fleming BM: Mallory-Weiss tear complicating intraoperative transesophageal echocardiography in a patient undergoing aortic valve replacement. *Anesthesiology* 1991; **73:**77-778.

59. Spahn DR, Schmid S, Carrel T, et al: Hypopharynx perforation by a transesophageal echocardiography probe. *Anesthesiology* 1995; **82:**581-583.

60. Hogue CW, Lappas GD, Creswell LL, et al: Swallowing dysfunction after cardiac operations. Associated adverse outcomes and risk factors including intraoperative transesophageal echocardiography. *J Thorac Cardiovasc Surg* 1995; **110:**517-522.

61. Frommelt PC, Stuth EAE: Transesophageal echocardiography in totally anomalous pulmonary venous drainage: Hypotension caused by compression of the pulmonary venous confluence during probe passage. *J Am Soc Echocardiogr* 1995; **7:**652-654.

62. Lunn RJ, Oliver WC, Hagler DJ, et al: Aortic compression by transesophageal echocardiographic probe in infants and children undergoing cardiac surgery. *Anesthesiology* 1992; **77:**587-590.

63. Gilbert TB, Panico FG, McGill WA, et al: Bronchial obstruction by transesophageal echocardiography probe in a pediatric cardiac patient. *Anesth Analg* 1992; **74:**156-158.

64. Suriani RJ, Tzou N: Bradycardia during transesophageal echocardiographic probe manipulation. *J Cardiothorac Vasc Anesth* 1995; **9:**347.

65. Steckelberg JM, Khandheria BK, Anhalt JP, et al: Prospective evaluation of the risk of bacteremia associated with transesophageal echocardiography. *Circulation* 1991; **84:**177-180.

66. Daniel WG, Erbel R, Kasper W, et al: Safety of transesophageal echocardiography: A multicenter survey of 10,419 examinations. *Circulation* 1991; **83:**817-821.

67. Sellden H, Nilsson K, Larsson LE, Ekstrom-Jodal B: Radial artery catheters in children and neonates: A prospective study. *Crit Care Med* 1987; **15:**1106-1109.

68. Slogoff S, Keats AS, Arlund C: On the safety of radial artery cannulation. *Anesthesiology* 1983; **59:**42-47.

69. Marshall AG, Erwin DC, Wyse RKH, Hatch DJ: Percutaneous arterial cannulation in children. *Anesthesia* 1984; **39:**27-31.

70. Glenski JA, Beynen FM, Brady J: A prospective evaluation of femoral artery monitoring in pediatric patients. *Anesthesiology* 1987; **66:**227-229.

71. Ersoz CJ, Hedden M, Lain L: Prolonged femoral artery catheterization for intensive care. *Anesth Analg* 1973; **49:**160-164.

72. Metz S, Horrow JC, Balcar I: A controlled comparison of techniques for localizing the internal jugular vein using ultrasonography. *Anesth Analg* 1984; **63:**673-679.

73. Kaplan JA, Miller ED: Internal jugular vein catheterization. *Anesth Rev* 1976; May: 21-23.

74. Cote CJ, Jobes DR, Schwartz AJ, Ellison N: Two approaches to cannulation of a child's internal jugular vein. *Anesthesiology* 1979; **50:**371-373.

75. Mosteret JW, Kenny GM, Murphy GP: Safe placement of cardiovascular catheters into the internal jugular vein. *Arch Surg* 1970; **101:**431-432.

76. Jerigan WR, Gardner WC, Mahr MM: Use of the internal jugular vein for placement of central venous catheters. *Surg Gynecol Obstet* 1973; **130:**520-524.

77. Troianos CA, Kuwik RJ, Pasqual JR, et al: Internal jugular vein and carotid artery anatomic relation as determined by ultrasonography. *Anesthesiology* 1996; **85:**43-48.

78. Targ AG, Neumayr P, Cahalan MD, et al: Anatomic relationship of the right carotid artery and internal jugular vein in pediatric patients with congenital heart disease. *Anesthesiology* 1993; **79:**A1186.

79. Sulek CA, Gravenstein N, Blackshear RH, et al: Head rotation during internal jugular vein cannulation and the risk of carotid artery puncture. *Anesth Analg* 1996; **82:**125-128.

80. Mangar D, Turnage WS, Mohamed SA: Is the internal jugular vein cannulated during insertion or withdrawal of the needle during central vein cannulation. *Anesth Analg* 1993; **76:**1375.

81. Troianos CA, Jobes DR, Ellison N: Ultrasound-guided cannulation of the internal jugular vein: A prospective randomized study. *Anesth Analg* 1991; **72:**823-826.

82. Mallory DL, McGee WT, Shawker TH, et al: Ultrasound guidance improves the success rate of internal jugular vein cannulation. *Chest* 1990; **98:**157-60.

83. Denys BG, Uretsky BF, Reddy PS: Ultrasound-assisted cannulation of the internal jugular vein: A prospective comparison to the external landmark-guided technique. *Circulation* 1993; **87:**1557-1562.

84. Reeves ST, Roy RC, Dorman BH, et al: The incidence of complications after the double-catheter technique for cannulation of the right internal jugular vein in a university teaching hospital. *Anesth Analg* 1995; **81:**1073-1076.

85. Marini JJ: Pulmonary artery occlusion pressure: Clinical physiology, measurement, and interpretation. *Am Rev Respir Dis* 1983; **128:**319-326.

86. Benumof JL, Saidman LJ, Arkin DB, Diamant M: Where pulmonary artery catheters go: Intrathoracic distribution. *Anesthesiology* 1977; **48:**336-338.

87. Sharkey SW: Beyond the wedge: Clinical physiology and the Swan-Ganz catheter. *Am J Med* 1987; **83:**111-122.

88. Fuchs RM, Heuser RR, Yin FCP, Prinker JA: Limitations of pulmonary wedge V waves in diagnosing mitral regurgitation. *Am J Cardiol* 1982; **49:**849-854.

89. Moore RA, Neary MJ, Gallagher JD, Clark DL: Determination of the pulmonary capillary wedge position in patients with giant left atrial V waves. *J Cardiothorax Anesth* 1987; **1:**108-113.

90. Chapin JC, Downs JB, Douglas ME, et al: Lung expansion, airway pressure transmission, and positive end-expiratory pressure. *Arch Surg* 1979; **114:**1193-1197.

91. Yelderman ML, Ramsay MA, Quinn MD, et al: Continuous cardiac output measurements in intensive care unit patients. *J Cardiothorac Vasc Anesth* 1992; **6:**270-274.

92. Boldt J, Menges T, Wolbruck M, et al: Is continuous cardiac output measurement using thermodilution reliable in the critically ill patient? *Crit Care Med* 1994; **22:**1913-1918.

93. Yelderman M, Ramsay MA, Quinn MD, et al: Continuous cardiac output measurement in intensive care unit patients. *J Cardiothorac Vasc Anesth* 1992; **6:**270-274.

94. Seigel LC, Hennessy MM, Pearl RG: Delayed time response of the continuous cardiac output pulmonary artery catheter. *Anesth Analg* 1996; **83:**1173-1177.

95. Haller M, Zollner C, Forst H: Evaluation of a new continuous thermodilution cardiac output monitor in critically ill patients: A prospective criterion standard study. *Crit Care Med* 1995; **23:**860-866.

96. Levett JM, Replogle RL: Thermodilution cardiac output: A critical analysis and review of the literature. *J Surg Res* 1979; **27:**392-404.

97. Stevens JH, Raffin TA, Mihm FG, et al: Thermodilution cardiac output measurement. Effects of the respiratory cycle on its reproducibility. *JAMA* 1985; **253:**2240-2422.

98. Okamoto K, Komatsu T, Kumar V, et al: Effects of intermittent positive-pressure ventilation on cardiac output measurements by thermodilution. *Crit Care Med* 1986; **14:**977-980.

99. Jansen JRC, Versprille A: Improvement of cardiac output estimation by the thermodilution method during mechanical ventilation. *Intensive Care Med* 1986; **12:**71-79.

100. Pearl RG, Rosenthal MH, Nielson L, et al: Effect of injectate volume and temperature on thermodilution cardiac output determination. *Anesthesiology* 1986; **64:**798-801.

101. Hickey PR, Hansen DD, Cramolini GM, et al: Pulmonary and systemic hemodynamic responses to ketamine in infants with normal and elevated pulmonary vascular resistance. *Anesthesiology* 1985; **62:**287-293.

102. Colgan FJ, Stewart S: An assessment of cardiac output by thermodilution in infants and children following cardiac surgery. *Crit Care Med* 1977; **5:**220-225.

103. Freed MD, Keane JF: Cardiac output measured by thermodilution in infants and children. *J Pediatr* 1978; **92:**39-42.

104. Nishikawa T, Dohi S: Slowing of heart rate during cardiac output measurements by thermodilution. *Anesthesiology* 1982; **57:**538-539.

105. Harris AP, Miller CF, Beattie C, et al: The slowing of sinus rhythm during thermodilution cardiac output determination and the effect of altering injectate temperature. *Anesthesiology* 1985; **63:**540-541.

106. Todd MM: Atrial fibrillation induced by the right atrial injection of cold fluids during thermodilution cardiac output determination: A case report. *Anesthesiology* 1983; **59:**253-255.

107. Nishikawa T, Namiki A: Mechanism for slowing of heart rate and associated changes in pulmonary circulation elicited by cold injectate during thermodilution cardiac output determination in dogs. *Anesthesiology* 1988; **68:**221-225.

108. Morady F, Brundage BH, Gelberg HJ: Rapid method for determination of shunt ratio using thermodilution technique. *Am Heart J* 1983; **106:**369-373.

109. Wetzel RC, Latson TW: Major errors in thermodilution cardiac output measurement during rapid volume infusion. *Anesthesiology* 1985; **62:**684-687.

110. Bazarai MG, Petre J, Novoa R: Errors in thermodilution cardiac output measurements caused by rapid pulmonary artery temperature decreases after cardiopulmonary bypass. *Anesthesiology* 1992; **77:**31-37.

111. Latson TW, Whitten CW, O'Flaherty D: Ventilation, thermal noise, and errors in cardiac output measurements after cardiopulmonary bypass. *Anesthesiology* 1993; **79:**1233-1243.

112. Bottiger BW, Rauch H, Bohrer H, et al: Continuous versus intermittent cardiac output measurement in cardiac surgical patients undergoing hypothermic cardiopulmonary bypass. *J Cardiothorac Vasc Anesth* 1995; **9**:405-411.

113. Salmenpera M, Peltola K, Ronsenberg P: Does prophylactic lidocaine control cardiac arrhythmias associated with pulmonary artery catheterization? *Anesthesiology* 1982; **56**:210-212.

114. Shah KB, Rao TLK, Laughlin S, El-Etr AA: A review of pulmonary artery catheterization in 6,245 patients. *Anesthesiology* 1984; **61**:271-275.

115. Johnston WE, Royster RL, Vinten-Johansen J, et al: Influence of balloon inflation and deflation on location of pulmonary artery catheter tip. *Anesthesiology* 1987; **67**:110-115.

116. Leman R, Jones JG, Cowan G: A mechanism of pulmonary artery-perforation by Swan-Ganz catheters. *N Engl J Med* 1975; **292**:211-212.

117. Barash PG, Nardi D, Hammond G, et al: Catheter-induced pulmonary artery perforation. *J Thorac Cardiovasc Surg* 1981; **82**:5-12.

118. Keeler DK, Johnson WE, Vinten-Johansen J, et al: Pulmonary artery wedge pressure measurements during experimental pulmonary hypertension: Comparison of techniques in relation to catheter-induced hemorrhage. *J Cardiothorac Anesth* 1987; **1**:305-308.

119. Boscoe MJ, deLange S: Damage to the tricuspid valve with a Swan-Ganz catheter. *Br Med J* 1981; **283**:346-347.

120. O'Toole JD, Wurtzbacher JJ, Wearner NE, Jain AC: Pulmonary valve injury and insufficiency during pulmonary-artery catheterization. *N Engl J Med* 1979; **301**:1167-1168.

121. Rowley KM, Clubb S, Smith GJW, Cabin HS: Right-sided endocarditis as a consequence of flow-directed pulmonary-artery catheterization. *N Engl J Med* 1984; **311**:1152-1156.

122. Greeley WJ, Kates RA, Bushman GA, et al: Intraoperative esophageal electrocardiography for dysrhythmia analysis and therapy in pediatric cardiac surgical patients. *Anesthesiology* 1986; **65**:669-672.

123. Kates RA, Zaidan JR, Kaplan JA: Esophageal lead for intraoperative electrocardiographic monitoring. *Anesth Analg* 1982; **61**:781-785.

124. Trager MA, Feinberg BI, Kaplan JA: Right ventricular ischemia diagnosed by an esophageal electrocardiogram and right atrial pressure trace. *J Cardiothorac Anesth* 1987; **1**:123-125.

125. Blackburn H, Katigbak R: What electrocardiographic leads to take after exercise? *Am Heart J* 1964; **67**:184-185.

126. Kaplan JA, King SB: The precordial electrocardiographic lead (V5) in patients who have coronary artery disease. *Anesthesiology* 1976; **45**: 570-574.

127. Roy WL, Edelist G, Gilbert B: Myocardial ischemia during noncardiac surgical procedures in patients with coronary artery disease. *Anesthesiology* 1979; **51**:393-397.

128. Griffin RM, Kaplan JA: Comparison of ECG leads V5, CS5, CB5, and II by computerized ST segment analysis. *Anesth Analg* 1986; **65**:S65.

129. London MJ, Hollenberg M, Wong MG, et al: Intraoperative myocardial ischemia: Localization by continuous 12-lead electrocardiography. *Anesthesiology* 1988; **69**:232-241.

130. London MJ, Felipe E, Wong M, et al: Perioperative myocardial ischemia: Detection using continuous 12-lead microcomputer-augmented electrocardiography *Anesthesiology* 1986; **65**:A138.

131. Corait P, Daloz M, Bousseau D, et al: Prevention of intraoperative myocardial ischemia during noncardiac surgery with intravenous nitroglycerin. *Anesthesiology* 1984; **61**:193-196.

132. Ellis JE, Shah MN, Briller JE, et al: A comparison of methods for the detection of myocardial ischemia during noncardiac surgery: automated ST-segment analysis systems, electrocardiography, and transesophageal echocardiography. *Anesth Analg* 1992; **75**: 764-772.

133. Speiss BD: Thromboelastography and cardiopulmonary bypass. *Semin Thromb Hemost* 1995; **21**(suppl 4): 27-33.

134. Essell JH, Martin TJ, Salinas J, et al: Comparison of thromboelastography to bleeding time and standard coagulation tests in patients. *J Cardiothorac Vasc Anesth* 1993; **7**:410-415.

135. Wang JS, Lin CY, Hung WT, et al: Thromboelastogram fails to predict postoperative hemorrhage in cardiac patients. *Ann Thorac Surg* 1992; **53**:435-439.

136. Chandler WL: The thromboelastograph and the thromboelastograph technique. *Semin Thromb Hemost* 1995; **21**(suppl 4):1-6.

137. Tuman KJ, McCarthy RJ, Ivankovich AD: The thromboelastograph: Is it the solution to coagulation problems? *Cardiovasc Thorac Vasc Anesth* 1991; 1-13.

138. Tuman KJ, McCarthy RJ, Dijuric M, et al: Evaluation of coagulation during cardiopulmonary bypass with a heparinase-modified thromboelastographic assay. *J Cardiothorac Vasc Anesth* 1994; **8**:144-149.

4

Anesthesia for Myocardial Revascularization

James A. DiNardo

A firm understanding of the dynamics of coronary blood flow, the determinants of myocardial oxygen balance, and the consequences and treatment of ischemia are necessary to safely and efficiently provide anesthesia for patients undergoing coronary revascularization.

■ CONTROL OF CORONARY BLOOD FLOW

Coronary Perfusion Pressure

Coronary perfusion can only occur in the time intervals when aortic root pressure exceeds subepicardial and subendocardial pressure. Myocardial back pressure, which is the summation of factors that tend to collapse microvessels, has been determined to be important in determining coronary perfusion pressure (CPP).[1] For practical, clinical purposes, myocardial back pressure can be assumed to be equal to myocardial tissue pressure. The best estimate of myocardial tissue pressure is the ventricular intracavitary pressure. In diastole, this will be the ventricular end-diastolic pressure. The best clinical estimate of left ventricular end-diastolic pressure is the pulmonary capillary wedge pressure (PCWP), whereas the best estimate of right ventricular end-diastolic pressure is the central venous or right atrial pressure (RAP).

CPP will differ during systole and diastole. In the left ventricle, intracavitary pressure during systole is equal to or, in the case of aortic stenosis, greater than aortic root pressure. For this reason, most coronary blood flow to the left ventricle occurs during ventricular diastole. Aortic blood pressure gradually fails during diastole due to peripheral runoff, and thus, reference to mean aortic diastolic blood pressure (MADBP) is often made. In the absence of obstruction to flow within the coronary arterial system, left ventricular CPP = MADBP – PCWP (*see* Fig. 4-1). In the right ventricle, in which intracavitary systolic and diastolic pressures are both considerably less than aortic root pressure, coronary blood flow is more evenly distributed between systole and diastole.

Autoregulation

Changes in coronary vascular resistance are necessary if the myocardium is to be able to regulate coronary blood flow in response to changes in myocardial oxygen consumption. When myocardial oxygen consumption is constant, it is desirable for the myocardium to maintain coronary blood flow constant. The intrinsic ability of the myocardium to maintain coronary blood flow constant over a variety of perfusion pressures when myocardial oxygen consumption is constant is referred to as *coronary autoregulation.*[2] As illustrated in Figure 4-2, coronary autoregulation maintains coronary blood flow constant between perfusion pressures of 60 and 140 mm Hg. Below and above these pressures, myocardial blood

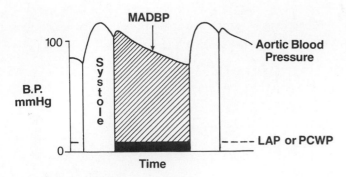

Figure 4–1. Left ventricular coronary perfusion pressure (CPP) is the difference between aortic diastolic blood pressure and left ventricular end-diastolic pressure (LVEDP). Clinically, LVEDP is estimated by left atrial pressure (LAP) or pulmonary capillary wedge pressure (PCWP). Diastolic CPP is represented by cross-hatched area and can be seen to decrease as diastole progresses. Average diastolic CPP can be obtained by taking difference between mean aortic diastolic blood pressure (MADBP) and LAP or PCWP. Length of time available for perfusion of left ventricle is dependent on length of diastole. Shortening diastole by increasing length of systole per beat or by increasing heart rate will decrease the time available for left ventricular perfusion.

flow is said to be pressure-dependent; that is, myocardial blood flow will vary linearly with pressure and with the time available for perfusion (diastole for the left ventricle, systole and diastole for the right ventricle).

Autoregulation is dependent on changes in coronary vascular resistance. The primary source of resistance in the coronary arterial system is the intramyocardial arterioles. Currently, the stimulus for changes in resistance is poorly understood. It seems that autoregulation is tied to myocardial oxygen metabolism and

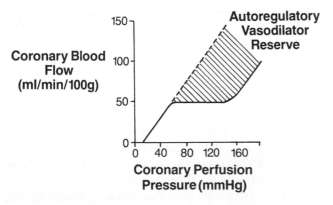

Figure 4–2. Coronary blood flow is seen to be constant (autoregulated) over coronary perfusion pressures from 60 to 140 mm Hg. When coronary perfusion pressure reaches 60 mm Hg, there will be maximal autoregulatory vasodilation to maintain coronary blood flow. Further decreases in coronary perfusion pressure will result in decreases in coronary blood flow. At pressures higher than 60 mm Hg, maximal autoregulatory vasodilation will provide autoregulatory vasodilator reserve. This reserve provides the increased coronary blood flow necessary to meet increases in myocardial oxygen consumption such as those induced by exercise.

coronary venous pO_2, although the exact mediators at the vascular level are unknown.[2] During exercise, reductions in coronary vascular resistance result in increased coronary blood flow (up to six times normal). Likewise, as CPP falls, coronary vascular resistance decreases so that coronary blood flow is maintained. At the lower pressure limits of autoregulated coronary blood flow, coronary vascular resistance is minimal. This is referred to as exhaustion of autoregulatory coronary vasodilator reserve. Because further reductions in coronary vascular resistance are impossible through the autoregulatory process, coronary blood flow decreases linearly with coronary perfusion pressure after the lower pressure limits of autoregulation are reached. The autoregulatory vasodilator reserve of the subendocardium seems to be exhausted before that of the subepicardium.[2]

Collateral Blood Flow

The development of collateral blood flow in humans is dependent on enlargement of preexisting anastomoses between coronary arteries. These anastomoses may be either serial (prestenosis to poststenosis from the same artery) or parallel (one artery to another). It is important to emphasize that these existing collateral pathways enlarge in response to pressure gradients. After the collateral pathways have enlarged, the direction and magnitude of collateral blood flow remain pressure-dependent. For this reason, collateral blood flow to a poststenotic segment can be drastically reduced if perfusion pressure at the origin of the collateral is reduced.

■ CAUSES OF INCREASED MYOCARDIAL OXYGEN DEMAND

Three factors are primarily responsible for determining myocardial oxygen consumption (MVo_2): wall tension, contractility, and heart rate.

Wall Tension

Myocardial wall tension (T) is determined by the relationship between intraventricular radius (r), intraventricular pressure (P), and ventricular wall thickness (h) according to Laplace's law: $T = Pr/h$. Ventricular wall tension is constantly changing during the cardiac cycle. For example, during isovolumic contraction, intraventricular pressure and wall thickness will be increasing while ventricular radius remains unchanged. During ventricular ejection, ventricular pressure will remain relatively constant while radius decreases and wall thickness increases. Inherent in the analysis of wall tension are the concepts of preload, afterload, and hypertrophy. Increases in end-diastolic volume (preload) will increase ventricular radius and will reduce wall thickness if dilation is severe. These changes will increase wall tension. Increases in the impedance to ventricular ejection (afterload) will necessarily increase intraventricular pressure and will also increase wall tension. Concentric ventricular hypertrophy will increase wall thickness and reduce wall tension.

There are important differences between the increase in MVO_2 induced by increases in preload and by those induced by increases in afterload. Work done in the isovolumic phase of ventricular contraction is very energy-consumptive. Increases in the impedance to ventricular ejection increase the pressure required to begin ventricular ejection and thus increase the work done in the isovolumic contraction phase. The ejection phase of ventricular contraction, on the other hand, is a more energy-efficient process. Increases in preload induce ejection of a larger stroke volume and an increase in the work done in the ejection phase. For these reasons, when equal quantities of work are compared, the increase in MVO_2 induced by an increase in preload (volume work) is much less than that induced by an increase in afterload (pressure work).[3]

Contractility

Contractility is defined as the state of myocardial performance independent of preload and afterload. Increasing the contractile state of the heart increases MVO_2. However, an increase in contractility may actually result in an MVO_2 that is reduced or unchanged under certain conditions. For example, if ventricular dilation (increased ventricular radius) exists to maintain cardiac output, wall tension and MVO_2 will be high. Improving contractility through use of an inotropic agent can reduce ventricular radius while maintaining cardiac output. The reduction in MUO_2 that accompanies the reduction in ventricular radius may more than offset the increase that accompanies an increase in contractility.

Heart Rate

It is important to review the manner in which increases in heart rate affect myocardial oxygen balance. Myocardial oxygen balance must be examined on a beat-to-beat basis. Myocardial ischemia is not induced with tachycardia simply because there are more beats per minute but because supply per beat is inadequate to meet demand per beat. Increases in heart rate increase MVO_2 per beat by increasing contractility via the Bowditch effect. Normally, an increase in heart rate is accompanied by a decrease in end-diastolic volume. This reduction in preload reduces wall tension and MVO_2 per beat. Thus, with tachycardia, the increase in MVO_2 per beat caused by enhanced contractility is in large part offset by the reduction in MVO_2 per beat that accompanies reduced wall tension. On the other hand, oxygen delivery may be compromised by tachycardia-induced reductions in the length of diastole per beat (discussed later).

■ CAUSES OF REDUCED MYOCARDIAL OXYGEN DELIVERY

Adequate myocardial oxygen supply is dependent on delivery of the appropriate volume of oxygenated coronary blood flow. The following sections describe factors that may compromise myocardial oxygen delivery.

Reduction in CPP

Left ventricular CPP can be reduced either by a reduction in MADBP or an increase in left ventricular end-diastolic pressure. A commonly overlooked cause of reduced CPP is bradycardia. Bradycardia encourages diastolic runoff from the proximal aorta and may result in a wide pulse pressure and reduced MADBP. Furthermore, maintenance of cardiac output with bradycardia requires an increased stroke volume. The increased stroke volume will be maintained primarily by an increase in left ventricular end-diastolic volume and pressure. This further reduces CPP.

Reduction in Time Available for Coronary Perfusion

Because the left ventricle receives most its perfusion during diastole, reductions in the time per beat spent in diastole are potentially detrimental. Figure 4–3 illustrates that, as heart rate increases, the length of time per beat spent in diastole is diminished while the length of systole remains more constant. Because MVO_2 per beat is minimally affected by tachycardia, the primary disadvantage of tachycardia is a reduction in diastolic perfusion time per beat.

Obstruction to Flow Within the Coronary Artery

Any obstruction to flow in a coronary artery results in a pressure drop across the obstruction. The high velocity of blood flow in the area of a stenosis or spasmotic segment necessarily results in the conversion of pressure energy to kinetic energy. On the distal side of the obstruction, turbulent eddies form and dissipate. The transfer of kinetic energy to this turbulent energy and the subsequent dissipation of the turbulence reduces the quantity of kinetic energy available for conversion to pressure energy.[4] This results in a pressure drop across the obstruction. The pressure drop will increase in direct proportion to any increase in flow across the obstruction as a greater proportion of kinetic energy is dissipated as turbulence. For this reason, requirements for

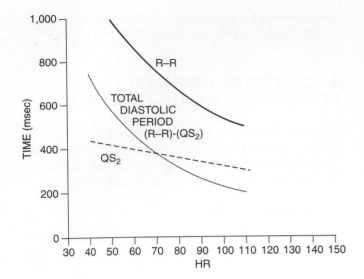

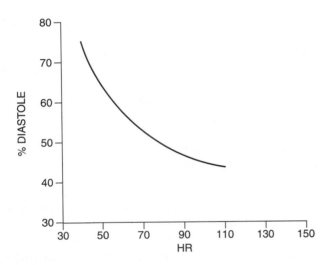

Figure 4–3. Top. Increases in heart rate cause decreases in length of each cardiac cycle (R-R interval). Decreases in length of systole (QS₂) with increases in heart rate are far less dramatic than decreases in length of diastole (R-R − QS₂). **Bottom.** Percent of each cardiac cycle (R-R interval) spent in diastole at various heart rates. Small changes in heart rate are seen to cause large decreases in percent of time spent in diastole. *(From: Boudoulas H: Changes in diastolic time with various pharmacologic agents.* Circulation *1979;* **60***:165. Reprinted by permission.)*

increased coronary blood flow such as those that accompany exercise will increase the hemodynamic significance of any obstructive lesion.

Arteriolar dilatation distal to the obstruction will help compensate for this pressure loss until the stenosis becomes critical. A stenosis is said to be critical when the autoregulatory vasodilator reserve distal to it is nearly exhausted to maintain coronary blood flow at rest. Some vasodilatory reserve is needed to maintain basal coronary blood flow with stenoses as small as 30 to 45%, and this reserve is exhausted with stenoses greater than 90%.[5] When reserve is exhausted and the

pressure distal to the stenosis falls below 55 to 60 mm Hg, coronary blood flow will fall linearly with further decreases in perfusion pressure and the subendocardium will be at risk for developing ischemia. It follows that in the presence of an obstructive coronary lesion, proximal coronary artery pressure (MADBP) will have to be greater than 60 mm Hg to ensure a distal pressure higher than 60 mm Hg.

The factors described in the following sections deserve attention.[6]

Atherosclerotic Disease. Early atheromatous lesions are believed to be the result of chronic minimal vascular injury to the arterial endothelium. Lesions are classified as:[6]

- Type I — these involve functional endothelial cell changes with no morphologic damage.
- Type II — these involve endothelial denudation and intimal damage.
- Type III — these involve endothelial denudation with damage to both the intima and media.

The fate of these early atheromatous lesions is dependent on three factors:[6]

- Plaque disruption — type III lesions are lipid rich, soft, and prone to disruption from mechanical forces. Plaque rupture may result in exposure of superficial vascular wall elements or of deep fibrillar collagen.
- Thrombosis — exposure of vascular wall elements is a stimulus for thrombus formation. Platelet deposition occurs at the site of disruption. Superficial plaque disruption is a much milder thrombogenic stimulus than deep plaque disruption. Thrombus formation at the site of a superficial injury is likely to be labile and transient, whereas thrombus formation associated with deep plaque disruption is likely to be stable and permanent.
- Vasoconstriction — transient vasoconstriction accompanies plaque disruption and thrombus formation. Injury to the endothelium produces thrombin-mediated vasoconstriction, whereas subsequent platelet deposition mediates vasoconstriction via release of thromboxane A₂ and serotonin. In addition, endothelial injury may impair the release of nitric oxide (NO) containing endothelium-derived relaxation factor (EDRF).

The spectrum of coronary artery disease from chronic stable angina to acute myocardial infarction can be explained using these concepts.[6] Chronic stable stenotic lesions that cause angina develop as the result of progression of atherosclerotic lesions. Progression of early lesions is more rapid in patients with coronary risk factors. Progression is the result of mural thrombus formation and fibrotic organization, which follows minor plaque disruption in type III lesions. Initially, platelet thrombi form on the disruption. This is followed by migration of smooth muscle cells from the media into the intima. During the final phase, intimal thickening and progression of the lesion occur. Repetition of this process leads to gradual progression of the lesion. Ultimately, it may lead to a chronic fibrotic vessel occlusion. The slow progression of the lesion allows time and provides stimulus for distal collaterization. This explains why thrombotic occlusion is frequent in patients with high-grade stenoses but does not lead to infarction.

In unstable angina, a small plaque disruption may change plaque morphology such that coronary blood flow is reduced and angina intensifies. Alternatively, plaque disruption may be associated with labile thrombus, temporary vessel occlusion, and angina at rest. Coronary blood flow is further compromised by release of vasoconstrictor substances and impaired endothelial relaxation.

In non-Q-wave myocardial infarction (MI), the process is similar to that in unstable angina, except that the duration of vessel occlusion by labile thrombus is longer. Spontaneous thrombolysis or resolution of arterial spasm ultimately limits occlusion and prevents Q-wave MI. This process is responsible for 75% of non-Q-wave MIs. The other 25% are caused by complete occlusion of the infarct-related vessel with distal collateralization.

In Q-wave MI, plaque disruption is associated with formation of a fixed, persistent thrombus. This leads to cessation of blood flow and myocardial necrosis. The coronary lesion involved usually is mild to moderate in severity with limited distal collateralization. Thus, it is the intensity of plaque disruption and subsequent thrombus formation rather than the severity of the lesion that is the determining factor.

Some further discussion is necessary to explain the spectrum of anginal symptoms that can accompany a chronic, stable stenotic coronary lesion. The main coronary artery epicardial branches have lumens that are 2 to 4 mm in diameter. In the absence of collaterals, exertional angina occurs when lumen area is reduced to 1.0 mm^2 (50–60% reduction in lumen diameter or 75% reduction in cross-sectional area) and angina at rest occurs when lumen area is reduced to 0.65 mm^2 (75% reduction in lumen diameter or 90% in cross-sectional area).

Figure 4–4 illustrates how changes in coronary vascular tone can alter the clinical characteristics of a chronic stable stenotic lesion. Atheromatous lesions may be localized to one area of the arterial wall. As these eccentrically located lesions enlarge, they encroach upon the arterial lumen. Because the remainder of the arterial wall is free of plaque, it remains responsive to vasoactive stimuli and is capable of contraction. Such contraction will cause the fixed atheromatous lesion to occupy a greater portion of the arterial lumen and will result in a larger pressure drop across the lesion. Therefore, the severity of the stenosis is not static but is dynamic and dependent on the vasomotor activity of the free arterial wall. This phenomenon is known as dynamic coronary stenosis.[4,7] As illustrated in Figure 4–4, a normal change

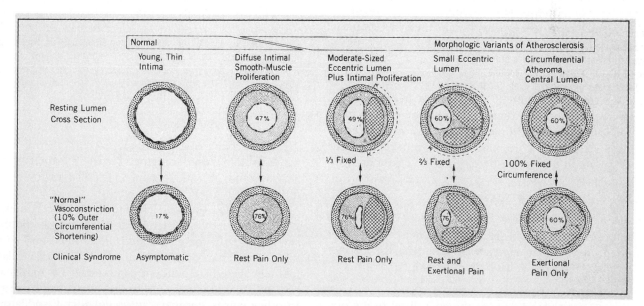

Figure 4–4. Cross sections of normal and diseased coronary arteries. Morphologic state of arteries is illustrated. Percent reduction in lumen diameter for each morphologic state at rest and following normal degree of vasoconstriction is also shown. Clinical syndromes associated with both resting and vasoconstricted state of normal and diseased arteries are summarized at bottom of diagram. *(From: Brown BG: Dynamic mechanisms in human coronary stenosis. Circulation 1985:* **70:***921. Reprinted by permission.)*

in coronary vasomotor tone resulting in a 10% circumferential shortening of the outer arterial wall can convert a nonsignificant 49% eccentric stenosis to a 76% stenosis, which will result in rest ischemia. Likewise, Figure 4–4 illustrates that a normal increase in arterial tone can convert an eccentric stenosis, which causes ischemia on exertion (60% stenosis), to one that also causes ischemia at rest (76% stenosis).

Atheromatous lesions may be static if the atheromatous changes involve the entire circumference of the arterial wall. In this instance, the lumen area is fixed and is unaltered by changes in arterial vasomotor activity. Figure 4–4 illustrates that a lesion that occupies the entire circumference of the arterial wall and causes exertional ischemia (60% stenosis) will be unaffected by changes in arterial vasoconstriction.

Variations in Coronary Vasomotor Tone.

There is large variation in the extent of coronary vasomotor activity manifest by patients. At one end of the spectrum is the normal 10% reduction in outer arterial wall circumference that occurs with alpha-adrenergic stimulation such as that induced by isometric hand grip, hand emersion in ice water, or emotional upset.[4,7] At the other end of the spectrum is the intense vasoconstriction or spasm that occurs with variant or Prinzmetal's angina. Spasm is defined as inappropriate active vasoconstriction of a segment of coronary artery resulting in total or subtotal occlusion in response to stimuli that cause only minimal constriction in individuals who do not have variant angina.[8] For patients with physiologic coronary vasoconstriction, myocardial ischemia will occur only if coronary stenoses also exist. For patients with coronary spasm, myocardial ischemia may develop in the absence of coronary stenoses.

Coronary Steal

Recently, the phenomenon of coronary steal has received a great deal of attention. It must be emphasized that for patients with coronary artery disease to develop coronary steal, their coronary anatomy must meet certain criteria and they must be exposed to a potent arteriolar dilator. Two types of coronary steal exist,[9] described in the following two sections.

Collateral Dependent to Collateral Independent.

For this type of steal (also known as *pressure dependent to pressure independent*) to exist, the following anatomical criteria must be met (*see* Fig. 4–5):[9,10]

- An occluded coronary artery.
- Collateral blood flow to the area distal to the occlusion.
- A hemodynamically significant stenosis of the vessel supplying the collaterals.

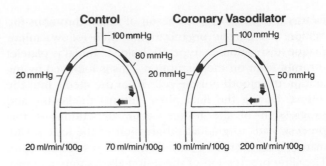

Figure 4–5. Schematic representation of coronary anatomy present in patients at risk for coronary-vasodilator-induced coronary steal. **Control.** In control state, myocardium distal to completely obstructed vessel is supplied via collaterals from partially stenosed vessel. In this collateral-dependent myocardium, autoregulatory vasodilation is maximal and perfusion to this zone is pressure-dependent. Pressure gradient for perfusion of this area is 60 mm Hg (80–20 mm Hg) and flow is 20 mL/min/100 g in direction of arrows. Myocardium distal to partially stenosed vessel retains coronary vasodilator reserve. Flow to this area is 70 mL/min/100 g, and this flow is distributed evenly between subepicardium and subendocardium. **Coronary vasodilator.** Myocardium distal to partially stenosed vessel retains autoregulatory vasodilator reserve, whereas myocardium distal to the completely obstructed vessel does not. In the presence of coronary arteriolar dilator, blood flow to area distal to partial stenosis increases. Increased flow across the stenosis results in larger pressure drop across stenosis than that seen in control state. Because autoregulatory vasodilator reserve is exhausted in collateral-dependent myocardium, perfusion to this area remains pressure-dependent. Pressure gradient for perfusion of this area is 30 mm Hg (50–20 mm Hg) and flow decreases to 10 mL/min/100 g with resulting ischemia. Flow to myocardium distal to partially stenosed vessel increases to 200 mL/min/100 g, but there is greater distribution of flow to subepicardium (300 mL/min/100 g) at the expense of subendocardium (100 mL/min/100 g). Distal to coronary stenosis subendocardial coronary autoregulatory vasodilation may be nearly maximal while subepicardium will retain autoregulatory vasodilator reserve. Exposure to coronary vasodilator will enhance flow to the subendocardium only slightly while subepicardial flow will be greatly enhanced. In the setting in which subendocardial autoregulatory vasodilator reserve is exhausted and perfusion is pressure-dependent, exposure to a coronary vasodilator may enhance subepicardial flow at expense of subendocardial ischemia. *(Used by permission of the American Journal of Cardiology. From: Gross GJ, Warltier DC: Coronary Steal in four models of single or multiple vessel obstruction in dogs. Am J Cardiol 1981; **48**:84–92.)*

It has been demonstrated that 23% of the 16,249 patient angiograms contained in the Coronary Artery Surgery Study (CASS) registry met these anatomical criteria.[11]

After these anatomical criteria have been met, the administration of an agent that is an arteriolar dilator, such as dipyridamole or adenosine, is necessary to produce a steal. Autoregulation-induced arteriolar dilation in the collateral-dependent region will be maximal at rest to maintain blood flow to this compromised region. In other words, coronary autoregulatory vasodilator reserve will be exhausted in this region and perfusion will be pressure-dependent. Exposure to an arteriolar dilator will have little additional effect on collateral-dependent arteriolar tone but will dilate arterioles in the collateral-independent region. This will cause an increase in flow across the stenosis and a reduction in the perfusion pressure distal to the stenosis. The result will be a reduction in flow to the pressure-dependent collateralized region. Blood will be shunted from this collaterized region to the region supplied by the stenosed vessel that provides the collaterals (see Fig. 4–5). Ischemia in the collateral-dependent region may then develop.

Subendocardial to Subepicardial (Transmural). For this type of steal to exist, only a severe stenosis in a coronary artery and exposure to an arteriolar dilator such as dipyridamole or adenosine is required.[9] Autoregulation-induced arteriolar dilatation in the subendocardium distal to a stenosis will be maximal at rest to maintain subendocardial blood flow. When this occurs, subendocardial perfusion will be pressure-dependent. Exposure to an arteriolar dilator will have little additional effect on subendocardial arteriolar tone but will dilate arterioles in the subepicardium. This will cause an increase in flow across the stenosis and a reduction in the perfusion pressure distal to the stenosis. The result will be a shunting of blood away from the subendocardium toward the subepicardium with resultant subendocardial ischemia (see Fig. 4–5).

Controversy exists regarding whether isoflurane is a potent enough coronary arteriolar dilator to cause coronary steal in humans when administered in the presence of the appropriate coronary anatomy. Evidence derived from animal and human studies is currently available.

Animal Studies. Isoflurane (1.2 to 1.8%) has been demonstrated to reduce coronary vascular resistance in the nonstenotic coronary arteries of canines.[12] This isoflurane-induced reduction in coronary vascular resistance has been shown to occur at the level of the intramyocardial arterioles.[13] In swine, to the contrary, isoflurane caused less blunting of the maximal coronary vasodilation induced by occlusive hyperemia than did halothane. This has been interpreted as evidence that isoflurane is not a potent coronary vasodilator.[14]

Isoflurane can induce a steal from the collateral-dependent region to the collateral-independent region under the appropriate conditions. In a canine model in which coronary blood flow was artificially held constant below the autoregulated control level, isoflurane (0.94%) reduced CPP from 80 to 55 mm Hg, and induced a collateral-dependent to collateral-independent steal with resultant ischemia in the collateral-dependent zone.[15] In this model, isoflurane was found to decrease coronary vascular resistance and alter coronary blood flow distribution in a manner similar to the potent coronary arteriolar dilator adenosine.[15] In a similar canine model in which CPP was held constant and coronary

blood flow was not controlled, isoflurane and halothane (0.5 and 1.5 MAC) both slightly decreased coronary vascular resistance but neither induced a collateral-dependent to collateral-independent steal.[16] Both models used radiolabeled microspheres to quantitate myocardial blood flow distribution.

In a canine model, isoflurane-induced hypotension to a mean aortic pressure (MAP) of 55 mm Hg caused regional myocardial dysfunction suggestive of ischemia in the distribution of a single severe left anterior descending artery stenosis.[17] A subsequent study in the same model demonstrated that isoflurane-associated-hypotension (MAP = 55 mm Hg) was more likely to induce regional myocardial dysfunction than comparable degrees of halothane-associated hypotension.[18] Because these studies did not quantitate subepicardial and subendocardial blood flow, it is not possible to prove that isoflurane induced myocardial dysfunction by inducing a transmural steal in the distribution of the stenosis.

With the use of radiolabeled microspheres, isoflurane has been demonstrated to induce a transmural steal in the distribution of a single coronary stenosis in a canine model.[19,20] Isoflurane induction of this transmural steal caused ischemic dysfunction in the distribution of the stenosis, which resolved after restoration of blood pressure to baseline levels with phenylephrine.[19] In the same canine model, isoflurane was found to decrease myocardial oxygen consumption and to induce a transmural steal in the distribution of a single coronary stenosis.[20] When MAP was maintained at 80 mm Hg, ischemic dysfunction did not develop in the distribution of the transmural steal. This led the authors to conclude that maintenance of perfusion pressure allowed blood flow to remain at or above the reduced energy needs of the myocardium despite induction of a transmural steal.

Human Studies. No direct evidence that isoflurane is a coronary arteriolar dilator capable of inducing coronary steal has yet been demonstrated in humans. However, indirect evidence is available. Despite large reductions in myocardial oxygen consumption and a relative increase in coronary blood flow, there was electrocardiogram (ECG) and metabolic evidence (lactate production) of myocardial ischemia in 10 of 21 patients with coronary artery disease anesthetized with 1% isoflurane as the primary anesthetic agent.[21] Three of five patients continued to exhibit ECG and metabolic evidence of ischemia despite normalization of CPP and heart rate in this same study.[21] Induction of anesthesia with isoflurane (0.67 to 3.8%) for coronary revascularization resulted in lactate production in three of ten patients despite large reductions in myocardial oxygen consumption and a relative increase in coronary blood flow.[22] Under isoflurane anesthesia (1.2%), 10 patients with left anterior descending coronary artery stenoses were seen to develop reductions in regional coronary blood flow while global coronary blood flow increased.[23] Four of these patients went on to exhibit metabolic and ECG evidence of ischemia. In contrast, patients with coronary artery disease anesthetized with halothane or enflurane as the primary agents demonstrate large decreases in myocardial oxygen demand coupled with "appropriate" decreases in coronary blood flow without ECG or metabolic evidence of ischemia.[23,24]

These studies have been interpreted by some as evidence that isoflurane is a coronary arteriolar dilator that initiates a steal of blood flow from susceptible regions of myocardium despite a relative increase in coronary blood flow. Others point to the fact that in these studies, isoflurane anesthesia (in contrast to halothane and enflurane anesthesia) has been consistently associated with reductions in mean arterial pressure and increases in heart rate. This combination can potentially reduce coronary blood flow by reducing both the time and pressure available for myocardial perfusion. It is therefore not surprising that criticism of these studies has focused on the role of these hemodynamic changes in the production of myocardial ischemia independent of a steal phenomenon.

To the contrary, low-dose isoflurane (0.5%) has been demonstrated to improve tolerance to pacing-induced ischemia in adults with coronary artery disease.[25] Likewise, studies of patients with coronary artery disease in which isoflurane is used to supplement narcotic anesthesia intraoperatively have been favorable. Isoflurane (1.5 to 2.0%) has been used successfully to control intraoperative hypertension in patients undergoing coronary revascularization under flunitrazepam/fentanyl anesthesia.[26] In a more comprehensive analysis, no increases in either regional or global coronary blood flow or lactate production were seen when isoflurane (0.75 to 1.0%) was used to control intraoperative hypertension during coronary artery bypass surgery under sufentanil anesthesia.[27]

Transesophageal echocardiographic (TEE) detection of regional systolic wall motion abnormalities is four times more sensitive than ECG changes as an indicator of myocardial ischemia.[28] TEE and ECG analysis revealed no difference in the incidence of myocardial ischemia between patients receiving sufentanil or isoflurane anesthesia for coronary revascularization when hemodynamics were carefully controlled.[29] This remained true when the study was repeated in a subset of patients with documented steal-prone coronary antatomy.[30] Sevoflurane and desflurane have not been implicated in causing coronary steal.[31,32]

Anemia

Myocardial oxygen delivery is the product of coronary blood flow and the oxygen content of the transported blood. Anemia may reduce myocardial oxygen delivery by reducing the oxygen-carrying capacity of blood. The degree of anemia that an area of myocardium can tolerate without developing ischemia will be determined by the relationship between regional MV_{O_2} and regional coronary blood flow. In the absence of coronary stenoses, hematocrit levels lower than 15% result in subendocardial ischemia in anesthetized canines.[33] In the presence of the increased MV_{O_2} that accompanies large increases in afterload, hematocrit levels lower than 30% produce subendocardial ischemia in the same canine model.[33] The presence of coronary stenoses and the awake state will further reduce the ability of the subendocardium to tolerate anemia.

Hematocrit levels must be individualized for each patient, but it should be kept in mind that low hematocrit levels (lower than 30%) are potentially dangerous for awake patients with coronary artery disease for the following reasons:

- Increased cardiac output necessarily accompanies normovolumic anemia to maintain systemic oxygen transport; this cardiac output increases results in an increased MV_{O_2}.
- Increases in coronary blood flow to maintain coronary oxygen delivery result in increased pressure drops across stenoses and potential for subendocardial hypoperfusion.

■ MYOCARDIAL ISCHEMIA

Regional or global imbalances in myocardial oxygen supply and demand result in the production of myocardial ischemia. The metabolic consequences of ischemia are discussed in detail in Chapter 12. The clinical manifestations of myocardial ischemia are varied. Angina pectoris with or without signs of ventricular failure or dysrhythmias is assumed to be the classic manifestation of myocardial ischemia. However, more recent evidence demonstrates that angina is not a universal manifestation of ischemia. In fact, myocardial ischemia may present as ventricular failure or dysrhythmias without angina or may remain clinically silent.[8] Furthermore, it also must be emphasized that patients have varying thresholds for the development of ischemia during the course of a day.[34] The dynamic nature of coronary stenoses accounts for the changes in the caliber of a stenosis that may produce rest pain at one time and angina with varying degrees of exercise at other times.

Despite these varied clinical presentations, the progression of hemodynamic and electrocardiographic changes with ischemia tends to follow a consistent pattern in a given patient. Myocardial ischemia is heralded by a decrease in regional ventricular diastolic distensibility (see Chapter 2), which usually results in an elevation in left ventricular end-diastolic pressure (PCWP) or right ventricular end-diastolic pressure (EDP) (central venous pressure [CVP]). This is followed by systolic dysfunction, ECG changes, and finally by angina during symptomatic episodes.[35] Patients manifesting elevations in PCWP with symptomatic episodes are likely to do so with asymptomatic episodes as well.[36] Some patients will not manifest wedge pressure changes with either symptomatic or asymptomatic episodes.[35,36]

Symptomatic Versus Asymptomatic Myocardial Ischemia

Ambulatory holter monitoring of patients with chronic stable angina has demonstrated that 83% of ischemic episodes with ST segment depression of 1 to 2 mm are asymptomatic, whereas 63% of ischemic episodes with ST segment depression of 3 mm or more are asymptomatic.[37] Other studies report similar incidences for asymptomatic ischemia in ambulatory patients.[38,39] Recently, patients have been studied in the preoperative period. Of the ischemic ECG changes seen in elective coronary artery bypass surgery patients monitored for 48 hours in the preoperative period, 87% were asymptomatic.[40] The reasons why some episodes of ischemia are symptomatic while others are not remain unclear. There is some suggestion that asymptomatic episodes are of shorter duration and lesser severity than symptomatic episodes, but this is not consistently true.[8,36] There is also evidence to suggest that patients with asymptomatic episodes have a higher pain tolerance, but this is not uniformly true.[41]

Incidence of Perioperative Ischemia

Preoperative Ischemia. Efforts to prevent myocardial ischemia have historically been directed toward careful control of the readily obtainable hemodynamic determinants of myocardial oxygen demand such as heart rate and blood pressure. Recent evidence demonstrates that most ischemic episodes that occur during daily activities are not preceded by increases in heart rate[36,42,43] or rate-pressure product (the product of heart rate and systolic blood pressure) and are clinically silent.[44] Similar observations have been made in cardiac surgical patients in the preoperative period.[40] Of 50 patients monitored with holter monitors for 48 hours before coronary artery bypass surgery, 21 demonstrated ECG evidence of ischemia despite maximal medical therapy. Only 23% of these ischemic episodes were preceded by a heart rate increase of 20% or more (mean arterial pressure was not measured).

Most of these episodes were clinically silent. A recent investigation confirmed these findings and indicated that the subset of patients with steal-prone anatomy had longer and more frequent episodes.[45] Other studies have examined the incidence of myocardial ischemia upon arrival in the operating room in patients undergoing coronary revascularization. The incidence varies from 0.3 to 27%; a large proportion of the episodes are hemodynamically unrelated.[46-49]

Intraoperative Ischemia. As with preoperative ischemic events, a large percentage of intraoperative ischemic events are not preceded by changes in heart rate and blood pressure. In a study of 1023 patients undergoing coronary revascularization, intraoperative hemodynamic abnormalities were common, occurring in 83% of patients.[47] Some 282 patients (28%) developed intraoperative ischemia; however, 51% of the intraoperative ischemic events were not temporally related to a hemodynamic abnormality. A hemodynamic abnormality was defined as any or all of the following: heart rate higher than 100 beats per minute, systolic blood pressure lower than 90 mm Hg, or systolic blood pressure higher than 180 mm Hg. This study has been criticized because the criteria for heart rate increase may have been too stringent for patients with low baseline heart rates, thereby underestimating the true incidence of significant hemodynamic abnormalities.[50]

This criticism was addressed in a subsequent study of 495 coronary revascularization patients.[48] Defining tachycardia as an increase in heart rate of 10 beats per minute, hypotension as a 20% decrease in systolic pressure, and hypertension as a 20% increase in systolic pressure, the authors found that 43% of patients suffered an intraoperative ischemic event. Of these ischemic episodes, 70 to 80% occurred while heart rate and blood pressure were in the patients' in-hospital resting range.

More recent studies have confirmed that most intraoperative ischemic events are unrelated to hemodynamic perturbations, suggesting that decreases in myocardial oxygen supply may be important in the genesis of intraoperative ischemia.[40,50-52]

In summary, although the reported incidence of intraoperative myocardial ischemia during coronary revascularization is variable, it is clear that a large proportion (50% or greater) of these episodes occur without readily measurable changes in myocardial oxygen consumption. This supports the conclusion that the ischemia seen during coronary revascularization consists of a background of hemodynamically unrelated, silent ischemia, upon which is superimposed episodes of hemodynamically related ischemia.[49] Others have suggested that rigorous intraoperative hemodynamic control will not worsen the preoperative ischemic pattern and may actually improve it.[53] Future efforts to reduce the incidence of ischemic episodes will likely be directed toward ameliorating reductions in myocardial blood flow due to dynamic alterations in the caliber of coronary stenoses or to alterations in platelet function and plaque morphology.

Outcome After Myocardial Ischemia

Obviously the most feared of consequences of pre- and intraoperative ischemia is postoperative myocardial infarction (PMI). In a landmark study, it was demonstrated that the risk of PMI was 6.9% in coronary revascularization patients who had preoperative ischemia, intraoperative ischemia, or both, and 2.5% in patients who did not have ischemia.[47] The risk of PMI also was correlated with the severity of ischemia. Those patients who had ST segment depressions greater than 2 mV had a 9.3% incidence of PMI, whereas those who had ST segment depressions between 1.0 and 1.9 mV had a 6.2% incidence. All of these observations were confirmed in a later study by the same authors.[48] Other investigators have reported an association between intraoperative ischemia and PMI.[40]

Factors well beyond the control of the anesthesiologist also are responsible for increasing the incidence of PMI.[47] An aortic cross-clamp time in excess of 40 minutes increased the incidence of PMI from 2.6 to 10.9%. PMI occurred in 14.3% of patients in whom the distal anastomoses were rated by the surgeon as poor as compared with 3.4% of patients in whom the anastomoses were considered of good quality. Again, these findings were confirmed in a later study.[48]

Recent investigations have focused on the significance of postoperative myocardial ischemia in patients undergoing coronary revascularization. The highest incidence of both TEE- and ECG-detected ischemia is in the postcardiopulmonary bypass (post-CPB) and immediate postoperative periods.[54-56]

Both post-CPB ECG- and TEE-detected ischemia have been correlated with adverse clinical outcomes (MI, congestive heart failure, death). This topic is discussed in detail later in this chapter.

Diagnosing Myocardial Ischemia

ECG Changes.   The gold standard for diagnosis of myocardial ischemia is the presence of ECG changes. As previously discussed, ECG changes occur relatively late in the temporal sequence of myocardial ischemia after deterioration of ventricular diastolic and systolic function. For ECG monitoring to be effective in detecting ischemia, the appropriate leads must be monitored. Simultaneous monitoring of leads II and V_5 is commonly used because of the high sensitivity of this combination in detecting myocardial ischemia (*see* Chapter 3). Monitoring of leads II and V_5 will not detect true posterior ischemia, and for this reason, use of an esophageal ECG

lead has been suggested[57,58] to monitor right ventricular and posterior left ventricular ischemia (*see* Chapter 3).

PCWP Traces.   The PCWP trace of the pulmonary artery catheter has been described as a tool to make early diagnosis of left ventricular (LV) ischemia.[59] Similar observations have been made regarding the CVP trace and RV ischemia.[60] Reduction in LV distensibility occurs in the early stages of LV ischemia because of diastolic dysfunction (*see* Chapter 2). In particular, LVEDP is elevated. Under these circumstances, left arterial pressure (LAP) will be elevated to maintain LV diastolic filling. Movement of the left atrium (LA) to a steeper portion of its pressure–volume relationship will result in magnification of the normal LAP waveforms. In addition, dilation of the LA may result in a more forceful atrial contraction and production of an enlarged A wave. The peak of this A wave will reflect LVEDP. LV ischemia, which produces LV dilation or papillary muscle dysfunction, may cause mitral regurgitation with generation of a prominent V wave.

The PCWP trace is a reflection of LAP. However, because the PCWP waveform is transmitted through the compliant pulmonary venous system, it is a damped version of the LAP. In particular, the LA A wave may be poorly seen. As a result, it has been demonstrated that mean PCWP reflects mean LV diastolic pressure and may underestimate LVEDP by 10 to 15 mm Hg during ischemia.[61]

Changes in PCWP and the PCWP waveform have poor sensitivity and specificity in detecting episodes of myocardial ischemia.[52,62-64] This is true for a number of reasons:

- PCWP does not necessarily reflect LVEDP as previously described.
- When only a small region of LV wall develops diminished distensibility with an ischemic episode, the distensibility of the LV as a whole changes only slightly and subsequent changes in LVEDP as reflected by the PCWP are difficult to detect.
- The quantitative change in PCWP and the qualitative change in the PCWP waveform necessary to define an ischemic event have not been systematically defined.[64]
- Acute elevations in afterload in the absence of ischemia can produce elevations in PCWP.[64]

Because PCWP trace changes are not seen in all episodes of myocardial ischemia, they cannot be relied upon as the sole indicator of ischemia. For this reason, it is important to emphasize that suspicious ECG or TEE changes cannot be ignored simply because there is no change in the PCWP or the PCWP waveform.

Transesophageal Echocardiography (TEE).
Regional wall motion abnormalities (RWMA) during sys-

tole (diminished inward excursion and thickening) are known to occur as a result of ischemia, and these wall motion and thickening abnormalities are known to precede ECG changes. The development of severe hypokineses, akinesis, or dyskinesis (*see* Chapter 3) is more specific for ischemia than mild hypokinesis.[65] Changes in wall thickening are more sensitive for detecting ischemia than changes in wall excursion.[66] In the instance of complete coronary occlusion, wall motion abnormalities and ECG changes occur within 60 seconds of each other.[67] For cases in which ischemia is less severe, RWMA may precede ECG changes by several minutes.[68] In fact, numerous studies have shown intraoperative TEE qualitative analysis of regional wall excursion and thickening to be a more sensitive detector of myocardial ischemia than ECG changes and to be capable of detecting ischemia before ECG changes.[68]

Recent data demonstrate a lack of concordance between ischemia detected by ECG and that detected by TEE.[65,69] There are both TEE-detected ischemic episodes not detected by EGC and ECG-detected ischemic episodes not detected by TEE. This may be due to several factors:

- Normally, the TEE probe is placed at the mid left ventricular level (level of the papillary muscles), at which wall segments in the distribution of all three coronary arteries can be monitored.[68] Because a short-axis view of the left ventricle can only be obtained at one level at a time, ischemic changes occurring in the basal or apical ventricular levels will be missed. Biplane and multiplane probes allow visualization of the apex and base of the heart. Recent evidence demonstrates better concordance between ECG and TEE detected ischemia when biplane TEE is used and RWMA are detected in both the short-axis and long-axis views.[70]
- Ischemic episodes may be missed because qualitative wall motion analysis is difficult for patients with preexisting wall motion abnormalities. Likewise, all RWMAs (particularly in areas tethered to scar) may not be ischemic in origin. Changes in afterload may unmask areas of previous scarring. Ventricular pacing or a bundle-branch block may make detection of RWMA more difficult because of asynchronous contraction. Stunned myocardium may exhibit continued RWMA despite adequate perfusion.
- The ECG may detect ischemia with small areas of subendocardial ischemia undetectable by TEE.

These observations, combined with the fact that no evidence exists to support the contention that early detection and treatment of ischemia alters outcome, temper enthusiasm for TEE as the ideal ischemia monitor.

Predicting Myocardial Ischemia

The ability to predict hemodynamic alterations that are likely to result in myocardial ischemia in individual patients would allow prompt treatment and avoidance of events initiating ischemia. Unfortunately, the diverse nature of myocardial oxygen imbalance in patients leaves the anesthesiologist with no predictor of myocardial ischemia that is reliable in all circumstances. The indices described in the next sections all have limited usefulness.

Rate-Pressure Product (RPP) and Triple Index (TI).   The RPP is the product of heart rate and systolic blood pressure, whereas the TI is the product of heart rate, systolic blood pressure, and PCWP. The RPP has been shown to provide a useful assessment of MV_{O_2} and to predict ischemia in patients undergoing stress testing. Most patients experience the onset of ischemia at an RPP of 20,000. However, its usefulness in assessing MV_{O_2} and predicting ischemia in anesthetized patients is not reliable. For patients anesthetized with halothane, RPP does not provide a good assessment of MV_{O_2} because halothane-induced reductions in MV_{O_2} are not reflected in the RPP.[71] Of greater importance is the fact that RPP is a poor predictor of myocardial ischemia in anesthetized patients. Episodes of hypertension and tachycardia leading to ischemia will be predicted by an RPP greater than 12,000 in patients with coronary artery disease.[72] However, under anesthesia, it is possible for a patient to have a combination of hemodynamic parameters (tachycardia and hypotension) particularly deleterious to myocardial oxygen delivery that will not result in an elevated RPP. It has been demonstrated in animals that RPP does not correlate with the onset of myocardial ischemia when a wide variety of heart rates and systolic blood pressures are examined.[73] Similarly, RPP was not a useful predictor of myocardial ischemia in patients undergoing coronary revascularization with halothane anesthesia, because tachycardia and hypotension were the hemodynamic alterations most often associated with intraoperative ischemia.[74]

The TI is subject to the same criticisms as the RPP. The addition of PCWP to the product adds the variable of wall radius to the assessment of MV_{O_2}. However, the TI still fails to account for large reductions in myocardial oxygen delivery in the genesis of ischemia.

Myocardial Supply–Demand Ratio (DPTI: SPTI).   Efforts to account for beat-to-beat variations in both myocardial supply and demand in the genesis of ischemia led to development of the supply–demand ratio. Supply is defined as the diastolic pressure time index (DPTI). DPTI = (mean diastolic pressure − left ventricular end-diastolic pressure) × duration of diastole. Demand is defined as the systolic pressure time index (SPTI). SPTI = mean arterial pressure × duration of systole. Ratios below 0.5 have been found to result in development of subendocardial ischemia.[75] Unfortunately, use of this ratio is unreliable for several reasons:[75]

- Increases in MV_{O_2} due to increased contractility are not reflected in blood pressure and heart rate changes and therefore are not accounted for by SPTI.
- A higher ratio will be needed in the presence of anemia to compensate for the reduced oxygen-carrying capacity of blood.
- The presence of pressure drops across coronary stenoses makes the DPTI an unreliable index of distal coronary perfusion.
- Changes in coronary vascular resistance make DPTI an unreliable index of distal coronary perfusion.
- Use of the ratio is cumbersome because it requires calculation of the areas under the diastolic and systolic pressure curves, respectively.

Mean Arterial Blood Pressure–Heart Rate Quotient. Recent animal work demonstrates that ischemia occurs in the distribution of a critical coronary stenosis[76] and in collateral-dependent myocardium[77] when the pressure rate quotient (PRQ), defined as MAP/HR, is less than 1. This relationship seems to be valid over a wide range of pressures and heart rates. An increase in heart rate can cause or worsen ischemic dysfunction at any mean arterial blood pressure; however, the absolute heart rate at which ischemia occurs is dependent on the preexisting mean arterial pressure. In other words, higher heart rates are tolerated without ischemia at higher mean arterial pressures. For patients undergoing coronary revascularization, PRQ < 1.0 has poor sensitivity and specificity in predicting myocardial ischemia as detected by both ECG and TEE.[51,52,78,79]

In summary:

- The combination of hypertension and tachycardia may result in myocardial ischemia by increasing myocardial oxygen demand.
- The combination of hypotension and tachycardia is particularly detrimental to myocardial oxygen balance because it reduces both the time and the pressure gradient available for myocardial perfusion.
- Tachycardia, in and of itself, is detrimental to myocardial oxygen balance. Experimentally, tachycardia causes or worsens ischemic dysfunction at any given mean arterial blood pressure.[76] Clinically, tachycardia is associated with the development of ischemia in patients undergoing coronary revascularization whereas hypertension per se is not a risk factor.[48-50] In particular, heart rates greater than 110 beats per minute are asso-

ciated with a dramatically increased incidence of intraoperative ischemia in patients undergoing coronary revascularization.[49]

Treatment of Ischemia

Because the genesis of myocardial ischemia is multifactorial, treatment must be aimed at the specific causes at work in each instance.

Tachycardia. No single value of heart rate is uniformly detrimental to myocardial oxygen balance in a given patient. As already discussed, the heart rate at which ischemia is likely to occur will vary with mean arterial blood pressure and the other determinants of myocardial oxygen balance. When an increase in heart rate results in ischemia or is likely to result in ischemia, immediate therapy is necessary.

Immediate steps should be taken to eliminate inadequate anesthetic depth as a cause. Efforts to ensure that preload is adequate also must be taken. This is particularly important for patients with diminished ventricular distensibility, for when a higher-than-normal end-diastolic pressure will be necessary to ensure an adequate ventricular end-diastolic volume. When these measures fail, treatment with a beta blocker may be necessary in patients with and without preoperative beta-blocker therapy. Many patients taking beta blockers preoperatively will have plasma concentrations that are too low to blunt the hemodynamic responses to surgery and will require supplemental beta blockage.[80] Propranolol in incremental doses of 0.5 to 1.0 mg to a total of 0.1 mg/kg may be used for patients without severe ventricular systolic dysfunction. For patients with a history of bronchospasm or reactive airway disease, a beta-1-selective agent such as metoprolol is useful. Incremental doses of 2.5 to 5.0 mg to a total of 0.5 mg/kg can be used. Because elevations in PCWP will reduce CPP, concomitant therapy with nitroglycerin 0.5 to 1.0 μg/kg/min is indicated in the presence of an elevated PCWP.

In some instances, the ultra-short-acting beta blocker esmolol may be useful. Esmolol has an elimination half-life of 9 minutes due to metabolism by red-cell esterases and is relatively beta-1-selective.[81] Esmolol is started with a bolus of 0.5 mg/kg given over several minutes followed by an infusion of 50 μg/kg/min and titrated up to 300 μg/kg/min as necessary. Esmolol is useful for patients with poor ventricular function or bronchospastic disease, because if it is not tolerated, therapy can be quickly terminated. Furthermore, unlike longer-acting beta blockers, esmolol can be used aggressively in the pre-CPB period without fear that it will compromise termination of CPB.[82]

Hypotension. The extent of hypotension that can be tolerated before ischemia develops is dependent on several variables. For example, a reduction in arterial blood pressure may reduce MVo_2 by reducing afterload but may, at the same time, reduce proximal perfusion pressure and drastically reduce myocardial blood flow distal to a stenosis. Furthermore, as discussed previously, at higher heart rates, lesser degrees of hypotension will be tolerated. The source of hypotension must be quickly and accurately determined. Determination of cardiac output and systemic vascular resistance (SVR) will help direct therapy.

When hypotension is due to a reduction in cardiac output, heart rate and preload should be optimized. If these measures fail to correct the fall in cardiac output, any inhalational anesthetic agents should be discontinued to eliminate their negative inotropic properties. A fall in SVR can be treated with an alpha-adrenergic agonist such as phenylephrine in incremental doses of 40 to 100 µg. It should be kept in mind that alpha-adrenergic agonists may constrict coronary arteries with dynamic stenoses and should therefore be titrated carefully. Because elevations in PCWP will reduce CPP, concomitant therapy with nitroglycerin 0.5 to 1.0 µg/kg/min is indicated in the presence of an elevated PCWP.

Hypertension. Hypertension is classically associated with tachycardia in the genesis of myocardial ischemia. Treatment, in this instance, is directed toward deepening of anesthesia. If hypertension is persistent despite adequate anesthetic depth, vasodilator therapy is warranted. Sodium nitroprusside is a readily titratable, potent arteriolar dilator and can be used effectively to treat hypertension. An infusion can be started at 0.25 µg/kg/min and titrated upward. However, because sodium nitroprusside is a potent arteriolar dilator, it has the potential to induce a coronary steal in the presence of the appropriate anatomy[83] (coronary steal was discussed earlier in the chapter).

Nitroglycerin dilates large coronary vessels and not arterioles and therefore is not implicated in the steal phenomenon. Nitroglycerin has its greatest dilating effect on the venous beds and arterial dilatation occurs only at higher doses. Despite this, when used in appropriate doses nitroglycerin and nitroprusside have been shown to be equally effective in treatment of hypertension associated with coronary artery bypass surgery.[84,85] Both agents have comparable effects on heart rate, cardiac output, and PCWP.[84,85] With comparable reductions in systolic blood pressure, nitroglycerin causes less reduction in diastolic blood pressure than does nitroprusside.[85] Therefore, CPP may be better preserved with nitroglycerin than with nitroprusside. For these reasons, nitroglycerin may be the preferred agent for treatment of hypertension associated with myocardial ischemia. For treatment of hypertension, nitroglycerin is started at

0.5 µg/kg/min and may have to be increased up to 20 µg/kg/min.

Dynamic Stenoses. Evidence of myocardial ischemia may occur with little or no initial change in heart rate or blood pressure. In these instances, acute reductions in coronary blood flow may occur due to vasoconstriction in the area of a coronary stenosis or due to true coronary spasm in an area free of a stenosis. The mainstays of therapy are nitroglycerin and calcium channel blockers to reduce coronary vasomotor tone.[86] Nitroglycerin can be started at 0.5 µg/kg/min and titrated upward. When an elevated PCWP accompanies one of these episodes nitroglycerin is effective in reducing PCWP through both venodilation and treatment of the underlying ischemia. Nipedipine is a calcium channel blocker and systemic vasodilator that can be administered sublingually in a 10-mg dose to reduce coronary vasomotor tone. Intravenous verapamil 7.5 mg also has been used to terminate an episode of intraoperative coronary vasospasm.[87]

Care must be taken to avoid systemic hypotension with administration of these agents. CPP is improved when the pressure drop across the stenosis diminishes with vasodilation in the area of the stenosis and when venodilation reduces PCWP. However, extreme diastolic hypotension will offset any potential improvement of CPP. For this reason, phenylephrine augmentation of diastolic blood pressure may be necessary to preserve CPP.[88]

■ ANESTHETIC MANAGEMENT

Goals

1. Avoid increases in myocardial oxygen consumption; hypertension and tachycardia leading to ischemia will be heralded by a rising RPP.
2. Avoid tachycardia; it compromises oxygen delivery at any mean arterial pressure.
3. Appreciate that the patient's baseline ischemic pattern will continue into the preoperative and intraoperative periods; these episodes must be treated when recognized.

Preoperative Cardiac Assessment

Preoperative evaluation is discussed in detail in Chapter 1. Careful review of the cardiac catheterization data is also an essential part of the preoperative visit. The important features of the catheterization report are reviewed here and discussed in detail in Chapter 2.

Diastolic Function. To varying degrees, patients with coronary artery disease will manifest diminished ventricular distensibility. This will require that an elevated LVEDP be maintained to provide adequate LV end-diastolic volume (EDV). The measurement of LVEDP at the time of cardiac catheterization will provide some index of the degree of diastolic impairment. In addition to diminished distensibility, patients with long-standing systemic hypertension may have concentric hypertrophy and diminished ventricular compliance. Patients functioning on the steep portion of their diastolic pressure–volume curve will be dependent on a well-timed atrial systole (the A wave in the atrial pressure trace) to adequately fill the ventricle at end diastole.

For patients undergoing repeat coronary revascularization procedures ("redos"), elevated right heart pressures increase the risk of inadvertent right atriotomies and ventriculotomies during sternotomy.[89] Similarly, if the pericardium was left open after the original surgical procedure, the anterior surface of the right ventricle is more likely to be adherent to the sternum. The hemorrhage induced by these traumatic atriotomies, and ventriculotomies can be life threatening. A femoral vein and artery usually are exposed before sternotomy in redo patients so that partial bypass (*see* Chapter 10) can be initiated emergently if hemorrhage occurs with sternotomy. Partial bypass provides the circulatory support and the decompression of the right heart that may be necessary for surgical repair.

Systolic Function.   Ejection fraction (EF) and assessment of wall motion are the most commonly obtained assessments of systolic function. Because EF is an ejection-phase index, it is dependent on loading conditions. For this reason, the presence of a low-impedance outflow tract, such as that which exists via the mitral valve in mitral insufficiency, will cause the EF to overestimate systolic function. EF is an assessment of global systolic function and will not be depressed until a relatively large portion of ventricle exhibits compromised systolic function. An EF lower than 40% is believed to represent poor systolic function. Wall motion abnormalities are analyzed during ventriculography. When large areas of akinesis and dyskinesis exist, systolic function will be severely compromised.

Right ventricular EF and wall motion analysis generally are not obtained at the time of catheterization. For patients with suspected right ventricular systolic dysfunction, either first-pass or equilibrium noninvasive radionuclear imaging can be used to determine EF.

Coronary Anatomy and Coronary Lesions. The extent of coronary disease and the presence or absence of collateral flow to jeopardized areas should be assessed. This will allow intelligent assessment of the areas most at risk for developing ischemia. Knowledge of these areas will allow monitoring such as ECG and TEE to be directed appropriately.

The coronary angiograms also will provide insight into the likelihood that a given area can be revascular-

ized successfully. Distal disease in small vessels makes the technical success of the operative procedure less likely. Furthermore, bypassing a vessel supplying a dyskinetic or aneurysmal area of ventricle may yield little in terms of improved systolic function postoperatively because such areas have little salvageable myocardium.

The term "left main equivalent" is commonly used and deserves clarification. A high-grade left main coronary artery lesion potentially jeopardizes most of the LV muscle mass. Likewise, high-grade stenoses of both the left anterior descending (LAD) and circumflex arteries jeopardize the same territory. As a result, this combination of lesions is considered a left main equivalent. The difference is that with the true left main lesion, only one vessel (the left main) must become completely occluded to compromise LV blood flow. In the case of the LAD and circumflex lesions, both vessels would have to be occluded to produce the same effect. Another high-risk combination of lesions occurs when myocardium distal to an occluded vessel is supplied by collaterals from a vessel with a high-grade stenosis. An example would be myocardial distal to an occluded LAD supplied by collaterals from a right coronary artery (RCA) with a high-grade proximal stenosis. In this setting, complete occlusion of the remaining vessel (RCA) compromises most of the LV.

For patients undergoing redo procedures, evaluation of the extracardiac conduits (internal mammary arteries and reverse saphenous veins) should be made as well. A determination of how much myocardium is supplied by the conduits that are patent should be made. Nicking or cutting of these conduits during the difficult dissection that often accompanies redos may severely compromise myocardial perfusion. Likewise, surgical manipulation of these conduits may result in embolization of atherosclerotic plaques into the distal coronary vascular bed with subsequent transmural myocardial ischemia.[90,91]

Premedication

Ample time should be taken during the preoperative period to reassure patients and address their concerns. Patients with preserved ventricular function are premedicated with morphine 0.10 to 0.15 mg/kg IM, scopolamine 0.005 mg/kg IM, and diazepam 0.15 mg/kg or lorazepam 0.04 mg/kg PO approximately 1.5 hours before scheduled induction time. Alternatively, morphine 0.10 to 0.15 mg/kg IM and midazolam 0.03 to 0.05 mg/kg IM may be used. The dysphoric effects of scopolamine may be troublesome for elderly patients. For elderly patients or patients with poor ventricular function, the doses can be reduced and supplemental premedication can be given in the operating room holding area under direct observation. Supplemental O_2 with a face mask is started at the time of premedication. Ranitidine 150 mg PO or a similar H_2 blocker is given at the time of premedication and the evening before surgery.

All cardiac medications are continued on schedule until the time of surgery and are taken with sips of water. Preoperative beta-blocker therapy has been shown to blunt the hemodynamic responses to surgical stimulation during coronary revascularization[80] and to reduce the incidence of heart-rate-related intraoperative ischemic events.[49,80,92] Continuation of preoperative beta-blockade therapy does not compromise myocardial performance during the post-CPB period.[93,94] Furthermore, abrupt withdrawal of beta-blockade therapy has been associated with myocardial ischemia, hypertension, and tachydysrhythmias secondary to a beta-blockade-induced increase in beta-receptor density.[95]

Continuation of preoperative nifedipine therapy does not exacerbate the decreases in blood pressure seen with fentanyl–pancuronium and fentanyl–diazepam pancuronium inductions in patients undergoing coronary revascularization.[96] Likewise, continuation of preoperative diltiazem therapy in combination with fentanyl–pancuronium anesthesia is not associated with a reduced SVR or a requirement for additional vasopressor or inotropic support in the pre- or post-CPB period.[97] To the contrary, withdrawal of calcium channel blockers may be associated with an increased need for vasodilator therapy in the post-CPB period.[98] Patients treated with diltiazem and nifedipine preoperatively do demonstrate a diminished but intact response to phenylephrine.[99] Thus, treatment of intraoperative hypotension may require higher-than-usual doses of phenylephrine for patients continued on preoperative calcium channel blockers.[99] The incidence of perioperative ischemia during coronary revascularization is greater in patients receiving just calcium channel blockers (nifedipine, diltiazem, or verapamil) preoperatively than in patients receiving beta blockers or a combination of calcium channel and beta blockers.[49,92] This is probably due to better attenuation of tachycardia-induced ischemia in patients receiving beta blockers.

Preinduction

After arrival in the operating room, all patients should be attached to an ECG system capable of monitoring leads I, II, III, aVR, aVL, AVF, and V_5. Baseline recording of all seven leads should be obtained for comparative purposes. Normally, two leads (II and V_5) are monitored simultaneously intraoperatively. However, if the areas of myocardium at risk are better assessed in other leads, then it is those leads that should be monitored.

All patients should have radial arterial catheters and two large-bore (14-gauge) peripheral IVs placed with local anesthesia. Alternatively, if peripheral IV access is poor, a peripheral IV suitable for induction can be started and a large-bore double-lumen (16- or 14-gauge) central venous line can be placed at the same time as the pulmonary artery catheter (see Chapter 3). For patients who are to have an internal mammary artery (IMA) harvested, the arterial waveform obtained in the ipsilateral radial or brachial artery may be compromised during IMA dissection.[100] This occurs when the patient's arm is tucked at the side and is compressed between the body and the Favarloro retractor used for IMA dissection. This results in compression of the brachial artery against the humerus and is particularly common in large patients. The arterial line may be placed in the contralateral arm or the ipsilateral arm can be abducted to avoid this problem. Needless to say, when the arm is to be tucked at the side, care should be taken to provide ample padding between the arm and the retractor.

The use of pulmonary artery catheters for all patients undergoing coronary revascularization is controversial.[101,102] Pulmonary artery catheters allow measurement of thermodilution cardiac outputs; pulmonary artery, right atrial, and pulmonary capillary wedge pressures; systemic and pulmonary vascular resistances; and left and right ventricular stroke work. In addition, as discussed previously, analysis of the PCWP and RAP traces may be helpful in the early diagnosis of ischemia. Critics of pulmonary artery catheters point out that for patients with good left ventricular function (EF higher than 40% with minimal wall motion abnormalities), RAP provides as good an assessment of left ventricular end-diastolic volume as PCWP. In addition, they point out that early diagnosis of ischemia by the use of a pulmonary artery catheter has never been shown to improve patient outcome. Furthermore, evidence suggests that outcome in both low- and high-risk patients undergoing coronary revascularization is not influenced by use of a pulmonary artery catheter in place of a CVP catheter.[103]

Nonetheless, the following are commonly considered indications for use of a pulmonary artery catheter:

- LV diastolic dysfunction; this will make the correlation between LVEDV and RAP less accurate than that between PCWP and LVEDV.
- LV systolic dysfunction; this can be defined in a number of ways: EF less than 40%, large areas of hypokinesis, more limited areas of akinesis and dyskinesis, presence of a ventricular aneurysm, or recent myocardial infarction. Management of these patients may be simplified by the ability to determine and manipulate cardiac output, preload, and systemic vascular resistance.
- Unstable angina, left main coronary disease, or severe three-vessel coronary disease; with a very large area of myocardium at risk, careful control

of the factors involved in initiating an ischemic process is imperative.

- Associated valvular lesions; this includes mitral regurgitation secondary to papillary muscle dysfunction or ventricular dysfunction.
- Pulmonary hypertension; determination and manipulation of pulmonary vascular resistance will be useful for these patients.
- Right ventricular diastolic and systolic dysfunction.
- Emergency cases such as revascularization after failed percutaneous coronary transluminal angioplasty (PCTA) or in association with a postinfarct ventricular septal defect.

If a pulmonary artery catheter is to be placed, certain precautions should be taken. All of the equipment and medications for treatment of dysrhythymias should be on hand before placement of the catheter is attempted. In particular, a defibrillator with demonstrated consistent synchronization to the patient's ECG signal must be in the room in case cardioversion is necessary.

There is concern that the placement of intravascular catheters before induction of anesthesia may predispose patients to the risk of stress-induced myocardial ischemia. It has been demonstrated that in well-premedicated, beta-blocked patients, catheter placement can be accomplished without hemodynamic abnormalities or myocardial ischemia.[104] It should be kept in mind that the preoperative myocardial ischemic pattern of a patient tends to continue into the preinduction and intraoperative period.[40]

The information obtained at cardiac catheterization about LV diastolic function and LV end-diastolic pressure should be used in conjunction with the PCWP to optimize LV preload. Patients with reduced distensibility may require a PCWP in the range of 12 to 15 mm Hg to ensure an adequate preload (LVEDV). When preload is inadequate, stroke volume and cardiac output will be reduced and systemic blood pressure and CPP will be maintained by increases in SVR. Subsequent reductions in SVR (as with induction) may lead to hypotension and potentially to tachycardia. In this setting, any advantage of a low PCWP in terms of CPP will be offset by systemic hypotension.

For patients with poor systolic function, preload reserve will be limited or exhausted to meet baseline cardiac output demands (*see* Chapter 2). Any increase in afterload will produce afterload mismatch and result in progressive reductions in stroke volume and cardiac output. Because poor systolic function associated with ischemic heart disease is accompanied by reduced diastolic distensibility, maintenance of an adequate preload will require a PCWP in the range of 12 to 18 mm Hg.

All episodes of ischemia in the preinduction period should be treated aggressively. Therapy as described previously will have to be directed toward the specific causes at hand. Because such a high proportion of ischemic episodes are likely to be asymptomatic and to occur in the absence of hemodynamic changes, the ECG, RAP, and PCWP traces must be monitored with vigilance. The use of prophylactic IV nitroglycerin in the preinduction period has not been investigated, but prophylactic administration of IV nitroglycerin at doses of 0.5 mg/kg/min[105] and 1.0 mg/kg/min[106] have not been shown to be effective in reducing the incidence of myocardial ischemia during the induction and maintenance of anesthesia for coronary revascularization.

Induction and Maintenance

A variety of anesthetic techniques using both intravenous and inhalational agents have been shown to result in comparable outcomes after coronary revascularization surgery.[107-110] Two types of techniques will be discussed here: a traditional high dose narcotic technique and a "fast-track" technique geared toward shorter postoperative ventilation and earlier discharge from the intensive care unit (ICU).

High-dose Narcotic Technique. Fentanyl and sufentanil generally provide the stable hemodynamics essential in preventing imbalance in myocardial oxygen supply and demand. These agents have no effect on myocardial contractility and cause a reduction in peripheral vascular resistance only through a diminution in central sympathetic tone.[111-114] Generally, 50 to 75 µg/kg of fentanyl or 10 to 15 µg/kg of sufentanyl can be used as the primary anesthetic for induction and maintenance before cardiopulmonary bypass. A benzodiazapine should be included as a part of the premedication or should be administered intraoperatively to avoid awareness.

It has been suggested that, for patients undergoing coronary revascularization, sufentanil causes greater decreases in arterial blood pressure and SVR on induction than does fentanyl,[115,116] and that sufentanil is more effective than fentanyl in blunting the hypertensive responses to skin incision, sternotomy, sternal spread, and aortic manipulation.[115] Other clinical comparisons of fentanyl and sufentanil for coronary revascularization have not clearly demonstrated these differences.[111,114] Variability in the preload and beta-blockade status of patients in the different studies may account for these apparent discrepancies. Optimization of preload before induction may blunt the induction-induced decreases in arterial pressure seen with sufentanil.[114-116] The need for vasodilator therapy to treat hypertensive responses is reduced by the presence of preoperative and intraoperative beta blockade, regardless of which narcotic is used.[80,81,115] Finally, the use of sufentanil has been shown to result in more rapid induction and earlier emergence and extubation in coronary artery surgery patients than fentanyl.[117]

The choice of muscle relaxant influences the hemodynamic stability of a high-dose narcotic anesthetic. Pancuronium has a vagolytic effect as well as the capacity to enhance sympathetic outflow by blockade of sympathetic postganglionic muscarinic receptors, inhibition of catecholamine reuptake, and stimulation of release of catecholamine from nerve terminals.[118] Vecuronium and cis-atracurium are devoid of these effects. Induction with fentanyl–pancuronium has been shown to result in a high incidence of tachycardia-induced ischemia on induction[119,120] and to provide stable induction hemodynamics without ischemia.[111,112,122] Induction with fentanyl–vecuronium or sufentanil–vecuronium has been shown to result in bradycardia and hypotension[122] and to provide stable induction hemodynamics.[123] Induction with sufentanil–pancuronium has been shown to result in tachycardia[122,124] that may progress to ischemia[121] and to provide stable induction hemodynamics.[125]

These discrepancies seem to be due to differences in the preoperative extent of beta and calcium channel blockade as well as in the type of premedication. For patients who are clinically well beta blocked, sufentanil–pancuronium or fentanyl–pancuronium provides stable induction hemodynamics, whereas for poorly beta-blocked patients, sufentanil–vecuronium or fentanyl–vecuronium provides similar hemodynamic stability.[126-128] Severe bradycardia has been seen in patients who are clinically well beta blocked and who subsequently receive vecuronium in combination with high-dose fentanyl[120] or sufentanil.[129] Calcium channel blockade alone does not seem to protect against pancuronium-induced tachycardia,[124] and the use of vagolytic agents such as scopolamine as part of the premedication augments the vagolytic actions of pancuronium.[125-127]

The extent of beta blockade can be assessed clinically before surgery by noting the patient's baseline pulse rate and response to daily activity. Further assessment can be made in the operating room by observation of the patient's pulse rate during movement from stretcher to operating table and during placement of peripheral lines. Combinations containing pancuronium are best avoided in patients not receiving beta blockade and in patients on beta blockers who have a baseline heart rate higher than 70 or who are capable of increasing their heart rates by 15 to 20 beats per minute with mild exertion.

After several minutes of preoxygenation and with the patient breathing 100% oxygen, induction begins with an infusion of fentanyl 550 µg/min or sufentanil 100 µg/min over 5 to 10 minutes. A system of graded stimulation is used to individualize the narcotic dose for each patient. After loss of consciousness, the hemodynamic response to insertion of an oral airway, followed by insertion of a urinary catheter, is used to gauge the need for additional narcotic to blunt the hemodynamic response to tracheal intubation. Laryngoscopy is performed carefully and should not be prolonged. If an upward trend in heart rate or blood pressure is noted as laryngoscopy commences, laryngoscopy should be terminated and additional narcotic should be titrated. If there is poor visualization of the trachea, laryngoscopy should be terminated and intubating conditions should be improved by changing head position, using a stylet, or changing blades. This approach will help prevent long, stimulating laryngoscopies that compromise hemodynamics. A TEE probe (see Chapter 3) is placed after tracheal intubation and verification of tube position.

Vecuronium or pancuronium 0.02 mg/kg or cis-atracurium 0.04 mg/kg is administered approximately 1 to 2 minutes before starting the narcotic infusion. As the patient loses consciousness, the remainder of the total dose of 0.1 mg/kg of vecuronium or pancuronium or 0.2 mg/kg of cis-atracurium is administered and controlled ventilation with 100% O_2 is initiated. This regime minimizes the risk of narcotic-induced rigidity without undue stress to the patient.

Bradycardia with hemodynamic compromise must be treated promptly. A small dose of pancuronium (1 to 3 mg) is often effective if vecuronium or cis-atracurium has been used. Atropine should be used cautiously. Atropine administration may initiate tachycardia and atropine, unlike beta-1-adrenergic agents, increases heart rate without any reduction in the duration of systole. Thus, for equal increases in heart rate, atropine will cause a greater reduction in the duration of diastole and will compromise subendocardial perfusion to a greater degree than a beta-1-adrenergic agent. Ephedrine (a direct- and indirect-acting beta and alpha agonist), 5 mg, is a reliable agent to increase heart rate without compromising diastole. In addition, the augmentation in diastolic blood pressure obtained is beneficial when hypotension accompanies bradycardia.

Tachycardia must be treated aggressively to avoid subendocardial ischemia and hemodynamic compromise. The first strategy should be to terminate any noxious stimuli and increase the depth of anesthesia when necessary. Failing this, a short- or long-acting beta blocker may be used, as described previously.

Should hypotension due to reduced SVR occur during the narcotic infusion, the infusion should be stopped. Small doses of phenylephrine (40 to 120 µg) and volume infusion to increase preload to preinduction levels usually will correct the problem. A dose of phenylephrine very reliably causes an increase in SVR with a concomitant increase in wall stress and a reduction in ejection phase indices of contractility in CABG patients.[130] The peak effect of a phenylephrine dose occurs 30 to 40 seconds after injection.[131]

If surgical stimulation (skin incision, sternotomy, sternal spreading, and aortic manipulation) produces hypertension, additional doses of sufentanil (1 to 5 μg/kg) or fentanyl (5 to 25 μg/kg) may be necessary. Recent data calls this practice into question. Once a patient has received high doses of sufentanil (10 to 30 μg/kg) or fentanyl (50 to 100 μg/kg) administration of addition agent as an infusion or a bolus will not reliably blunt the hemodynamic response to noxious stimuli.[132] If this fails to control the hypertension, the use of additional agents will be necessary. As discussed previously, treatment of hypertension with vasodilator therapy must take into account the effect of these agents on regional myocardial blood flow and on their ability to improve concomitant ischemia. It may also become necessary to administer supplemental narcotic anesthesia with additional anesthetic agents:

1. Benzodiazepines. Diazepam, midazolam, and lorazepam administered in conjunction with fentanyl or sufentanil have been implicated in causing decreases in peripheral vascular resistance with subsequent hypotension.[133-135] Therefore, they must be titrated with caution. Midazolam in increments of 1 to 2 mg or lorazepam in increments of 0.5 to 1 mg are reasonable.

2. Inhalational anesthetics. N_2O in association with high-dose opiates causes systolic dysfunction in patients with coronary artery disease, particularly those with an LVEDP greater than 15 mm Hg.[136,137] An animal model of coronary stenosis suggests that this may be secondary to ischemia-induced segmental contraction abnormalities.[138] No such contraction abnormalities have been observed in humans with preserved LV function and ischemic heart disease exposed to high-dose opiates and N_2O.[139] N_2O combined with high-dose opiates also elevates pulmonary vascular resistance, particularly in the presence of preexisting pulmonary hypertension.[140] Because of the potential for altered myocardial oxygen balance in all patients with coronary artery disease, N_2O must be used with caution. Isoflurane, as discussed in detail previously, may be safely used as an adjuvant with little risk of ischemia in steal-prone anatomy patients. Sevoflurane and desflurane may be used as well.[31,141] Enflurane causes both vasodilation and depression of systolic function.[142] Nonetheless, enflurane in combination with 50% N_2O has been shown to provide comparable hemodynamics to sufentanil-O_2 in patients undergoing coronary revascularization.[143]

Fast-track Technique

The "fast track" is a comprehensive program designed to reduce costs by reducing hospital stay for patients undergoing coronary revascularization.[144] Early extubation (<12 hours) is an intregral part of this program. A number of anesthetic techniques have been reported that allow early extubation without increasing the risk of adverse cardiac and noncardiac outcomes. Generally, patients selected for inclusion in the protocol are considered to be low-risk coronary revascularization patients, but more and more centers are including all cardiac surgical patients. Risk factors that seem to contribute to the need for prolonged postoperative ventilation in coronary revascularization patients are female sex, advanced age, congestive heart failure (CHF) requiring preoperative diuretic therapy, and unstable angina.[145]

The following is an example of a fast-track protocol. It should be kept in mind that there are many approaches, including continuous infusions of sufentanil-propofol and sufentanil-midazolam, bolus administration of fentanyl, or sufentanil in conjunction with either a propofol infusion or administration of an inhalation agent.[146]

Premedication is most commonly midazolam 0.015 to 0.07 mg/kg IV because the patients are morning admissions.

Fentanyl 15 to 20 μg/kg and etomidate 0.20 to 0.30 mg/kg are used for induction in combination with cis-atracurium, vecuronium, or pancuronium. The considerations used in choosing a relaxant are the same used in the high-dose opoid technique. Anesthesia is maintained with isoflurane 0.5 to 1.0% and addition of fentanyl to a total dose of 25 μg/kg. Hemodynamic changes and myocardial ischemia are managed as described in the high-dose narcotic protocol. Propofol 75 to 100 μg/kg/min is administered while on CPB and is discontinued and replaced with isoflurane 0.5 to 1.0% once ejection through the pulmonary circuit and ventilation commences. No additional fentanyl is given. Isoflurane is discontinued after the skin is closed and propofol 33 to 50 μg/kg/min is started for transport to the ICU. Propofol has been shown to provide satisfactory sedation after coronary revascularization without deleterious hemodynamic effects.[147]

Emergency Coronary Artery Bypass Surgery

Anesthesia for emergency coronary artery bypass surgery provides some unique challenges. The patients to be considered here are those suffering from complications of cardiac catheterization or of catheter-based interventional techniques to treat coronary stenoses. Currently, several catheter-based techniques are in use:

percutaneous transluminal coronary angioplasty (PTCA), directional coronary atherectomy (DCA), laser angioplasty, and transluminal extraction catheter (TEC). All of these techniques have the potential to acutely compromise or terminate myocardial blood flow.

PTCA is the most commonly used method. This technique involves placement of a small, steerable guidewire across a coronary stenosis. Subsequently, a balloon-tipped catheter is placed over the guidewire. The balloon is then inflated to dilate the stenosis. Abrupt coronary closure after PCTA is the result of a coronary dissection with intimal flap obstruction of the vessel lumen or thrombus formation on the damaged endothelium. Use of a perfusion balloon catheter (PBC) or "bail-out" catheter can be lifesaving in this instance. This catheter has multiple side holes both proximal and distal to the balloon. After the balloon is in place across the dissection, perfusion across the lesion takes place via the side holes and the central lumen of the catheter. Alternatively, a stent can be placed across the lesion. A rarer complication of PCTA is vessel perforation.

Patients presenting with failed coronary angioplasty procedures fall into three categories:

1. Hemodynamically stable, nonischemic patients — some of these patients will have sustained no endothelial damage and can be managed as elective coronary revascularization patients. Some patients will have sustained endothelial damage and are at risk for subsequent thrombus formation and vessel closure. These patients may require surgical revascularization but can afford to wait several hours. This is time enough to complete a comprehensive anesthetic evaluation and to allow further gastric emptying if necessary.

2. Hemodynamically stable, ischemic patients — these patients require urgent revascularization. The ischemic interval should be limited to <6 hours to avoid infarction. Temporizing measures in the form of an IABP, PBC, or stent will likely have taken place. Anesthetic evaluation should be concise and focused. Communication with the cardiologist is essential to determine the extent of jeopardized myocarium, current vasoactive agents, anticoagulation methods (heparin, streptokinase, tissue plasminogen activator [tPA], NPO status, current laboratory values, and vascular access. The arterial access used for the catheterization procedure (femoral artery) should be left in place and used for monitoring in the operating room. Femoral vein sheaths can be used for venous access. A pulmonary artery catheter is commonly placed via the femoral

vein and can be used as well. Induction can be accomplished easily and safely using the high-dose narcotic technique described previously. For patients deemed at high risk for aspiration, a nonparticulate antacid and metaclopromide 10 to 20 mg IV should be administered. A rapid sequence induction can be accomplished with etomidate 0.15 to 0.3 mg/kg and succinylcholine 1.0 to 1.5 mg/kg, in conjunction with fentanyl (10 µg/kg) or sufentanil (1 µg/kg). Etomidate produces minimal cardiovascular effects at this dosage when administered in conjunction with narcotics.[148] Alternatively, sufentanil 5 µg/kg and succinylcholine 1.0 to 1.5 mg/kg can be used in a rapid-sequence technique.[149] Hypotension and ischemia must be aggressively and promptly treated as outlined previously in this chapter.

After the patient is induced, placement of additional intravascular catheters can be accomplished in parallel with the surgical preparation. In particular, a pulmonary artery (PA) catheter can be placed via the right internal jugular vein. This substantially improves the ability to manipulate and position the PA catheter and to infuse vasoactive agents at a proximal site. The femoral vein PA catheter often is not in a sterile sheath and is distant from the head of the bed. If peripheral venous access is poor, a large-bore double lumen (16- or 14-gauge) central venous line can be placed at the same time as the pulmonary artery catheter. Because these patients usually are anticoagulated with at least heparin, placement of these catheters using ultrasonic guidance is desirable (*see* Chapter 3).

3. Hemodynamically unstable, ischemic patients — these patients require emergent revascularization. Evaluation must often be performed in the hallway on the way to the operating room. Again, communication with the cardiac catheterization team is essential. Some of these patients are mildly hypotensive, requiring minimal cardiovascular pharmacologic support, whereas others will be intubated and will receive cardiopulmonary resuscitation (CPR). The goal is to establish CPB as expeditiously as possible. Vascular access for monitoring and volume infusion can be obtained on the surgical field if necessary. All existing intravascular access should be used. For more stable patients, the induction techniques described above are applicable. For patients receiving CPR, scopolamine 0.005 mg/kg or midazolam 0.05 to 0.1 mg/kg in conjunction with a nondepolarizing muscle relaxant may be all that is necessary.

Post-cardiopulmonary Bypass Management

The assumption that coronary revascularization will produce a patient with normal myocardial function after CPB is erroneous. Immediate improvements in LV systolic and diastolic function occur within the first 10 minutes after termination of CPB.[150] However, after this initial period, abnormalities in systolic and diastolic performance are apparent. Even in patients with successful revascularization, abnormalities in LV chamber stiffness (*see* Chapter 2) exist post-CPB such that at a given PCWP LV end-diastolic area or volume will be 15% smaller in the post-CPB period as compared with the pre-CPB period.[151] This is due to a leftward shift of the LV pressure–volume relationship. Preload recruitable stroke work is reduced.[152] In addition, depression of both RV and LV systolic function (reduced EF, LV stroke work index [SWI], cardiac index [CI]) is seen with the nadir occurring approximately 4 hours after termination of CPB.[153] Complete recovery is seen by 48 hours with substantial improvements by 7 to 8 hours. Others have described a recovery pattern that includes two types of patients: one subset shows complete recovery of biventricular function in the first 4 hours, the other subset demonstrates biventricular dysfunction with no recovery for 24 hours.[154]

Coronary revascularization may be less than complete for technical reasons, such as small distal vessels or nonbypassable lesions. Communication with the surgeon is necessary to determine the success of the operative procedure. The sense of security that accompanies a "successful" operative procedure must be tempered with the knowledge that a significant number of patients (35 to 50%) continue to have evidence of myocardial ischemia in the postbypass period after apparently successful revascularization.[40,54-56] Most episodes occur in the immediate (0 to 8 hours) postoperative period. The development of post-CPB RWMA and the development of ECG-detected ischemia in the immediate postoperative period are both associated with adverse clinical outcome.

There may be alterations in the vascular tone of the native coronary circulation during the post-CPB period.[155,156] Coronary vasospasm may occur distal to bypass grafts or in segments of artery that have not been bypassed. This usually is heralded by the presence of elevated ST segments in the absence of a precipitating hemodynamic event. IV nitroglycerin should be titrated and sublingual nifedipine (10 mg) may be added if necessary. If these measures fail, nitroglycerin or papaverine can be injected directly into the coronary artery by the surgeon.

Flow-through IMA and saphenous vein grafts may be affected by vasoactive substances used during the post-CPB period. In humans, infusion of epinephrine to increase systemic blood pressure during the post-CPB period increases IMA graft flow, norepinephrine infusion does not change IMA graft flow, and phenylephrine infusion reduces IMA graft flow.[157] One canine model suggests that such changes are due to the effects of vasoactive substances on IMA vascular tone,[158] whereas another canine model implicates changes in systemic blood pressure.[159] In humans, vasopressor-associated increases in systemic blood pressure are accompanied by increases in saphenous vein graft flows.[157] Additional work must be done to determine more precisely how changes in graft vascular resistance, systemic blood pressure, and myocardial oxygen consumption contribute to these flow variations. Nonetheless, it should be kept in mind that the choice of vasopressor may affect flow through engrafted arteries and veins.

LV systolic function may be compromised by inadequate myocardial protection during bypass. This is particularly likely if the patient has suffered a preoperative ischemic event or has poor preoperative ventricular function. In these patients, optimization of preload and heart rate are necessary first steps in obtaining hemodynamic stability. It must be remembered that patients with compromised systolic function will be dependent on heart rate for cardiac output increases. In addition, patients with reduced ventricular compliance and distensibility will be dependent on atrial systole to provide an adequate LVEDV without a high mean PCWP. For these reasons, pacing of the atrium (with intrinsic conduction via the atrioventricular [AV] node) or of the atrium and ventricle (when AV nodal dysfunction exists) may be necessary.

Optimization of preload after termination of CPB requires careful attention and is facilitated by use of TEE and/or PCWP and CVP. Preload reserve can be assessed by infusion of blood from the CPB circuit in increments of 10 to 15 mL/kg. One of three distinct hemodynamic responses will be observed:

1. Intact preload reserve — infusion of volume will produce an increase in MAP with little or no change in PCWP or CVP. TEE will demonstrate a nondistended LV and RV. Cardiac output should increase, but the response time of the thermodilution method to this intervention may be on the order of minutes. For this subset of patients, further infusion of volume to improve hemodynamics is warranted.

2. Optimized preload — infusion of volume will produce little or no change in mean arterial pressure (MAP) with no change or a small increase in PCWP or CVP. TEE will demonstrate a LV or RV at the upper limits of size for the particular patient. Obviously, pre-CPB assessment of LV and RV dimensions is necessary to take full

advantage of this modality. Cardiac output should increase slightly or should remain unchanged. For this subset of patients, no further infusion of volume to improve hemodynamics is warranted.

3. Exhausted preload reserve — infusion of volume will produce no change or a fall in MAP with a substantial increase in PCWP or CVP. TEE will demonstrate a distended LV or RV. Cardiac output should decrease slightly or should remain unchanged. For this subset of patients, no further infusion of volume to improve hemodynamics is warranted and initiation of inotropic support is indicated to improve hemodynamics and reduce ventricular dimensions.

Several factors seem to be associated with an increased incidence of inotropic agent use to terminate CPB.[160] Factors related to inotrope use are low EF (<55%), older age, cardiac enlargement, female sex, and higher baseline and post-contrast LVEDP. For patients with an EF > 55%, the presence of preoperative wall motion abnormalities and an elevation of >10 mm Hg in LVEDP with contrast injection was associated with the need for inotropes. In addition, for patients with an EF > 46%, prolonged duration of CPB was associated with the need for inotropes.

The most commonly used inotropic agents are described below. Use of inotropic agents post-CPB should be used with the knowledge that both adults and children exhibit uncoupling of beta adrenoceptors from the Gs-protein-adenylate cyclase complex after CPB.[161,162] This desensitization may contribute to a relative catecholamine resistance in the post-CPB period.

Dopamine. Dopamine possesses beta-1-adrenergic, alpha-1-adrenergic, and dopaminergic activities. Some of the alpha activity is due to release of endogenous norepinephrine. At doses of 2 to 3 µg/kg/min the dopaminergic activity is maximal, which results in preferential dilation of renal, mesenteric, and coronary vasculature. This dopaminergic activity is not antagonized by alpha agonists. This makes dopamine a useful agent for preservation of renal blood flow in the presence of alpha agonists. Beta-1-induced enhanced inotropy is seen at doses between 1 and 10 µg/kg/min; however, at doses above 4 to 6 µg/kg/min dopamine's alpha-adrenergic activity increases such that SVR, PVR, and PCWP increase with little concomitant increase in cardiac output.[163] This combination of increased ventricular wall radius and afterload may cause detrimental increases in myocardial oxygen consumption. At doses higher than 10 µg/kg/min, the alpha-adrenergic effects of dopamine predominate, producing vasoconstriction. Dopamine's chronotropic and dysrhythymic effects increase as the dose increases.

Dobutamine. Dobutamine possesses beta-1-, beta-2-, and alpha-1-adrenergic activities. The predominant effect is enhanced inotropy through beta-1 stimulation. The beta-2 and alpha-1 activities are balanced such that mild vasodilation occurs at the commonly used doses from 5 to 20 µg/kg/min. Dobutamine decreases pulmonary vascular resistance,[164] blunts hypoxic pulmonary vasoconstriction,[165] and increases coronary blood flow.[166] Dobutamine may actually reduce myocardial oxygen consumption in the failing heart, because although it increases contractility, it reduces LV radius and end-diastolic pressure while increasing arterial pressure and maintaining heart rate.[167] Dobutamine seems to have less of a chronotropic effect than dopamine.[168]

Epinephrine. Epinephrine possesses beta-1-, beta-2-, and alpha-1-adrenergic activities. At doses of 1 to 3 µg/min, epinephrine has a potent inotropic effect mediated through beta-1 stimulation, with little effect on vasomotor tone due to the balance of beta-2 and alpha-1 stimulation. As the dose increases above 3 µg/min, progressively more alpha-1 activity occurs, with resultant mixed inotropic and vasoconstrictive effects. Doses above 3 µg/min also cause progressive decreases in renal blood flow.[169] Above 10 µg/min, epinephrine is primarily a vasoconstrictor. Epinephrine's vasoconstrictive effects also reduce venous capacitance. Although coronary blood flow is maintained, epinephrine may not be favorable to myocardial energetics, because in addition to increasing contractility, it increases systolic blood pressure, increases LV end-diastolic volume and pressure, and reduces diastolic blood pressure while increasing heart rate.

Epinephrine 10 and 30 ng/kg/min is as effective as dobutamine 2.5 and 5 µg/kg/min in increasing stroke volume in coronary revascularization patients post-CPB and produces less tachycardia than dobutamine. The increase in CI with epinephrine was less than that seen with dobutamine and SVR was significantly lower with the higher dose of dobutamine as compared with the higher dose of epinephrine.[170]

Epinephrine 15 to 40 ng/kg/min has been described as the agent of choice to terminate CPB. The potent inotropic and balanced peripheral vascular effects allow prompt, reliable termination of CPB while avoiding the ventricular distension and systemic hypotension that compromise subendocardial perfusion. Critics point out that the potent inotropic effects of epinephrine may not be necessary in every instance, and thus, epinephrine's potentially deleterious effects on myocardial energetics and renal blood flow can be avoided.

Norepinephrine. Norepinephrine possesses beta-1- and alpha-1-adrenergic activity. The alpha-1 effects of norepinephrine are manifest at low doses (1 to 2 µg/min) and predominate as the dose increases. Norepinephrine reduces renal blood flow, elevates both systolic and diastolic blood pressure, reduces venous capacitance, and generally causes a reflex decrease in heart rate. Although coronary blood flow is maintained, norepinephrine may not be favorable to myocardial energetics, because in addition to increasing contractility, it increases systolic and diastolic blood pressure.

Amrinone. Amrinone is a potent inotropic agent that acts not by beta-1-adrenergic stimulation but by inhibiting phosphodiesterase III (PDE III) to increase intracellular cyclic adenosine monophosphate (cAMP).[171] In addition, amrinone possesses vasodilator activity by virtue of PDE III inhibition in vascular smooth muscle.[171] Amrinone increases cardiac index, reduces LVEDP and LVEDV, reduces systolic blood pressure, and has little effect on heart rate. Like dobutamine, in the failing heart, this increase in cardiac index may be associated with a decrease in myocardial oxygen consumption due to the concomitant reduction in wall stress.[172] Amrinone's vasodilator activity also reduces pulmonary vascular resistance.

Because amrinone does not act via beta-1 receptors, it is potentially synergistic with beta-1 agents in augmenting inotropy.[173,174] Evidence to date in cardiac surgical patients demonstrates that amrinone (1.5 mg/kg) is at least as effective as epinephrine (30 ng/kg/min) in improving post-CPB function and that the combination of the two agents produces effects at least as large as the sum of the two agents individually.[175] The benefit of the two agents together was particularly marked for the RV. In addition amrinone (1.5 mg/kg) has been shown to be as effective as dobutamine (5 μg/kg/min) in cardiac surgical patients.[176] Amrinone also has been shown to be as effective as epinephrine in improving post-CPB ventricular function in patients with preoperative LV dysfunction.[177]

Amrinone is administered using a loading dose of 1.5 mg/kg followed by an infusion of 10 to 20 μg/kg/min.[171] The loading dose can be administered on CPB just before termination to attenuate the effects of the acute vasodilation the loading dose can cause.

Long-term oral use of amrinone has been associated with thrombocytopenia due to decreased platelet survival time. Amrinone and milrinone (see below) increase cAMP concentrations in platelets. This can impair platelet function by inhibiting platelet activation, inhibiting release of arachondonic acid, and inhibiting cyclooxygenase.[178] Despite this, there does not seem to be any further impairment of platelet function other than that expected with CPB when these agents are used.[178]

Milrinone. Milrinone is an analog of amrinone that is 10 to 30 times more potent than amrinone. Like amrinone, milrinone increases cardiac index, reduces LVEDP and LVEDV, reduces systolic blood pressure, and has lit-

tle effect on heart rate. In the failing heart, this increase in cardiac index may be associated with a decrease in myocardial oxygen consumption due to the concomitant reduction in wall stress. Milrinone's vasodilator activity also reduces pulmonary vascular resistance.[179] Milrinone has been shown to be effective for treatment of low cardiac output after cardiac surgery.[180,181] Milrinone, like amrinone, may be particularly useful for patients with RV failure for whom the combination of inotropy and RV afterload reduction are desirable.[182]

Milrinone is administered using a loading dose of 50 μg/kg as a loading dose followed by an infusion of 0.5 to 0.75 μg/kg/min.[183,184] The loading dose can be administered on CPB just before termination to attenuate the effects of the acute vasodilation the loading dose can cause.

Calcium. Calcium chloride 5 to 10 mg/kg is a commonly used adjuvant during termination of CPB. Recent evidence suggests that calcium administration may be no better than placebo in augmenting LV function, RV function, and CI after emergence from CPB.[185,186] Calcium administration does increase MAP, however.

The higher doses of calcium (10 mg/kg) can attenuate the effects of inotropic agents that are beta-adrenergic receptor agonists, such as dobutamine and epinephrine.[187,188] No such effects are seen with amrinone. A recent investigation suggests that entry of calcium ions through calcium channels attenuates adenylyl cyclase, which may explain the observation.[189]

Ionized calcium levels decrease during CPB but approach normal before separation from CPB.[190] Thus, hypocalcemia is rarely present as an indication for calcium administration, except perhaps in neonates and infants, who are more prone to hypocalcemia. In addition, because loss of calcium homeostasis is one of the hallmarks of ischemia (*see* Chapter 12), the administration of calcium in the vulnerable reperfusion interval after aortic cross-clamp removal may exacerbate cell injury and death.

For routine termination of CPB in which SVR is in the normal range and inotropic support is needed, epinephrine, 0.015 to 0.05 μg/kg/min, dopamine, 1 to 5 μg/kg/min, or dobutamine, 5 to 10 μg/kg/min, are reasonable choices because they provide inotropic support with little concomitant vasoconstriction and afterload increase. For situations in which cardiac index is low and SVR is elevated, therapy with a vasodilator such as nitroprusside may be all that is necessary to relieve afterload mismatch. If an inotrope is found to be necessary in this situation, dobutamine is a good choice because it possesses some vasodilatory activity.

For instances in which CI remains low (less than 2.0 L/min/m²), it may be necessary to increase the dose of the chosen inotrope. Dobutamine may be increased to 15 to 20 µg/kg/min; however, the progressive decrease in SVR may require the addition of a small dose (0.5 to 1.0 µg/min) of norepinephrine to normalize SVR. As the doses of epinephrine and dopamine are increased, SVR may increase, and the addition of nitroprusside to the inotropic regime may be necessary to reduce afterload and improve systolic performance. Epinephrine in combination with nitroprusside is a reliable approach to severe ventricular failure. In all instances, elevations of PCWP above 15 to 18 mm Hg should be treated with nitroglycerin to prevent ventricular dilatation and pulmonary congestion and to improve subendocardial blood flow.

The addition of amrinone or milrinone may be useful when these measures fail to produce acceptable hemodynamics (CI > 2 L/min/m^2, PCWP < 18 mm Hg, CVP < 15 mm Hg, systolic BP > 90 mm Hg, or MAP > 50 mm Hg). More specific guidelines for treatment of RV dysfunction are addressed in Chapter 7. Continued LV and RV dysfunction in the setting of aggressive inotropic and vasodilator support is an indication for placement of a mechanical circulatory assist device, as discussed in Chapter 11.

■ REFERENCES

1. Klocke FJ, Weinstein IR, Klocke JF, et al: Zero-flow pressures and pressure-flow relationships during single long diastoles in the canine coronary bed before and during maximal vasodilation. *J Clin Invest* 1981; **68**:970-980.
2. Dole WP: Autoregulation of the coronary circulation. *Prog Cardiovasc Dis* 1987; **29**:293-323.
3. Suga H, Hayashi T, Suehiro S, et al: Equal oxygen consumption rates of isovolumic and ejecting contractions with equal systolic pressure-volume areas in canine left ventricle. *Circ Res* 1981; **49**:1082-1091.
4. Brown BG, Bolson EL, Dodge HT: Dynamic mechanisms in human coronary stenosis. *Circulation* 1984; **70**:917-922.
5. Gould KL, Lipscomb K: Effects of coronary stenoses on coronary blood flow reserve and resistance. *Am J Cardiol* 1974; **34**:48-55.
6. Fuster V, Badimon L, Badimon JJ, et al: The pathogenesis of coronary artery disease and the acute coronary syndromes. Part 1 and Part 2. *N Engl J Med* 1992; **326**:242-250, 310-318.
7. Brown BG, Lee AB, Bolson EL, Dodge HT: Reflex constriction of significant coronary stenosis as a mechanism contributing to ischemic left ventricular dysfunction during isometric exercise. *Circulation* 1984; **70**:18-24.
8. Maseri A: Role of coronary artery spasm in symptomatic and silent myocardial ischemia. *J Am Coll Cardiol* 1987; **9**:249-262.
9. Gross GJ, Warltier DC: Coronary steal in four models of single or multiple vessel obstruction in dogs. *Am J Cardiol* 1981; **48**:84-92.
10. Becker LC: Conditions for vasodilator-induced coronary steal in experimental myocardial ischemia. *Circulation* 1978; **57**:1103-1110.
11. Buffington CW, Davis KB, Gillispie S, Pettinger M: The prevalance of steal-prone coronary anatomy in patients with coronary artery disease: An analysis of the Coronary Artery Surgery Study registry. *Anesthesiology* 1988; **69**:721-727.
12. Preibe H-J: Differential effects of isoflurane on regional right and left ventricular performances, and on the coronary, systemic, and pulmonary hemodynamics in the dog. *Anesthesiology* 1987; **66**:262-272.
13. Sill JC, Bove AA, Nugent M, et al: Effects of isoflurane on coronary arteries and coronary arterioles in the intact dog. *Anesthesiology* 1987; **66**:273-279.
14. Gilbert M, Roberts SL, Mori M, et al: Comparative coronary vascular reactivity and hemodynamics during halothane and isoflurane anesthesia in swine. *Anesthesiology* 1988; **68**:243-253.
15. Buffington C, Romson JL, Levine A, et al: Isoflurane induces coronary steal in a canine model of chronic coronary occlusion. *Anesthesiology* 1987; **66**:280-292.
16. Cason BA, Verrier ED, London MJ, et al: Effects of isoflurane and halothane on coronary vascular resistance and collateral myocardial blood flow: Their capacity to induce coronary steal. *Anesthesiology* 1987; **67**:665-675.
17. Preibe H-J, Foex P: Isoflurane causes regional myocardial dysfunction in dogs with critical coronary artery stenoses. *Anesthesiology* 1987; **66**:293-300.
18. Preibe H-J: Isoflurane causes more severe regional myocardial dysfunction than halothane in dogs with a critical coronary artery stenosis. *Anesthesiology* 1988; **69**:72-83.
19. Wilton NC, Knight PR, Ullrich K, et al: Transmural redistribution of myocardial blood flow during isoflurane anesthesia and its effects on regional myocardial function in a canine model of fixed coronary stenosis. *Anesthesiology* 1993; **78**:510-523.
20. Tatekawa S, Traber KB, Hantler CB, et al: Effects of isoflurane on myocardial blood flow, function, and oxygen consumption in the presence of a critical coronary stenosis in dogs. *Anesth Analg* 1987; **66**:1073-1082.
21. Reiz S, Balfors E, Sorensen MB, et al: Isoflurane — A powerful coronary vasodilator in patients with coronary artery disease. *Anesthesiology* 1983; **59**:91-97.
22. Moffitt E, Baker RA, Glenn JJ, et al: Myocardial metabolism and hemodynamic responses with isoflurane anesthesia for coronary arterial surgery. *Anesth Analg* 1986; **65**:53-61.
23. Khambatta HJ, Sonntag H, Larsen R, et al: Global and regional myocardial blood flow and metabolism during equipotent halothane and isoflurane anesthesia in patients with coronary artery disease. *Anesth Analg* 1988; **67**:936-942.
24. Moffitt EA, Sethna DH: The coronary circulation and myocardial oxygenation in coronary artery disease: Effects of anesthesia. *Anesth Analg* 1986; **65**:395-410.
25. Tarnow J, Markschies-Hornung A, Schulte-Sasse U: Isoflurane improves the tolerance to pacing-induced myocardial ischemia. *Anesthesiology* 1986; **64**:147-156.
26. Hess W, Arnold B, Schulte-Sasse U, Tarnow J: Comparison of isoflurane and halothane when used to control intraoperative hypertension in patients undergoing coronary artery bypass surgery. *Anesth Analg* 1983; **62**:15-20.
27. O'Young J, Mastrocostopoulos G, Hilgenberg A, et al: Myocardial circulatory and metabolic effects of isoflurane and sufentanil during coronary artery bypass surgery. *Anesthesiology* 1987; **66**:653-658.
28. Smith JS, Cahalan MK, Benefeil DJ, et al: Intraoperative detection of myocardial ischemia in high risk patients: Electrocardiography versus two-dimensional transesophageal echocardiography. *Circulation* 1985; **72**:1015-1021.
29. Leung JM, Goehner P, O'Kelly BF, et al: Isoflurane anesthesia and myocardial ischemia: Comparative risk versus sufentanil anesthesia in patients undergoing coronary artery bypass graft surgery. *Anesthesiology* 1991; **74**:838-847.
30. Leung JM, Hollenberg M, O'Kelly BF, et al: Effects of steal-prone anatomy on intraoperative myocardial ischemia. *J Am Coll Cardiol* 1992; **20**:1205-1212.

31. Ebert TJ, Harkin CP, Muzi M: Cardiovascular responses to sevoflurane: A review. *Anesth Analg* 1995; **81:**S11-S22.

32. Warltier DC, Pagel PS: Cardiovascular and respiratory actions of desflurane: Is desflurane different from isoflurane? *Anesth Analg* 1992; **75:**S17-S31.

33. Brazier J, Cooper N, Buckberg G: The adequacy of subendocardial oxygen delivery. The interaction of flow, arterial oxygen content and myocardial oxygen need. *Circulation* 1974; **69:**968-977.

34. Maseri A, Chierchia S, Kaski JC: Mixed angina pectoris. *Am J Cardiol* 1985; **56:**30E-33E.

35. Nesto RW, Kowalchuk GJ: The ischemic cascade: Temporal sequence of hemodynamic, electrocardiographic and symptomatic expressions of ischemia. *Am J Cardiol* 1987; **57:**23C-30C.

36. Singh BN, Nademanee K, Figuras J, Josephson MA: Hemodynamic and electrocardiographic correlates of symptomatic and silent myocardial ischemia: Pathophysiologic and therapeutic implications. *Am J Cardiol* 1986; **58:**3B-10B.

37. Deanfield JE, Selwyn AP, Chierchia A, et al: Myocardial ischemia during daily life in patients with stable angina: Its relationship to symptoms and heart rate changes. *Lancet* 1983; **2:**753-758.

38. Cecchi AC, Dovellini EV, Marchi F, et al: Silent myocardial ischemia during ambulatory electrocardiographic monitoring in patients with effort angina. *J Am Coll Cardiol* 1983; **1:**934-939.

39. Rocco MB, Barry J, Campbell S, et al: Circadian variation of transient myocardial ischemia in patients with coronary artery disease. *Circulation* 1987; **75:**395-400.

40. Knight AA, Hollenberg M, London MJ, et al: Perioperative myocardial ischemia: Importance of the preoperative ischemic pattern. *Anesthesiology* 1988; **68:**681-688.

41. Glazier JJ, Chierchia S, Brown MJ, Maseri A: Generalized defective perception of painful stimuli: A cause of silent myocardial ischemia in chronic stable angina. *Am J Cardiol* 1986; **58:**667-672.

42. Pepine CJ, Imperi G, Lambert C: Relationship of transient ischemic episodes to daily activities. *Circulation* 1987; **75**(suppl 2):28-30.

43. Campbell S, Barry J, Rebecca GS, et al: Active transient myocardial ischemia during daily life in asymptomatic patients with positive exercise tests and coronary-artery disease. *Am J Cardiol* 1986; **57:**1010-1016.

44. Chierchia S, Muijesan L, Balasubramanian V, et al: Ambulatory ECG and blood pressure monitoring in patients with chronic stable angina. Relationship between myocardial demand and acute ischemia. *Circulation* 1984; **70**(suppl 2):452.

45. Hogue CW, Herbst TJ, Pond C, et al: Perioperative myocardial ischemia. Its relationship to anatomic pattern of coronary artery stenosis. *Anesthesiology* 1993; **79:**514-524.

46. Kotter GS, Kotrly KJ, Kalbfleisch JH, et al: Myocardial ischemia during cardiovascular surgery as detected by an ST segment trend monitoring system. *J Cardiothorac Anesth* 1987; **1:**190-199.

47. Slogoff S, Keats AS: Does perioperative myocardial ischemia lead to postoperative myocardial infarction? *Anesthesiology* 1985; **62:**107-114.

48. Slogoff S, Keats AS: Further observations on perioperative myocardial ischemia. *Anesthesiology* 1986; **65:**539-542.

49. Slogoff S, Keats AS: Does chronic treatment with calcium entry blocking drugs reduce perioperative myocardial ischemia? *Anesthesiology* 1988; **68:**676-680.

50. Lowenstein E: Perioperative ischemic episodes cause myocardial infarction in humans — A hypothesis confirmed. *Anesthesiology* 1985; **62:**103-106.

51. Urban MK, Gordon MA, Harris SN, et al: Intraoperative hemodynamic changes are not good indicators of myocardial ischemia. *Anesth Analg* 1993; **76:**942-949.

52. Leung JM, O'Kelly BF, Mangano DT: Relationship of regional wall motion abnormalities to hemodynamic indices of myocardial oxygen supply and demand in patients undergoing CABG surgery. *Anesthesiology* 1990; **73:**802-814.

53. Goehner P, Hollenberg M, Mangano DT: Perioperative myocardial ischemia in CABG patients: Effect of anesthesia and hemodynamics (abstract). In: Proceedings of the 10th annual meeting of the Society of Cardiovascular Anesthesia. Society of Cardiovascular Anesthesia, 1988.

54. Leung J, O'Kelly B, Browner W, et al: Prognostic importance of postbypass regional wall-motion abnormalities in patients undergoing coronary artery bypass graft surgery. *Anesthesiology* 1989; **71:**16-25.

55. Mangano DT, Siliciano D, Hollenberg M, et al: Postoperative myocardial ischemia: Theraputic trials using intensive analgesia following surgery. *Anesthesiology* 1992; **76:**342-353.

56. Smith R, Leung J, Mangano D, et al: Postoperative myocardial ischemia in patients undergoing coronary artery bypass graft surgery. *Anesthesiology* 1991; **74:**464-473.

57. Kates RA, Zaidan JR, Kaplan JA: Esophageal lead for intraoperative electrocardiographic monitoring. *Anesth Analg* 1982; **61:**781-785.

58. Trager MA, Feinberg BI, Kaplan JA: Right ventricular ischemia diagnosed by an esophageal electrocardiogram and right atrial pressure trace. *J Cardiothorac Anesth* 1987; **1:**123-125.

59. Kaplan JA, Wells PH: Early diagnosis of myocardial ischemia using the pulmonary artery catheter. *Anesth Analg* 1981; **60:**789-793.

60. Trager MA, Feinberg BI, Kaplan JA: Right ventricular ischemia diagnosed by an esophageal electrocardiogram and right atrial pressure trace. *J Cardiothorac Anesth* 1987; **1:**123-125.

61. Rahimtoola S, Loeb HS, Ehsani A, et al: Relationship of pulmonary artery to left ventricular diastolic pressures in acute myocardial infarction. *Circulation* 1972; **46:**283-290.

62. Haggmark S, Hohner P, Ostman M, et al: Comparison of hemodynamic, electrocardiographic, mechanical, and metabolic indicators of intraoperative myocardial ischemia in vascular surgical patients with coronary artery disease. *Anesthesiology* 1989; **70:**19-25.

63. Kleinman B, Henkin RE, Glisson SN, et al: Qualitative evaluation of coronary flow during anesthetic induction using thallium-201 perfusion scans. *Anesthesiology* 1986; **64:**157-164.

64. van Daele MERM, Sutherland GR, Mitchell MM, et al: Do changes in pulmonary capillary wedge pressure adequately reflect myocardial ischemia during anesthesia? A correlative preoperative hemodynamic, electrocardiographic, and transesophageal echocardiographic study. *Circulation* 1990; **81:**865-871.

65. London MJ, Tubau JF, Wong MG, et al: The "natural history" of segmental wall motion abnormalities in patients undergoing non cardiac surgery. *Anesthesiology* 1990; **73:**644-655.

66. Voci P, Bilotta F, Aronson S, et al: Echocardiographic analysis of dysfunctional and normal myocardial segments before and immediately after coronary artery bypass graft surgery. *Anesth Analg* 1992; **75:**312-318.

67. Wohlgelernter D, Cleman M, Highman HA, et al: Regional myocardial dysfunction during coronary angioplasty: Evaluation by two-dimensional echocardiography and 12 lead electrocardiography. *J Am Coll Cardiol* 1986; **7:**1245-1254.

68. Clements F, de Bruijn NP: Perioperative evaluation of regional wall motion by transesophageal two-dimensional echocardiography. *Anesth Analg* 1987; **66:**249-261.

69. Eisenberg MJ, London MJ, Leung JM, et al: Monitoring for myocardial ischemia during noncardiac surgery. A technology assessment of transesophageal echocardiography and 12-lead electrocardiography. *JAMA* 1992; **268:**210-216.

70. Koide Y, Keehan L, Nomura T, et al: Relationship of regional wall motion abnormalities detected by biplane transesophageal echocardiography and electrocardiographic changes in patients undergoing coronary artery bypass graft surgery. *J Cardiothorac Vasc Anesth* 1996; **10:**719-727.

71. Sonntag H, Merin RG, Donath U, et al: Myocardial metabolism and oxygenation in man awake and during halothane anesthesia. *Anesthesiology* 1979; **51**:204-210.

72. Kaplan JA: Hemodynamic Monitoring, in Kaplan JA (ed): *Cardiac Anesthesia.* New York, Grune and Stratton, 1979.

73. Kissin I, Reves JG, Mardis M: Is rate-pressure product a misleading guide? *Anesthesiology* 1980; **52**:373-374.

74. Lieberman RW, Orkin FK, Jobes DR, Schwartz AJ: Hemodynamic predictors of myocardial ischemia during halothane anesthesia for coronary revascularization. *Anesthesiology* 1983; **59**:36-41.

75. Hoffman JIE, Buckberg GD: The myocardial supply: Demand ratio — A critical review. *Am J Cardiol* 1978; **41**:327-332.

76. Buffington CW: Hemodynamic determinants of ischemic myocardial dysfunction in the presence of coronary stenosis in dogs. *Anesthesiology* 1985; **63**:651-662.

77. Buffington CW, Bashein G, Sivarajan M: Blood pressure and heart rate predict ischemia in collateral-dependent myocardium. *Anesthesiology* 1987; **67**:A5.

78. Gordon MA, Urban MK, O'Connor T, et al: Is the pressure rate quotient a predictor or indicator of myocardial ischemia as measured by ST-segment changes in patients undergoing coronary artery bypass surgery? *Anesthesiology* 1991; **74**:848-853.

79. Harris SN, Gordon MA, Urban MK, et al: The pressure rate quotient is not an indicator of myocardial ischemia in humans. *Anesthesiology* 1993; **78**:242-250.

80. Sill JC, Nugent M, Moyer TP, et al: Influence of propranolol plasma levels on hemodynamics during coronary artery bypass surgery. *Anesthesiology* 1984; **60**:455-463.

81. Newsome LR, Roth JV, Hug CC, Nagle D: Esmolol attenuates hemodynamic responses during fentanyl–pancuronium anesthesia for aortocoronary bypass surgery. *Anesth Analg* 1986; **65**:451-456.

82. Girard D, Shulman BJ, Thys DM, et al: The safety and efficacy of esmolol during myocardial revascularization. *Anesthesiology* 1986; **65**:157-164.

83. Mann T, Cohn PF, Holman BL, et al: Effect of nitroprusside on regional myocardial blood flow in coronary artery disease. Results in 25 patients and comparison with nitroglycerin. *Circulation* 1978; **57**:732-737.

84. Flaherty JT, Magee PA, Gardner TL, et al: Comparison of intravenous nitroglycerin and sodium nitroprusside for treatment of acute hypertension developing after coronary artery bypass surgery. *Circulation* 1982; **65**:1072-1077.

85. Kaplan JA, Jones EL: Vasodilator therapy during coronary artery surgery. Comparison of nitroglycerin and nitroprusside. *J Thorac Cardiovasc Surg* 1977; **77**:301-309.

86. Conti CR: Large vessel coronary vasospasm: Diagnosis, natural history and treatment. *Am J Cardiol* 1985; **55**:41B-49B.

87. Nussmeier NA, Slogoff S: Verapamil treatment of intraoperative coronary artery spasm. *Anesthesiology* 1985; **62**:539-541.

88. Miller RR, Awan NA, DeMaria AN, et al: Importance of maintaining systemic blood pressure during nitroglycerin administration for reducing ischemic injury in patients with coronary disease. *Am J Cardiol* 1977; **40**:504-508.

89. Dobell ARC, Jain AK: Catastrophic hemorrhage during redo sternotomy. *Ann Thorac Surg* 1984; **37**:273-278.

90. Keon WJ, Heggtveit HA, Leduc J: Perioperative myocardial infarction caused by atheroembolism. *J Thorac Cardiovasc Surg* 1982; **84**:849-855.

91. Grondin CM, Pomar JL, Herbert Y: Re-operation in patients with patent atherosclerotic coronary vein grafts. *J Thorac Cardiovasc Surg* 1984; **87**:379-385.

92. Chung F, Houston PL, Cheng DCH, et al: Calcium channel blockade does not offer adequate protection from perioperative myocardial ischemia. *Anesthesiology* 1988; **69**:343-347.

93. Heikkila H, Jalonen J, Laaksonen V: Metoprolol medication and coronary artery bypass grafting operation. *Acta Anaesthesiol Scand* 1984; **28**:677-682.

94. Stanley TH, deLange S, Boxcoe MJ: The influence of chronic preoperative propranolol therapy on cardiovascular dynamics and narcotic requirements during operation in patients with coronary artery disease. *Can Anaesth Soc J* 1982; **29**:319-324.

95. Miller RR, Olson HG, Amsterdam EA: Propranolol-withdrawal-rebound phenomenon. Exacerbation of coronary events after abrupt cessation of anti-anginal therapy. *N Engl J Med* 1975; **293**:416-418.

96. Roach GW, Moldenhauser CC, Hug CC, et al: Hemodynamic responses to fentanyl or diazepam–fentanyl anesthesia in patients on chronic nifedipine therapy. *Anesthesiology* 1984; **61**:A374.

97. Larach DD, Hensley FA, Pae LR, et al: A randomized study of diltiazem withdrawal prior to coronary artery bypass surgery. *Anesthesiology* 1985; **63**:A23.

98. Casson WR, Jones RM, Parsons RS: Nifedipine and cardiopulmonary bypass. *Anaesthesia* 1984; **39**:1197-1201.

99. Massagee JT, McIntyre RW, Kates RA, et al: Effects of preoperative calcium entry blocker therapy on alpha-adrenergic responsiveness in patients undergoing coronary revascularization. *Anesthesiology* 1987; **67**:485-491.

100. Kinzer JB, Lichtenthal PR, Wade LD: Loss of radial arterial trace during internal mammary artery dissection for coronary artery bypass graft surgery. *Anesth Analg* 1985; **64**:1134-1136.

101. Weintraub AC, Barash PG: Pro: A pulmonary catheter is indicated in all patients for coronary artery surgery. *J Cardiothorac Anesth* 1987; **1**:358-361.

102. Bashein G, Ivey TD: Con: A pulmonary artery catheter is not indicated for all coronary artery surgery. *J Cardiothorac Anesth* 1987; **1**:362-365.

103. Tuman KJ, McCarthy RJ, Spiess BD, et al: Effect of pulmonary artery catheterization on outcome in patients undergoing coronary artery surgery. *Anesthesiology* 1989; **70**:199-206.

104. Waller JL, Zaidan JR, Kaplan JA, Bauman DI: Hemodynamic responses to preoperative vascular cannulation in patients with coronary artery disease. *Anesthesiology* 1982; **56**:219-221.

105. Thomson IR, Mutch WAC, Culligan JD: Failure of intravenous nitroglycerin to prevent myocardial ischemia during fentanyl–pancuronium anesthesia. *Anesthesiology* 1984; **61**:385-393.

106. Gallagher JD, Moore RA, Jose AB, et al: Prophylactic nitroglycerin infusion during coronary artery bypass surgery. *Anesthesiology* 1986; **64**:785-789.

107. Slogoff S, Keats AS: Randomized trial of primary anesthetic agents on outcome of coronary artery bypass operations. *Anesthesiology* 1989; **70**:179-188.

108. Tuman KJ, McCarthy RJ, Spiess BD, et al: Does choice of anesthetic agent significantly affect outcome after coronary artery surgery. *Anesthesiology* 1989; **70**:189-198.

109. Mora CT, Dudek C, Torjman MC, et al: The effects of anesthetic technique on the hemodynamic response and recovery profile in coronary revascularization patients. *Anesth Analg* 1995; **81**:900-910.

110. Jain U, Body SC, Bellows W, et al: Multicenter study of target controlled infusion of propofol-sufentanil or sufentanil–midazolam for coronary artery bypass graft surgery. *Anesthesiology* 1996; **85**:522-535.

111. Rosow CE, Philbin DM, Keegan CR, Moss J: Hemodynamics and histamine release during induction with sufentanil or fentanyl. *Anesthesiology* 1984; **60**:489-491.

112. Stanley TH, Webster LR: Anesthesia requirements and cardiovascular effects of fentanyl-oxygen and fentanyl–diazepam–oxygen anesthesia in man. *Anesth Analg* 1978; **57**:411-426.

113. Sebel PS, Bovil JB: Cardiovascular effects of sufentanil anesthesia. *Anesth Analg* 1982; **61**:115-119.

114. Howie MB, McSweeney TD, Lingam Maschke SP: A comparison of fentanyl-O_2 and sufentanil-O_2 for cardiac anesthesia. *Anesth Analg* 1985; **64**:877–887.

115. deLange S, Boscoe MJ, Stanley TH, Pace N: Comparison of sufentanil-O_2 and fentanyl-O_2 for coronary artery surgery. *Anesthesiology* 1982; **56**:112–118.

116. Komatsu T, Shibutani K, Okamoto K, et al: Is sufentanil superior to fentanyl as an induction agent? *Anesthesiology* 1985; **63**:A378.

117. Sanford TJ, Smith NT, Dec-Silver H, Harrison WK: A comparison of morphine, fentanyl, and sufentanil anesthesia for cardiac surgery: Induction, emergence, and extubation. *Anesth Analg* 1986; **65**:259–266.

118. Savarese JJ, Lowenstein E: The name of the game: No anesthesia by cookbook. *Anesthesiology* 1985; **62**:703–705.

119. Thomson IR, Putnins CL: Adverse effects of pancuronium during high dose fentanyl anesthesia for coronary artery bypass grafting. *Anesthesiology* 1985; **62**:708–713.

120. Paulissan R, Mahdi M, Joseph N, et al: Hemodynamic responses to pancuronium and vecuronium during high dose fentanyl anesthesia for coronary artery bypass grafting. *Anesthesiology* 1986; **65**:A523.

121. Quintin L, Whalley DG, Wynands JE, et al: High dose fentanyl anesthesia with oxygen for aorto-coronary bypass surgery. *Can Anaesth Soc J* 1981; **28**:314–320.

122. Gravlee GP, Ramsey FM, Roy R, et al: Rapid administration of a narcotic and neuromuscular blocker: A hemodynamic comparison of fentanyl, sufentanyl, pancuronium, and vecuronium. *Anesth Analg* 1988; **67**:39–47.

123. McDonnell TE, Lefever GS, Zebrowski ME: Comparison of fentanyl-vecuronium and sufentanil-vecuronium inductions for coronary artery surgery. *Anesthesiology* 1986; **65**:A522.

124. Estafanous FG, Williams G, Sethna D, Starr N: Effects of preoperative Ca channel blockers, beta blockers, and pancuronium or vecuronium on hemodynamics of induction of anesthesia in patients with coronary disease receiving sufentanil anesthesia. *Anesthesiology* 1986; **65**:A524.

125. Gravlee GP, Ramsey FM, Roy R, Angert KC, Rogers AT, Pauca AL: Rapid administration of a narcotic and neuromuscular blocker: A hemodynamic comparison of fentanyl, sufentanyl, pancuronium, and vecuronium. *Anesth Analg* 1988; **67**:39–47.

126. Thomson IR, Bergstrom RG, Rosenbloom M, Meatherall RC: Premedication and high dose fentanyl anesthesia for myocardial revascularization: A comparison of lorazepam versus morphine-scopolamine. *Anesthesiology* 1988; **68**:194–200.

127. Thompson IR, MacAdams CL, Hudson RJ, et al: Drug interactions with sufentanil. Hemodynamic effects of premedication and muscle relaxants. *Anesthesiology* 1992; **76**:922–929.

128. Zahl K, Ellison N: Influence of beta-blockers on vecuronium/sufentanil or pancuronium/sufentanil combinations for rapid induction and intubation of cardiac surgical patients. *J Cardiothoracic Anesth* 1988; **2**:607–614.

129. Starr NJ, Sethna DH, Estafanous FG: Bradycardia and asystole following rapid administration of sufentanil with vecuronium. *Anesthesiology* 1986; **64**:521–523.

130. Goertz AW, Lindner KH, Seefelder C, et al: Effect of phenylephrine bolus administration on global left ventricular function in patients with coronary artery disease and patients with valvular aortic stenosis. *Anesthesiology* 1993; **78**:834–841.

131. Schwinn DA, Clements F, Hawkins E, Kates RA, Reves JG: Time course and hemodynamic effect of alpha 1 adrenergic administration in anesthetized patients. *Anesthesiology* 1987; **67**:A72.

132. Philbin DM, Roscow CE, Schneider RC, et al: Fentanyl and sufentanil anesthesia revisited: How much is enough? *Anesthesiology* 1990; **73**:5–11.

133. Tomicheck RC, Rosow CE, Philbin DA, et al: Diazepam-fentanyl interaction — Hemodynamic and hormonal effects in coronary artery surgery. *Anesth Analg* 1983; **62**:881–884.

134. Heikkila H, Jalonen J, Arola M: Midazolam as adjunct to high-dose fentanyl anesthesia for coronary artery bypass grafting operation. *Acta Anaesthesiol Scand* 1984; **28**:683–689.

135. Heikkila H, Jalonen J, Laaksonen V: Lorazepam and high-dose fentanyl anaesthesia: Effects on hemodynamics and oxygen transportation in patients undergoing coronary revascularization. *Acta Anaesthesiol Scand* 1984; **28**:357–361.

136. Balasaraswathi K, Kumar P, Rao TLK, El-Etr AA: Left ventricular end-diastolic pressure (LVEDP) as an index for nitrous oxide use during coronary artery bypass surgery. *Anesthesiology* 1981; **55**:708–709.

137. Meretoja OA, Takkunen O, Heikkila H: Hemodynamic response to nitrous oxide during high-dose fentanyl pancuronium anaesthesia. *Acta Anaesthesiol Scand* 1985; **29**:137–141.

138. Philbin DM, Foex P, Drummond G, et al: Postsystolic shortening of canine left ventricle supplied by stenotic coronary artery when nitrous oxide is added in the presence of narcotics. *Anesthesiology* 1985; **62**:166–174.

139. Cahalan MK, Praksah O, Rulf ENR, et al: Addition of nitrous oxide to fentanyl anesthesia does not induce myocardial ischemia in patients with ischemic heart disease. *Anesthesiology* 1987; **67**:925–929.

140. Schulte-Sasse U, Hess W, Tarnow J: Pulmonary vascular response to nitrous oxide in patients with normal and high pulmonary vascular resistance. *Anesthesiology* 1982; **57**:9–13.

141. Thompson IR, Bowering JB, Hudson RJ, et al: A comparison of desflurane and isoflurane in patients undergoing coronary artery surgery. *Anesthesiology* 1991; **75**:776–781.

142. Eger EI: Isoflurane: A review. *Anesthesiology* 1981; **55**:559–576.

143. Samuelson PN, Reves JG, Kirklin JK, et al: Comparison of sufentanil and enflurane-nitrous oxide anesthesia for myocardial revascularization. *Anesth Analg* 1986; **65**:217–226.

144. Velasco FT, Tarlow LS, Thomas SJ: Economic rationale for early extubation. *J Cardiothorac Vasc Anesth* 1995; **9**:2–9.

145. Arom KV, Emery RW, Peterson RJ, et al: Cost-effectiveness and predictors of early extubation. *Ann Thorac Surg* 1995; **60**:127–132.

146. Higgins TL: Safety issues regarding early extubation after coronary artery bypass surgery. *J Cardiothorac Vasc Anesth* 1995; **9**:24–29.

147. Wahr JA, Plunkett JJ, Ramsay JG, et al: Cardiovascular responses during sedation after coronary revascularization. Incidence of myocardial ischemia and hemodynamic episodes with propofol versus midazolam. *Anesthesiology* 1996; **84**:1350–1360.

148. Waterman PM, Bjerke R: Rapid sequence induction in patients with severe ventricular dysfunction. *J Cardiothorac Anesth* 1988; **2**:602–606.

149. Butterworth JF, Bean E, Royster RL: Sufentanil is preferable to etomidate during rapid-sequence anesthesia induction for aortocoronary bypass surgery. *J Cardiothorac Anesth* 1989; **3**:396–400.

150. De Hert SG, Rodrigus IE, Haenen LR, et al: Recovery of systolic and diastolic left ventricular function early after cardiopulmonary bypass. *Anesthesiology* 1996; **85**:1063–1075.

151. McKenney PA, Apstein CS, Mendes LA, et al: Increased left ventricular diastolic chamber stiffness immediately after coronary artery bypass surgery. *J Am Coll Cardiol* 1994; **24**:1189–1194.

152. Gorcsan J, Gasior TA, Mandarino WA, et al: Assessment of immediate effects of cardiopulmonary bypass on left ventricular performance by on-line pressure-area relations. *Circulation* 1994; **89**:180–190.

153. Breisblatt WM, Stein KL, Wolfe CJ, et al: Acute myocardial dysfunction and recovery: A common occurrence after coronary bypass surgery. *J Am Coll Cardiol* 1990; **15**:1261–1269.

154. Mangano DT: Biventricular function after myocardial revascularization: Deterioration and recovery patterns during the first 24 hours. *Anesthesiology* 1985; **62**:571–577.

155. Skaravan K, Graedel E, Hasse J, et al: Coronary artery spasm after coronary artery bypass surgery. *Anesthesiology* 1984; **61**:323-327.

156. Lemmer JH, Kirsh MM: Coronary artery spasm following coronary artery surgery. *Ann Thorac Surg* 1988; **46**:108-115.

157. DiNardo JA, Bert A, Schwartz MJ, et al: Effects of vasoactive drugs on flows through left internal mammary artery and saphenous vein grafts in man. *J Thorac Cardiovasc Surg* 1991; **102**:730-735.

158. Jett GK, Arcidi JM, Dorsey LMA, et al: Vasoactive drug effects on blood flow in internal mammary artery and saphenous vein grafts. *J Thorac Cardiovasc Surg* 1987; **94**:2-11.

159. Beavis RE, Mullany CJ, Cronin KD, et al: An experimental in vivo study of canine internal mammary artery and its response to vasoactive drugs. *J Thorac Cardiovasc Surg* 1988; **95**:1058-1066.

160. Poyster RL, Butterworth JF 4th, Prough DS, et al: Preoperative and intraoperative predictors of inotropic support and long-term outcome in patients having coronary artery bypass grafting. *Anesth Analg* 1991; **72**:729-736.

161. Smiley RM, Pantuck CB, Chadburn A, et al: Down-regulation and desesitization of the β-adrenergic receptor system of human lymphocytes after cardiac surgery. *Anesth Analg* 1993; **77**:653-661.

162. Schranz D, Droege A, Broede A, et al: Uncoupling of human cariac beta-adrenoceptors during cardiopulmonary bypass with cardioplegic cardiac arrest. *Circulation* 1993; **87**:422-426.

163. Leier CV, Heban PT, Huss P, et al: Comparative systemic and regional hemodynamic effects of dopamine and dobutamine in patients with cardiomyopathic heart failure. *Circulation* 1978; **58**:466-475.

164. Makabali C, Weil MH, Henning RJ: Dobutamine and other sympathomimetic drugs for the treatment of low cardiac output failure. *Sem Anesth* 1982; **1**:62-69.

165. Furman WR, Summer WR, Kennedy TP, Sylvester JT: Comparison of the effects of dobutamine dopamine and isoproterenol on hypoxic pulmonary vasoconstriction in the pig. *Crit Care Med* 1982; **10**:371-374.

166. Fowler MB, Alderman EL, Oesterle SN: Dobutamine and dopamine after cardiac surgery: Greater augmentation of myocardial blood flow with dobutamine. *Circulation* 1985; **70**(suppl 1):105-111.

167. Amin DK, Shah PK, Shellock FG: Comparative hemodynamic effects of intravenous dobutamine and MDL-17,043, a new cardioactive drug in severe congestive heart failure. *Am Heart J* 1985; **109**:91-98.

168. Benoti JR, McCue JE, Alpert JS: Comparative vasoactive therapy for heart failure. *Am J Cardiol* 1985; **56**:19B-24B.

169. Weiner N: Norepinephrine, epinephrine, and the sympathomimetic amines, in Gilman AG, Goodman LS, Gilman A (eds): *The Pharmacological Basis of Therapeutics.* 6th ed. New York, Macmillan, 1980.

170. Butterworth JF 4th, Prielipp RC, Royster RL, et al: Dobutamine increases heart rate more than epinephrine in patients recovering from aortocoronary bypass surgery. *J Cardiothorac Vasc Anesth* 1992; **6**:535-541.

171. Mancini D, LeJemtel T, Sonnenblick E: Intravenous use of amrinone for treatment of the failing heart. *Am J Cardiol* 1985; **56**:8B-15B.

172. Baim DS: Effects of amrinone on myocardial energetics in severe congestive heart failure. *Am J Cardiol* 1985; **56**:16B-18B.

173. Goenen M, Pedemonte O, Baele P, Col J: Amrinone in the management of low cardiac output after open heart surgery. *Am J Cardiol* 1985; **56**:33B-38B.

174. Gage J, Rutman H, Lucido D, LeJemtel T: Additive effects of dobutamine and amrinone on myocardial contractility and ventricular performance in patients with severe congestive heart failure. *Circulation* 1986; **74**(suppl 2):367-373.

175. Royster RL, Butterworth JF 4th, Prielipp RC, et al: Combined inotropic effects of amrinone and epinephrine after cardiopulmonary bypass in humans. *Anesth Analg* 1993; **77**:662-672.

176. Butterworth JF 4th: Use of amrinone in cardiac surgery. *J Cardiothorac Vasc Anesth* 1993; **7**:1-7.

177. Butterworth JF 4th, Royster RL, Prielipp RC, et al: Amrinone in cardiac surgical patients with left-ventricular dysfunction. A prospective, randomized placebo-controlled trial. *Chest* 1993; **104**:1660-1667.

178. Kikura M, Lee MK, Safon RA, et al: The effect of milrinone on platelets in patients undergoing cardiac surgery. *Anesth Analg* 1995; **81**:44-48.

179. Sherry KM, Locke TJ: Use of milrinone in cardiac surgical patients. *Cardiovasc Drugs Ther* 1993; **7**:671-675.

180. Feneck RO, the European Milrinone Multicentre Trial Group: Intravenous milrinone following cardiac surgery: I. Effects of bolus infusion followed by variable dose maintenance infusion. *J Cardiothorac Vasc Anesth* 1992; **6**:554-562.

181. Feneck RO, the European Milrinone Multicentre Trial Group: Intravenous milrinone following cardiac surgery: II. Influence of baseline hemodynamics and patient factors on theraputic response. *J Cardiothorac Vasc Anesth* 1992; **6**:563-567.

182. Feneck RO: Milrinone and postoperative pulmonary hypertension. *J Cardiothorac Vasc Anesth* 1993; **7**:21-23.

183. Butterworth JF, Hines RL, Royster RL, et al: A pharmacodynamic evaluation of milrinone in adults undergoing cardiac surgery. *Anesth Analg* 1995; **81**:783-792.

184. Bailey JM, Levy JH, Kikura M, et al: Pharmacokinetics of intravenous milrinone in patients undergoing cardiac surgery. *Anesthesiology* 1994; **81**:616-622.

185. Johnston WE, Robertie PG, Butterworth JF, et al: Is calcium or ephedrine superior to placebo for emergence from cardiopulmonary bypass? *J Cardiothorac Vasc Anesth* 1992; **6**:528-534.

186. Royster RL, Butterworth JF 4th, et al: A randomized, blinded, placebo-controlled evaluation of calcium chloride and epinephrine for inotropic support after emergence from cardiopulmonary bypass. *Anesth Analg* 1992; **74**:3-13.

187. Zaloga GP, Strickland RA, Butterworth JF 4th, et al: Calcium attenuates epinephrine's β-adrenergic effects in postoperative heart surgery patients. *Circulation* 1990; **81**:196-200.

188. Butterworth JF 4th, Zaloga GP, Prielipp RC, et al: Calcium inhibits the cardiac stimulating properties of dobutamine but not of amrinone. *Chest* 1992; **101**:174-180.

189. Abernethy WB, Butterworth JF 4th, Prielipp RC, et al: Calcium entry attenuates adenylyl cyclase activity. A possible mechanism for calcium-induced catecholamine resistance. *Chest* 1995; **107**:1420-1425.

190. Robertie PG, Butterworth JF 4th, Royster RL, et al: Normal parathyroid hormone responses to hypocalcemia during cardiopulmonary bypass. *Anesthesiology* 1991; **75**:43-48.

Anesthesia for Valve Replacement in Patients With Acquired Valvular Heart Disease

James A. DiNardo

This chapter deals with four valvular heart lesions: aortic stenosis (AS), aortic regurgitation (AR), mitral stenosis (MS), and mitral regurgitation (MR). When this chapter is read in its entirety, the reader will notice some repetition in the sections on Anesthetic Technique. This was done intentionally so that the section on each lesion could be referred to independently. Rational management of each lesion depends on systematic analysis of all the determinants of hemodynamic function.

Transesophageal echocardiography (TEE) is a valuable tool in managing patients with valvular heart disease for valve replacement and repair. Details of the use of TEE for these patients is discussed in Chapter 3.

A modification of a scheme originally proposed by Chambers[1] will be used to analyze each lesion:

1. *Pathophysiology and adaptation.* In this section, ventricular loading will be considered, as well as acute versus chronic and mechanical versus functional lesions.

   The nature of left ventricular loading. Mitral regurgitation and aortic regurgitation present the left ventricle with volume overload, whereas aortic stenosis results in left ventricular pressure overload. Mitral stenosis is unique in that it results in left ventricular volume underload secondary to compromise of diastolic filling.

   Acute versus chronic lesions. The hemodynamic sequelae of acute valvular lesions generally are more severe than where gradual adaptation has occurred.

   Mechanical versus functional lesions. Mechanical valvular lesions are those in which the valve leaflets or supporting structures are damaged. These lesions may be chronic, as in calcification of aortic and mitral valves, or acute, as in papillary muscle rupture or bacterial endocarditis. Functional lesions are those in which the valve apparatus is not damaged but where valve function is compromised acutely and reversibly. Examples include acute ventricular dilation leading to mitral regurgitation, papillary muscle dysfunction leading to mitral regurgitation, and proximal aortic dissection leading to aortic regurgitation.

2. *Ventricular diastolic function and the atrial transport mechanism.* Atrial transport via sinus rhythm is important for lesions in which diastolic function is impaired.

3. *Myocardial oxygen balance.* It is necessary to be familiar with the unique relationship between myocardial oxygen supply and demand in each valve lesion.

4. *Left ventricular systolic function.* Careful assessment of ventricular systolic function is necessary to identify high-risk patients and to screen for patients who are unlikely to have improved ventricular function after valve replace-

ment. The anesthetic management of patients with valvular heart disease and poor ventricular function is a demanding challenge.

5. *Right ventricular function and the pulmonary vasculature.* Pulmonary artery hypertension may exist secondary to the primary valve lesion. It is important to know the extent of the pulmonary artery hypertension because this will affect right ventricular function. It also is necessary to know whether the pulmonary artery hypertension is likely to be reversible after surgery.

6. *Effect of heart rate alterations on hemodynamics.* Small alterations in heart rate may profoundly affect the hemodynamics of a particular lesion. For example, in aortic regurgitation bradycardia may drastically increase the regurgitant fraction.

7. *Effect of afterload alterations on hemodynamics.* Alterations in afterload may worsen or improve the hemodynamics of a particular lesion. For example, in mitral regurgitation, an increase in the impedance to ejection via the aorta may dramatically increase the regurgitant fraction.

■ AORTIC STENOSIS

Isolated AS in adults is more common in males and almost always is nonrheumatic in origin. It usually is degenerative and thus mechanical in nature. The valve cusps are partially immobilized by calcific deposits developing on the aortic surface of the valve. The flexion lines at the base of the valve and the valve cusps are involved; there is little or no involvement of the commissures. The result is progressive stenosis of the aortic valve orifice. Congenitally bicuspid valves develop the same changes seen in the calcific degeneration of tricuspid aortic valves. However, secondary to the turbulent flow across the bicuspid orifice, these changes occur several decades earlier. Atherosclerotic, rheumatoid, and ochronotic processes are other less common causes of isolated AS in adults.

Rheumatic AS is mechanical in nature but differs in several aspects from degenerative AS. In rheumatic AS, the valve commissures are fused such that aortic valve leaflet excursion is limited. The result is a stenotic valve orifice. Isolated aortic stenosis is rare; most of these patients exhibit some degree of aortic regurgitation as well. In addition, some degree of mitral valve involvement is also common.

Pathophysiology and Adaptation

Aortic stenosis is a chronic left ventricular pressure overload lesion. The natural history of the lesion is a gradual reduction in the aortic valve area from the nor-

mal 2.6 to 3.5 cm² to less than 1.0 cm² occurring over five to six decades. Replacement generally is considered before the aortic valve area <0.7 cm² or the peak systolic pressure gradient >50 mm Hg. Thus, the left ventricle is faced with a gradual increase in the impedance to ejection, and a pressure gradient develops across the valve such that peak intraventricular pressure exceeds aortic systolic pressure. Under these circumstances, left ventricular wall stress (which equals $Pr/2h$) is greatly elevated (P = peak intraventricular pressure, r = inner ventricular radius, and h = wall thickness). This stimulus results in concentric ventricular hypertrophy or wall thickening. The degree of thickening parallels the increased ventricular pressure demands. The result is normalization of ventricular wall stress despite greatly elevated peak ventricular pressure (*see* Fig. 5-1). This normalization of wall stress allows ejection fraction (EF) to be maintained despite the high impedance to ejection found in critical aortic stenosis.[2,3] Eventually, the valve orifice narrows to the point at which stroke volume and EF can no longer be maintained (*see* Fig. 5-2).

Ventricular Diastolic Function and the Atrial Transport Mechanism

The concentric hypertrophy that accompanies AS is not without hemodynamic consequences. Concentric hypertrophy results in reduced ventricular compliance (*see* Chapter 2). One result is compromise of early diastolic filling of the ventricle.[4] However, even for patients with severe aortic stenosis, normal end-diastolic volumes can be obtained with the well-timed atrial systole present in sinus rhythm.[4,5] In these patients, atrial systole contributes 29% of the left ventricular end-diastolic volume (LVEDV), whereas in normal patients, it contributes 20%.[4] This late diastolic filling occurs on the steep portion of the diastolic pressure–volume curve. The well-timed atrial systole allows this late diastolic filling to occur with minimal elevation in mean left atrial pressure (*see* Chapter 2). With acute loss of atrial systole, normal end-diastolic volume can only be maintained by increasing mean left atrial pressure to equal or exceed left ventricular end-diastolic pressure. When compliance is poor, a normal LVEDV may occur at a left ventricular end-diastolic pressure in excess of 25 mm Hg. Obviously, an acute increase in mean left atrial pressure is prohibitive because it results in severe pulmonary congestion. With a lower mean left atrial pressure, LVEDV and stroke volume will be diminished.

Diminished ventricular compliance also limits the use of preload reserve. With the ventricle operating on the steep portion of its diastolic pressure–volume curve, incremental increases in end-diastolic volume result in prohibitive increases in end-diastolic pressure. Even with

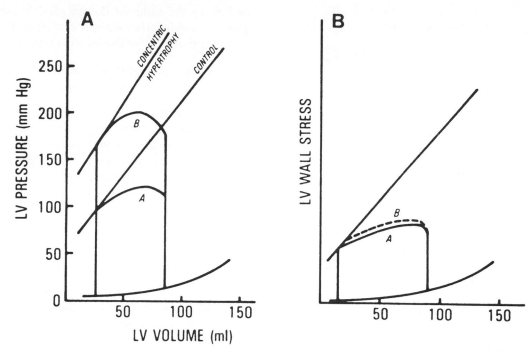

FIGURE 5–1. A. Left ventricular pressure–volume loops demonstrating adaptation to chronic pressure overload. Loop A represents normal ventricle before development of aortic stenosis. Loop B represents the same ventricle after prolonged exposure to elevated afterload and development of concentric hypertrophy. End-systolic and end-diastolic volumes in loop B are unchanged from those in loop A, but left ventricular systolic pressure is greatly elevated. **B.** The same loops illustrated in **A** are shown again here, except that wall stress is plotted against volume. It is obvious that elevated ventricular systolic pressure seen in loop A does not result in elevated wall stress compared with loop B. Development of concentric hypertrophy allows normalization of wall stress in face of chronically elevated left ventricular systolic pressure. *(Reprinted with permission from: the American College of Cardiology. J Am Coll Cardiol 1985; **5**:811–826.)*

preserved atrial systole, it may be possible to augment preload only with an elevation of mean left atrial pressure above 20 to 25 mm Hg with subsequent pulmonary congestion. The result is that stroke volume can be augmented minimally by increases in preload. Thus, for a given contractile state, stroke volume is nearly fixed.

Myocardial Oxygen Balance

Several factors are responsible for the unique myocardial oxygen supply demand imbalance that places the subendocardium at particular risk in AS.[6,7] Myocardial oxygen consumption is increased by:

1. The increased mass of myocardium that must be supplied with oxygen.
2. The demands of left ventricular pressure work, which is much more energy-consumptive than volume work.[8] A large portion of the total myocardial workload is devoted to the isovolumic contraction phase because of the high intraventricular pressures necessary to commence the ejection phase (*see* Fig. 5–1). Recall that the isovolumic contraction phase is a very energy-consumptive process.
3. The prolonged ejection phase.

Myocardial oxygen delivery is compromised by:

1. Elevated left ventricular end-diastolic pressure secondary to diminished ventricular compliance.
2. An aortic diastolic pressure that is low relative to the elevated left ventricular end-diastolic pressure.
3. Diminished diastolic coronary perfusion time secondary to the prolonged ejection phase.
4. Compression of subendocardial vessels by hypertrophied myocardium.
5. Absence of any systolic coronary perfusion because left ventricular systolic pressure greatly exceeds aortic systolic pressure.

This combination of factors explains why 30% of patients with critical AS experience angina in the absence of significant coronary artery disease.[9]

Left Ventricular Systolic Function

Generally speaking, global ventricular function as determined by EF is well preserved in aortic stenosis. The mechanism for depressed EF in patients with severe AS is not entirely clear. Concentric hypertrophy inadequate to normalize wall stress will result in excessive afterload and reduced EF; subendocardial ischemia may play a role as well.[10] In patients without myocardial infarction,

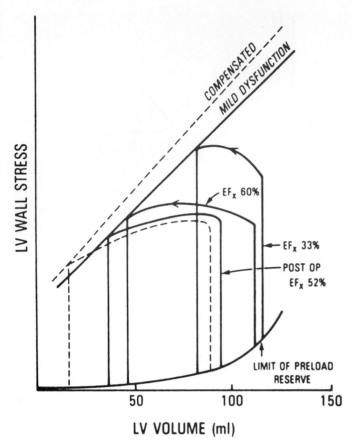

FIGURE 5–2. Left ventricular wall stress–volume loops in progressive AS. Dotted loop represents ventricle with concentric hypertrophy and preserved systolic function. As systolic dysfunction develops, SV and EF can be maintained by making use of the preload reserve (EF_x 60%). Further progression of systolic dysfunction results in exhaustion of preload reserve. At this point further progression of AS results in afterload mismatch and reduction in SV and EF (EF_x 33%). Surgical therapy for replacement of stenotic aortic valve results in reduction in afterload, the abolition of afterload mismatch, and the ability of ventricle to deliver nearly normal SV and EF despite the presence of systolic dysfunction (EF_x 52%). (*Reprinted with permission from: the American College of Cardiology.* J Am Coll Cardiol *1985;* **5**:811–826.)

irreversible myocardial damage is relatively uncommon, and there is remarkable improvement in EF after uncomplicated aortic valve replacement.[11] Most patients with severely depressed function preoperatively exhibit a normal EF postoperatively.[12]

In patients with systolic dysfunction, there is a progressive increase in LVEDV so that stroke volume and EF are maintained through use of preload reserve (*see* Fig. 5–2). Reduced ventricular compliance limits the increase in end-diastolic volume and pressure that can be tolerated without pulmonary congestion. With severe systolic dysfunction, the maximal wall stress that the ventricle can generate is severely limited. In this situation, afterload mismatch may limit maintenance of stroke volume and EF despite use of preload reserve. In these patients, the aortic valve gradient may be low sec-

ondary to the reduced flow across the stenotic valve. The calculated valve area will give a much better indication of the severity of the stenosis (*see* Chapter 2).

Right Ventricular Function and the Pulmonary Vasculature

Right ventricular function is not directly affected by severe AS until secondary pulmonary artery hypertension intercedes. In patients with severe AS and an EF less than 50%, a reduced stroke volume and cardiac output is maintained at the expense of elevated left atrial and pulmonary artery pressures. Pulmonary artery pressures begin to rise through passive pulmonary venous congestion when left atrial pressures exceed 18 mm Hg.[13] Ultimately, pulmonary artery fibroelastosis develops and secondary pulmonary artery hypertension follows. When the mean pulmonary artery pressure gradually rises to exceed 50 mm Hg, the right ventricle, which normally functions with low impedance to ejection, begins to fail.[14] Patients with critical AS and an EF less than 40% have very low cardiac outputs maintained by a gradual increase in mean left atrial pressure to 25 to 30 mm Hg, with mean pulmonary artery pressure in excess of 50 mm Hg. These patients may have clinical evidence of right ventricular failure with peripheral edema and liver congestion.

Effect of Heart Rate Alterations on Hemodynamics

Increases in heart rate normally result in a marked decrease in the length of diastole, whereas the length of systole remains much more constant[15] (*see* Fig. 5–3). Over the heart rate range of 50 to 110 beats per minute, the length of systole decreases from 441 to 315 msec, whereas the length of diastole decreases from 759 to 230 msec. Tachycardia in patients with AS is detrimental because, although there is adequate time in systole to allow ejection across the stenotic valve, diastolic time and subendocardial perfusion are drastically reduced.

Bradycardia in these patients is detrimental as well. Recall that the valve gradient increases as the square of the flow across the valve (*see* Chapter 2). If cardiac output is to be maintained at a reduced heart rate, stroke volume or the flow across the aortic valve will have to increase and the gradient will increase by the square of the flow. Figure 5–4 demonstrates that for a given cardiac output, progressive decreases in heart rate result in large increases in the transvalvular gradient. With aortic valve areas less than 0.5 cm², gradients in excess of 150 mm Hg are possible, even with low normal stroke volumes.[16] Because the left ventricle is capable of generating peak pressures in the range of 250 to 300 mm Hg,[16,17] maximal intraventricular pressures are needed to maintain a systolic blood pressure greater than 100

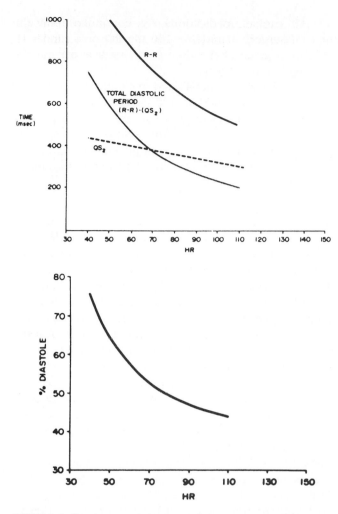

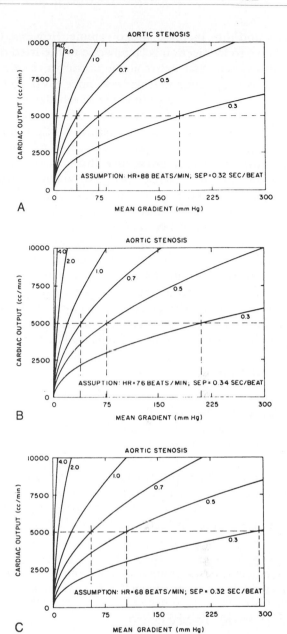

FIGURE 5–3. Top. Increases in heart rate cause decreases in length of each cardiac cycle (R-R interval). Decreases in length of systole (QS_2) with increases in heart rate are far less dramatic than decreases in the length of diastole (R-R – QS_2). **Bottom.** Percent of each cardiac cycle (R-R interval) spent in diastole at various heart rates. Small changes in heart rate are seen to cause large decreases in percent of time spent in diastole. *From: Boudoulas H: Changes in diastolic time with various pharmacologic agents.* Circulation *1979;* **60:***165. Reprinted with permission.)*

FIGURE 5–4. Relationship of heart rate, cardiac output, aortic valve area, and systolic pressure gradient across aortic valve is illustrated for patients with AS. Cardiac output is plotted against the systolic pressure gradient for aortic valve areas ranging from 0.3 to 4.0 cm². Plot **A** illustrates these relationships for heart rate of 88 bpm and systolic ejection period (SEP) of 0.32 sec/beat. Plot **B** illustrates these relationships for heart rate of 76 bpm and SEP of 0.34 sec/beat. Plot **C** illustrates these relationships for heart rate of 68 bpm and SEP of 0.32 sec/beat.

Clearly, for a given cardiac output and heart rate, systolic pressure gradient increases as aortic valve area decreases. Furthermore, for a given cardiac output and aortic valve area, systolic pressure gradient increases as heart rate decreases. Increases in heart rate in the range examined here have little effect on length of SEP. Therefore, for cardiac output to remain constant as heart rate decreases, larger SV must be ejected across stenotic aortic valve in relatively constant time period. This results in larger systolic pressure gradient. *(From: Grossman W:* Cardiac Catheterization and Angiography. *3rd ed. Philadelphia, Lea & Febiger, 1986, p 149.)*

mm Hg. In this setting, bradycardia with an increase in the gradient will result in systemic hypotension. The result is poor subendocardial perfusion and ischemia. In addition, diminished diastolic compliance may prohibit the increase in end-diastolic volume necessary to augment stroke volume in bradycardic states without prohibitive increases in mean left atrial pressure.

Effect of Afterload Alterations on Hemodynamics

Contrary to what might be expected, decreasing afterload by reducing systemic vascular resistance does not always have a beneficial effect for patients with AS. A reduction in afterload should enhance left ventricular ejection and thus increase stroke volume. However, the impedance to LV ejection is largely due to the fixed outflow obstruction that exists at the aortic valve orifice. Reductions in systemic vascular resistance (SVR) will be offset by the large increases in the transvalvular gradient that accompany increased flow across the stenotic valve orifice. Thus, SVR reduction results in very little augmentation of cardiac output in patients with significant AS. Furthermore, agents used to reduce afterload, such as nitroprusside and hydralazine, decrease aortic diastolic pressure and compromise the tenuous subendocardial blood flow in these patients. Increases in afterload result in an elevation of left ventricular end-diastolic volume and pressure with maintenance of stroke volume in patients with good ventricular function and some preload reserve.[3] In patients with poor ventricular function, in whom preload reserve is exhausted to maintain basal cardiac output demands, further increases in afterload result in a progressive decline in stroke volume and EF secondary to afterload mismatch[3] (*see* Fig. 5–2).

Critical Aortic Stenosis

The term "critical aortic stenosis" commonly is used in association with aortic valve disease. Typically, it is used to describe patients with aortic valve areas <0.7 cm^2 or 0.5 cm^2/m^2. In truth, critical aortic stenosis should be used to describe a specific pathophysiologic state. Critical aortic stenosis exists when preload reserve is exhausted and ejection fraction is reduced such that further reductions in aortic valve area will produce increased pulmonary vascular congestion or further reductions in stroke volume. It is conceivable that critical aortic stenosis can exist with a larger valve area in patients with severe concomitant diastolic or systolic dysfunction or in patients who are unable to be maintained in sinus rhythm.

Anesthetic Technique

Goals

1. Sinus rhythm is essential.
2. Maintain heart rate at 70 to 90 bpm.
3. Maintain a pulmonary capillary wedge pressure (PCWP) A-wave pressure high enough to guarantee adequate LVEDV.
4. Maintain afterload; decreases in diastolic blood pressure are to be avoided.
5. Maintain contractility.

Premedication

Patients with preserved LV function are premedicated with morphine sulfate 0.1 mg/kg IM, and lorazepam 1 to 2 mg PO approximately 1.5 hours before scheduled incision time. Supplemental O$_2$ with a face mask is begun at the time of premedication.

All cardiac medications are continued until the time of surgery. Ranitidine 150 mg PO or a similar H$_2$ blocker is given at the time of premedication and the evening before surgery.

For elderly or debilitated patients, patients with poor ventricular function, and patients with poor pulmonary function, smaller doses are used. Err on the side of undermedicating these patients and reassuring them preoperatively. If necessary, supplemental premedication can be administered when the patient is seen in the operating room (OR) holding area.

Preinduction

All patients should have two large-bore peripheral IV lines (14 gauge). Alternatively, if peripheral IV access is poor, a peripheral IV suitable for induction can be started and a large-bore double-lumen (16- or 14-gauge) central venous line can be placed at the same time as the pulmonary artery catheter (*see* Chapter 3). ECG monitoring should allow assessment of V$_5$, I, II, III, aVR, aVL, and aVF. Baseline recording of all seven leads should be obtained for comparative purposes. Normally, two leads (II and V$_5$) are monitored simultaneously intraoperatively.

A radial artery catheter is placed with local anesthesia and adequate sedation before induction of anesthesia. A pulmonary artery catheter can be placed before or after induction of anesthesia. All of the equipment and medications necessary for treatment of dysrythmias are available before placement of the pulmonary artery catheter. In particular, a defibrillator with demonstrated consistent synchronization to the patient's electrocardiogram (ECG) signal must be in the room if loss of sinus rhythm requires immediate cardioversion. Placement of the pulmonary artery catheter before induction allows preload and afterload to be optimized before induction of anesthesia.

The presence of compensatory left ventricular concentric hypertrophy will cause left ventricular compliance to be considerably less than right ventricular compliance. This will cause the right atrial pressure to greatly underestimate the PCWP and LVEDP. Therefore, the peak A-wave pressure of the PCWP trace is used. The LVEDP measured at the time of cardiac catheterization is a useful guide as to the PCWP that will be necessary to obtain the end-diastolic volume that will optimize stroke volume. In general, for patients with significant AS, a PCWP A-wave pressure of 15 to 20 mm Hg and often as high as 25 mm Hg is needed. In the absence of right ventricular failure, the mean right atrial pressure will be in the 5 to 8 mm Hg range. If necessary, volume infusion is used before induction to optimize LVEDV.

Induction and Maintenance

Generally, 50 to 75 μg/kg of fentanyl or 10 to 15 μg/kg of sufentanil can be used as the primary anesthetic for induction and maintenance before cardiopulmonary bypass. These agents are chosen because they have no effects on myocardial contractility and cause a reduction in peripheral vascular resistance only through a diminution in central sympathetic tone.[18,19] Compared with fentanyl, sufentanil is more likely to cause a fall in mean arterial pressure secondary to a reduced peripheral vascular resistance in patients with valvular heart disease.[20,21] On the other hand, patients with valvular heart disease receiving sufentanil in these doses are less likely to require supplemental anesthesia or vasodilator therapy for skin incision, sternotomy, sternal spread, or aortic manipulation.[20,21]

After several minutes of preoxygenation and with the patient breathing 100% oxygen, induction begins with an infusion of fentanyl 500 µg/min or sufentanil 100 µg/min over 5 to 10 minutes. A system of graded stimulation is used to individualize the narcotic dose for each patient. Compared with patients with coronary artery disease, patients with valvular heart disease have a lower narcotic requirement to achieve unconsciousness.[21] This is probably due to a lower cardiac output with a relative greater distribution of output to the brain and spinal cord.[21] After loss of consciousness, the hemodynamic response to insertion of an oral airway followed by insertion of a urinary catheter is used to gauge the need for additional narcotic to blunt the hemodynamic response to tracheal intubation. Laryngoscopy is performed carefully and should not be prolonged. If an upward trend in heart rate or blood pressure is noted as laryngoscopy commences, laryngoscopy should be terminated and additional narcotic should be titrated. If there is poor visualization of the larynx, laryngoscopy should be terminated and intubating conditions improved by changing head position, using a stylet, or changing blades. This approach will help prevent long stimulating larnygoscopies that compromise hemodynammics. If the entire narcotic dose is not used for induction, the remainder is infused slowly in anticipation of the skin incision. A TEE probe (*see* Chapter 3) is placed after tracheal intubation and verification of tube position.

To optimize heart rate, the choice of muscle relaxant is critical (*see* Chapter 4). For patients who are poorly beta blocked and for those not taking beta blockers, fentanyl or sufentanil in combination with vecuronium is a good choice. Bradycardia is rare in patients who are not beta blocked, and tachycardia secondary to pancuronium is avoided. Vecuronium 0.02 mg/kg or cis-atracurium 0.04 mg/kg is administered approximately 1 to 2 minutes before starting the narcotic infusion. As the patient loses consciousness, the remainder of the total dose of 0.1 mg/kg of vecuronium or 0.2 mg/kg of cis-atracurium is administered and controlled ventilation with 100% O_2 is initiated. For patients who are well beta blocked, fentanyl or sufentanil in combination with pan-

curonium is the best choice. The incidence of bradycardia in these patients when sufentanil or fentanyl is used in combination with vecuronium or cis-atracurium makes them a poor choice. Pancuronium 0.02 mg/kg is administered approximately 1 to 2 minutes before starting the narcotic infusion. As the patient loses consciousness, the remainder of the 0.1 mg/kg dose is administered and controlled ventilation is initiated. These regimes minimize the risk of narcotic-induced rigidity without undue stress to the patient.

If bradycardia with hemodynamic compromise occurs, it must be treated promptly. A small dose of pancuronium (1 to 3 mg) is often effective if vecuronium has been used. Atropine is not a good choice for two reasons: its effect on heart rate, even in small doses (0.2 mg), is unpredictable and a tachycardia may be initiated by larger doses. Atropine, unlike beta-1-adrenergic agents, increases heart rate without any reduction in the duration of systole. Thus, for equal increases in heart rate, atropine will cause a greater reduction in the duration of diastole and will compromise subendocardial perfusion to a greater degree than a beta-1-adrenergic agent. Ephedrine (a direct- and indirect-acting beta and alpha agonist) 5 mg is a reliable agent to increase heart rate without compromising diastole. In addition, the augmentation in diastolic blood pressure obtained is beneficial when hypotension accompanies bradycardia.

Tachycardia must be treated aggressively to avoid subendocardial ischemia and hemodynamic compromise. The first strategy should be to terminate any noxious stimuli and increase the depth of anesthesia when necessary. Propranolol in increments of 0.5 mg is given for two to three doses to get the heart rate in the desired range. If this fails, the incremental dose can be increased to 1.0 mg. For patients with poor ventricular function, doses greater than 0.1 mg/kg over less than a 1-hour period must be used with caution to avoid compromise of systolic function. In some instances, the ultra-short-acting beta blocker esmolol may be useful. Esmolol has an elimination half-life of 9 minutes due to metabolism by red cell esterases and is relatively beta-1-selective. Esmolol is started with a bolus of 0.5 mg/kg given over several minutes followed by an infusion of 50 µg/kg/min and titrated up to 300 µg/kg/min as necessary. Esmolol is useful for patients with poor ventricular function or bronchospastic disease because, if it is not tolerated, therapy can be terminated quickly. Furthermore, unlike longer-acting beta blockers, esmolol can be used aggressively in the pre-CPB period without fear that it will compromise termination of CPB.

If hypotension due to reduced peripheral vascular resistance occurs during the narcotic infusion, the infusion should be stopped. Small doses of phenylephrine (40 to 120 µg) and volume infusion to increase preload to preinduction levels usually will correct the problem.

TEE is very useful at this point. If TEE reveals a dilated, hypokinetic LV or if the patient fails to respond with a prompt increase in aortic blood pressure, an inotropic agent should be started to avoid a downward spiral of hypotension-initiating subendocardial ischemia, depressed systolic function, and further hypotension. Dobutamine 5 to 10 μg/kg/min is a reasonable choice because it is unlikely to cause tachycardia. IV nitroglycerin should be started to treat the elevated PCWP that inevitably accompanies this downward spiral. The infusion can be started at 0.15 to 0.3 μg/kg/min and titrated as necessary (*see* Chapter 4).

If surgical stimulation (skin incision, sternotomy, sternal spreading, or aortic manipulation) produces hypertension, additional doses of sufentanil (1 to 5 μg/kg) or fentanyl (5 to 25 μg/kg) may be necessary. Recent data call this practice into question. After a patient has received high doses of sufentanil (10 to 30 μg/kg) or fentanyl (50 to 100 μg/kg), administration of an additional agent as an infusion or a bolus will not reliably blunt the hemodynamic response to noxious stimuli.[22] If this fails to control the hypertension, the use of additional agents will be necessary. Vasodilation with sodium nitroprusside can be titrated easily and terminated quickly. This makes it an ideal choice for treatment of transient elevations in peripheral vascular resistance during high-dose narcotic anesthesia. Although relatively large doses of nitroglycerin may be needed to control systemic hypertension, nitroglycerin is a better choice than nitroprusside for cases in which myocardial ischemia exists (*see* Chapter 4).

It may also become necessary to supplement narcotic anesthesia with additional anesthetic agents:

1. Benzodiazepines. Diazepam, midazolam, and lorazepam administered in conjunction with fentanyl or sufentanil have been implicated in causing decreases in peripheral vascular resistance with subsequent hypotension.[23-26] Therefore, they must be titrated with caution. Midazolam in increments of 1 to 2 mg or lorazepam in increments of 0.5 to 1.0 mg are reasonable.
2. Inhalation anesthetics. N_2O in association with high-dose opiates causes systolic dysfunction in patients with coronary artery disease, particularly those with an LVEDP higher than 15 mm Hg.[27,28] An animal model of coronary stenosis suggests that this may be secondary to ischemia-induced segmental contraction abnormalities.[29] No such contraction abnormalities have been observed in humans with preserved left ventricular function and ischemic heart disease exposed to high-dose opiates and N_2O.[30] N_2O, combined with high-dose opiates, also elevates pulmonary vascular resistance, particularly in

the presence of preexisting pulmonary hypertension.[31] Because of the potential for altered myocardial oxygen balance in all patients with AS, and the presence of an elevated pulmonary vascular resistance in some patients, N_2O must be used with caution. Isoflurane is a potent vasodilator that causes little depression of systolic function.[32] Sevoflurane and desflurane have similar effects.[33,34] However, care must be taken to avoid decreases in peripheral vascular resistance and hypotension when they are used in patients with AS. Controversy exists regarding whether isoflurane in the presence of coronary stenosis is responsible for producing a coronary steal phenomena leading to ischemia (*see* Chapter 4). Enflurane causes both vasodilation and depression of systolic function[32] and must be titrated with caution as well.

Post-Cardiopulmonary Bypass Management

After aortic valve replacement, most impedance to ventricular ejection is abolished. A small peak gradient of 10 to 20 mm Hg exists across most aortic valve prostheses. This reduction in the transvalvular gradient will allow the hypertrophied LV to significantly decrease left ventricular end-systolic volume (LVESV) and thus augment stroke volume and EF (*see* Fig. 5-2). In addition, the ventricle can now respond to further reductions in afterload with an increase in stroke volume.

Mechanical (nontissue) valves in the aortic position exhibit some regurgitant flow in diastole. This small amount of regurgitant flow may cause problems in the period immediately after removal of the aortic cross-clamp. The regurgitation may lead to ventricular distention if the heart is not vented or beating.

LV systolic function may be compromised by inadequate myocardial protection during cardiopulmonary bypass (CPB). It may therefore be necessary to rely on inotropic agents for augmentation of systolic function despite the dramatic reduction in afterload. This is particularly true if there is coexisting coronary artery disease. Epinephrine 0.015 to 0.03 μg/kg/min, dopamine 1 to 5 μg/kg/min, or dobutamine 5 to 10 μg/kg/min are reasonable choices because they provide inotropic support with little concomitant vasoconstriction and afterload increase (*see* Chapter 4).

Because there is no significant regression of concentric hypertrophy for 6 to 12 months after aortic valve replacement,[3,35] the compliance characteristics of the LV will be unchanged in the postbypass period. In fact, poor subendocardial myocardial protection during aortic cross-clamping may result in ischemic diastolic dysfunction and diminished ventricular distensibility. Sinus rhythm must be maintained. The peak A-wave pressure must be high enough to ensure adequate LVEDV. In general, because LVESV will be lower because of the reduction in impedance to ventricular ejection, LVEDV and therefore the A-wave pressure need not be as high in the postbypass period. An A-wave pressure of 10 to 20 mm Hg usually is adequate. Subendocardial perfusion will remain compromised in diastole and, therefore, aortic diastolic blood pressure must remain high enough to ensure perfusion.

Tachycardia remains detrimental because of its effects on subendocardial perfusion. Bradycardia, however, is better tolerated because of the dramatic reduction in the transvalvular gradient with surgery.

Because the surgical procedure requires an aortotomy with subsequent repair, it is helpful to avoid a wide pulse pressure, which places undue stress on the aortic suture line. The AV node lies proximal to the aortic valve annulus and may be transiently or permanently damaged after valve replacement. Ventricular pacing may be necessary.

Goals

1. Maintain sinus rhythm; use atrioventricular (AV) sequential pacing if necessary.
2. Avoid tachycardia; bradycardia is well tolerated.
3. Maintain PCWP A-wave pressure high enough to ensure adequate LVEDV.
4. Maintain aortic diastolic pressure.
5. Avoid a wide pulse pressure.
6. Support ventricular systolic function with inotropes if necessary.

■ AORTIC REGURGITATION

Aortic regurgitation (AR) may result from damage to the aortic valve leaflets or from dilatation of the aortic root. Damage to the aortic valve leaflets results in a mechanical valve defect, whereas aortic root dilatation results in functional aortic valve impairment. In addition, AR may be acute or chronic in nature.

Infective endocarditis with destruction of the valve leaflets is a cause of acute aortic regurgitation. There may be actual destruction of the valve leaflet by the infective process. Alternatively, the infective process may cause perforation of a leaflet or the presence of vegetations may prevent proper apposition of the leaflets.

Trauma may result in acute aortic regurgitation. Rupture and/or laceration of the aortic valve cusps results in mechanical valve dysfunction. Aortic dissection may cause aortic regurgitation through a variety of mechanisms. Dilation of the proximal aortic root and valve annulus results in poor apposition of the leaflets and functional valvular incompetence. Dissection also may cause functional incompetence when hematoma

formation causes poor apposition of the valve leaflets. Dissection can result in mechanical incompetence when the valvular annulus is destroyed.

Connective tissue diseases such as Marfan's syndrome, Ehlers-Danlos syndrome, and pseudoxanthoma elasticum produce chronic AR. Progressive aortic root dilation with subsequent dilation of the valve annulus results in functional AR. As time passes, the poorly apposed valve leaflets begin to bow, thicken, and shorten, resulting in worsening regurgitation. These patients may suffer from mitral valve incompetence as well.

Inflammatory diseases of the aorta, such as syphilis, rheumatoid disease, ankylosing spondylitis, and Takayasu's aortitis, may produce chronic AR. These diseases cause distortion of the aortic root as well as destruction of valve cusps and annular support structures. Mitral regurgitation may exist as well.

Aortic valve leaflet damage due to rheumatic fever is a common cause of chronic mechanical aortic regurgitation. However, isolated AR secondary to rheumatic fever is rare. In rheumatic fever, the valve cusps become infiltrated with fibrous tissue and retract. This results in poor valve apposition in diastole with subsequent regurgitation. Commissure fusion results in some degree of aortic stenosis. Some mitral valve involvement is common as well.

Pathophysiology and Adaptation

AR is a volume-overload lesion that may be acute or chronic in nature. The extent of regurgitation is determined by the diastolic pressure gradient between the aorta and the left ventricle, the time available for regurgitation (diastole), and the aortic valve area. The pressure gradient, in turn, is determined by aortic diastolic pressure, ventricular early diastolic pressure, and ventricular compliance. Regurgitation ceases when the ventricular diastolic and aortic diastolic pressures equalize. The duration of diastole is inversely related to heart rate as demonstrated in Figure 5–3.

Chronic volume overloading of the left ventricle results in eccentric ventricular hypertrophy or increased ventricular radius. The details of this process are summarized in Figure 5–5A. Whereas both LVESV and LVEDV increase, LVEDV increases to a greater extent. This results in an enhanced stroke volume (SV) with no need for an increased EF. The slope of the diastolic pressure–volume curve is little changed and, thus, compliance in the true sense of the concept is only slightly increased. However, the entire pressure–volume loop is shifted to the right, a phenomenon known as *creep*. This rightward shift of the diastolic pressure–volume curve allows low diastolic pressures to be maintained at very large end-diastolic volumes. The large increase in ventricular radius that accompanies eccentric hypertrophy elevates wall stress and stimulates some degree of con-

AORTIC REGURGITATION

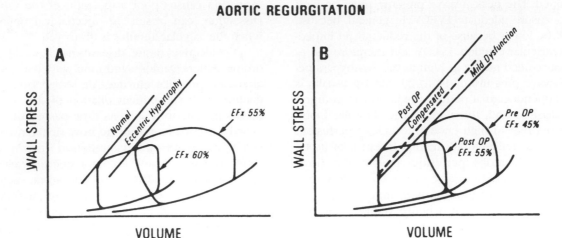

FIGURE 5–5. Left ventricular wall stress–volume loops for patient with progressive AR. **A.** Wall stress–volume loops of normal ventricle and of ventricle having developed eccentric hypertrophy in response to chronic volume overload of AR are shown. The ventricle with eccentric hypertrophy has a reduced isovolumic contraction phase and has its entire wall stress–volume relationship shifted to the right. These adaptations allow the ventricle to deliver large stroke volume with nearly normal EF despite elevation of end-systolic wall stress. **B:** Wall stress–volume relationships in ventricle with chronic aortic regurgitation and mild systolic dysfunction. Progressive systolic dysfunction leads to exhaustion of preload reserve and elevation of wall stress due to large ventricular radius. This, in turn, results in reduced SV and EF (EF$_x$ 45%). After surgical replacement of aortic valve, ventricular radius and wall stress are reduced and near-normal SV and EF exist despite the presence of systolic dysfunction (EF$_x$ 55%). *(From Hurst JW: The Heart. 5th ed. New York, McGraw-Hill, 1985, p 818. Reprinted with permission.)*

centric hypertrophy as well. This compensation is not complete and wall stress remains elevated both in end systole and end diastole (*see* Fig. 5-5A).

Unique LV pressure loading exists in AR, as illustrated in Figure 5-5A. The isovolumic phase of ventricular systole is of very short duration and limited pressure generation. This allows a greater portion of myocardial energy expenditure to be directed toward ejecting a large volume and less toward overcoming impedance to begin ejection.

In acute AR, there is not ample time for compensatory eccentric hypertrophy to occur. Without increased diastolic compliance and ventricular creep, the regurgitated volume results in a very high LVEDP. Because LVEDP rises rapidly to equal aortic end-diastolic pressure, the gradient for regurgitation is abolished quickly. As a result, the aortic end-diastolic pressure generally is higher and the regurgitant volume generally is smaller in acute versus chronic AR. Ventricular dilation from acute AR may result in functional mitral regurgitation. For other patients, the rapid rise in diastolic pressure may result in early diastolic equalization of left atrial and left ventricular pressures such that premature mitral valve closure occurs. In this setting, the PCWP or left atrial pressure (LAP) will greatly underestimate the LVEDP.

Ventricular Diastolic Function and the Atrial Transport Mechanism

In chronic AR, the increased compliance and the rightward shift of the diastolic pressure–volume curve allows passive filling of the left ventricle in early and mid-diastole via the left atrium. Therefore, LVEDV can be maintained without an atrial kick, except in end-stage AR, in which preload reserve is exhausted and the ventricle operates on the steep portion of its diastolic pressure–volume curve (*see* Fig. 5-5B).

In acute AR, increased ventricular compliance and a rightward shift of the diastolic pressure–volume curve are absent. In this setting, an atrial systole may be necessary to increase the left atrial to left ventricular pressure gradient enough to allow filling of the left ventricle via the left atrium. If premature mitral valve closure occurs due to rapid rise of left ventricular diastolic pressure, atrial transport will be entirely ineffective.

Eccentric hypertrophy and creep allow large increases in LVEDV with minimal increases in LVEDP in patients with chronic AR. This affords a great deal of preload reserve. Stroke volume can be increased by preload augmentation without pulmonary congestion.

In contrast, in acute AR preload reserve is nearly exhausted. Without adequate time for adaptation the left ventricle operates on the steep portion of its diastolic pressure–volume curve.

Myocardial Oxygen Balance

Myocardial oxygen consumption is increased by:

1. The large mass of myocardium that must be supplied with oxygen.

2. The enormous volume of work done by the left ventricle. Volume work increases oxygen consumption, but to a much lesser extent than pressure work.[8] The isovolumic contraction phase is highly energy consumptive. Because of the low aortic diastolic blood pressures present in AR, the isovolumic contraction phase is very brief and represents only a small portion of the total work done by the ventricle (*see* Fig. 5–5A). A greater portion of the total workload is devoted to the generation of volume ejection, which is an energy-efficient process.

3. Despite the development of eccentric hypertrophy and some degree of concentric hypertrophy, wall stress remains slightly elevated in both systole and diastole (*see* Fig. 5–5A). Recall that wall stress determines oxygen consumption in the ejection phase of ventricular contraction.

Myocardial oxygen delivery is compromised by the following factors:

1. The low diastolic aortic pressure characteristic of AR reduces the gradient for coronary blood flow (aortic diastolic blood pressure — LVEDP). This is particularly true in acute AR, in which precipitous increases in LVEDP occur. It also is true when bradycardia occurs in the acute or chronic situation. Bradycardia increases the regurgitant volume and thus increases LVEDP.

2. In acute AR due to aortic dissection, one or both of the coronary ostia may be involved in the dissection. This may acutely and drastically reduce coronary blood flow.

Left Ventricular Systolic Function

Patients with chronic AR may remain symptom-free for long periods of time despite progressive decreases in systolic function. The enormous preload reserve available to these patients allows stroke volume (SV) to be maintained by progressive increases in LVEDV in the face of declining contractile function. When preload reserve is exhausted, further diminution in systolic function cannot be compensated for and SV falls. At this point, symptoms of reduced cardiac output appear and systolic function is already seriously compromised (*see* Fig. 5–5B).

As contractility decreases, LVEDV increases in the face of the increasing LVESV. SV is maintained but EF falls. EF will remain in the low normal range until significant systolic dysfunction occurs. In fact, valve replacement is recommended for patients with AR without symptoms when ventricular dilation and a depressed EF are present.[3,36]

Right Ventricular Function and the Pulmonary Vasculature

As with aortic stenosis, right ventricular function is not directly affected by AR until secondary pulmonary hypertension intercedes. In chronic AR, ventricular dilation may lead to functional mitral regurgitation. This, in turn, may lead to a gradual elevation in left atrial and pulmonary artery pressures. If this situation persists, secondary pulmonary artery hypertension will begin to develop. Right ventricular failure develops if the pulmonary artery hypertension becomes severe.

In acute AR, functional mitral regurgitation from ventricular dilation is likely to be poorly tolerated. Acute ventricular dilation and functional mitral regurgitation leads to an immediate and profound elevation in LAP. Pulmonary vascular congestion with interstitial pulmonary edema rather than secondary pulmonary artery hypertension and right ventricular failure is the consequence here.

Effect of Heart Rate Alterations on Hemodynamics

The relationship between heart rate and cardiac output in AR is complex. Recall that the regurgitant volume is in large part determined by the length of diastole. Figure 5–3 illustrates the inverse relationship between heart rate and the length of diastole.

Bradycardia (heart rate less than 60 bpm) is detrimental in AR for several reasons. It increases the regurgitant volume per beat, which tends to lower aortic diastolic blood pressure and increase LVEDP. This decreases the gradient for subendocardial oxygen delivery. Simultaneously, the large SVs that accompany bradycardia increase wall tension and per-beat oxygen consumption. Forward SV and cardiac output are compromised because the regurgitant volume represents a large portion of the total SV (the regurgitant fraction is high).

With an increase in heart rate, the regurgitant volume per beat falls, whereas the regurgitant volume per minute may remain unchanged. The relationship between regurgitant volume and total SV (the regurgitant fraction) does not remain constant as heart rate increases. Therefore, cardiac output may decrease, remain unchanged, or increase with a heart rate increase. Latson and Lappas reviewed the literature and concluded that when going from bradycardia to rates of 75 to 85 bpm cardiac output increased significantly.[37] Further increases in heart rate from 85 to 110 bpm showed a trend toward a slight additional increase in cardiac output.[37] Little additional change, or a slight decrease in cardiac output, was noted when heart rate was in excess of 110 to 120 bpm.[37] Therefore, extremes of tachycardia offer no advantage over more moderate rates of

75 to 85 bpm in improving cardiac output and are deleterious to myocardial oxygen supply by limiting diastolic perfusion time.

Effect of Afterload Alterations on Hemodynamics

Increased afterload is detrimental to patients with both acute and chronic AR because it increases the regurgitant volume per beat. Recall that one of the determinants of the regurgitant volume is the gradient between the aorta and the left ventricle in early diastole. It is important, then, to avoid agents and to blunt stimuli that will increase afterload.

Contrary to what might be expected, efforts to actively decrease afterload in patients with AR are not uniformly helpful. In chronic AR, vasodilators benefit patients who have a depressed ejection fraction, high LVEDP, decreased forward cardiac output, and high arterial pressure.[36] Patients who do not meet these criteria may actually experience diminished forward cardiac output with vasodilator therapy due to preload reduction from venodilation.

In acute AR, vasodilator therapy is warranted. Recall that the absence of adequate ventricular compensation creates a very high LVEDP and that a low forward cardiac output exists despite preserved systolic function. Afterload reduction will reduce LVEDP and increase forward cardiac output. In addition, functional mitral regurgitation due to ventricular dilation can be dramatically improved in these patients with a reduction in ventricular size by vasodilators.

In properly selected patients, vasodilator therapy enhances ventricular performance in two ways. Systolic performance is enhanced by reducing aortic impedance, which allows generation of a larger SV. The regurgitant volume is reduced by a reduction in the diastolic aortic to left ventricular gradient. Care must be taken to ensure that the reduction in aortic diastolic blood pressure that accompanies vasodilator therapy is not so severe as to jeopardize subendocardial perfusion.

Anesthetic Technique

Goals

1. Maintain sinus rhythm; not as important as in AS.
2. Maintain heart rate at 75 to 85 bpm.
3. Avoid afterload increases; pursue afterload reduction in acute AR and in chronic AR when LVEDP and arterial blood pressure are elevated and cardiac output and EF are depressed.
4. Maintain a PCWP high enough to guarantee adequate LVEDP.
5. Maintain contractility.

Premedication

Patients with preserved LV function are premedicated with morphine sulfate 0.1 mg/kg IM, and lorazepam 1 to 2 mg PO approximately 1.5 hours before scheduled incision time. Supplemental O_2 with a face mask is begun at the time of premedication. All cardiac medications are continued until the time of surgery. Ranitidine 150 mg PO or a similar H_2 blocker is given at the time of premedication and the evening before surgery.

For elderly or debilitated patients, patients with poor ventricular function, and patients with poor pulmonary function, smaller doses are used. Err on the side of undermedicating these patients and reassuring them preoperatively. If necessary, supplemental premedication can be administered when the patient is seen in the OR holding area.

For patients with acute AR, severe hemodynamic compromise usually is the rule. It is dangerous to sedate these patients before surgery. All sedatives and narcotics should be given with careful observation of the fully monitored patient. Antiaspiration prophylaxis with an H_2 blocker and metoclopramide should be initiated.

Preinduction

All patients should have two large-bore peripheral IV lines (14 gauge). Alternatively, if peripheral IV access is poor, a peripheral IV suitable for induction can be started and a large-bore double-lumen (16- or 14-gauge) central venous line can be placed at the same time as the pulmonary artery catheter (see Chapter 3). ECG monitoring should allow assessment of V_5, I, II, III, aVR, aVL, and aVF. Baseline recording of all seven leads should be obtained for comparative purposes. Normally two leads (II and V_5) are monitored simultaneously intraoperatively. A radial artery catheter is placed with local anesthesia and adequate sedation before the induction of anesthesia. A pulmonary artery catheter can be placed before or after induction of anesthesia. All of the equipment and medications necessary for treatment of dysrhythmias are available before placement of the pulmonary artery catheter. Placement of the pulmonary artery catheter before induction allows preload and afterload to be optimized before induction of anesthesia.

In chronic AR, a large LVEDV is necessary to ensure an adequate forward cardiac output in the face of regurgitation. Because of the increased ventricular compliance and the phenomenon of creep, the peak A-wave pressure will differ little from mean PCWP. Likewise, LVEDV will be supplemented with only small increases in the mean PCWP. For patients with preserved LV function, a mean PCWP in the range of 10 to 15 mm Hg will ensure optimal LVEDV. Serial cardiac outputs obtained in conjunction with volume infusion will help with optimization of preload.

For patients with depressed ventricular function who have exhausted preload reserve, peak A-wave pressure will be in the range of 20 to 25 mm Hg when preload is optimized. For these patients, afterload reduction is indicated. Sodium nitroprusside is the agent of choice. It is easily titratable with a very short half-life. The infusion can be started at 0.15 to 0.3 µg/kg/min and titrated with careful attention paid to forward cardiac output, arterial blood pressure, and LVEDP. Although nitroprusside is primarily an arterial vasodilator, it has vasodilatory effects on the venous system as well. It is important not to let reductions in preload offset the beneficial effects of arterial dilation. If necessary, volume infusion should be used to maintain PCWP in the range of 10 to 15 mm Hg.

In acute AR in which premature closure of the mitral valve occurs, mean PCWP will underestimate LVEDP. When mitral incompetence from ventricular dilation occurs, mean PCWP will overestimate LVEDP in direct proportion to the amplitude and duration of the regurgitant V wave. These patients are very ill and may require pharmacologic stabilization before induction. Due to the lack of compensatory creep, these patients may have a PCWP in the range of 20 to 25 mm Hg to maintain a low normal cardiac index. Afterload reduction with nitroprusside (as described previously) is indicated. Inotropic support should be added if cardiac index remains depressed (less than 2.2 L/min/m²) or functional mitral regurgitation persists due to a dilated ventricle. Either dopamine (1 to 5 µg/kg/min) or dobutamine (5 to 10 µg/kg/min) can be used; neither will cause an elevation of afterload.

Use of an intra-aortic balloon pump is contraindicated in AR because balloon inflation and augmentation of diastolic blood pressure will worsen the regurgitation.

Induction and Maintenance

Generally, 50 to 75 µg/kg of fentanyl or 10 to 15 µg/kg of sufentanil can be used as the primary anesthetic for induction and maintenance before cardiopulmonary bypass. These agents are chosen because they have minimal effects on myocardial contractility and peripheral vascular resistance.[18,19] Compared with fentanyl, sufentanil is more likely to cause a fall in mean arterial pressure secondary to a reduced peripheral vascular resistance in patients with valvular heart disease.[20,21] On the other hand, patients with valvular heart disease receiving sufentanil in these doses are less likely to require supplemental anesthesia or vasodilator therapy for skin incision, sternotomy, sternal spread, or aortic manipulation.[20,21]

After several minutes of preoxygenation and with the patient breathing 100% oxygen, induction begins with an infusion of fentanyl 500 µg/min or sufentanil 100 µg/min over 5 to 10 minutes. A system of graded stimulation is used to individualize the narcotic dose for each patient. Compared with patients with coronary artery disease, patients with valvular heart disease have a lower narcotic requirement to achieve unconsciousness.[21] This probably is due to a lower cardiac output with a relative greater distribution of output to the brain and spinal cord.[21] After loss of consciousness, the hemodynamic response to insertion of an oral airway followed by insertion of a urinary catheter is used to gauge the need for additional narcotic to blunt the hemodynamic response to tracheal intubation. Laryngoscopy is performed carefully and should not be prolonged. If an upward trend in heart rate or blood pressure is noted as laryngoscopy commences, laryngoscopy should be terminated and additional narcotic should be titrated. If there is poor visualization of the larynx, laryngoscopy should be terminated and intubating conditions should be improved by changing head position, using a stylet, or changing blades. This approach will help prevent long stimulating larnygoscopies that compromise hemodynamics. If the entire narcotic dose is not used for induction, the remainder is infused slowly in anticipation of the skin incision. A TEE probe (see Chapter 3) is placed after tracheal intubation and verification of tube position.

Muscle relaxants are chosen with optimization of heart rate in mind (see Chapter 4). In the absence of beta blockade, the vecuronium–fentanyl or vecuronium–sufentanil combination is a good choice if a small heart rate decrease is desired. The pancuronium-fentanyl or pancuronium–sufentanil combination is more likely to cause a heart rate increase, which is advantageous for those patients who are relatively bradycardic. Vecuronium or pancuronium 0.02 mg/kg is administered approximately 1 to 2 minutes before starting the fentanyl infusion. As the patient loses consciousness the remainder of the total dose of 0.1 mg/kg is administered and controlled ventilation with 100% O_2 initiated. An alternative to vecuronium is cis-atracurium 0.04 mg/kg as the priming dose and 0.2 mg/kg as the total dose. These regimes minimize the risk of narcotic-induced rigidity without undue stress to the patient.

Bradycardia with hemodynamic compromise must be treated promptly. A small dose of pancuronium (1 to 3 mg) is often effective if vecuronium or cis-atracurium has been used. Atropine 0.4 to 0.8 mg is a reasonable choice despite the risk of tachycardia because tachycardia is well tolerated by these patients. Ephedrine is a poor choice because the concomitant increase in afterload is detrimental.

Hypotension must not be treated routinely with vasopressors because an increase in the regurgitant volume will worsen the situation. If heart rate and preload are optimized, then augmentation of stroke volume with an inotropic agent should be initiated. Dopamine 1 to 5 µg/kg/min or dobutamine 5 to 10 µg/kg/min will both augment cardiac output without increasing afterload (*see* Chapter 4). When AR is caused by an aortic dissection, it must be appreciated that in theory, agents that increase contractility may worsen an aortic dissection by increasing shear forces on the aortic wall.

If surgical stimulation (skin incision, sternotomy, sternal spreading, or aortic manipulation) produces hypertension additional doses of sufentanil (1 to 5 µg/kg) or fentanyl (5 to 25 µg/kg) may be necessary. Recent data call this practice into question. After a patient has received high doses of sufentanil (10 to 30 µg/kg) or fentanyl (50 to 100 µg/kg), administration of an additional agent as an infusion or a bolus will not reliably blunt the hemodynamic response to noxious stimuli.[22] If this fails to control the hypertension, the use of additional agents will be necessary. Vasodilation with sodium nitroprusside can be titrated easily and terminated quickly. This makes it an ideal choice for treatment of transient elevations in peripheral vascular resistance during high-dose narcotic anesthesia. It also may become necessary to supplement narcotic anesthesia with additional anesthetic agents:

1. Benzodiazepines. Diazepam, midazolam, and lorazepam administered in conjunction with fentanyl or sufentanil have been implicated in causing decreases in peripheral vascular resistance with subsequent hypotension.[23-26] Therefore, they must be titrated with caution. Midazolam in increments of 1 to 2 mg or lorazepam in increments of 0.5 to 1.0 mg is reasonable.
2. Inhalation anesthetics. N_2O in association with high-dose opiates causes systolic dysfunction in patients with coronary artery disease, particularly those with an LVEDP above 15 mm Hg.[27,28] An animal model of coronary stenosis suggests that this may be secondary to ischemia-induced segmental contraction abnormalities.[29] No such contraction abnormalities have been observed in humans with preserved left ventricular function and ischemic heart disease exposed to high-dose opiates and N_2O.[30] N_2O combined with high-dose opiates also elevates pulmonary vascular resistance, particularly in the presence of preexisting pulmonary hypertension.[31] Because of the potential for altered myocardial oxygen balance and the presence of an elevated pulmonary vascular resistance in some patients with AR, N_2O must be used with caution. Isoflurane is a potent vasodilator that causes little depression of systolic function[32] and is potentially useful for the subset of patients who will benefit from afterload reduction. Sevoflurane and desflurane have similar effects.[33,34] However, care must be taken to avoid decreases in peripheral vascular resistance and hypotension. Enflurane causes both vasodilation and depression of systolic function[32] and must be titrated with caution as well.

The induction sequence should be modified for emergency patients deemed at high risk for aspiration. After preoxygenation and with cricoid pressure applied, etomidate 0.15 to 0.3 mg/kg, succinylcholine 1.0 to 1.5 mg/kg, in conjunction with fentanyl 10 µg/kg or sufentanil 1 µg/kg can be administered. Alternatively, sufentanil 5 µg/kg and succinylcholine 1.0 to 1.5 mg/kg can be used.

Post-Cardiopulmonary Bypass Management

Replacement of the aortic valve will result in a small residual peak gradient (10 to 20 mm Hg). Mechanical (nontissue) valves in the aortic position exhibit some regurgitant flow in diastole. This small amount of regurgitant flow may cause problems in the period immediately after removal of the aortic cross-clamp. The regurgitation may lead to ventricular distention if the heart is not vented or beating.

After aortic valve replacement for chronic AR, the impedance to ventricular ejection will be increased. The ventricle that has undergone compensation for a volume overload lesion is now faced with a relative pressure overload. The competent aortic valve causes an elevation of intraventricular pressure during the isovolumic contraction phase (*see* Fig. 5-5B). The elimination of regurgitation via the competent valve greatly reduces the need for a large total SV. Therefore, a greater proportion of total myocardial oxygen consumption goes toward the more energy-consumptive process of pressure generation to begin ejection and less toward volume ejection. Although there is an increase in LV pressure generation, wall stress does not increase substantially because ventricular radius is greatly reduced by elimination of the regurgitant volume. Nonetheless, if poor myocardial protection is obtained during bypass and aortic cross-clamping, or if depressed systolic function exists preoperatively, inotropic support of systolic function may be necessary in the postbypass period. Epinephrine 0.015 to 0.03 µg/kg/min, dopamine 1 to 5 µg/kg/min, or dobutamine 5 to 10 µg/kg/min are good choices because they provide inotropic support with little vasoconstrictor activity at these doses (*see* Chapter 4).

After valve replacement in acute AR, the elimination of the regurgitant fraction allows the ventricle to maintain cardiac output with a much lower LVEDV and therefore LVEDP drops precipitously. Wall stress is diminished as well. Inotropic support may be necessary when preoperative systolic and diastolic dysfunction exists due to subendocardial ischemia or where myocardial preservation on bypass is poor. Again, epinephrine, dopamine, or dobutamine are good choices.

All LV diastolic filling must occur via the mitral valve when both acute and chronic regurgitation is abolished. Therefore, atrial systole becomes more important in ensuring adequate LVEDV. Maintenance of sinus rhythm or AV sequential pacing becomes necessary. Bradycardia will be better tolerated in the postbypass period.

In chronic AR, there is no significant regression of ventricular creep and eccentric hypertrophy for 6 to 12 months after valve replacement[3,35] (see Fig. 5–5B). Therefore, LVEDP will remain low, even for large LVEDVs. This low LVEDP in combination with the elevation in aortic diastolic blood pressure will greatly improve myocardial oxygen delivery. The temptation when cardiac output is low will be to use the large preload reserve available in these patients. Because intraventricular pressure is elevated during the prolonged isovolumic contraction phase, wall stress for a given LVEDV will be greater in the postbypass period. Efforts to increase preload to contend with poor systolic function or high afterload states will result in afterload mismatch and declining systolic function. A mean PCWP or LAP of 10 to 15 mm Hg usually is adequate. A better approach would be inotropic support with epinephrine or afterload reduction with sodium nitroprusside as described previously.

In acute AR, little or no creep or eccentric hypertrophy exists and postoperative preload reserve will resemble that of a normal ventricle.

Because the surgical procedure requires an aortotomy with subsequent repair, it is helpful to avoid a wide pulse pressure, which places undue stress on the aortic suture line. The AV node lies proximal to the aortic valve annulus and may be transiently or permanently damaged after valve replacement. Ventricular pacing may be necessary.

Goals

1. Maintain sinus rhythm; use AV sequential pacing if necessary.
2. Avoid reliance on a large LVEDV; wall stress will be greatly elevated and systolic function may deteriorate.
3. Support ventricular function with inotropes if necessary.
4. Decrease wall stress with afterload reduction if necessary.
5. Avoid a wide pulse pressure.

■ MITRAL STENOSIS

Mitral stenosis (MS) is almost always rheumatic in origin. Rheumatic fever results in fusion of the mitral valve apparatus in various locations. The site of valve appara-

tus involvement determines whether the valve will be primarily stenotic or incompetent in nature. Fusion of the cusps and commissures results in a stenotic valve orifice. The valve leaflets may become so rigid that they are incapable of closing, in which case MS and incompetence coexist. When only the chordae tendinae contract and fuse, pure mitral incompetence exists. Pure MS only exists in approximately one-fourth of patients with rheumatic mitral involvement; most patients have some degree of mitral incompetence as well.

Pathophysiology and Adaptation

MS is a chronic left ventricular volume underload lesion. The natural history of the disease is a gradual reduction in the mitral valve area from a normal of 4 to 6 cm² to less than 1 cm² over three to four decades. Left ventricular filling occurs in diastole via the left atrium across the mitral valve. Therefore, left ventricular filling is determined by the length of diastole, the pressure gradient between the left atrium and the left ventricle, and the mitral valve area. As the mitral valve orifice decreases in size, the left atrium is faced with a gradual increase in impedance to left ventricular filling, and a pressure gradient develops across the valve such that LAP exceeds left ventricular diastolic pressure.

Early on in the disease process, complete LV filling can be accomplished without an elevation of mean LAP if diastole is long enough and if an atrial systole exists. As the valve area decreases further and the transvalvular gradient rises, a long diastole and an elevated mean left atrial pressure are necessary to ensure ventricular filling. Eventually, the valve orifice narrows to the point at which a long diastole and an elevated mean left atrial pressure are no longer adequate to maintain a normal LVEDV and the LV remains underloaded. The pressure-volume loop for MS is illustrated in Figure 5–6.

Ventricular Diastolic Function and the Atrial Transport Mechanism

Because MS presents a fixed resistance to ventricular inflow and because the atrial systole is of short duration, a large portion of the kinetic energy produced by atrial systole is dissipated in overcoming resistance to inflow. The role of atrial systole in augmenting LVEDV in MS is less dramatic than in aortic stenosis but important nonetheless. At heart rates of 80 to 110 bpm, the loss of atrial systole results in a 20% decrease in diastolic flow per beat and cardiac output in patients with moderate and severe MS.[38] However, in moderate and severe MS, the presence of an atrial systole alone will not maximize left ventricular filling and an elevation of mean LAP is necessary as well.[38]

The high LAPs that develop as a result of the stenotic mitral valve orifice result in left atrial hypertro-

Mitral Stenosis

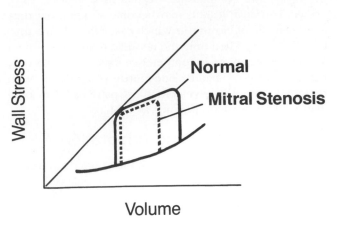

FIGURE 5–6. Pressure–volume loop from patient with MS. LVEDV is severely limited compared to normal. This results in reduction in SV.

phy and eventually left atrial distention. This distension results in the development of atrial dysrhythmias, the most common of which is atrial fibrillation. In severe MS, atrial fibrillation rather than sinus rhythm generally is the rule. When atrial systole is lost, diastolic flow per beat and cardiac output can only be maintained with a further elevation of mean LAP. The higher the mean LAP that can be tolerated, the more complete the left ventricular filling. Mean LAP is limited by the development of pulmonary congestion and pressures greater than 25 mm Hg are rarely tolerated without symptoms. For a given valve area, after mean LAP is maximized, ventricular inflow is determined by the length of diastole.

Ventricular diastolic function and compliance remains unchanged in MS. Despite this, preload reserve is severely limited in this lesion. Maximal LVEDV in moderate and severe MS is well below that seen in normals. Mean LAP must be elevated (often to the point of pulmonary congestion) to obtain an LVEDV large enough to meet baseline cardiac output demands. Further increases in mean LAP only slightly augment LVEDV due to the large pressure gradient across the valve. In addition, this further elevation of mean LAP leads to progressive pulmonary congestion and frank pulmonary edema.

Myocardial Oxygen Balance

There are no special considerations regarding myocardial oxygen balance in patients with MS. It is important, however, to keep in mind the relationship between the length of diastole, aortic diastolic pressure, and LVEDP on subendocardial perfusion. It is also important to determine the extent of coronary artery disease in patients with MS and angina pectoris.

Left Ventricular Systolic Function

Whether LV systolic function is compromised in MS is controversial. Rheumatic myocardial fibrosis in the posterobasal region of the LV may result in segmental wall motion abnormalities and reduced systolic performance.[39] It has been demonstrated, as well, that patients with MS have normal indices of LV contractility but have a reduced ejection fraction due to an elevated afterload with no compensatory increase in preload.[40] Therefore, patients with MS may have intrinsically impaired contractile function, afterload mismatch, or both.

Right Ventricular Function and the Pulmonary Vasculature

The prolonged elevations of LAP seen in progressive MS have profound effects on the pulmonary vasculature and right ventricular function. Early in the disease, elevated LAP is transmitted to the pulmonary venous system, and there is reversible passive elevation of the pulmonary artery pressures while pulmonary vascular resistance remains normal (*see* Fig. 5–7). Right ventricular function remains unchanged.

As the disease progresses, reactive changes occur in the pulmonary vasculature. Prolonged perivascular edema results in arterial intima fibroelastosis and nonreversible elevations in pulmonary vascular resistance. Progression of this process presents a large increase in right ventricular afterload or a "second stenosis" (*see* Fig. 5–7). The RV is poorly adapted to generate pressures that approach systemic. As a result, afterload mismatch occurs, the RV invariably fails, and the RV output falls. Peripheral edema and hepatic congestion ensue. Right ventricular failure and dilation also may lead to functional tricuspid regurgitation and worsening symptoms of right heart failure. In the steady state, RV output and LV output must be equal. Therefore, LV output is limited by RV failure. Efforts to reduce RV afterload and improve RV output with nitroprusside have been shown to significantly improve systemic output in patients with elevated pulmonary vascular resistance.[41]

Effect of Heart Rate Alterations on Hemodynamics

Figure 5–3 illustrates the reduction in diastolic filling time that accompanies an increase in heart rate. If cardiac output is to remain constant as heart rate increases, then the flow rate across the mitral valve in diastole must increase. Recall that as flow rate increases across the stenotic valve, the gradient across the valve will increase by the square of the flow increase (*see* Chapter 2). Thus, the requirement for increased flow can result in prohibitive increases in mean LAP.

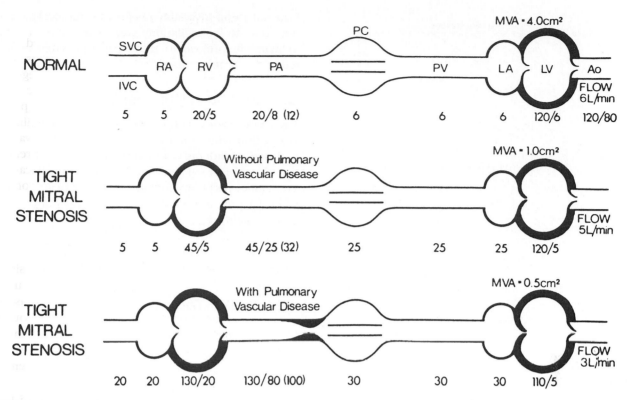

FIGURE 5–7. Illustration of changes seen with progression of MS. SVC, superior vena cava; IVC, inferior vena cava; RA, right atrium; RV, right ventricle; PA, pulmonary artery; PC, pulmonary capillary; PV, pulmonary vein; LA, left atrium; LV, left ventricle; Ao, aorta; MVA, mitral valve area. Pressure in each of cardiac chambers and great vessels is indicated.

In MS without pulmonary vascular disease, there is reversible passive elevation of PV, PC, and PA pressures while pulmonary vascular resistance remains normal. These elevations are secondary to elevation of LA pressure, which is necessary to maintain LV filling across stenotic mitral valve. RV pressure is elevated in response to elevated PA pressure, and RV concentric hypertrophy may result. RV systolic dysfunction usually is not present.

In MS with pulmonary vascular disease, PA pressure is elevated far in excess of LA, PC, and PV pressures because of the presence of pulmonary arterial occlusive disease with elevated pulmonary vascular resistance. This results in a second stenosis at the level of the PA. This second stenosis causes dramatic elevations in RV pressure. This RV pressure elevation may result in reduced RV stroke volume due to afterload mismatch and to tricuspid regurgitation due to RV dilation. Reduction in RV stroke volume results directly in decrease in systemic cardiac output. *(From Grossman W: Cardiac Catheterization and Angiography. 3rd ed. Philadelphia, Lea & Febiger, 1986, p 361. Reprinted by permission.)*

Figure 5–8 illustrates the effect of heart rate changes in MS. Higher heart rates can potentially improve cardiac output when SV is small. However, in MS, the transvalvular gradient increases so dramatically with tachycardia that prohibitive increases in mean LAP ensue. At slower rates, more diastolic filling time is available to augment LVEDV, but cardiac output is compromised by bradycardia unless LVEDV is large. Large LVEDVs require a further increase in mean LAP as ventricular compliance diminishes at higher LVEDVs. For these reasons, heart rates between 70 and 90 bpm are optimal.

Most patients with moderate and severe MS are in atrial fibrillation. In these patients, control of heart rate is dependent on adequate control of the ventricular response rate to the fibrillating atrium. Drugs used to control the ventricular response rate by producing AV nodal block such as digoxin, verapamil, and beta blockers must be continued.

Effect of Afterload Alterations on Hemodynamics

Patients with MS have severely limited preload reserve, as discussed previously. Some patients may have depressed systolic function due to posterobasal wall motion abnormalities.[39,40] In addition, high base-line afterload states may limit SV in other patients.[40] For these reasons, patients with MS tolerate large increases in afterload poorly because it is likely to cause afterload mismatch.

LV afterload reduction is fraught with hazard because of the limited preload reserve in these patients. Recall that afterload reduction will increase SV by reducing LVESV if LVEDV is maintained. Recall also that LVEDV is below normal in these patients and that small decreases in mean LAP will result in large decreases in LVEDV due to the mitral valve gradient. Because after-

A
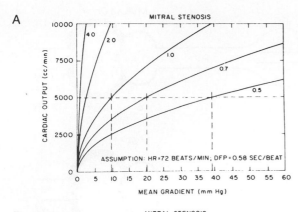

B

C
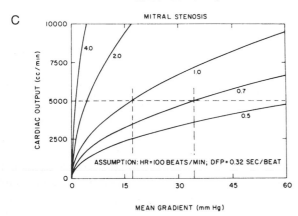

FIGURE 5–8. The relationship of heart rate, cardiac output, mitral valve area, and diastolic pressure gradient across the mitral valve is illustrated for patients with MS. Cardiac output is plotted against diastolic pressure gradient for mitral valve areas ranging from 0.5 to 4.0 cm². Plot **A** illustrates these relationships for heart rate of 72 bpm and diastolic filling period (DFP) of 0.58 sec/beat. Plot **B** illustrates these relationships for heart rate of 88 bpm and DFP of 0.43 sec/beat. Plot **C** illustrates these relationships for heart rate of 100 bpm and DFP of 0.32 sec/beat.

It is clear that for given cardiac output and heart rate, diastolic pressure gradient increases as mitral valve area decreases. Furthermore, for a given cardiac output and mitral valve area, the diastolic pressure gradient increases as heart rate increases. With cardiac output constant, an increase in heart rate requires smaller volume to cross the stenotic mitral valve during the DFP. This should result in reduction in diastolic pressure gradient. However, increases in heart rate in the range examined here progressively shorten the length of DFP. Reduction in DFP requires that volume be translocated across stenotic mitral valve in less time, which increases diastolic pressure gradient. Shortening of DFP is the more important determinant of diastolic pressure gradient at heart rates illustrated here.

load reduction invariably results in some preload reduction due to venodilation, great care must be taken to maintain preload in these patients when afterload-reducing agents are used.

Critical Mitral Stenosis

The term "critical mitral stenosis" is used commonly in association with mitral valve disease. Typically, it is used to describe patients with mitral valve areas <1.0 cm². In truth, critical mitral stenosis should be used to describe a specific pathophysiologic state. Critical MS exists when LA pressure is elevated, producing pulmonary venous congestion at rest to maintain a normal or reduced stroke volume. In the presence of diastolic and systolic dysfunction or poorly controlled atrial fibrillation or flutter, critical MS may exist with larger valve areas.

Anesthetic Technique

Goals

1. Maintain sinus rhythm where possible.
2. Maintain heart rate at 70 to 90 bpm.
3. Maintain PCWP high enough to guarantee as large an LVEDV as possible without pulmonary edema.
4. Maintain LV afterload; increases are poorly tolerated. Decreasing afterload is warranted when LV systolic function is poor and afterload is high. In this instance, preload *must* be maintained.
5. Maintain contractility.
6. When pulmonary vascular resistance is high and RV systolic performance is compromised (second stenosis), RV afterload reduction will improve RV and subsequently LV output. Caution must be exercised so that excessive systemic vasodilation does not result.
7. Avoid hypercarbia, hypoxemia, and acidemia, which tend to cause pulmonary hypertension and may result in acute RV decompensation.

Premedication

Patients with MS must be premedicated with caution, particularly when pulmonary artery hypertension and compromised LV performance exist. Hypercarbia, hypoxemia, and vasodilation may accompany overzealous use of narcotics and sedatives. Morphine sulfate 0.05 mg/kg IM, and lorazepam 1 mg PO approximately 1.5 hours before scheduled incision time will prevent undue anxiety in the fittest of these patients. For elderly or debilitated patients with RV failure and pulmonary congestion, 1 to 3 mg of morphine sulfate IM will suffice. All patients should have supplemental O_2 started at the time of premedication.

All cardiac medications are continued until the time of surgery. Ranitidine 150 mg PO or a similar H_2 blocker is given at the time of premedication and the evening before surgery.

Preinduction

All patients should have two large-bore peripheral IV lines (14 gauge). Alternatively, if peripheral IV access is poor, a peripheral IV suitable for induction can be started and a large-bore double-lumen (16- or 14-gauge) central venous line can be placed at the same time as the pulmonary artery catheter (see Chapter 3). ECG monitoring should allow assessment of V_5, I, II, III, aVR, aVL, and aVF. Baseline recording of all seven leads should be obtained for comparative purposes. Normally, two leads (II and V_5) are monitored simultaneously intraoperatively. A radial artery catheter is placed with local anesthesia and adequate sedation before the induction of anesthesia. A pulmonary artery catheter can be placed before or after induction of anesthesia. All of the equipment and medications necessary for treatment of dysrhythmias are available before placement of the pulmonary artery catheter. Placement of the pulmonary artery catheter before induction allows preload and afterload to be optimized before induction of anesthesia. The insertion distance necessary to obtain a wedge pressure trace is greater (5 cm more via the right internal jugular route) in patients with pulmonary hypertension than in normals.[42] The risk of pulmonary artery perforation is greater in patients with pulmonary hypertension.[43,44] This may be due to eccentric balloon inflation forcing the catheter tip into the wall of vessel,[43,44] direct vessel disruption during balloon inflation in a distal arterial branch,[44] or distal catheter migration during balloon deflation.[42] Locating the catheter tip in the proximal pulmonary artery and readvancing the catheter for each wedge pressure measurement has been shown to greatly reduce the risk of pulmonary artery perforation in an animal model of pulmonary hypertension.[45]

Patients in sinus rhythm will have a very large A wave on the PCWP trace, which can be used to estimate LVEDP. Patients in atrial fibrillation will have no A wave, and mean PCWP can be used. It must be remembered that both the A wave pressure and the mean PCWP will overestimate the LVEDP. The smaller the valve area and the greater the heart rate, the larger the overestimation. The cardiac catheterization report will provide information as to the relationship between mean PCWP and LVEDP in a given patient. In general, for patients with moderate to severe MS, a mean PCWP of 20 to 30 mm Hg will be needed to optimize LVEDV. Volume infusion may be necessary if overvigorous preoperative diuresis has occurred.

The pulmonary artery catheter allows pulmonary vascular resistance to be calculated and central venous pressure (CVP) to be measured. Therapy to reduce RV afterload and to improve RV systolic performance cannot be initiated safely without this information.

For patients with severe RV failure, pulmonary congestion, and systemic hypotension (systolic blood pressure below 90 mm Hg), efforts to improve RV function with vasodilator therapy may be unsuccessful due to worsening systemic hypotension. For these patients, the addition of inotropic support of the RV and LV is necessary. Dobutamine 5 to 10 µg/kg/min is a good choice because it has no alpha-adrenergic activity and little chronotropic activity and it tends to reduce pulmonary artery pressures (see Chapter 4). Therefore, it will not exacerbate pulmonary artery hypertension or cause tachycardia.

Induction and Maintenance

Generally, 50 to 75 µg/kg of fentanyl or 10 to 15 µg/kg of sufentanil can be used as the primary anesthetic for induction and maintenance before cardiopulmonary bypass. These agents are chosen because they have minimal effects on myocardial contractility and peripheral vascular resistance.[18,19] Compared with fentanyl, sufentanil is more likely to cause a fall in mean arterial pressure secondary to a reduced peripheral vascular resistance in patients with valvular heart disease.[20,21] On the other hand, patients with valvular heart disease receiving sufentanil in these doses are less likely to require supplemental anesthesia or vasodilator therapy for skin incision, sternotomy, sternal spread, or aortic manipulation.[20,21]

After several minutes of preoxygenation and with the patient breathing 100% oxygen, induction begins with an infusion of fentanyl 500 µg/min or sufentanil 100 µg/min over 5 to 10 minutes. A system of graded stimulation is used to individualize the narcotic dose for each patient. Compared with patients with coronary artery disease, patients with valvular heart disease have a lower narcotic requirement to achieve unconsciousness.[21] This is probably due to a lower cardiac output with a relative greater distribution of output to the brain and spinal cord.[21] After loss of consciousness, the hemodynamic response to insertion of an oral airway, followed by insertion of a urinary catheter, is used to gauge the need for additional narcotic to blunt the hemodynamic response to tracheal intubation. Laryngoscopy is performed carefully and should not be prolonged. If an upward trend in heart rate or blood pressure is noted as laryngoscopy commences, laryngoscopy should be terminated and additional narcotic should be titrated. If there is poor visualization of the larynx, laryngoscopy should be terminated and intubating conditions should be improved by changing head position, using a stylet, or changing blades. This approach will help prevent long stimulating laryngoscopies that compromise hemodynamics. If the entire narcotic dose is not used for induction, the remainder is infused slowly in anticipation of the skin incision. A TEE probe (*see* Chapter 3) is placed after tracheal intubation and verification of tube position.

Muscle relaxants are chosen with optimization of heart rate in mind (*see* Chapter 4). In the absence of beta blockade, the vecuronium–fentanyl or vecuronium–sufentanil combination is a good choice if a small heart rate decrease is desired. The pancuronium-fentanyl or pancuronium-sufentanil combination is more likely to cause a heart rate increase, which is advantageous for patients who are relatively bradycardic. Vecuronium or pancuronium 0.02 mg/kg is administered approximately 1 to 2 minutes before starting the fentanyl infusion. As the patient loses consciousness, the remainder of the total dose of 0.1 mg/kg is administered and controlled ventilation with 100% O_2 is initiated. An alternative to vecuronium is cis-atracurium 0.04 mg/kg as the priming dose and 0.2 mg/kg as the total dose. These regimes minimize the risk of narcotic-induced rigidity without undue stress to the patient.

Bradycardia with hemodynamic compromise should be treated promptly. Pancuronium 1 to 3 mg IV often is effective if vecuronium or cis-atracurium has been used. Atropine 0.4 to 0.8 mg IV is effective as well, but the possibility that the ventricular response to atrial fibrillation will increase must be appreciated.

Tachycardia must be treated aggressively to avoid the large increases in mean LAP that will be necessary to maintain cardiac output. The first strategy should be to terminate any noxious stimuli and increase the depth of anesthesia when necessary. Propranolol in increments of 0.5 mg is given for two to three doses to get the heart rate in the desired range. If this fails, the incremental dose can be increased to 1.0 mg. For patients with poor ventricular function, doses greater than 0.1 mg/kg over less than a 1-hour period must be used with caution to avoid compromise to systolic function. In some instances, the ultra-short-acting beta blocker esmolol may be useful. Esmolol has an elimination half-life of 9 minutes due to metabolism by red cell esterases and is relatively beta-1 selective. Esmolol is started with a bolus of 0.5 mg/kg given over several minutes, followed by an infusion of 50 µg/kg/min and titrated up to 300 µg/kg/min as necessary. Esmolol is useful for patients with poor ventricular function or bronchospastic disease, because if it is not tolerated, therapy can be quickly terminated. Furthermore, unlike longer-acting beta blockers, esmolol can be used aggressively in the pre-CPB period, without fear that it will compromise termination of CPB.

Hypotension may be treated initially with volume infusion if PCWP has decreased and with cautious use of phenylephrine 40 to 80 µg. Continued hypotension is best handled without the use of vasopressors, particularly if pulmonary artery hypertension exists. After preload and heart rate have been optimized, it may be necessary to use an inotropic agent to reduce LVESV and increase stroke volume. As discussed previously, dobutamine 5 to 10 µg/kg/min is a good choice.

If surgical stimulation (skin incision, sternotomy, sternal spreading, or aortic manipulation) produces hypertension, additional doses of sufentanil (1 to 5 µg/kg) or fentanyl (5 to 25 µg/kg) may be necessary. Recent data call this practice into question. After a patient has received high doses of sufentanil (10 to 30 µg/kg) or fentanyl (50 to 100 µg/kg), administration of an additional agent as an infusion or a bolus will not reliably blunt the hemodynamic response to noxious stimuli.[22] If this fails to control the hypertension, the use of additional agents will be necessary. Vasodilation with sodium nitroprusside can be titrated easily and terminated quickly. This makes it an ideal choice for treatment of transient elevations in peripheral vascular resistance during high-dose narcotic anesthesia. It also may become necessary to supplement narcotic anesthesia with additional anesthetic agents:

1. Benzodiazepines. Diazepam, midazolam, and lorazepam administered in conjunction with fentanyl or sufentanil have been implicated in causing decreases in peripheral vascular resistance with subsequent hypotension.[23-26] Therefore, they must be titrated with caution. Midazolam in increments of 1 to 2 mg or lorazepam in increments of 0.5 to 1.0 mg is reasonable.

2. Inhalation anesthetics. N_2O combined with high-dose opiates elevates pulmonary vascular resistance, particularly in the presence of preexisting pulmonary hypertension.[31] Because of the existence of pulmonary hypertension in most patients with MS, N_2O should be avoided. Isoflurane is a potent vasodilator that causes little depression of systolic function and is potentially useful for patients with MS, where systolic function[32] is preserved and LV afterload is high. Sevoflurane and desflurane have similar effects.[33,34] However, care must be taken to avoid decreases in peripheral vascular resistance and hypotension. Enflurane causes both vasodilation and depression of systolic function[32] and must be titrated with caution as well.

Post-Cardiopulmonary Bypass Management

After mitral valve replacement for MS, a small mean gradient of 2 to 5 mm Hg exists across the prosthetic valve.

Mechanical (nontissue) valves exhibit a small amount of regurgitant flow in systole. Repaired mitral valves may exhibit some residual mild regurgitation and stenosis. This is assessed with TEE (*see* Chapter 3). Nonetheless, there is a dramatic improvement in LV filling via the LA after replacement or repair. As a result, preload reserve is greatly improved. This makes LV afterload mismatch less likely and allows cardiac output to be augmented via increases in preload even when preoperative systolic dysfunction exists. A mean PCWP or LAP of 10 to 15 mm Hg usually is adequate to take advantage of this increased preload reserve.

Patients in atrial fibrillation with large left atrial will only rarely convert to sinus rhythm postoperatively. The reduction in the transvalvular gradient allows tachycardia to be better tolerated; nonetheless, control of the ventricular response rate is important to allow adequate time in diastole to fill the LV.

The management of RV function and the pulmonary vasculature can be problematic in the postbypass period. For all patients with elevated pulmonary artery pressures, there will be a dramatic reduction in pulmonary artery pressures due to the reductions in the mean LAP and passive pulmonary congestion after valve replacement.[46] Despite this, some patients will continue to have elevated pulmonary vascular resistances due to reversible (reactive pulmonary vasoconstriction) and nonreversible (morphologic changes in the pulmonary vasculature) causes.[46] For these patients, careful management is necessary. The increased preload reserve of the LV will not be realized if the RV fails and is unable to deliver volume to the LA via the pulmonary system. The hallmarks of this syndrome are a high RAP (above 10 mm Hg) and pulmonary vascular resistance (above 150 dynes sec/cm[5]) coupled with a low LAP (under 5 mm Hg) and cardiac index (less than 2.0 L/min/m[2]). Aggressive efforts must be made to keep pulmonary vascular resistance as low as possible by avoiding hypercarbia, hypoxemia, and acidemia, and by avoiding pulmonary vasoconstrictors. If pulmonary hypertension persists despite these efforts, then active pulmonary vasodilation will be necessary. Nitroglycerin has been shown to be effective in reducing pulmonary artery pressures[47] and increasing pulmonary blood flow[48] after mitral valve replacement. The nitroglycerin can be started at 0.15 to 0.30 µg/kg/min and titrated upward as needed. Sodium nitroprusside started at the same dosage and titrated upward also is effective.

If poor RV protection has occurred during bypass and aortic cross-clamping, then inotropic support of the RV may be necessary in addition to pulmonary vasodilation. Inotropic support should be chosen with an eye toward avoiding increased pulmonary vascular resistance. Epinephrine 0.015 to 0.03 µg/kg/min, dopamine 1 to 5 µg/kg/min, or dobutamine 5 to 10 µg/kg/min, all

meet this requirement. However, when increased doses of epinephrine and dopamine are used, progressive pulmonary vasoconstriction from increased alpha-adrenergic activity results (*see* Chapter 4). In situations in which increasing demand for inotropic support is demonstrated amrinone 5 to 10 µg/kg/min following a loading dose of 0.75 to 1.5 µg/kg or milrinone 0.5 to 0.75 µg/kg/min after a loading dose of 50 to 75 mg/kg may be added (*see* Chapter 4). They provide potent inotropic support and pulmonary vasodilation.[49] Isoproterenol is a drug that often is suggested for use in patients who require inotropic support and pulmonary vasodilation.[50] Isoproterenol causes an increase in heart rate, myocardial oxygen consumption, and the incidence of ventricular dysrhythmias,[51] all of which may limit its usefulness. Recently, the combination of prostoglandin E_1 (PGE$_1$) and norepinephrine has been shown to be effective in treating refractory pulmonary hypertension and right ventricular failure after mitral valve replacement.[52] PGE$_1$ is a potent pulmonary and systemic vasodilator. PGE$_1$ 30 to 150 µg/kg/min is infused into the right heart in combination with norepinephrine in doses up to 1 µg/kg/min infused via a left atrial line. The norepinephrine is infused via the left atrial line to minimize its vasoconstrictive effects on the pulmonary vasculature, provide inotropic support, and counteract the profound systemic vasodilatory effects of PGE$_1$. Management of RV dysfunction, including TEE findings, are discussed in detail in Chapter 7.

A rare but potentially lethal complication of mitral valve replacement is ventricular disruption. This complication has been described after mitral valve replacement for a variety of lesions but is most common in patients undergoing replacement for chronic MS.[53,54] Three types of ventricular rupture have been described.[54] Type 1 involves rupture of the mitral annulus or of the ventricle at the atrioventricular junction due to a diseased annulus or posterior ventricular wall. Type 2 rupture occurs at the site of the excised papillary muscle due to surgically induced thinning of the ventricular wall. Type 3 rupture or transverse midventricular disruption (TMD) occurs midway between type 1 and 2 ruptures. Type 3 ruptures seem to be secondary to a variety of causes. Endocardial injury from inadvertent surgical trauma or the valve prosthesis itself has been implicated. Total excision of the mitral valve apparatus may result in loss of longitudinal support, which predisposes the ventricle to transverse disruption when ventricular dilation occurs.[54,55]

Ventricular rupture may present upon termination of CPB or up to 5 days postoperatively. In the immediate postoperative period, these lesions present with hypotension and copious arterialized blood welling up in the pericardium or issuing forth from the chest tubes. Repair of these lesions requires prompt reinstitution of

CPB, and the mortality is high.[54] Treatment of TMD may require sacrificing the circumflex artery to incorporate enough posterior myocardium for an adequate repair.[54]

Although the primary responsibility for prevention of this complication lies with the surgeon, preventative measures must be made by the anesthesiologist. If the mitral apparatus has been excised or if the posterior ventricular wall is diseased, efforts must be made to minimize ventricular dilatation and intraventricular pressures. Left ventricular afterload should be normalized or reduced to prevent high intraventricular pressures and left ventricular dilatation. Likewise, reliance on large left ventricular end-diastolic volumes should be avoided.

Goals

1. Maintain the ventricular response rate to atrial fibrillation below 100 bpm if sinus rhythm cannot be maintained.
2. Maintain LAP high enough to take advantage of the increased preload reserve.
3. Avoid pulmonary artery hypertension by treating hypercarbia, hypoxemia, and acidemia.
4. Aggressively treat pulmonary artery hypertension with vasodilator therapy to avoid RV failure. If RV failure does occur, inotropic support of the RV and pulmonary vasodilation may be necessary.
5. Maintain awareness of potential for left ventricular rupture.

■ MITRAL REGURGITATION

Mitral regurgitation (MR) may be caused by any number of processes that affect the components of the mitral valve apparatus. Valve leaflet involvement may cause regurgitation from mechanical impairment due to rheumatic fever, trauma, or infective endocarditis. The valve annulus may become calcified, causing mechanical impairment of leaflet apposition. Functional impairment of leaflet apposition due to annular dilation may result from ventricular dilation caused by ischemia or a dilated cardiomyopathy. Mechanical impairment may result from rupture of the chordae tendinae. Infective endocarditis, rheumatic, fever, trauma, or long-standing strain from mitral valve prolapse may result in chordae tendinae rupture.

Ischemia may cause asynergy of the ventricular wall and papillary muscle leading to functional impairment and regurgitation.[56] The posterior papillary muscles are more vulnerable to ischemia than the anterior papillary muscles. This is due to the fact that the posterior papillary muscle is supplied with blood solely from the posterior descending artery, whereas the anterior papillary muscle derives its blood supply from branches of both the left anterior descending and circumflex arteries. With continued ischemia, papillary muscle asynergy may progress to necrosis and rupture of the papillary muscle. Classically, rupture of one or more of the papillary muscle heads from necrosis occurs 2 to 7 days after an inferior myocardial infarction. This leads to mechanical impairment and severe acute MR.

Pathophysiology and Adaptation

MR is an LV volume overload lesion that can be acute or chronic in nature. In essence, a double-outlet left ventricle exists. There is a low-impedance outflow tract into the low-pressure left atrium via the incompetent mitral valve and a high-impedance outflow tract into the high-pressure aorta via the aortic valve. The extent of regurgitation is determined by the size of the mitral valve orifice, time available for regurgitation (systole), and pressure gradient between the LA and LV. The area of the mitral valve orifice is, in large part, determined by the size of the LV.[57,58] Dilation of the LV will result in distortion and enlargement of the valve orifice. The pressure gradient is determined by ventricular systolic pressure, LA pressure, and LA compliance. The length of ventricular systole is inversely related to heart rate, as illustrated in Figure 5-3.

Regurgitant flow ceases when the LV and LA pressures equalize. Equalization of pressure will occur more rapidly when a small, noncompliant LA exists, because LA pressure will rise more rapidly than in a large, compliant atrium. Equalization of pressure also occurs more rapidly when the impedance to LV ejection via the aorta is low. When aortic impedance is low, a larger forward stroke volume can be ejected and equalization of pressure will occur quickly.

Chronic volume overloading of the left ventricle results in eccentric ventricular hypertrophy similar to that seen in AR. The results of this process are summarized in Figure 5-9A. As in AR, both LVESV and LVEDV increase, but LVEDV increases to a greater extent. This results in an enhanced SV with no need for an increased EF. The slope of the diastolic pressure–volume curve is little changed, and thus, compliance, in the true sense of the concept, is only slightly increased. However, the entire pressure–volume loop is shifted to the right, a phenomenon known as "creep." This rightward shift of the diastolic pressure–volume curve allows low diastolic pressures to be maintained at very large end-diastolic volumes. The large increase in ventricular radius that accompanies eccentric hypertrophy elevates wall stress and stimulates some degree of concentric hypertrophy as well. Unlike AR, this compensation is complete and wall stress is normalized in both end systole and end diastole (see Fig. 5-9A).

Unique LV pressure loading exists in chronic MR, as illustrated in Figure 5-9A. The isovolumic phase of ven-

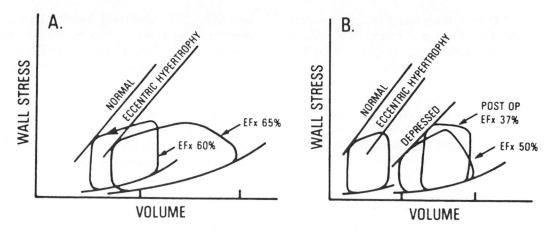

FIGURE 5–9. Left ventricular wall stress–volume loops for patient with progressive MR. **A.** Wall stress–volume loops of normal ventricle and of ventricle having developed eccentric hypertrophy in response to chronic volume overload of MR. Ventricle with eccentric hypertrophy has reduced isovolumic contraction phase and has its entire wall stress–volume relationship shifted to the right. Isovolumic contraction phase is even shorter than seen in AR (*see* Fig. 5–5). In addition, end-systolic wall stress is normalized. These adaptations allow the ventricle to deliver large SV with high normal EF. **B.** Wall stress–volume relationships in ventricle with chronic mitral regurgitation and systolic dysfunction. Low-impedance outflow tract to the left atrium provided by incompetent mitral valve allows wall stress to remain low during early and late ventricular systole. Thus despite presence of systolic dysfunction, EF is maintained near normal (EF$_x$ 50%). After surgical replacement of mitral valve, low-impedance outflow tract to left atrium is abolished. This results in elevation of wall stress during early and late systole. Under these loading conditions, afterload mismatch occurs and ventricular systolic dysfunction manifests as reduced ejection fraction (EF$_x$ 37%). *(From Ross J: Left ventricular function and the timing of surgical treatment in valvular heart disease. Ann Inter Med 1981; 94:502. Reprinted with permission.)*

tricular systole is of very short duration and limited pressure generation. In fact, because the impedance to ejection into the LA is so low, the isovolumic phase is shorter and lower in pressure than that seen in AR. This allows a greater portion of myocardial energy expenditure to be directed toward ejecting a large volume and less toward overcoming impedance to begin ejection.

In chronic MR, the sustained high LAPs result in left atrial hypertrophy and eventually left atrial distension. This distension results in the development of atrial dysrhythmias, the most common of which is atrial fibrillation. In severe MR, atrial fibrillation rather than sinus rhythm generally is the rule.

In acute MR, there is not ample time for ventricular eccentric hypertrophy to occur. As a result, the ventricle does not have the enormous preload reserve available in chronic MR. Of greater importance is the status of the left atrium. In acute MR, a small, noncompliant LA exists. Regurgitation of volume into a small LA results in high LA pressures, which manifests as a regurgitant V wave. As discussed in Chapter 2, the height of the V wave is not a good quantifier of the regurgitant volume but rather of the relationship between regurgitant volume and LA compliance. Nonetheless, this elevation of LA pressure results in acute pulmonary congestion.

Ventricular Diastolic Function and the Atrial Transport Mechanism

In chronic MR, as in AR, a large total stroke volume is necessary if forward SV is to be maintained when the regurgitant volume is large. An atrial kick is helpful in aug-

menting LVEDV. However, the increased compliance and rightward shift of the diastolic pressure–volume curve allows passive filling of the LV in early and mid-diastole via the LA when atrial fibrillation exists.

In acute MR, increased ventricular compliance and a rightward shift of the diastolic pressure–volume curve are absent. In this setting, an atrial systole may be necessary to increase the left atrial to left ventricular pressure gradient enough to complete filling of the left ventricle via the left atrium.

In chronic MR, eccentric hypertrophy and creep allow large increases in LVEDV with minimal increases in LVEDP. This affords a great deal of preload reserve. However, it must be kept in mind that the ventricular dilation that accompanies increases in LVEDV results in enlargement of the mitral annulus and an increase in the regurgitant fraction.

In contrast, in acute MR preload reserve is nearly exhausted. Without adequate time for adaptation, the left ventricle operates on the steep portion of its diastolic pressure–volume curve. Again, preload augmentation may result in ventricular dilation and a worsening of the regurgitation.

Myocardial Oxygen Balance

Myocardial oxygen consumption is increased by:

1. The large mass of myocardium that must be supplied with oxygen.
2. The enormous volume work done by the left ventricle. Volume work increases oxygen con-

sumption but to a much lesser extent than pressure work.[8] The isovolumic contraction phase is highly energy-consumptive. Because of the low impedance to ejection into the LA, the isovolumic contraction phase is very brief and represents only a small portion of the total work done by the ventricle (*see* Fig. 5–9A). A greater portion of the total work load is devoted to the generation of volume ejection, which is an energy-efficient process.

Myocardial oxygen delivery is compromised by:

1. The presence of coexistent coronary artery stenoses. This is particularly important for patients with acute MR from papillary muscle rupture or dysfunction. Unlike AR, aortic diastolic blood pressure is preserved, which helps maintain the gradient for coronary blood flow.
2. The high left ventricular end-diastolic pressures that accompany acute MR. In acute MR, eccentric hypertrophy has not had time to occur and large LVEDVs are accompanied by large LVEDPs.

Left Ventricular Systolic Function

Patients with chronic MR may remain symptom-free for long periods of time despite progressive decreases in systolic function. The enormous preload reserve available to these patients allows SV to be maintained by progressive increases in LVEDV in the face of declining contractile function and increasing LVESV. When preload reserve is exhausted, further diminution in systolic function cannot be compensated for and SV falls. At this point, symptoms of reduced cardiac output appear and systolic function is already seriously compromised (*see* Fig. 5–9B). In patients with acute MR secondary to ischemia, systolic function may be seriously compromised by acute myocardial ischemia or infarction.

Ejection fraction will greatly overestimate systolic function in MR because of the unique loading conditions present. Recall that EF determinations are very afterload-dependent (*see* Chapter 2). In MR, the impedance to ejection via the incompetent mitral valve is low. Therefore, EF may remain in the normal range despite severe systolic dysfunction. This severe dysfunction may only become apparent after mitral valve replacement when the low-impedance outflow tract is repaired (*see* Fig. 5–9B).

Right Ventricular Function and the Pulmonary Vasculature

The large, compliant LA that develops in chronic MR tends to shield the pulmonary circulation from elevated LA pressures. With time, however, pulmonary artery hypertension will develop from passive pulmonary venous

distension. If LA pressures remain elevated over a long period of time, reactive changes occur in the pulmonary vasculature. Prolonged perivascular edema results in arterial intima fibroelastosis and nonreversible elevations in pulmonary artery pressures and pulmonary vascular resistance. RV dysfunction from afterload mismatch may develop, as occurs in MS. In the most severe instances, tricuspid regurgitation from RV distension will complicate the picture. As in MS, efforts to reduce RV afterload and improve RV output with nitroprusside have been shown to significantly improve systemic output in patients with elevated pulmonary vascular resistance.[41]

In acute MR, the small, noncompliant LA is poorly adapted to shield the pulmonary vasculature from the regurgitated volume. Regurgitation of volume into the noncompliant LA results in profound and immediate elevation of LAP with a very large V wave. Pulmonary vascular congestion with interstitial pulmonary edema rather than secondary pulmonary artery hypertension is the issue here. RV systolic dysfunction may exist because reductions in posterior descending coronary artery perfusion severe enough to produce posterior papillary muscle dysfunction or infarction also may produce RV ischemia or infarction.

Effect of Heart Rate Alterations on Hemodynamics

Bradycardia (heart rate below 60 bpm) is detrimental in MR for several reasons:

1. It prolongs systole, which increases the time available for regurgitation.
2. It prolongs diastole (to a greater extent than systole), which allows a large LVEDV to develop. This may result in LV distension, particularly in acute MR, in which eccentric hypertrophy and creep are absent. LV distension leads to enlargement of the mitral annulus and worsening regurgitation.[57,58]
3. When the regurgitant fraction is large (50 to 60%), total SV will be large but forward SV will be compromised. Forward cardiac output can only be enhanced in this setting by an increase in heart rate.

Efforts to increase heart rate into the optimal range of 80 to 100 bpm must be tempered by the knowledge that faster heart rates compromise myocardial oxygen delivery by shortening diastole. This is particularly important for patients who have MR secondary to papillary muscle rupture or dysfunction from ischemia.

Most patients with moderate and severe MR are in atrial fibrillation. In these patients, control of heart rate is dependent on adequate control of the ventricular response rate to the fibrillating atrium. Drugs used to control the ventricular response rate at the AV node, such as digoxin, verapamil, and beta blockers, must be continued.

Effect of Afterload Alterations on Hemodynamics

Increased afterload is poorly tolerated by patients with acute and chronic MR because it increases the regurgitant fraction. Increased afterload tends to increase the size of the LV by increasing LVESV, followed by a compensatory increase in LVEDV. This LV dilation increases the size of the mitral orifice. Increased afterload also increases the impedance to ejection via the aorta. This favors ejection into the LA via the lower impedance outflow tract.

Unlike AR, in which afterload reduction must be used selectively, afterload reduction is uniformly advantageous in both acute and chronic MR. Afterload reduction improves forward cardiac output by promoting ejection via the aorta and reducing the regurgitant fraction. This is because the incompetent mitral valve provides such low impedance to ejection that any decrease in the impedance to ejection via the aortic valve will augment forward flow.

Anesthetic Technique

Goals

1. Maintain sinus rhythm where possible.
2. Maintain heart rate at 80 to 100 bpm.
3. Maintain end-diastolic PCWP high enough to guarantee a large LVEDV without ventricular distension and increased valve area.
4. Decrease LV afterload; increases are poorly tolerated. Decreasing afterload will improve cardiac output by decreasing regurgitation but preload *must* be maintained.
5. Maintain contractility.
6. When pulmonary vascular resistance is high or when RV systolic dysfunction exists, RV afterload reduction will improve RV and subsequently LV output. The concurrent systemic vasodilation also will directly reduce regurgitation.
7. Avoid hypercarbia, hypoxemia, and acidemia, which tend to cause pulmonary hypertension and may result in acute RV decompensation.

Premedication

Patients with chronic MR must be premedicated with caution, particularly when pulmonary artery hypertension and compromised LV performance exist. Hypercarbia, hypoxemia, and vasodilation may accompany overzealous use of narcotics and sedatives. Morphine sulfate 0.05 mg/kg IM and lorazepam 1 mg PO approximately 1.5 hours before scheduled incision time will prevent undue anxiety in the fittest of these patients. For elderly or debilitated patients with RV failure and pulmonary congestion, 1 to 3 mg of morphine sulfate IM will suffice. All patients should have supplemental O_2 started at the time of premedication. All cardiac medications are continued until the time of surgery. Ranitidine 150 mg PO or a similar H_2 blocker is given at the time of premedication and the evening before surgery.

For patients with acute MR, severe hemodynamic compromise usually is the rule. It is dangerous to sedate these patients before surgery. All sedatives and narcotics should be given with careful observation of the fully monitored patient. Antiaspiration prophylaxis with an H_2 blocker and metoclopramide should be initiated.

Preinduction

All patients should have two large-bore peripheral IV lines (14 gauge). Alternatively, if peripheral IV access is poor, a peripheral IV suitable for induction can be started and a large-bore double-lumen (16- or 14-gauge) central venous line can be placed at the same time as the pulmonary artery catheter (*see* Chapter 3). ECG monitoring should allow assessment of V_5, I, II, III, aVR, aVL, and aVF. Baseline recording of all seven leads should be obtained for comparative purposes. Normally, two leads (II and V_5) are monitored simultaneously intraoperatively. A radial artery catheter is placed with local anesthesia and adequate sedation before the induction of anesthesia. A pulmonary artery catheter can be placed before or after induction of anesthesia. All of the equipment and medications necessary for treatment of dysrhythmias are available before placement of the pulmonary artery catheter. Placement of the pulmonary artery catheter before induction allows preload and afterload to be optimized before induction of anesthesia. The insertion distance necessary to obtain a wedge pressure trace is greater (5 cm more via the right internal jugular route) in patients with pulmonary hypertension than in normals.[42] The risk of pulmonary artery perforation is greater in patients with pulmonary hypertension.[43,44] This may be due to eccentric balloon inflation forcing the catheter tip into the wall of vessel,[43,44] direct vessel disruption during balloon inflation in a distal arterial branch,[44] or distal catheter migration during balloon deflation.[44] Locating the catheter tip in the proximal pulmonary artery and readvancing the catheter for each wedge pressure measurement has been shown to greatly reduce the risk of pulmonary artery perforation in an animal model of pulmonary hypertension.[45]

The V wave and the mean PCWP are *not* good estimates of LVEDP in patients with MR. Recall that the V wave occurs during early ventricular systole and quantifies the relationship between the regurgitant volume and left atrial compliance. The mean PCWP will be skewed upward by a large V wave and will, therefore, overestimate the LVEDP by an amount proportional to the amplitude and duration of the V wave. The best estimate of LVEDP is the end-diastolic PCWP. In patients in sinus rhythm, this will be the A-wave pressure. In patients in atrial fibrillation, it will be the PCWP just before the onset of the V wave (*see* Chapter 3). The cardiac catheterization report will provide information regarding the optimal LVEDP in a given patient. The pulmonary artery catheter allows pulmonary vascular resistance to be calculated and CVP to be measured. Therapy to reduce RV afterload and improve RV systolic performance cannot be initiated safely without this information.

In chronic MR, because of the increased ventricular compliance and the phenomenon of creep, LVEDV will be supplemented with only small increases in the mean PCWP. In patients with preserved LV function, a mean PCWP in the range of 10 to 15 mm Hg will ensure optimal LVEDV. Serial cardiac outputs obtained in conjunction with volume infusion will help with optimization of preload. In patients with depressed ventricular function who have exhausted preload reserve, PCWP will be in the range of 20 to 25 mm Hg when preload is optimized.

In acute MR, there will be large V waves and LVEDP will be elevated because of the lack of compensatory atrial and ventricular enlargement. It may be necessary to have an end-diastolic PCWP of 20 to 25 mm Hg to ensure an adequate LVEDV in patients with acute MR.

For patients in whom afterload reduction is sought before induction, sodium nitroprusside is the agent of choice. It is easily titratable with a very short half-life. The infusion can be started at 0.15 to 0.3 µ/kg/min and titrated with careful attention paid to cardiac output, arterial blood pressure, and PCWP. Although nitroprusside is primarily an arterial vasodilator, it has vasodilatory effects on the venous system as well. It is important not to let reductions in preload offset the beneficial effects of arterial dilation. If necessary, volume infusion should be used to maintain PCWP in the optimal range.

For patients with severe RV failure, pulmonary congestion, and systemic hypotension (systolic blood pressure lower than 90 mm Hg), efforts to improve RV function and reduce regurgitation with vasodilator therapy may be unsuccessful due to worsening systemic hypotension. For these patients, the addition of inotropic support of the RV and LV is necessary. Dobutamine 5 to 10 µg/kg/min is a good choice because it has no alpha-adrenergic activity and little chronotropic activity and it tends to reduce pulmonary artery pressures (*see* Chapter 4). Therefore, it will not exacerbate pulmonary artery hypertension or increase LV afterload and regurgitation.

In patients with myocardial ischemia, efforts must be directed toward lowering LVEDP, decreasing ventric-

ular radius, improving aortic diastolic blood pressure, and decreasing heart rate as much as is possible without worsening the regurgitant process. IV nitroglycerin is a mainstay of therapy. Dobutamine 5 to 10 µg/kg/min is a good choice if an inotropic agent is necessary. It reduces LV radius and end-diastolic pressure while increasing aortic blood pressure and causing little change in heart rate (*see* Chapter 4). In patients with MR, the resultant reduction in wall stress and the valve orifice area will serve to decrease both myocardial oxygen consumption and the regurgitant volume. When pharmacologic interventions fail, the use of the intra-aortic balloon pump (IABP) may be indicated (*see* Chapter 11).

Induction and Maintenance

Generally, 50 to 75 µg/kg of fentanyl or 10 to 15 µg/kg of sufentanil can be used as the primary anesthetic for induction and maintenance before cardiopulmonary bypass. These agents are chosen because they have minimal effects on myocardial contractility and peripheral vascular resistance.[18,19] Compared with fentanyl, sufentanil is more likely to cause a fall in mean arterial pressure secondary to a reduced peripheral vascular resistance in patients with valvular heart disease.[20,21] On the other hand, patients with valvular heart disease receiving sufentanil in these doses are less likely to require supplemental anesthesia or vasodilator therapy for skin incision, sternotomy, sternal spread, or aortic manipulation.[20,21]

After several minutes of preoxygenation and with the patient breathing 100% oxygen, induction begins with an infusion of fentanyl 500 µg/min or sufentanil 100 µg/min over 5 to 10 minutes. A system of graded stimulation is used to individualize the narcotic dose for each patient. Compared with patients with coronary artery disease, patients with valvular heart disease have a lower narcotic requirement to achieve unconsciousness.[21] This is probably caused by a lower cardiac output with a relative greater distribution of output to the brain and spinal cord.[21] After loss of consciousness, the hemodynamic response to insertion of an oral airway followed by insertion of a urinary catheter is used to gauge the need for additional narcotic to blunt the hemodynamic response to tracheal intubation. Laryngoscopy is performed carefully and should not be prolonged. If an upward trend in heart rate or blood pressure is noted as laryngoscopy commences, laryngoscopy should be terminated and additional narcotic should be titrated. If there is poor visualization of the larynx, laryngoscopy should be terminated and intubating conditions should be improved by changing head position, using a stylet, or changing blades. This approach will help prevent long stimulating laryngoscopies that compromise hemodynamics. If the entire narcotic dose is not used for induction, the remainder is infused slowly in anticipation of the skin incision. A TEE probe (*see* Chapter 3) is placed after tracheal intubation and verification of tube position.

Muscle relaxants are chosen with optimization of heart rate in mind (*see* Chapter 4). In the absence of beta blockade, the vecuronium–fentanyl or vecuronium–sufentanil combination is a good choice if a small heart rate decrease is desired. The pancuronium–fentanyl or pancuronium–sufentanil combination is more likely to cause a heart rate increase, which is advantageous for patients who are relatively bradycardic. Vecuronium or pancuronium 0.02 mg/kg is administered approximately 1 to 2 minutes before starting the fentanyl infusion. As the patient loses consciousness, the remainder of the total dose of 0.1 mg/kg is administered and controlled ventilation with 100% O_2 is initiated. An alternative to vecuronium is cis-atracurium 0.04 mg/kg as the priming dose and 0.2 mg/kg as the total dose. These regimens minimize the risk of narcotic-induced rigidity without undue stress to the patient.

If tachycardia develops and is determined to be detrimental, immediate treatment is required. The first strategy should be to terminate any noxious stimuli and increase the depth of anesthesia when necessary. Propranolol in increments of 0.5 mg is given for two to three doses to get the heart rate in the desired range. If this fails, the incremental dose can be increased to 1.0 mg. In patients with poor ventricular function, doses greater than 0.1 mg/kg over less than a 1-hour period must be used with caution to avoid compromise of systolic function. In some instances, the ultra-short-acting beta blocker esmolol may be useful. Esmolol has an elimination half-life of 9 minutes due to metabolism by red cell esterases and is relatively beta-1 selective. Esmolol is started with a bolus of 0.5 mg/kg given over several minutes followed by an infusion of 50 µg/kg/min and titrated up to 300 µg/kg/min as necessary. Esmolol is useful for patients with poor ventricular function or bronchospastic disease, because if it is not tolerated, therapy can be terminated quickly. Furthermore, unlike longer-acting beta blockers, esmolol can be used aggressively in the pre-CPB period without fear that it will compromise termination of CPB.

Bradycardia with hemodynamic compromise must be treated promptly. A small dose of pancuronium (1 to 3 mg) is often effective if vecuronium or cis-atracurium has been used. Atropine 0.4 to 0.8 mg is a reasonable choice despite the risk of tachycardia because tachycardia is well tolerated by these patients. Ephedrine is a poor choice because the concomitant increase in afterload is detrimental.

Hypotension must not be treated routinely with vasopressors because an increase in the regurgitant volume will worsen the situation. If heart rate and preload are optimized, then augmentation of SV with an inotropic agent should be initiated. Dobutamine 5 to 10 µg/kg/min will augment cardiac output without increasing afterload or worsening pulmonary artery hypertension.

If surgical stimulation (skin incision, sternotomy, sternal spreading, or aortic manipulation) produces hypertension, additional doses of sufentanil (1 to 5 µg/kg) or fentanyl (5 to 25 µg/kg) may be necessary. Recent data call this practice into question. After a patient has received high doses of sufentanil (10 to 30 µg/kg) or fentanyl (50 to 100 µg/kg), administration of an additional agent as an infusion or a bolus will not reliably blunt the hemodynamic response to noxious stimuli.[22] If this fails to control the hypertension, the use of additional agents will be necessary. Vasodilation with sodium nitroprusside can be titrated easily and terminated quickly. This makes it an ideal choice for treatment of transient elevations in peripheral vascular resistance during high-dose narcotic anesthesia. Although relatively large doses of nitroglycerin may be needed to control systemic hypertension, nitroglycerin is a better choice than nitroprusside in cases in which myocardial ischemia exists (*see* Chapter 4). It also may become necessary to supplement narcotic anesthesia with additional anesthetic agents:

1. Benzodiazepines. Diazepam, midazolam, and lorazepam administered in conjunction with fentanyl or sufentanil have been implicated in causing decreases in peripheral vascular resistance with subsequent hypotension.[23-26] Therefore, they must be titrated with caution. Midazolam in increments of 1 to 2 mg or lorazepam in increments of 0.5 to 1.0 mg are reasonable.

2. Inhalation anesthetics. N_2O combined with high-dose opiates elevates pulmonary vascular resistance, particularly in presence of preexisting pulmonary hypertension.[31] Because of the existence of pulmonary hypertension in most patients with MR, N_2O should be avoided. N_2O in association with high-dose opiates causes systolic dysfunction in patients with coronary artery disease, particularly those with an LVEDP > 15 mm Hg.[27,28] An animal model of coronary stenosis suggests that this may be secondary to ischemia-induced segmental contraction abnormalities.[29] No such contraction abnormalities have been observed in humans with preserved left ventricular function and ischemic heart disease exposed to high-dose opiates and N_2O.[30] Nonetheless, in patients with MR secondary to myocardial ischemia, N_2O should be avoided even in the absence of pulmonary hypertension. Isoflurane is a potent vasodilator that causes little depression of systolic function[32] and is potentially useful for patients with MR in which

systolic function is preserved and LV afterload reduction is sought. Sevoflurane and desflurane have similar effects.[33,34] However, care must be taken to avoid decreases in peripheral vascular resistance and hypotension. Controversy exists regarding whether isoflurane in the presence of coronary stenoses is responsible for producing a coronary steal phenomenon leading to ischemia (*see* Chapter 4). Enflurane causes both vasodilation and depression of systolic function[32] and must be titrated with caution as well.

Many patients with acute MR from myocardial ischemia or infarction will be in cardiogenic shock with impending respiratory distress from pulmonary vascular congestion. These patients may arrive from the cardiac catheterization laboratory intubated, ventilated, and supported with an IABP. In addition, these patients may be at high risk for aspiration. The induction sequence should be modified for nonintubated patients. After preoxygenation and with cricoid pressure applied, etomidate 0.15 to 0.3 mg/kg, succinylcholine 1.0 to 1.5 mg/kg, in conjunction with fentanyl 10 μg/kg or sufentanil 1 μg/kg can be administered. Alternatively, sufentanil 5 μg/kg and succinylcholine 1.0 to 1.5 mg/kg can be used.

Post-Cardiopulmonary Bypass Management

After mitral valve replacement, a small residual mean gradient (2 to 5 mm Hg) exists across the prosthetic valve. Mechanical (nontissue) valves exhibit a small amount of regurgitant flow in systole. Repaired mitral valves may exhibit some residual mild regurgitation and stenosis. This is assessed with TEE (*see* Chapter 3).

After mitral valve replacement or repair for chronic MR, the ventricle that has undergone compensation for a volume overload lesion is now faced with a relative pressure overload. The competent mitral valve eliminates the low-impedance outflow tract into the LA. The very favorable loading conditions have been eliminated and all volume must be ejected via the high-impedance outflow tract into the aorta. This causes a substantial elevation of intraventricular pressure during the isovolumic contraction phase. The elimination of regurgitation by the competent valve greatly reduces the need for a large total stroke volume. Therefore, a greater proportion of total myocardial oxygen consumption goes toward the more energy-consumptive process of pressure generation to begin ejection and less toward volume ejection. In MR in contrast to AR, postoperatively, there is an elevation of early and late systolic wall stress, despite the dramatic reduction in ventricular radius that accompanies elimination of the regurgitant volume (*see* Fig. 5–9B). This results in a state of afterload mismatch

such that postoperative systolic function is compromised. The temptation when cardiac output is low will be to use the large preload reserve available in these patients. Because intraventricular pressure is already elevated, during the prolonged isovolumic contraction phase wall stress for a given LVEDV will be greater in the postbypass period. Efforts to increase preload to contend with poor systolic function or high afterload states will only worsen afterload mismatch. A mean PCWP or LAP or 10 to 15 mm Hg usually is adequate.

For these reasons, and particularly if poor myocardial protection is obtained during bypass and aortic cross-clamping or if depressed systolic function exists preoperatively, management of these patients post-CPB is challenging. The mainstays of therapy are afterload reduction and inotropic support of systolic function. The goal of vasodilator therapy is to reduce the impedance to ejection via the aorta as much as possible to avoid afterload mismatch.

When systolic blood pressure is low (below 90 mm Hg) and the cardiac index is low (less than 2.0 L/min/m[2]), an inotrope is started first. Epinephrine 0.015 to 0.03 μg/kg/min is a good choice because it is a potent inotrope with little vasoconstrictor activity at this dose. When afterload reduction is needed, as determined by a high SVR or mean aortic pressure, nitroprusside is added. It is easily titratable with a short half-life. The infusion can be started at 0.15 to 0.3 μg/kg/min and titrated with careful attention paid to cardiac index, arterial blood pressure, and PCWP. Volume infusion may be necessary to keep PCWP in the optimal range. If the PCWP remains elevated (over 18 mm Hg) with inotrope infusion, then nitroglycerin started at 0.15 to 0.3 μg/kg/min and titrated upward is the vasodilator of choice.

In acute MR, little or no creep or eccentric hypertrophy exists, and thus, postoperative preload reserve will resemble that of a normal ventricle. Nonetheless, inotropic support and afterload reduction may be necessary, particularly if MR was secondary to ischemia and systolic function was compromised preoperatively. The same strategy of inotrope and vasodilator therapy used in chronic MR is used here.

The management of RV function and the pulmonary vasculature can be problematic in the postbypass period. In all patients with elevated pulmonary artery pressures, there will be a dramatic reduction in pulmonary artery pressures due to the reductions in the mean LAP and passive pulmonary congestion after valve replacement.[46] Despite this, some patients will continue to have elevated pulmonary vascular resistances due to reversible (reactive pulmonary vasoconstriction) and nonreversible (morphologic changes in the pulmonary vasculature) causes.[46] For these patients, careful management is necessary. LV function may be seriously compromised by RV failure when the RV is unable to deliver volume to the LA via the pulmonary system. The hallmarks of this syndrome are a high RAP (above 10 mm Hg) and pulmonary vascular resistance (over 150 dynes sec/cm[5]), coupled with a low LAP (under 5 mm Hg) and cardiac index (less than 2.2 L/min/m²). Aggersive efforts must be made to keep pulmonary vascular resistance as low as possible by avoiding hypercarbia, hypoxemia, and acidemia and by avoiding pulmonary vasoconstrictors. If pulmonary hypertension persists despite these efforts, then active pulmonary vasodilation will be necessary. Nitroglycerin has been shown to be effective in reducing pulmonary artery pressures[47] and increasing pulmonary blood flow[48] after mitral valve replacement. The nitroglycerin can be started at 0.15 to 0.30 μg/kg/min and titrated upward as needed. Sodium nitroprusside started at the same dosage and titrated upward also is effective.

If poor RV protection has occurred during bypass and aortic cross-clamping, then inotropic support of the RV may be necessary, in addition to pulmonary vasodilation. Inotropic support should be chosen with an eye toward avoiding increased pulmonary vascular resistance. Epinephrine 0.015 to 0.03 μg/kg/min, dopamine 1 to 5 μg/kg/min, or dobutamine 5 to 10 μg/kg/min all meet this requirement. However, when increased doses of epinephrine and dopamine are used, progressive pulmonary vasoconstriction from increased alpha-adrenergic activity results (*see* Chapter 4). In situations in which increasing demand for inotropic support is demonstrated, amrinone 5 to 10 μg/kg/min after a loading dose of 0.75 to 1.5 mg/kg or milrinone 0.5 to 0.75 μg/kg/min after a loading dose of 50 to 75 μg/kg may be added (*see* Chapter 4). They provide potent inotropic support and pulmonary vasodilation.[49] Isoproterenol is a drug often suggested for use in patients who require inotropic support and pulmonary vasodilation.[50] Isoproterenol causes an increase in heart rate, myocardial oxygen consumption, and the incidence of ventricular dysrhythmias,[51] all of which may limit its usefulness. Recently, the combination of prostaglandin E$_1$ (PGE$_1$) and norepinephrine has been shown to be effective in treating refractory pulmonary hypertension and right ventricular failure after mitral valve replacement.[52] PGE$_1$ is a potent pulmonary and systemic vasodilator. PGE$_1$ 30 to 150 μg/kg/min is infused into the right heart in combination with norepinephrine in doses up to 1 μg/kg/min infused via a left atrial line. The norepinephrine is infused via the left atrial line to minimize its vasoconstrictive effects on the pulmonary vasculature, provide inotropic support, and counteract the profound systemic vasodilatory effects of PGE$_1$. Management of RV dysfunction, including TEE findings, are discussed in detail in Chapter 7.

Patients in atrial fibrillation with large left atria will only rarely convert to sinus rhythm postoperatively. Therefore, the ventricular response rate will have to be controlled. Bradycardia is better tolerated after replacement of the incompetent mitral valve than before replacement.

A rare but potentially lethal complication of mitral valve replacement is ventricular disruption. This complication has been described after mitral valve replacement for a variety of lesions but is most common in patients undergoing replacement for chronic MS.[53,54] Three types of ventricular rupture have been described.[54] Type 1 involves rupture of the mitral annulus or of the ventricle at the atrioventricular junction due to a diseased annulus or posterior ventricular wall. Type 2 rupture occurs at the site of the excised papillary muscle due to surgically induced thinning of the ventricular wall. Type 3 rupture or transverse midventricular disruption (TMD) occurs midway between type 1 and 2 ruptures. Type 3 ruptures seem to be secondary to a variety of causes. Endocardial injury from inadvertent surgical trauma or the valve prosthesis itself has been implicated. Total excision of the mitral valve apparatus may result in loss of longitudinal support, which predisposes the ventricle to transverse disruption when ventricular dilation occurs.[54,55]

Ventricular rupture may present upon termination of CPB or up to 5 days postoperatively. In the immediate postoperative period, these lesions present with hypotension and copious arterialized blood welling up in the pericardium or issuing forth from the chest tubes. Repair of these lesions requires prompt reinstitution of CPB and the mortality is high.[54] Treatment of TMD may require sacrificing the circumflex artery to incorporate enough posterior myocardium for an adequate repair.[54]

Although the primary responsibility for prevention of this complication lies with the surgeon, preventative measures must be made by the anesthesiologist. If the mitral apparatus has been excised or if the posterior ventricular wall is diseased, efforts must be made to minimize ventricular dilatation and intraventricular pressures. Left ventricular afterload should be normalized or reduced to prevent high intraventricular pressures and left ventricular dilatation. Likewise, reliance on large left ventricular end-diastolic volumes should be avoided.

Goals

1. Maintain the ventricular response rate to atrial fibrillation below 100 bpm if sinus rhythm cannot be maintained.
2. Avoid reliance on a large LVEDV; wall stress will be greatly elevated and systolic function may decline.
3. Aggressively use inotropic support and afterload reduction of the LV, particularly for patients in whom systolic function is compromised preoperatively or by CPB.

4. Avoid pulmonary artery hypertension by treating hypercarbia, hypoxemia, and acidemia.
5. Aggressively treat pulmonary artery hypertension with vasodilator therapy to avoid RV failure. If RV failure does occur, inotropic support of the RV and pulmonary vasodilation may be necessary.
6. Maintain awareness of potential for left ventricular rupture.

■ MULTIPLE VALVE LESIONS

It is not uncommon for patients with valvular heart disease to have both a stenotic and regurgitant process affecting one valve or to have involvement of two or more valves. There are several important points to keep in mind when evaluating patients with multiple valve lesions:

1. It is possible for a valve to be stenotic and incompetent; however, a severely stenotic valve can allow only minimal regurgitation because of the profound reduction in valve area. Likewise, a severely incompetent valve can offer only minimal impedance to flow across its large area. It is possible for a prosthetic valve to possess high-grade stenosis and regurgitation if it has a large perivalvular leak and is itself stenotic.
2. When a valve is not clearly primarily stenotic or incompetent, it is necessary to determine which lesion has the most pronounced effect on the patient's hemodynamics. If a patient with MS and MR is found to have a large LVEDV, it follows that MR is the predominant lesion. Likewise, if a patient with AS and AR is found to have a normal LVEDV with left atrial enlargement and a large A-wave pressure, it follows that AS is the predominant lesion.
3. When two valves are involved, it is necessary to know which features of each lesion exacerbate or ameliorate the effects of the other lesions. This is described in the subsequent sections.

AR and MS. The underloading of the LV characteristic of MS will be offset by the regurgitant aortic valve lesion. Passive filling of the LV via the LA and mitral valve will be compromised and the increased LAP and pulmonary artery hypertension characteristic of MS will be present. The increased heart rate so beneficial in AR will cause precipitous increases in LAP with subsequent pulmonary congestion. Therapy for both RV and LV afterload reduction will be necessary.

AS and MS. The LV underloading characteristic of MS will severely limit the preload reserve of the LV. Be-

cause LV compliance in AS will be diminished, LAP will have to be greatly elevated to ensure adequate filling of the LV with the gradient across the mitral valve. This will, in turn, exacerbate pulmonary congestion. LV afterload reduction will be poorly tolerated because of the large gradient across the aortic valve and the limited ability to increase LVEDV. Therefore, efforts to reduce RV afterload will be severely limited by the concomitant systemic vasodilation.

AR and MR. The pathophysiology of LV volume overload obviously will be predominant. Efforts to reduce LV afterload will be of benefit in the management of both lesions. Likewise, a relatively fast heart rate will be of benefit. High LAP and pulmonary artery hypertension not normally seen in AR may be a feature here. If the MR is secondary to ventricular dilation from AR, then only replacement of the aortic valve will be necessary.

AS and MR. The high intraventricular pressure seen in AS will cause dramatic MR if the mitral valve is incompetent. The combination of concentric and eccentric hypertrophy will allow the LV to maintain a relatively large stroke volume; the more severe the AS, the greater the regurgitant fraction. With a larger than normal preload reserve available, some LV afterload reduction might be tolerated in an effort to reduce regurgitation if the AS is mild. Efforts to increase heart rate to reduce the regurgitant process will have detrimental effects on the subendocardial perfusion of the hypertrophied LV. Pulmonary congestion and pulmonary artery hypertension with RV failure also are likely. Reduction of pulmonary arterial pressure will be difficult for patients with severe AS, because the concomitant systemic vasodilation will not be tolerated. In instances in which MR is mild to moderate and AS is severe, replacement of the aortic valve may reduce intraventricular pressures and ventricular dilatation such that mitral valve replacement or repair is unnecessary.

■ REFERENCES

1. Chambers DA: Acquired valvular heart disease, in Kaplin JA (ed): *Cardiac Anesthesia.* 1st ed. New York, Grune & Stratton, 1979.
2. Grossman W: Wall stress and patterns of hypertrophy in the human left ventricle. *J Clin Invest* 1975; **56**:56.
3. Ross J: Afterload mismatch in aortic and mitral valve disease: Implications for surgical therapy. *J Am Coll Cardiol* 1985; **5**:811–826.
4. Hanrath P, Mathey DG, Siegert R, Bleifeld W: Left ventricular relaxation and filling pattern in different forms of left ventricular hypertrophy: An echocardiographic study. *Am J Cardiol* 1980; **45**:15-23.
5. Stott DK, Marpole DGF, Bristow JD, et al: The role of left atrial transport in aortic and mitral stenosis. *Circulation* 1970; **41**:1031-1041.

6. Vinten-Johansen J, Weiss HR: Oxygen consumption in subepicardial and subendocardial regions of the canine left ventricle — The effect of experimental acute valvular aortic stenosis. *Circ Res* 1980; **46:**139.

7. Bertrand ME, LaBlanche JM, Tilmant PY, et al: Coronary sinus blood flow at rest and during isometric exercise in patients with aortic valve disease. Mechanism of angina pectoris in presence of normal coronary arteries. *Am J Cardiol* 1981; **47:**199.

8. Suga H, Hisano R, Hirata S, et al: Mechanism of higher oxygen consumption rate: Pressure-loaded vs. volume-loaded heart. *Am J Physiol* 1982; **242:**H942-H948.

9. Hakki AH, Kimbiris D, Iskandrian AS, et al: Angina pectoris and coronary artery disease in patients with severe aortic valvular disease. *Am Heart J* 1980; **100:**441.

10. Ross J: Left ventricular function and the timing of surgical treatment in valvular heart disease. *Ann Intern Med* 1981; **94:**498-504.

11. Croke RP, Pifarre R, Sullivan H, et al: Reversal of advanced left ventricular dysfunction following aortic valve replacement for aortic stenosis. *Ann Thorac Surg* 1977; **24:**38-43.

12. Smith N, McAnulty JH, Rahimtoola SH: Severe aortic stenosis with impaired left ventricular function and clinical heart failure: Results of valve replacement. *Circulation* 1978; **58:**255-264.

13. Dexter L: Pulmonary vascular disease in acquired and congenital heart disease. *Arch Intern Med* 1979; **139:**922-928.

14. Robotham JL: Cardiovascular disturbance in chronic respiratory insufficiency. *Am J Cardiol* 1981; **47:**941-949.

15. Boudoulas H, Rittgers SE, Lewis RP, et al: Changes in diastolic time with various pharmacologic agents. Implications for myocardial perfusion. *Circulation* 1979; **60:**164-169.

16. Rapaport E: Natural history of aortic and mitral valve disease. *Am J Cardiol* 1975; **35:**221-227.

17. Gorlin R, McMillan IKR, Medd WE, et al: Dynamics of the circulation in aortic valvular disease. *Am J Med* 1955; **18:**855-870.

18. Stanley TH, Webster LR: Anesthesia requirements and cardiovascular effects of fentanyl-oxygen and fentanyl-diazepam-oxygen anesthesia in man. *Anesth Analg* 1978; **57:**411-426.

19. Sebel PS, Bovil JG: Cardiovascular effects of sufentanil anesthesia. *Anesth Analg* 1982; **61:**115-119.

20. Bovill JG, Warren PJ, Schuller JL, et al: Comparison of fentanyl, sufentanil, and alfentanil anesthesia in patients undergoing valvular heart surgery. *Anesth Analg* 1984; **63:**1081-1086.

21. Stanley TH, de Lange S: Comparison of sufentanil-oxygen and fentanyl-oxygen anesthesia for mitral and aortic valvular surgery. *J Cardiothorac Anesth* 1987; **1:**6-11.

22. Philbin DM, Roscow CE, Schneider RC, et al: Fentanyl and sufentanil anesthesia revisited: How much is enough? *Anesthesiology* 1990; **73:**5-11.

23. George J, Samuelson PN, Lell WA, et al: Hemodynamic effects of diazepam-sufentanil compared to diazepamfentanyl. *Soc Cardiovasc Anesth* 1986, abstract 91.

24. Tomicheck RC, Rosow CE, Philbin DA, et al: Diazepam-fentanyl interaction — Hemodynamic and hormonal effects in coronary artery surgery. *Anesth Analg* 1983; **62:**881-884.

25. Heikkila H, Jalonen J, Arola M: Midazolam as adjunct to high-dose fentanyl anesthesia for coronary artery bypass grafting operation. *Acta Anaesthesiol Scand* 1984; **28:**683-689.

26. Heikkila H, Jalonen J, Laaksonen V: Lorazepam and high-dose fentanyl anaesthesia: Effects on hemodynamics and oxygen transportation in patients undergoing coronary revascularization. *Acta Anaesthesiol Scand* 1984; **28:**357-361.

27. Balasaraswathi K, Kumar P, Rao TLK, El-Etr AA: Left ventricular end-diastolic pressure (LVEDP) as an index for nitrous oxide use during coronary artery bypass surgery. *Anesthesiology* 1981; **55:**708-709.

28. Meretoja OA, Takkunen O, Heikkila H: Haemodynamic response to nitrous oxide during high-dose fentanyl pancuronium anaesthesia. *Acta Anaesthesiol Scand* 1985; **29:**137-141.

29. Philbin DM, Foex P, Drummond G, et al: Postsystolic shortening of canine left ventricle supplied by stenotic coronary artery when nitrous oxide is added in the presence of narcotics. *Anesthesiology* 1985; **62:**166-174.

30. Cahalan MK, Praksah O, Rulf ENR, et al: Addition of nitrous oxide to fentanyl anesthesia does not induce myocardial ischemia in patients with ischemic heart disease. *Anesthesiology* 1987; **67:**925-929.

31. Schulte-Sasse U, Hess W, Tarnow J: Pulmonary vascular response to nitrous oxide in patients with normal and high pulmonary vascular resistance. *Anesthesiology* 1982; **57:**9-13.

32. Eger EI: Isoflurane: A review. *Anesthesiology* 1981; **55:**559-576.

33. Ebert TJ, Harkin CP, Muzi M: Cardiovascular responses to sevoflurane: A review. *Anesth Analg* 1995; **81:**S11-22.

34. Warltier DC, Pagel PS: Cardiovascular and respiratory actions of desflurane: Is desflurane different from isoflurane. *Anesth Analg* 1992; **75:**S17-31.

35. Monrad ES, Hess OM, Murakami T, et al: Time course of regression of left ventricular hypertrophy after aortic valve replacement. *Circulation* 1988; **77:**1345-1355.

36. Hoshino PK, Gaasch WH: When to intervene in chronic aortic regurgitation. *Arch Intern Med* 1986; **146:**349-352.

37. Latson WL, Lappas DG: Use of a pacing catheter to control heart rate in a patient with aortic insufficiency and coronary artery disease. *Anesthesiology* 1985; **63:**712-715.

38. Thompson ME, Shaver JA, Leon DF: Effect of tachycardia on atrial transport in mitral stenosis. *Am Heart J* 1977; **94:**297-306.

39. Bolen JL, Lopes MG, Harrison DC, Alderman EL: Analysis of left ventricular function in response to afterload changes in patients with mitral stenosis. *Circulation* 1975; **52:**894.

40. Gash AK, Carabello BA, Cepin D, Spann JF: Left ventricular ejection performance and systolic muscle function in patients with mitral stenosis. *Circulation* 1983; **67:**148-154.

41. Stone JG, Hoar PF, Faltas AN, Khambatta HJ: Nitroprusside and mitral stenosis. *Anesth Analg* 1980; **59:**662-665.

42. Johnston WE, Royster RL, Vinten-Johansen J, et al: Influence of balloon inflation and deflation on location of pulmonary artery catheter tip. *Anesthesiology* 1987; **67:**110-115.

43. Leman R, Jones JG, Cowan G: A mechanism of pulmonary artery-perforation by Swan-Ganz catheters. *N Engl J Med* 1975; **292:**211-212.

44. Barash PG, Nardi D, Hammond G, et al: Catheter-induced pulmonary artery perforation. *J Thorac Cardiovasc Surg* 1981; **82:**5-12.

45. Keeler DK, Johnson WE, Vinten-Johansen J, et al: Pulmonary artery wedge pressure measurements during experimental pulmonary hypertension: Comparison of techniques in relation to catheter-induced hemorrhage. *J Cardiothorac Anesth* 1987; **1:**305-308.

46. Foltz BD, Hessel EA, Ivey TD: The early course of pulmonary artery hypertension in patients undergoing mitral valve replacement with cardioplegic arrest. *J Thorac Cardiovasc Surg* 1984; **88:**238-247.

47. Ziskind Z, Pohoryles L, Mohr R, et al: The effect of low dose intravenous nitroglycerin on pulmonary hypertension immediately after replacement of a stenotic mitral valve. *Circulation* 1985; **72**(suppl 2):164-169.

48. Halperin JL, Brooks KM, Rothlauf EB, et al: Effect of nitroglycerin on the pulmonary venous gradient in patients after mitral valve replacement. *J Am Coll Cardiol* 1985; **5:**34-39.

49. Doyle AR, Dhir AK, Moors AH, et al: Treatment of perioperative low cardiac output syndrome. *Ann Thorac Surg* 1995; **59:**S3-11.

50. Daoud FS, Reeves JT, Kelly DB: Isoproterenol as a potential pulmonary vasodilator in primary pulmonary hypertension. *Am J Cardiol* 1978; **42:**817-822.

51. Tinker JH, Tarhan S, White RD: Dobutamine for inotropic support during emergence from cardiopulmonary bypass. *Anesthesiology* 1976; **44:**281-286.

52. D'Ambra MN, LaRaia PJ, Philbin DM, et al: Prostaglandin E₁: A new therapy for refractory right heart failure and pulmonary hypertension after mitral valve replacement. *J Thorac Cardiovasc Surg* 1985; **89:**567-572.

53. Bjork VO, Henze A, Rodriguez L: Left ventricular rupture as a complication of mitral valve replacement. Surgical experience with eight cases and a review of the literature. *J Thorac Cardiovasc Surg* 1977; **73:**14-21.

54. Craver JM, Jones EL, Guyton RA, et al: Avoidance of transverse midventricular disruption following mitral valve replacement. *Ann Thorac Surg* 1985; **40:**163-171.

55. Cobbs BW, Hatcher CR, Craver JM: Transverse midventricular disruption after mitral valve replacement. *Am Heart J* 1980; **99:**33-50.

56. Gorman RC, McCaughan JS, Ratcliffe MB, et al: Pathogenesis of acute ischemic mitral regurgitation in three dimensions. *J Thorac Cardiovasc Surg* 1995; **109:**684-693.

57. Yoran C, Yellin EL, Becker RM, et al: Dynamic aspects of acute mitral regurgitation: Effects of ventricular volume, pressure and contractility on the effective regurgitant orifice area. *Circulation* 1979; **60:**170-176.

58. Borgenhagen DM, Serur JR, Gorlin R, et al: The effects of left ventricular load and contractility on mitral regurgitant orifice size and flow in the dog. *Circulation* 1977; **56:**106-113.

6

Anesthesia for Congenital Heart Disease

James A. DiNardo

■ INTRODUCTION

The anesthesiologist who cares for patients with congenital heart disease faces myriad challenges in the perioperative management of these often complex individuals. In major pediatric cardiac centers, almost every lesion is amenable to surgical intervention. Simplistic "recipe" approaches to these complicated patients will fall short of adequate management and will result in suboptimal outcome. Therefore, the anesthesiologist must understand the features that are unique to the pediatric cardiovascular system:

1. The dynamic transitional circulation of the neonate.
2. The functional limitations of the immature myocardium.
3. Age- and disease-related changes in the pulmonary vascular bed.
4. The effects of chronic hypoxemia, polycythemia, abnormal blood flow patterns, and pulmonary hypertension on the heart and other organ systems.

In addition, a detailed understanding of the surgical intervention planned is crucial. Every palliative or definitive operation has potential risks and complications that influence anesthetic management.

The pathophysiology of a wide variety of congenital heart defects can be best understood by applying certain basic principles to each patient. This chapter outlines those principles. The anesthesiologist who understands the dynamics of these lesions and the planned surgical intervention will be able to conduct an appropriate anesthetic. Although younger, smaller, and sicker patients are presenting for more complex, innovative surgical treatment, it is encouraging and impressive that there has been a concomitant decrease in surgical and anesthetic morbidity and mortality.[1]

Occurrence

Multiple studies have consistently shown the incidence of congenital heart disease to be approximately 7 to 10 births per 1000 live births.[2] Environmental factors such as drugs, viral infection, maternal diabetes, or maternal alcohol abuse may account for specific lesions. Genetic abnormalities including multiple syndromes may have cardiac disease as part of the clinical syndrome; most notably VATER and CHARGE syndromes. The chromosomal abnormalities also may be associated with cardiac disease, especially for patients with Trisomy 21, who have a 50% incidence of cardiac disease. However, most congenital heart defects are the result of an interaction of genetic predisposition and environmental factors.

■ PEDIATRIC CARDIOVASCULAR PHYSIOLOGY

Fetal Circulation and Postnatal Adjustments.
Although dramatic circulatory changes occur within minutes of birth, there continue to be more gradual changes over the first few days and weeks of life. These changes have profound effects on neonatal cardiovascular physiology. It is not coincidental that 50% of the neonates born with congenital heart disease will become ill enough during the first days or weeks of life to require medical or surgical intervention. Optimal anesthetic management of the neonate with congenital heart disease must be based on a firm understanding of these developmental changes.

Fetal Circulation

Most of the data on the physiology of fetal circulation have been obtained in fetal lambs, and although there may be species differences, important understanding of human fetal physiology has been derived from such studies.[3-5]

The placenta is the organ of gas exchange in the fetus, and fetal circulatory channels reflect this fact. Some of the dramatic changes that occur at birth are directly related to the exclusion of the placenta and the establishment of the lungs as the unit of gas exchange. Fetal circulatory channels shunt blood away from the lung, resulting in a parallel circuit in which both ventricles supply systemic circulation. It is also the presence of this parallel circulation that permits normal fetal growth and development in fetuses with cardiac malformations. Fetal shunts permit alternate pathways and provide adequate systemic blood flow to the fetus.

Oxygenated blood from the placenta returns to the fetus via the umbilical veins, which enter the portal venous system (*see* Fig. 6–1). Some of the blood from the portal venous sinus shunts via the ductus venosus directly into the inferior vena cava (IVC), bypassing the hepatic circulation. Inferior vena cava blood, containing blood from the lower fetal body, umbilical veins and portal vein, enters the right atrium (RA) while a smaller percentage of IVC blood shunts across the foramen ovale (FO) to the left atrium (LA). Superior vena caval (SVC) blood is shunted minimally across the FO and mainly flows into the right ventricle (RV) and pulmonary artery (PA). Most blood that enters the PA is shunted via the ductus arteriosus into the distal aorta. At birth, a series circulation is established in which each ventricle pumps into a specific vascular bed (RV → PA; LV → AO). The removal of the placenta and ventilation of the lungs at birth has the immediate effect of establishing this series circulation. To maintain the adult series circulation, the fetal channels must be closed. Com-

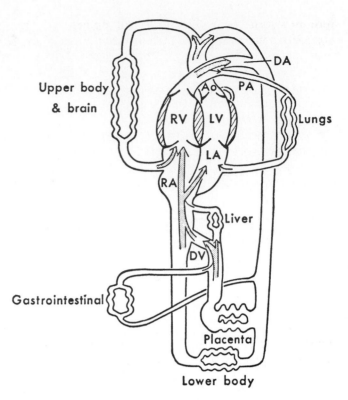

FIGURE 6–1. Schematic of the fetal circulation. (DA = ductus arteriosus; DV = ductus venosus; Ao = aorta; PA = pulmonary artery; RA = right atrium; RV = right ventricle; LA = left atrium; LV = left ventricle.) *(From: Rudolph AM: The fetal circulation, in* Congenital Diseases of the Heart. *Chicago, Mosby Year Book, 1974, p 2.)*

plex neurochemical and hormonal influences affect the closing of these fetal shunts. Acidosis, sepsis, hypothermia, hypoxia, and hypercarbia may cause reopening of the shunts and persistence of the fetal circulation (PFC). Most neonates who are critically ill from congenital heart disease have one or more of these inciting factors at the time of presentation, and in some instances persistence of fetal circulatory channels may be beneficial or even mandatory for survival.

Closure of the Ductus Arteriosus

In the fetus, patency of the ductus arteriosus is maintained by high levels of prostaglandin (PGI_2 and PGE_1).[6,7] There are two stages of ductal closure in the newborn: functional closure and permanent anatomic closure. Functional closure occurs by contraction of the smooth muscle of the ductal wall and usually occurs within the first day of life. An increase in Po_2 and a decrease in prostaglandins contribute to functional closure. Oxygen is a dose-dependent ductal constrictor that acts by increasing the rate of oxidative phosphorylation within smooth muscle cells. In addition, the response to oxygen may be age-related; full-term neonates have a more dramatic response to oxygen than an immature newborn. Norepinephrine and epinephrine, by changing pulmonary and systemic vascular resistances, may secondarily contribute to ductal closure. Acetylcholine has a direct constrictor effect on ductal tissue. Permanent anatomic closure of the duct usually is accomplished by 2 to 3 weeks of life in the normal full-term neonate. The lumen is sealed by fibrous connective tissue, leaving the vestigal structure, known as the *ligamentum arteriosum* (*see* Fig. 6–2).

Survival of some neonates with congenital cardiac lesions is dependent on ductal patency. Because functional closure is a reversible event, the use of PGE_1 infusions (0.05–0.1 µg/kg/min) has been one of the major medical advances in stabilization of neonates with ductal-dependent heart lesions. Preterm neonates are at risk of delayed ductal closure. This may be due to decreased degradation of PGE_1, increased production of PGE_1, or diminished sensitivity to the ductal constricting effects of oxygen. In instances in which delayed ductal closure is disadvantageous, prostaglandin inhibitors such as indomethacin (0.1 to 0.3 mg/kg PO or IV) have been used successfully to promote ductal closure and establish normal patterns of pulmonary blood flow.[8]

Closure of the Foramen Ovale

In the fetus, a flap-like valve known as the *foramen ovale* permits the right atrial and left atrial blood flow to mix. In utero, the right atrial pressure is higher than left atrial pressure, and IVC blood tends to flow in such a manner as to keep the foramen ovale open. Removal of the placenta causes a significant decrease in venous return to the right heart, causing a decrease in right atrial pressure. In addition, ventilation causes a marked increase in pulmonary arterial and venous blood flow and, therefore, an increase in left atrial pressure. This elevation of left atrial relative to right atrial pressure causes the flap-like valve of the foramen ovale to functionally close. In instances in which right atrial pressure remains elevated, right-to-left shunting may persist. Functional closure usually progresses to anatomic closure. However, probe patency of the foramen ovale may persist in 20% of normal adults and 50% of children younger than 5 years of age.[9,10]

Closure of the Ductus Venosus

The umbilical vessels constrict strongly after mechanical stimulation such as clamping and in response to high oxygen tensions. The resultant decrease in umbilical venous blood flow causes passive closure of the ductus venosus. The ductus venosus does not appear to be as sensitive as the ductus arteriosus to PO_2, PCO_2, or pH, although high levels of norepinephrine may cause constriction. The ductus venosus is functionally closed by 1 week of life and anatomically closed by 3 months, leaving the ligamentum venosum.

In addition to the establishment of the adult series circulation, dramatic alterations in pulmonary circulation, cardiac output and distribution, myocardial performance, and myocardial cell growth and hypertrophy continue to occur during the first weeks, months, and even years of life. In the presence of congenital heart disease, these changes may be pathologically affected. Furthermore, the physiologic consequences of a specific lesion may be very different for the neonate, infant, child, or adult.

Pulmonary Vascular Changes

The fetus has low pulmonary blood flow secondary to a high pulmonary vascular resistance. The minimal blood flow that does reach the pulmonary bed has a very low PO_2, which may cause hypoxic pulmonary vasoconstriction and contributes to the elevated pulmonary resistance seen in the fetus. In addition, morphologic examination of the small arteries of the fetal and newborn lung show a thick medial smooth muscle layer. The fetal pulmonary vasculature is reactive to a number of stimulants. Vasoconstriction is induced by decreases in PO_2 and pH, leukotrienes, and LTD_4. Acetylcholine, histamine, tolazoline, and beta-adrenergic catecholamines are potent vasodilators of fetal pulmonary vessels, as are bradykinin, PGE_1, PGE_2, PGI_2 (prostacyclin), and pros-taglandin D_2.[11-13]

At birth, alveolar ventilation commences. This reduces mechanical compression of small pulmonary vessels and increases PO_2. The result is a dramatic reduction in pulmonary vascular resistance (PVR). During the following weeks and months, remodeling of the pulmonary vessels occurs; the most notable change is a thinning of the medial smooth muscle layer. By 6 months of life, this process results in reduction of PVR to near normal adult levels. The normal process of postnatal pulmonary maturation may be altered significantly by pathologic conditions, such as those associated with congenital heart disease.

Myocardial Performance in the Neonate

In utero, the right ventricle (RV) has a cardiac output of approximately 330 mL/kg/min compared with the left ventricular (LV) output of 170 mL/kg/min. At birth, both RV and LV eject an output of approximately 350 mL/kg/min. This requires a minimal stroke volume increase for the RV but a considerable stroke volume increase for the LV. The high output state of the newborn effectively limits further increases in cardiac output.[14] This high output state decreases to about 150 mL/kg/min by 8 to 10 weeks of life.

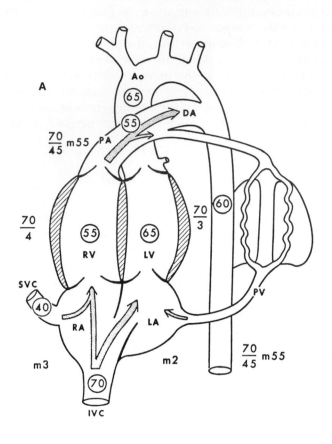

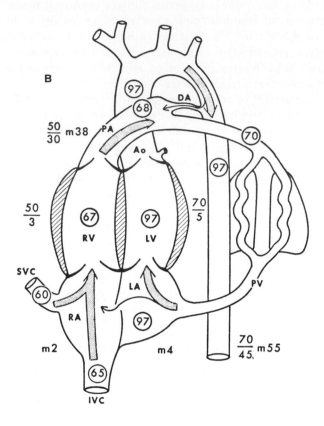

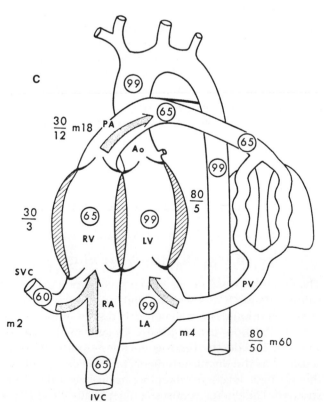

FIGURE 6–2. Hemodynamics of fetus and neonate. Circled figures are oxygen saturations. Systolic, diastolic, and mean (m) pressures appear near their respective chambers and vessels. **A.** Circulation of the term fetus. **B.** Transitional circulation less than 1 day after birth. **C.** Circulation several days after birth. (DA = ductus arteriosus: DV = ductus venosus; Ao = aorta; PA = pulmonary artery; RA = right atrium; RV = right ventricle; LA = left atrium; LV = left ventricle; SVC = superior vena cava; IVC = inferior vena cava; PV = pulmonary vein.) *(From: Rudolph AM: Changes in the circulation after birth, in* Congenital Diseases of the Heart. *Chicago, Mosby Year Book, 1974, pp 18–19.)*

Myocardial morphology and performance is notably different in the neonate.[15,16] These differences are summarized as follows:

1. *Afterload mismatch.* The neonatal heart is more susceptible to afterload mismatch (*see* Chapter 2), and therefore, stroke volume is poorly maintained in the face of increasing outflow resistance.

2. *Limited preload reserve.* The neonatal heart has limited preload reserve (*see* Chapter 2); thus, augmentation of stroke volume via the Frank–Starling mechanism is limited as compared with an adult.

3. *Reduced contractile capacity.* Neonatal cardiac cells contain more water and fewer contractile elements than mature myocardium. In fact, Friedman showed that fetal lamb myocardium contains about one-half the amount of contractile tissue per unit area of cross section compared with the adult.

4. *Reduced ventricular compliance.* The compliance of the neonatal myocardium is poor because a deficiency of elastic elements parallels the deficiency of contractile elements.

5. *Increased interventricular dependence.* Changes in ventricular pressure are transmitted to the opposite ventricle via the ventricular septum more readily in the immature myocardium. Left ventricular diastolic filling is disproportionately impaired in the neonate by high right ventricular end-diastolic pressure. This is due to a leftward shift of the interventricular septum and a reduction in left ventricular distensibility (*see* Chapter 2). Right ventricular diastolic filling is impaired to an equal extent by high left ventricular end-diastolic pressure in neonates and adults.[17] This enhanced ventricular interaction is caused by reduced ventricular compliance and because, at birth, the LV and RV are of equal mass. The increased volume and pressure load experienced by the LV after birth produces LV hypertrophy, and the normal adult LV to RV mass ratio of 2:1 is not seen until several months after birth.

6. *Incomplete autonomic innervation.* Sympathetic innervation, which is responsible for increasing heart rate and contractility, is incompletely developed at birth.[16] As a result, local myocardial release of norepinephrine contributes less to increases in contractility than do increases in circulating catecholamine levels. For this reason, inotropic agents such as dopamine, the effects of which are partially mediated through release of norepinephrine from myocardial nerve endings, may have to be used in higher doses to be effective for younger patients. On the other hand, the parasympathetic system, which reflexly slows the heart, is fully functional at birth.

7. *Immature myocardial metabolism.* The neonatal myocardium is more dependent on anaerobic metabolism than the adult heart (*see* Chapter 12). This may have a somewhat protective effect, making the neonatal myocardium more tolerant to the effects of hypoxia.

■ PATHOPHYSIOLOGY OF CONGENITAL HEART DISEASE

Although some congenital heart defects involve purely obstructive or regurgitant valvular lesions (*see* Chapter 5), the presence of shunts (both physiologic and anatomic) is the hallmark of congenital heart disease. Anesthetic management of the patient with congenital heart disease is dependent on a clear understanding of:

1. The concepts of shunting (both physiologic and anatomic), complete mixing, and intercirculatory mixing.
2. The types of anatomic shunts and the dynamics of the anatomic shunting process.
3. The effects of congenital lesions on the development of the pulmonary vascular system.
4. The factors that influence pulmonary and systemic vascular resistance.

The Concepts of Shunting, Complete Mixing, and Intercirculatory Mixing

Shunting. Shunting is the process whereby venous return into one circulatory system is recirculated through the arterial outflow of the same circulatory system.[18] Flow of blood from the systemic venous atrium (RA) to the aorta produces recirculation of systemic venous blood. Flow of blood from the pulmonary venous atrium (LA) to the pulmonary artery (PA) produces recirculation of pulmonary venous blood. Recirculation of blood produces a physiologic shunt. Recirculation of pulmonary venous blood produces a physiologic left-to-right (L-R), whereas recirculation of systemic venous blood produces a physiologic right-to-left (R-L) shunt. A physiologic R-L or L-R shunt commonly is the result of an anatomic R-L or L-R shunt. In an anatomic shunt, blood moves from one circulatory system to the other via a communication (orifice) at the level of the cardiac chambers or great vessels. Physiologic shunts can exist in the absence of an anatomic shunt.

Effective blood flow is the quantity of venous blood from one circulatory system reaching the arterial system of the other circulatory system. Effective pulmonary blood flow is the volume of systemic venous blood reaching the pulmonary circulation, whereas effective systemic blood flow is the volume of pulmonary venous blood reaching the systemic circulation. Effective pulmonary blood flow and effective systemic blood flows are the flows necessary to maintain life. Effective pulmonary blood flow and effective systemic blood flow are always equal, no matter how complex the lesions. Effective blood flow usually is the result of a normal pathway through the heart, but it may occur as the result of an anatomic R-L or L-R shunt.

Total pulmonary blood flow (Q_p) is the sum of effective pulmonary blood flow and recirculated pulmonary blood flow. Total systemic blood flow (Q_s) is the sum of effective systemic blood flow and recirculated systemic blood flow. Total pulmonary blood flow and total systemic blood flow do not have to be equal. Therefore, it is best to think of recirculated flow (physiologic shunt flow) as the extra, noneffective flow superimposed on the nutritive effective blood flow.

These concepts are illustrated in Figures 6–3 and 6-4.

Complete Mixing. Complete mixing or blending is the process whereby pulmonary and systemic venous blood mix completely in a cardiac chamber. Complete mixing can occur in a number of instances:

- when there is a single ventricle or atrium.
- when systemic venous and pulmonary venous blood return to the same atrium (totally anomalous pulmonary venous return).
- when all systemic venous blood is shunted from the systemic venous atrium into the pulmonary venous atrium due to the lack of a tricuspid valve (tricuspid atesia) or when all pulmonary venous blood is shunted from the pulmonary venous atrium into the systemic venous atrium due to the lack of a mitral valve (mitral atresia).
- when a common atrial or ventricular chamber exists due to bidirectional (both L-R and R-L) anatomic shunting across a large defect (atrial septal or ventricular septal).

In complete mixing, the arterial saturation (SaO_2) will be determined by the relative volumes and saturations of pulmonary venous and systemic venous blood flows that have mixed and reach the aorta. This is summarized in the following equation:

Aortic saturation = [(systemic venous saturation) (total systemic venous blood flow) + (pulmonary venous saturation) (total pulmonary venous blood flow)]/[total systemic venous blood flow + total pulmonary venous blood flow].

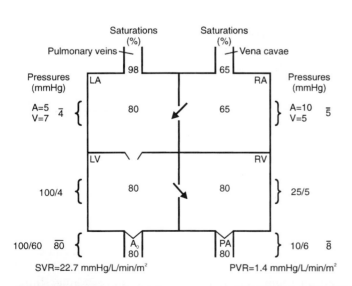

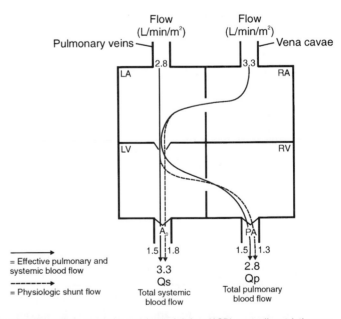

FIGURE 6–3. Depiction of saturations, pressures, and blood flows in tricuspid atresia with a mildly restrictive atrial septal defect (ASD), a small restrictive ventricular septal defect (VSD), and mild pulmonic stenosis (PS). Complete mixing or blending occurs at the atrial level. This complete mixing is the consequence of an obligatory physiologic and anatomic R-L shunting across the ASD. Effective pulmonary and effective systemic blood flow are equal (1.5 L/min/m²). Effective systemic blood flow occurs via a normal pathway through the heart. Effective pulmonary blood flow is the result of an anatomic R-L shunt at the atrial level and an anatomic L-R shunt at the ventricular level. This illustrates the concept that when complete outflow obstruction exists and there is obligatory anatomic shunting, a downstream anatomic shunt must exist to deliver blood back to the obstructed circuit. Q_p is 2.8 L/min/m² and is the sum of effective pulmonary blood flow (1.5 L/min/m²) and a physiologic and anatomic L-R shunt (1.3 L/min/m²) at the VSD. Q_s is 3.3 L/min/m² and is the sum of effective systemic blood flow (1.5 L/min/m²) and a physiologic and anatomic R-L shunt (1.8 L/min/m²) at the ASD.

In this depiction, there is a small pressure gradient at the atrial level and a large pressure gradient at the ventricular level. In addition, there is a small additional gradient at the level of the pulmonic valve.

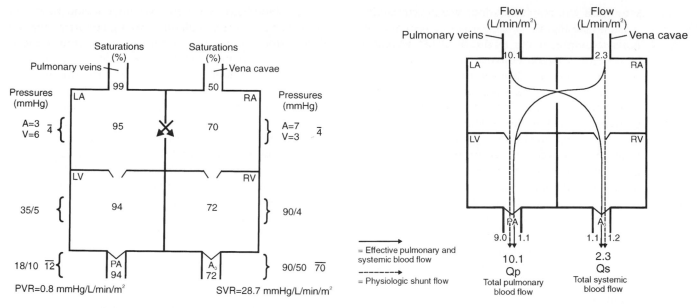

FIGURE 6–4. Depiction of saturations, pressures, and blood flows in complete transposition of the great vessels with a nonrestrictive ASD and a small left ventricular outflow tract gradient. Intercirculatory mixing occurs at the atrial level. Effective pulmonary and effective systemic blood flows are equal (1.1 L/min/m²) and are the result of a bidirectional anatomic shunt at the atrial level. The physiologic L-R shunt is 9.0 L/min/m²; this represents blood recirculated from the pulmonary veins to the pulmonary artery. The physiologic R-L shunt is 1.2 L/min/m²; this represents blood recirculated from the systemic veins to the aorta. It is apparent that total pulmonary blood flow (10.1 L/min/m²) is almost five times total systemic blood flow (2.3 L/min/m²) and that the bulk of pulmonary blood flow is recirculated pulmonary venous blood. In this depiction, pulmonary vascular resistance is low (approximately 1/35 of systemic vascular resistance) and there is a small (17 mm Hg peak to peak) gradient from the left ventricle to the pulmonary artery. These findings are compatible with the high pulmonary blood flow depicted.

This is illustrated in Figure 6–3, where $SaO_2 = [(65)(3.3) + (98)(2.8)]/(3.3 + 2.8) = 80\%$

From this equation, it is apparent that in complete mixing, three variables will determine arterial saturation:

1. The ratio of total pulmonary to total systemic blood flow (Q_p:Q_s). A greater proportion of the mixed blood will consist of saturated blood (pulmonary venous blood) than of desaturated blood (systemic venous blood) when Q_p:Q_s is high. Figure 6–5 demonstrates the increase in arterial saturation that occurs in complete mixing lesions with increases in pulmonary blood flow relative to systemic blood flow. Figure 6–5 also demonstrates that an arterial saturation approaching 100% is possible only with an extremely large Q_p:Q_s.

2. Systemic venous saturation. For a given total pulmonary blood flow and a given pulmonary venous saturation, a decrease in systemic venous

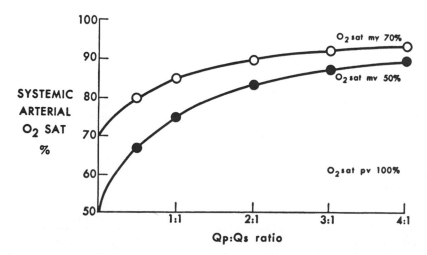

FIGURE 6–5. Influence of the Q_p:Q_s ratio, mixed venous (mv) oxygenation saturation, and pulmonary venous (pv) oxygen saturation on arterial oxygen saturation in complete mixing lesions. Note that Q_p:Q_s ratios higher than 3:1 do not substantially increase arterial oxygen saturation. *From: Rudolph AM: Congenital Diseases of the Heart. Chicago, Mosby Year Book, 1974, p 125.)*

saturation will result in a decrease in arterial saturation (*see* Fig. 6–5). Decreases in systemic venous saturation occur as the result of decreases in systemic oxygen delivery or increases in systemic oxygen consumption. Recall that systemic oxygen delivery is the product of cardiac output and arterial oxygen content. Arterial oxygen content, in turn, is dependent on the hemoglobin concentration and the arterial saturation.

3. Pulmonary venous saturation. In the absence of large intrapulmonary shunts and/or V/Q mismatch, pulmonary venous saturation should be close to 100%. In the presence of pulmonary parenchymal disease, pulmonary venous saturation may be reduced. In a complete mixing lesion, a reduction in pulmonary venous saturation will decrease arterial saturation for a given systemic venous saturation and total pulmonary blood flow.

Intercirculatory Mixing.   Intercirculatory mixing is the unique situation that exists in complete transposition of the great vessels (TGV). This lesion is depicted in detail in Figure 6–4. In TGV, two parallel circulations exist due to the existence of atrioventricular concordance (RA-RV, LA-LV) and ventriculoarterial discordance (RV-Aorta, LV-PA). This produces a parallel rather than a normal series circulation. In this arrangement, blood flow will consist of parallel recirculation of pulmonary venous blood in the pulmonary circuit and systemic venous blood in the systemic circuit. Therefore, the physiologic shunt or the percentage of venous blood from one system that recirculates in the arterial outflow of the same system is 100% for both circuits. Unless there are one or more communications between the parallel circuits to allow intercirculatory mixing, this arrangement is not compatible with life. In other words, one or more communications must exist so that effective pulmonary and systemic blood flow can be established.

An anatomic R-L shunt produces effective pulmonary blood flow, whereas an anatomic L-R shunt produces effective systemic blood flow. Effective pulmonary blood flow, effective systemic blood flow, and the volume of intercirculatory mixing are always equal. Total systemic blood flow is the sum of recirculated systemic venous blood plus effective systemic blood flow. Likewise, total pulmonary blood flow is the sum of recirculated pulmonary venous blood plus effective pulmonary blood flow. Recirculated blood makes up the largest portion of total pulmonary and total systemic blood flow with effective blood flows contributing only a small portion of the total flows. The net result is production of transposition physiology, in which the pulmonary artery oxygen saturation is greater than the aortic oxygen saturation.

Arterial saturation (SaO_2) will be determined by the relative volumes and saturations of the recirculated systemic and effective systemic venous blood flows reaching the aorta. This is summarized in the following equation:

Aortic saturation = [(systemic venous saturation) (recirculated systemic venous blood flow) + (pulmonary venous saturation)(effective systemic venous blood flow)]/[total systemic venous blood flow].

This is illustrated in Figure 6–4, where SaO_2 = $[(50)(1.2) + (99)(1.1)]/2.3 = 73\%$. Obviously, the greater the effective systemic blood flow (intercirculatory mixing) relative to the recirculated systemic blood flow, the greater the aortic saturation. For a given amount of intercirculatory mixing and total systemic blood flow, a decrease in systemic venous or pulmonary venous saturation will result in a decrease in arterial saturation.

Classification of Anatomic Shunts

Anatomic shunts can be characterized as simple or complex.

Simple Shunts.   In an anatomic shunt, a communication (orifice) exists between pulmonary and arterial vessels or heart chambers (*see* Table 6–1). In a simple shunt, there is no fixed obstruction to outflow from the vessels or chambers involved in the shunt.[19] When the shunt orifice is small (restrictive shunt), a large pressure gradient exists across the orifice, and variations in out-

TABLE 6–1. SIMPLE SHUNTS (NO OBSTRUCTIVE LESIONS)

Restrictive Shunts (Small Communications)	Nonrestrictive Shunts (Large Communications)	Common Chambers (Complete Mixing)
1. Large pressure gradient.	1. Small pressure gradient.	1. No pressure gradient.
2. Direction and magnitude more *independent* of PVR:SVR.	2. Direction and magnitude *dependent* on PVR:SVR.	2. Bidirectional shunting.
3. Less subject to control.	3. More subject to control.	3. Net Q_p:Q_s totally depends on PVR:SVR.
Examples: Small VSD, small PDA, Blalock-Taussig shunts, small ASD.	Examples: Large VSD, large PDA, large Waterston shunts.	Examples: Single ventricle, truncus arteriosus, single atrium.

Q_p = pulmonary blood flow; Q_s = systemic blood flow; PDA = patent ductus arteriosus.

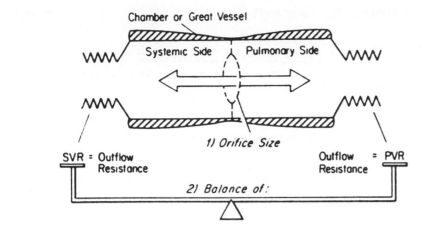

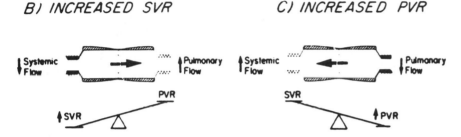

FIGURE 6–6. Influence of orifice size and the PVR:SVR ratio on the magnitude and direction of a simple shunt. **A.** PVR and SVR are balanced resulting in equal pulmonary and systemic blood flows. **B.** PVR is reduced relative to SVR, resulting in an increase in pulmonary blood flow and a decrease in systemic blood flow. **C.** PVR is elevated relative to SVR, resulting in a decrease in pulmonary blood flow and an increase in systemic blood flow.

flow resistance (pulmonary vascular resistance, PVR; and systemic vascular resistance, SVR) have little effect on shunt magnitude and direction. In this instance, the magnitude of the shunt is affected by the size of the shunt orifice. However, when the shunt orifice is large, the shunt becomes nonrestrictive, and the outflow resistance becomes the primary determinant of the magnitude and direction of shunting. These shunts, in which the ratio of PVR to SVR determines the magnitude of shunting, are known as *dependent shunts.* When the communication is very large, no pressure gradient exists between the vessels or chambers involved. In this instance, bidirectional shunting occurs, resulting in complete mixing and a functionally common chamber. Net systemic and pulmonary blood flow is then determined by the ratio of systemic to pulmonary vascular resistance (*see* Fig. 6–6).

Complex Shunts. In complex anatomic shunt lesions, obstruction to outflow is present, in addition to a shunt orifice (*see* Table 6–2). The obstruction may be at the valvular, subvalvular, or supravalvular level. Furthermore, the obstruction may be fixed (as with valvular or infundibular stenosis) or variable (as with dynamic infundibular obstruction). In complex shunts, outflow resistance is a combination of the resistance across the obstructive lesions and the resistance across the pulmonary or systemic vascular bed (*see* Fig. 6–7). When an obstruc-

tion is severe, the SVR or PVR distal to the obstruction will have little effect on shunt magnitude or direction.

Tetralogy of Fallot is a good example of a complex shunt in which there is partial obstruction to outflow. There is a fixed component of right ventricular outflow obstruction in tetralogy of Fallot secondary to infundibular, valvular, and possibly supravalvular obstruction. A dynamic component of right ventricular obstruction is produced by changes in the caliber of the right ventricular infundibulum. These two components of right ventricular outflow obstruction can produce a right-to-left shunt. Because right ventricular outflow obstruction is incomplete, increases in PVR will also increase the total right ventricular outflow resistance and increase right-to-left shunting. Similarly, a decrease in SVR relative to PVR will

TABLE 6–2. COMPLEX SHUNTS (SHUNT AND OBSTRUCTIVE LESION)

Partial Outflow Obstruction	Total Outflow Obstruction
1. Shunt magnitude and direction largely fixed by obstruction.	1. Shunt magnitude and direction totally fixed.
2. Shunt depends less on PVR:SVR.	2. All flow goes through shunt.
3. Orifice and obstruction determine pressure gradient.	3. Pressure gradient depends on orifice.
Examples: Tetralogy of Fallot, VSD and pulmonic stenosis, VSD with coarctation.	Examples: Tricuspid atresia, mitral atresia, pulmonary atresia, aortic atresia.

*SYSTEMIC OBSTRUCTION*_____

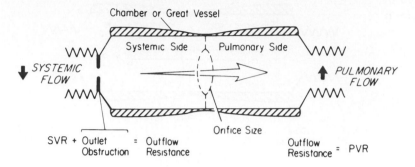

*PULMONARY OBSTRUCTION*_____

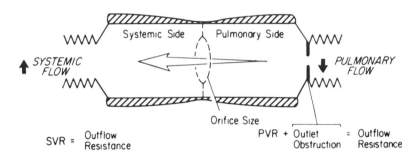

FIGURE 6–7. Influence of orifice size and total outflow resistance on the magnitude and direction of a complex shunt. Total outflow resistance will be a combination of PVR or SVR and the resistance offered by the obstructive lesion.

increase right-to-left shunting without any increase in right ventricular outflow resistance.

Another form of complex shunt is present in patients who have complete outflow obstruction, such as tricuspid, pulmonary, mitral, or aortic atresia. In these lesions, changes in SVR or PVR play no role in determining shunt magnitude or direction. The entire shunt flow is fixed and obligatory across the communication, and complete mixing results. For flow of this mixed blood to reach the obstructed circuit, an additional downstream shunt, such as a ventricular septal defect (VSD) or patent ductus arteriosus (PDA) must be present. The downstream shunt may be simple or complex.

These concepts are critical to a clear understanding of the pathophysiology involved in patients with congenital heart disease. Describing a lesion as cyanotic or acyanotic may be misleading and simplistic. For example, in a patient with tetralogy of Fallot, there may be minimal valvular or infundibular obstruction to pulmonary blood flow at baseline and the patient may not be cyanotic. In fact, this type of patient ("pink Tet") may have a large left-to-right shunt through the VSD with increased pulmonary blood flow. During induction, hypercarbia and hypoxemia may develop secondary to poor airway management. The result will be a dramatic increase in both PVR and the dynamic component of infundibular obstruction, with production of a net right-to-left shunt and cyanosis ("Tet spell"). Similarly, a cyanotic episode (a net right-to-left shunt) may be precipitated in the same patient by the SVR reduction that accompanies a febrile illness.

Pulmonary Vascular Pathophysiology

Pulmonary vascular occlusive disease (PVOD) may occur as the result of congenital heart lesions. PVOD produces obstruction to pulmonary blood flow due to structural changes in the pulmonary vasculature. The morphologic changes have three components: (1) increased muscularity of small pulmonary arteries; (2) small artery intimal hyperplasia, scarring, and thrombosis; and (3) reduced numbers of intra-acinar arteries.[20,21] These changes produce progressive obstruction to pulmonary blood flow and result in progressive and irreversible elevations of pulmonary vascular resistance and pulmonary artery pressure. These changes may be graded morphologically using lung biopsy[21] or angiographically using the pulmonary artery wedge angiogram (*see* Chapter 2). Ultimately, these changes elevate PVR so dramatically that they produce a reduction in pulmonary blood flow. In addition, the increased muscularity of the small pulmonary arteries that accompanies development of PVOD enhances the response of the pulmonary vasculature to pulmonary vasoconstrictors.

The stimulus for development of PVOD is exposure of the pulmonary vascular system (both in utero and after birth) to abnormal pressure and flow patterns associated with congenital heart disease. In particular, three categories of abnormalities predispose the development of PVOD:

1. Exposure of the pulmonary vascular circuit to systemic arterial pressures and high pulmonary blood flows. Patients for whom the pulmonary vasculature is exposed to high flows and systemic arterial pressures typically have very early development of PVOD. This classically occurs in the presence of a large (nonrestrictive) ventricular septal defect.

2. Exposure of the pulmonary vascular circuit to high pulmonary blood flow in the absence of high pulmonary artery pressures. The progression of PVOD is typically much slower in this situation than when pulmonary artery pressure is also elevated. A large atrial septal defect or a small (restrictive) patent ductus arteriosus are examples of this type of lesion.

3. Obstruction of pulmonary venous drainage. This will lead to elevation of pulmonary arterial pressure and will predispose development of PVOD. Pulmonary venous obstruction may result from stenotic pulmonary veins, which can exist in totally anomalous pulmonary venous return or cor triatrium. Pulmonary venous obstruction also may occur as the result of high left atrial pressures (mitral atresia, congenital aortic stenosis, severe coarctation of the aorta) or high right atrial pressures (totally anomalous pulmonary venous return).

Control of Pulmonary Vascular Resistance

As is obvious from the previous discussion, alterations in PVR may be an important determinant of shunt magnitude and direction in some shunt lesions. Furthermore, the patient with congenital heart disease is likely to have an enhanced response of the pulmonary vasculature to vasoconstricting substances. It is therefore necessary to be familiar with the interventions that will alter PVR in the patient with congenital heart disease:

1. P_{O_2}. Both alveolar hypoxia and arterial hypoxemia induce pulmonary vasoconstriction.[22] An arterial O_2 tension lower than 50 mm Hg increases PVR over a wide range of arterial pH; however, this effect is enhanced when pH is lower than 7.40.[23] Conversely, high levels of inspired O_2 can reduce an elevated PVR.[24]

2. P_{CO_2}. Hypercarbia increases PVR, independent of changes in arterial pH.[25] Hypocarbia, on the other hand, reduces PVR only through production of an alkalosis.[26] In fact, reliable reductions in PVR and increases in pulmonary blood flow and P_{O_2} are seen in children with right-to-left shunts when hyperventilation to a P_{CO_2} near 20 mm Hg and a pH near 7.60 is instituted.[27] Similarly, postbypass hyperventilation to a P_{CO_2} of 20 to 33 mm Hg and a pH of 7.50 to 7.56 in patients with preoperative pulmonary hypertension results in a reduction in PVR when compared with ventilation that produces normocarbia or hypercarbia.[28,29]

3. pH. Both respiratory and metabolic alkalosis reduce PVR,[22,25,26] whereas both respiratory and metabolic acidosis increase PVR.[22,23]

4. Variation in lung volumes. At small lung volumes, atelectasis results in compression of extra-alveolar vessels, whereas at high lung volumes, hyperinflation of alveoli results in compression of intra-alveolar vessels. Therefore, PVR is normally lowest at lung volumes at or near the functional residual capacity.[30] Positive end-expiratory pressure (PEEP) may cause an increase in PVR by increasing alveolar pressure through hyperinflation. However, in situations in which PEEP works to recruit atelectatic alveoli and increase arterial P_{O_2}, a decrease in PVR generally is seen.

5. Anesthetic agents. This topic will be discussed at length in the section on anesthetic agents.

6. Vasodilator agents. There is no intravenous drug that selectively acts as a pulmonary vasodilator. In general, intravenous drugs intended to induce pulmonary vasodilation (PGE_1, nitroglycerin, sodium nitroprusside, and tolazoline) induce systemic vasodilation as well. The use of inhaled pulmonary specific vasodilators is currently being evaluated. An endogenous vasodilator known as endothelium-derived relaxing factor (EDRF) has been described. This substance, derived from endothelium, is labile, diffusible, and capable of inducing vasodilation in response to a wide variety of substances that increase intracellular calcium.[31,32] In fact, an increase in intracellular calcium stimulates production of EDRF/NO from L-arginine. Recently, it has been determined that EDRF is nitric oxide (NO) or a NO-containing moiety.[33-35] After it has been formed, EDRF/NO diffuses from endothelium to vascular smooth muscle (VSM), where it binds to and activates guanylate cyclase to produce cyclic guanosine monophosphate (cGMP). cGMP acts as a second messenger to catalyze reactions that lead to a reduction of VSM calcium by reduced calcium influx, increased calcium efflux, and reduced release of intracellular cal-

cium.[36] This, in turn, produces relaxation of VSM and vasodilation. EDRF/NO is involved in modulation of basal VSM tone as well. This modulation capacity is lost in vessels in which entholethium is removed or damaged.

Inhaled NO selectively reduces pulmonary hypertension and improves ventilation/perfusion matching in a variety of disease states. Pulmonary selectivity is based on three characteristics of NO:[37]

- its gaseous state allows delivery to ventilated alveoli by inhalation.
- its small size and lipophilicity allows ready diffusion into the appropriate cells.
- its avid binding to and rapid inactivation by hemoglobin prevents systemic vasodilatation.

Recently inhaled NO has been used to treat pulmonary hypertension in both the pre- and post-CPB period in a variety of congenital heart lesions[38-44] and in treatment for persistent pulmonary hypertension of the newborn.[45,46] Generally, approximately 10 to 20 ppm inhaled NO has been used. Some caution is warranted because at least one instance of NO administration failing to provide sustained improvement in gas exchange and subsequent development of NO dependency has been reported.[41]

An alternative to inhaled NO is aerosolized prostacyclin (PGI$_2$). Prostacyclin acts by binding to prostacyclin receptors and activating cyclic adenosine monophosphate (cAMP). This, in turn, activates protein kinase A, which leads to a reduction of VSM intracellular calcium, causing vasorelaxation. PGI$_2$ also stimulates endothelial release of NO. Recently, aerosolized PGI$_2$ (2 to 50 ng/kg/min) has proved useful in selectively lowering PVR after congenital cardiac surgery[47] and is comparable to NO in children with acute respiratory distress syndrome (ARDS).[48] Neither drug is currently approved by the United States Food & Drug Administration (FDA).

7. Sympathetic nervous system stimulation. Sympathetic stimulation results in increases in both pulmonary and systemic vascular resistance. In children with pulmonary artery medial hypertrophy, this may result in a hyperactive pulmonary vasoconstrictor response. It has been demonstrated that blunting of sympathetic outflow during a stress response attenuates increases in PVR in children predisposed to pulmonary hypertension.[49]

In summary, control of ventilation with manipulation of Po$_2$, Pco$_2$, pH, and lung volumes is the best cur-

rently available method for altering PVR independently of SVR. A combination of a high inspired FIo$_2$, an arterial Po$_2$ higher than 60 mm Hg, an arterial Pco$_2$ of 20 to 30 mm Hg, a pH of 7.50 to 7.60, and low inspiratory pressures without high levels of PEEP, will produce reliable reductions in PVR. Conversely, a reduced FIo$_2$, an arterial Po$_2$ of 50 to 60 mm Hg, an arterial Pco$_2$ of 40 to 50 mm Hg, and the application of PEEP, can be used to increase PVR. There is enthusiasm for the use of inhaled NO and prostacyclin to selectively reduce PVR. These agents are currently being evaluated.

■ PREOPERATIVE EVALUATION

Psychological Considerations

The anesthesiologist who evaluates the patient with congenital heart disease must be aware of the considerable effect that appropriate psychological preparation may have during the preoperative and postoperative period. The pediatric patient has unique psychological concerns that depend on age and previous surgical and anesthetic experience. In addition, the profound effect that serious heart disease has on parents and other family members cannot be minimized and must be addressed sensitively during the preoperative evaluation. Although the neonate who requires urgent cardiac surgery does not require psychological preparation, the parents often are overwhelmed by the sophisticated technology, as well as the number of physicians and personnel involved in the diagnosis and management of their newborn child.

The preoperative psychological preparation must be appropriate to the age of the patient. Fear of separation from parents ("stranger anxiety") can be manifest in the infant at 8 to 12 months with an intense aversion to strangers. Very few toddlers, even if playful and cooperative in the presence of the parent, will leave their parent happily to go to the operating room. Older children have fears of disfigurement or that they will "wake up" or feel pain during and after surgery. Even the withdrawn, seemingly complacent adolescent often is in great turmoil regarding impending surgery. Previous surgery and anesthesia will influence even a young child's ability to cope with the newest operative experience. Just as excess stress is avoided in the anxious adult patient because of potential alterations in hemodynamics, the pediatric patient should have careful attention paid to these issues. In the preoperative evaluation of the pediatric patient, psychological issues influence not only the conduct of the physical examination but also how much detail is discussed with parents in the presence of the patient. Obtaining informed consent from the parent in the presence of a school-aged child may create undue stress for the child. On the other hand, weak promises of "no needles" or little discussion about what the child can expect is equally unpleasant and counterproductive. Most experienced pediatric anesthesiologists, aware of the spectrum and unpredictability of children's behavior, prudently plan for alternative approaches to physical examination and, most importantly, how to pleasantly and safely separate the child from the parent for the induction of anesthesia.

Clinical History

Clinical history should include medications, allergies, past hospitalizations and operations (including prior anesthetic experiences), and a thorough review of systems. Performance of age-appropriate activities will aid in the evaluation of cardiac function and reserve. The young infant in cardiac failure will manifest symptoms of low cardiac reserve during feeding, which is a strenuous activity, for even a normal newborn. A parent might report that sweating, tiring, dyspnea, and circumoral cyanosis occur during feeding. The observation by a parent that the patient cannot keep the same pace as siblings often is a reliable clinical sign that cyanosis or congestive heart failure is worsening. Frequent pulmonary infections may occur as a result of increased pulmonary blood flow in otherwise asymptomatic patients. These subtle points of the clinical history should not be minimized. Cardiac catheterization data may be several months old by the time the patient presents for surgery, and the newly observed clinical signs may more accurately reflect the patient's current cardiac status.

Physical Examination

Interpretation of vital signs also must be age-specific. Figures 6–8 and 6–9 illustrate that heart rate decreases and blood pressure increases with increasing age. Growth curves also are useful. Congestive heart failure will inhibit, sequentially, age-appropriate gains in weight, height, and head circumference. It is not unusual for patients with severe congestive heart failure to weigh less at 3 or 4 months of age than at birth. Interestingly, cyanotic children often do not manifest this failure to thrive.

Physical examination will reveal cyanosis, clubbing, or signs of congestive heart failure similar to those seen in adults, such as hepatomegaly, ascites, edema, or tachypnea. Rales may not be heard in infants and children with congestive heart failure, and the degree of heart failure may be determined more reliably by some of the signs and symptoms outlined above. The degree of cyanosis is

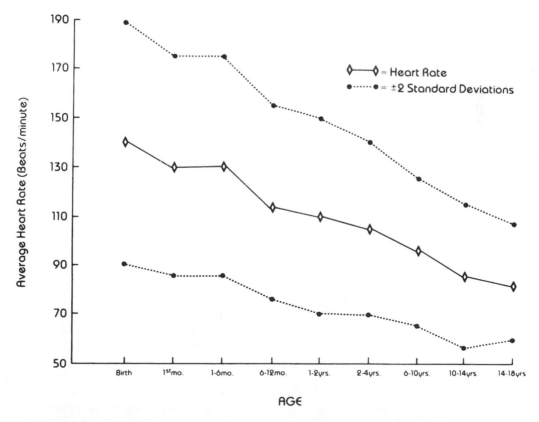

FIGURE 6–8. Variation in average heart rate with age. *(From: Moore RA: Anesthesia considerations for patients undergoing palliative or reoperative operations for congenital heart disease, in Swedlow DB, Russell RC (eds); Cardiovascular Problems in Pediatric Critical Care. New York, Churchill Livingstone, 1986, p 173.)*

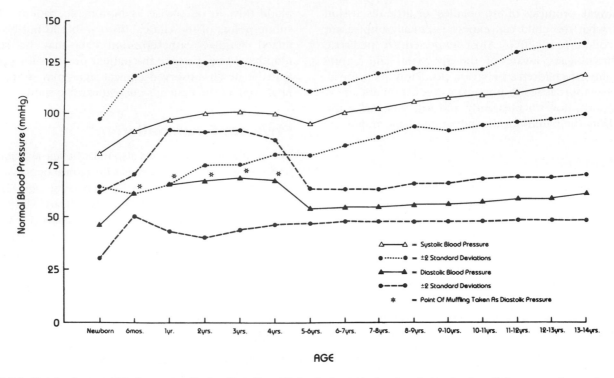

FIGURE 6–9. Variation in normal blood pressure with age. *(From: Moore RA: Anesthesia considerations for patients undergoing palliative or reoperative operations for congenital heart disease, in Swedlow DB, Russell RC (eds):* Cardiovascular Problems in Pediatric Critical Care. *New York, Churchill Livingstone, 1986, p 174.)*

related to the percentage of desaturated hemoglobin. A markedly hypoxemic child with baseline arterial saturations in the 60% range may be anemic and clinically appear less cyanotic than another child with similar arterial saturation and a more appropriate hematocrit of 65%.

Physical examination should include an evaluation of the limitations to vascular access and monitoring sites imposed by previous surgery. A child who has undergone a palliative shunt procedure may have a diminished pulse or unobtainable blood pressure in the arm in which the subclavian artery has been incorporated into the shunt. This obviously has implications for arterial catheter placement, sphygmomanometric blood pressure monitoring, and use of pulse oximetry during surgery. Finally, the child who has undergone multiple palliative procedures may have poor venous access, which may influence the mode of induction.

Because approximately 8% of children with congenital heart disease have other congenital abnormalities,[50] it is prudent to consider and define these defects. For example, patients with congenital heart defects may have associated craniofacial abnormalities (Treacher-Collins syndrome, Apert's syndrome). Tracheal stenosis may be a serious problem for patients with VATER syndrome who have undergone tracheoesophageal fistula repair. Patients with Down syndrome may present with problematic airways due to a large tongue and atlanto-occipital instability.

It often is difficult to differentiate clearly between signs and symptoms of congestive heart failure and a mild upper respiratory tract infection. Because increased pulmonary blood flow seems to predispose multiple respiratory tract infections, the physical examination may show mild tachypnea, wheezing, or upper airway congestion and, in the absence of abnormal laboratory findings or fever, may be impossible to distinguish from congestive heart failure. The decision to proceed to surgery may be necessary even when the differentiation between worsening congestive heart failure and a respiratory tract infection cannot be made with certainty.

Review of Laboratory Data

A review of pertinent laboratory data and correlation with the clinical findings is necessary. The child in congestive heart failure may have mild iron deficiency because of chronically increased metabolic needs. The cyanotic child will have polycythemia, which is a good reflection of the degree of arterial desaturation. Hematocrit levels higher than 65% are associated with a marked increase in blood viscosity. To avoid possible neurologic sequelae from such extreme viscosity, phlebotomy should be considered before surgery, especially if the proposed surgery is palliative and cardiopulmonary bypass with the potential for hemodilution will not be employed. Patients with severe cyanosis who are anemic may require transfusion because their diminished oxygen-carrying capacity may predispose them to hypoxic spells. Cyanosis also effects the coagulation process (*see* Chapter 1), and it is not unusual to observe prolongation of PT, aPTT, and bleeding times. Thrombocytopenia or functional platelet defects also may exist (*see* Chapter 1). In the face of reoperation with extensive dissection, the anesthesiologist should plan adequate blood component therapy for each patient (*see* Chapters 1 and 10). In addition, the use of anticoagulants for patients with artificial valves should be noted. The newborn with immature liver function may have bleeding problems, which the use of vitamin K and fresh whole blood transfusions may help correct.

Plasma electrolyte concentrations should be screened, especially in patients receiving digitalis and diuretic therapy. Hypocalcemia may be observed in patients with congestive heart failure as well as patients with DiGeorge's syndrome (aortic arch anomalies and thymic aplasia). Severe congestive heart failure may be accompanied by jitteriness and irritability. It is important to rule out hypoglycemia as an alternative cause of these findings.

The chest radiograph serves to confirm other clinical and diagnostic findings, such as cardiomegaly, the degree of pulmonary blood flow, previous surgical procedures, and the presence of acute pulmonary infections. The electrocardiogram similarly confirms chamber enlargement and the presence of dysrhythmias (*see* Chapter 1).

Review of the catheterization and echocardiographic data is critical to a clear understanding of the pathophysiology and surgical plan. Most pediatric cardiac centers review such data in a multidisciplinary catheterization conference. The combined perioperative planning of cardiologists, surgeons, and anesthesiologists is essential to the optimal care of patients with congenital heart disease. Pediatric cardiac catheterization is discussed in detail in Chapter 2; the following information should be obtained routinely from a review of the catheterization data:

1. Anatomic diagnosis.
2. Interpretation of saturation data. Saturation step-ups or step-downs between vessels and chambers are used to detect shunts. Likewise, saturation data are used to calculate the ratio of pulmonary to systemic blood flow (Q_p:Q_s). Saturation data also are used to differentiate intrapulmonary shunting and V/Q mismatch (atelectasis, hypoventilation, pulmonary disease) from intracardiac shunting.
3. Interpretation of pressure data. Pressure data are used to compare right and left heart pressures and systemic and pulmonary arterial pressures. In addition, pressure gradients across valve and shunt orifices are measured. Pressure data can be used to assess ventricular diastolic function (distensibility and compliance).
4. Interpretation of angiographic data. Cineangiograms can be used to assess ventricular wall motion (systolic function) and to assess intracardiac and great vessel blood flow patterns.
5. Functional status and location of prior surgical interventions. This information will allow intelligent decisions regarding monitor placement and anesthetic management to be made.
6. Effect of interventions. More interventions are made in the catheterization laboratory to palliate congenital heart lesions (balloon valvuloplasty, balloon septostomy, balloon angioplasty). The effects of these interventions on the underlying lesion must be assessed. Furthermore, a trial of 100% inspired oxygen may be used to assess the reversible component of pulmonary artery hypertension.

Two-dimensional echocardiography has revolutionized the field of pediatric cardiology over the last decade (*see* Chapters 1 and 3). Unlike adults, who may have a limited "echo" window, four-chamber assessment of the pediatric patient is routine. Many patients with straightforward lesions, including PDA, atrial septal defect (ASD), and coarctation of the aorta, may proceed to surgery without additional catheterization studies. In addition, critically ill neonates also may undergo surgery after a definitive echocardiographic study without catheterization. Although angiocardiographic studies often complement echo findings, it is not unusual for the echocardiographic data to be a superior diagnostic tool and offer the surgeon more valuable anatomic information. Furthermore, it should be noted that any congenital heart lesions, including those with surgical shunts, can be summarized using the "box" heart diagrams shown in Figures 6–3 and 6–4 (*see also* Fig. 6–21). This exercise is recommended for all lesions using the available catheterization and echocardiography data. In addition to clarifying the anatomy and pathophysiology, this exercise also delineates which chambers can be expected to be volume or pressure overloaded.

Preoperative Fluid Therapy

Preoperative fluid and NPO orders are routinely geared to the age-specific needs of the pediatric patient. In the absence of maintenance IV fluids, the following guidelines apply.

- 0 to 1 years: NPO for solids and milk at midnight. Clear liquids containing glucose as desired until 4 hours preoperatively.

- 1 to 5 years: NPO for solids and milk at midnight. Clear liquids containing glucose as desired until 6 hours preoperatively.
- 5 years and older: NPO for solids and milk at midnight. Offer clear liquids containing glucose until 8 hours preoperatively.

Because dehydration may have potentially deleterious effects on hemodynamics or on the degree of blood viscosity in the polycythemic patient, IV hydration with maintenance fluids before surgery should be considered for certain patients, especially severely cyanotic patients with hematocrit levels of 60% or higher.

Preoperative Medications

As with many issues in pediatric cardiac anesthesia, "recipes" for management are fraught with difficulties. There are a variety of proposed premedication regimens that will result in the desired goal of a calm, hemodynamically stable patient whose induction will proceed smoothly. Effective preoperative sedation that permits the older infant and child to separate easily from anxious parents need not preclude hemodynamic stability. Premedication may decrease the dose required for various induction agents. In addition, the deleterious effects of vagal stimulation and excess secretions may be minimized with premedication. The neonate and young infant may require no premedication. If desired, atropine may be given to avoid the bradycardia associated with vagal stimulation during induction. It often is necessary to supplement with additional atropine at the time of intubation, however. Atropine has the additional effect of decreasing airway secretions. For any child, excess secretions are a potent stimulus for laryngospasm or aspiration and should be avoided. Scopolamine is a potent antisialagogue and has sedative effects as well. Glycopyrrolate is a more potent antisialagogue than atropine but has less vagolytic activity.

Age-appropriate premedication dosages are outlined in Table 6-3. Premedication requires individualization of dosage to avoid respiratory depression. Lower doses are best used for smaller children and children in congestive heart failure. If there is any concern about potential respiratory depression, premedication should be omitted and the child should be evaluated and treated before induction in the presence of the anesthesiologist. Premedication with morphine/scopolamine or midazolam is associated with both hypercarbia and decreased SaO_2 in children with congenital heart disease, particularly those with pulmonary hypertension.[51] Older children may opt for placement of an IV rather than premedication by intramuscular injection.

Digoxin and diuretics are withheld the morning of surgery, except for those patients with poorly controlled congestive heart failure. When digoxin is used for dys-

TABLE 6–3. PREMEDICATION GUIDELINES

Age	Medication
0–6 months	Atropine 0.01–0.02 mg/kg IM (minimum 0.1 mg)
6–12 months	Atropine 0.01–0.02 mg/kg IM
	Morphine 0.1–0.15 mg/kg IM
Over 12 months	Atropine 0.02 mg/kg IM (maximum 0.4 mg), or
	Scopolamine 0.015 mg/kg IM (maximum 0.4 mg), or
	Glycopyrrolate 0.004 mg/kg IM (maximum 0.3 mg) plus
	Morphine 0.1–0.2 mg/kg IM
	Midazolam 0.5–1.0 mg/kg PO
	Ketamine 3 mg/kg
	Midazolam 0.1 mg/kg } IM
	Atropine 0.02 mg/kg
	Meperidine 3.0 mg/kg
	Pentobarbital 4.0 mg/kg } PO
	or
	Midazolam 0.5 mg/kg

rhythmia control, it should be continued during the perioperative period. Inotrope and prostaglandin infusions are continued into the operative period for critically ill neonates and children.

■ PREOPERATIVE PREPARATION

The routine preoperative preparation of the anesthesia equipment is not noticeably different for the pediatric patient. It is important to have various-sized airway equipment so that there can be quick selection of appropriate airways, masks, and endotracheal tubes. A pediatric circle system with humidification can be used for older children. The resistance to airflow created by the unidirectional valves is not an issue for patients receiving mechanical ventilation. Smaller children can be managed with a Bain modification of a Mapleson D circuit. A better approach is the use of a Siemens 900 series ventilator. This ventilator will provide either volume or pressure ventilation and can be used for all patients, from neonates to adults, simply by using the appropriate size of Y tubing. In addition, inhalational agents can be administered with minor modifications to the circuit.

Appropriate emergency medications should be available in doses consistent with the patient's weight. Tables 6-4, 6-5, and 6-6 summarize the use of inotropes and vasopressors, vasodilators, and antidysrhythmic agents for pediatric patients. For critically ill patients or patients with marginal reserve, selected infusions should be prepared in anticipation of their use. Careful attention should be paid to dosages because the dose per kg may vary significantly from those used for adults.

TABLE 6–4. INOTROPES AND VASOPRESSORS FOR CHILDREN

Agent	Doses (IV)
Calcium	
Chloride	10–20 mg/kg/dose (slowly)
Gluconate	30–60 mg/kg/dose (slowly)
Phenylephrine	0.1–0.5 µg/kg/min
Isoproterenol	0.1–0.5 µg/kg/min
Norepinephrine	0.1–0.5 µg/kg/min
Epinephrine	0.1 µg/kg/min
	0.2–0.5 µg/kg/min
Dopamine	2–4 µg/kg/min
	4–8 µg/kg/min
	>10 µg/kg/min
Dobutamine	2–10 µg/kg/min
Amrinone	loading dose, 3–5 mg/kg
	5–10 µg/kg/min

(From: Hickey PR, Crone RK: Cardiovascular physiology and pharmacology in children: Normal and diseased pediatric cardiovascular systems, in Ryan JF, Todres DI, Cote CJ, Goudsouzian NG (eds): A Practice of Anesthesia for Infants and Children. Orlando, FL, Grune & Stratton, 1986, p 185.)

Monitoring

If the infant or child is awake or minimally sedated, application of multiple monitors can prevent a smooth induction, even for an initially calm patient. Minimal stimulation, including distracting discussion in the operating room, will avoid disturbing the child. For these reasons, induction monitoring may include a precordial stethoscope and/or oxygen saturation monitor and nothing else. For adult cardiac anesthesiologists who are accustomed to intensive monitoring before induction, this lack of the usual monitoring may seem cavalier. However, an oxygen saturation monitor and precordial stethoscope can give the anesthesiologist critical information about perfusion, airway management, cardiac function, and status of shunting. The precordial stethoscope placed over the left precordium not only confirms adequate air exchange but allows monitoring of the cardiac impulse. An esophageal stethoscope can be placed after intubation.

TABLE 6–5. VASODILATORS FOR CHILDREN

Agent	Dose (IV)
Sodium nitroprusside	0.5–5.0 µg/kg/min
Hydralazine	0.1–0.3 mg/kg bolus
Nitroglycerin	0.25–1.0 µg/kg/min
Phentolamine	20 µg/kg/min
Prostaglandin E$_1$	0.1 µg/kg/min

(From: Hickey PR, Crone RK: Cardiovascular physiology and pharmacology in children: Normal and diseased pediatric cardiovascular systems, in Ryan JF, Todres DI, Cote CJ, Goudsouzian NG (eds): A Practice of Anesthesia for Infants and Children. Orlando, FL, Grune & Stratton, 1986, p 187.)

TABLE 6–6. ANTIARRHYTHMIA AGENTS FOR CHILDREN

Agent	IV Dose
Lidocaine	1 mg/kg
	20–50 µg/kg/min
Procainamide	2–5 mg/kg
Phenytoin	5 mg/kg
Bretylium	5–10 mg/kg
Propranolol	0.01–0.02 mg/kg
Verapamil	0.125–0.25 mg/kg
Esmolol	loading dose, 500 mg/kg
	50–300 µg/kg/min
Adenosine	50–200 µg/kg

(From: Hickey PR, Crone RK: Cardiovascular physiology and pharmacology in children: Normal and diseased pediatric cardiovascular systems in Ryan JF, Todres DI, Cote CJ, Goudsouzian NG (eds): A Practice of Anesthesia for Infants and Children. Orlando, FL, Grune & Stratton, 1986, p 188.)

Oxygen saturation monitors (*see* Chapter 3) are the most important contribution to monitoring in recent years. They provide reliable estimation of oxygen saturation, heart rate, and distal perfusion. Extensive use of pulse oximeters has recently taught pediatric cardiac anesthesiologists that dramatic changes in oxygen saturation often do not immediately affect blood pressure or heart rate until prolonged or profound decreases in saturation are present. Pulse oximeter probes should be placed in more than one location to provide a backup if one site fails during the operative procedure. The function of each probe should be verified before surgical prepping and draping.

Additional monitors can be placed quickly after the onset of induction. Electrocardiogram monitoring should include the ability to monitor two leads simultaneously, including both lead II for rhythm analysis and a V$_5$ lead. Blood pressure determination can be made with an automated blood pressure cuff. The presence of previous shunts or the anticipated creation of a shunt should guide the choice of the most appropriate limb for blood pressure measurement, including arterial cannulation. Arterial cannulation usually is performed after induction and intubation, except for older, more cooperative patients.

Appropriate IV catheters are placed with air-trap filters in line to avoid the potential for air embolism in every patient, not just those with right-to-left shunts. A double-lumen internal jugular vein catheter commonly is placed for central venous pressure (CVP) monitoring and drug infusion. Preoperative use of pulmonary artery catheters for pediatric patients is uncommon for anatomic reasons, including difficulty in placement and encroachment in the surgical field (*see* Chapter 3). Many surgeons will place right atrial, left atrial, and pulmonary artery catheters at the termination of cardiopulmonary bypass. In many instances, this will make preoperative placement of right atrial catheters unnecessary.

End-tidal (ET) CO_2 monitoring also is standard (*see* Chapter 3). After the airway has been secured and endotracheal tube position has been checked, an appropriately sized transesophageal echocardiography (TEE) probe is placed (*see* Chapter 3). The endotracheal tube must be secured carefully to prevent TEE manipulations from resulting in endotracheal tube position changes.

Airway Management

Fundamental to the anesthetic care of every patient with congenital heart disease is good airway management. As discussed previously, PVR is altered by changes in ventilatory pattern, Po_2, Pco_2, and pH. Changes in PVR may dramatically affect shunt magnitude and direction as well as cardiovascular function and stability. Therefore, prompt control of the airway and of ventilation will allow pulmonary blood flow to be optimized for each lesion. The mode of anesthetic induction should not complicate airway management and should be flexible enough to allow the anesthesiologist to deal with any unanticipated difficulties in controlling and securing the airway.

■ ANESTHETIC AGENTS

Interestingly, a variety of induction techniques have been shown to provide hemodynamic stability and improved arterial oxygen saturation in patients with cyanotic heart disease.[52-54] Nonetheless, it is prudent to individually tailor the choice of induction techniques to reduce metabolic needs, maintain airway control, and favorably manipulate pulmonary and systemic vascular resistances.

Intramuscular and Intravenous Agents

Ketamine. Ketamine is an extremely useful induction agent. In doses of 1 to 2 mg/kg IV or 3 to 5 mg/kg IM, ketamine has proved to be a reliable and safe induction agent in children with a variety of congenital heart lesions.[52,53] For patients with both normal and elevated baseline PVR, ketamine (2 mg/kg IV) causes minimal increases in pulmonary artery pressure as long as the airway and ventilation are supported.[55] Use of ketamine alone is associated with increased secretions, which may cause difficulties in airway management. For this reason, ketamine normally is combined with appropriate doses of atropine (0.02 mg/kg IM or IV). Succinylcholine (1 to 2 mg/kg IV or 2 to 4 mg/kg IM) added to ketamine and atropine in one syringe allows prompt control of the airway. Little change in cardiac output, heart rate, or blood pressure is seen after ketamine administration in children.[56] Smaller doses of ketamine

(0.2 to 0.5 mg/kg IV or 1 to 3 mg/kg IM) produce a dissociative state, which allows easy separation of the child from parents and also is useful in the catheterization laboratory, where brief periods of sedation without hemodynamic alteration are critical for interventional techniques.[57,58]

Narcotics. The hemodynamic stability that has been well documented in adult cardiac patients with high-dose narcotic techniques also is seen in pediatric patients. Morphine was the first narcotic to be used in high doses as the primary anesthetic agent for patients with congenital heart disease. Its use has been largely supplanted by the synthetic narcotics, fentanyl and sufentanil.

Fentanyl (25 to 100 µg/kg) and sufentanil (5 to 20 µg/kg), in combination with pancuronium and oxygen, provide stable induction and maintenance for infants and children undergoing correction of all types of congenital heart lesions.[59-62] These agents have minimal cardiovascular effects. In general, they induce only a slight decrease in SVR and PVR through a decrease in sympathetic outflow. In addition, these agents generally prevent or attenuate increases in SVR and PVR in response to intubation, incision, and sternotomy.[59,61,62] This attenuation of stress-induced increases in PVR is of particular importance considering the highly reactive nature of the pulmonary vasculature in patients with congenital heart disease. Despite the remarkable stability provided by these agents, in some instances, additional doses of fentanyl (5 to 15 µg/kg) or sufentanil (1 to 5 µg/kg) or supplementation with an inhalation agent may be necessary to attenuate hyperdynamic responses during maximal stimulation.[60,62]

Continuation of narcotic anesthesia may be useful in attenuating increases in PVR in response to routine postoperative manipulations. Increases in PVR are attenuated or ablated when fentanyl 25 µg/kg is administered before endotracheal suctioning.[49] Similarly, better attenuation of stress responses with sufentanil as compared with morphine/halothane may reduce the vulnerability of neonates undergoing cardiac surgery to complications and may even reduce mortality.[63]

Barbiturates. Because barbiturates are known to decrease blood pressure and to cause myocardial depression, they often are avoided for patients with poor cardiac reserve.

Benzodiazepines. Diazepam (0.15 mg/kg PO) is useful as a component of premedication for anxious older children. Diazepam (0.1 to 0.2 mg/kg IV) or midazolam (0.05 to 0.1 mg/kg IV) also can be used as an adjuvant to a high-dose narcotic anesthesia. Caution must be exercised because, as discussed in Chapters 4 and 5, the combination of narcotics and benzodiazepines is synergistic in reducing systemic vascular resistance. Midazolam provides reliable amnesia and does not produce pain when injected intravenously. This makes it a useful agent for preoperative sedation (0.025 to 0.05 mg/kg IV).

Inhalation Agents

Nitrous Oxide. The use of nitrous oxide (N_2O) for patients with congenital heart disease is somewhat controversial. Studies in adult patients show that use of N_2O is associated with decreases in blood pressure, heart rate, and cardiac output and with increases in PVR, particularly if baseline PVR is elevated.[64] However, postoperative administration of 50% N_2O to infants causes mild decreases in blood pressure, heart rate, and cardiac output with no significant increase in PVR, even if the baseline PVR is elevated.[65]

Every child with a shunt is at risk for systemic air embolism if air is introduced into the circulation under appropriate hemodynamic conditions. Because N_2O causes intravascular air bubbles to expand, its use has been criticized for patients with shunt lesions.

Halothane. Halothane is a well-recognized and widely used inhalational agent. Despite its well-accepted use in pediatric anesthesia, halothane has some potentially deleterious effects. Use of halothane for infants and children is associated with a decrease in echocardiographically assessed ventricular systolic function.[66-68] Recall that the immature myocardium contains fewer contractile elements than the mature myocardium, making it particularly sensitive to myocardial depressants. Furthermore, halothane causes a dose-dependent reduction in baroreceptor sensitivity, which is more pronounced in the immature cardiovascular system, with incomplete sympathetic innervation.[69] It is therefore not surprising that halothane administration predisposes normal infants and children to bradycardia and hypotension.[67,70,71] Hypotension and bradycardia may be attenuated by administration of atropine (0.02 mg/kg IM) before induction of halothane in infants.[71] Nonetheless, for children with limited cardiac reserve, halothane may be poorly tolerated and profound cardiovascular depression may result from its use.

Enflurane and Isoflurane. Inhalation induction with isoflurane causes decreases in systolic blood pressure similar to those seen with halothane inductions in infants.[72] Similarly, isoflurane anesthesia in preterm neonates produces depression of systolic blood pressure greater than that seen with halothane.[73] Isoflurane-induced systemic vasodilation plays an important role in the genesis of this systemic hypotension, because isoflurane has been shown to cause less echocardiographically assessed depression of ventricular systolic function than halothane in children.[68,69] However, like halothane, isoflurane does depress the baroreceptor response in

neonates.[74] Finally, inhalation induction with isoflurane may complicate airway management by producing copious secretions, airway irritation, and even laryngospasm.[72]

Enflurane use for children is less well studied than that of isoflurane and halothane. In isolated neonatal rat atria, enflurane causes significantly more depression of tension development than isoflurane or halothane.[75] Inhalation induction with enflurane seems to cause less airway irritation than isoflurane.[76]

Despite these limitations, infants and children with a variety of congenital lesions have safely undergone induction of anesthesia with halothane or isoflurane.[52-54,77] Isoflurane, by producing less myocardial depression, may offer some hemodynamic advantage over halothane when used for patients with marginal cardiac reserve. Patients with good cardiac reserve may be suitable candidates for inhalational induction and maintenance, especially when early extubation is planned. Likewise, inhalation anesthetic supplementation of narcotic anesthesia may be suitable for patients with less reserve.

Sevoflurane and Desflurane. Sevoflurane and desflurane are relatively new inhalational anesthetic agents with low blood–gas partition coefficients. Desflurane is not a good choice for inhalational induction because its pungency is responsible for a high incidence of airway complications in children.[78] Desflurane has hemodynamic effects similar to isoflurane[79] and may be useful as an adjuvant to narcotic anesthesia or as a primary maintenance agent after the airway has been secured. Sevoflurane has cardiovascular effects similar to isoflurane[80] and is a good agent for inhalational induction for children; the incidence of airway complications is similar to that of halothane.[81] Perhaps more important is the fact that inhalational induction with sevoflurane causes less myocardial depression than halothane in children.[82] Therefore, sevoflurane may have a role in both the induction and maintenance of anesthesia for children with congenital heart disease.

Muscle Relaxants

Nondepolarizing Agents. Pancuronium has vagolytic effects as well as sympathomimetic effects that can produce tachycardia and hypertension in children when given alone.[83] Pancuronium (0.1 mg/kg IV for intubation) commonly is used in combination with high doses of fentanyl or sufentanil. The vagolytic and sympathomimetic effects of pancuronium can be used to counteract the vagotonic effects of high doses of fentanyl or sufentanil.

Two intermediate duration nondepolarizing muscle relaxants that are relatively devoid of hemodynamic side effects are useful for children undergoing cardiac surgery: vecuronium (0.1 mg/kg for intubation) and rocuronium (0.6 mg/kg for intubation). Intubating doses of rocuronium have been associated with a slight increase in heart rate in children;[84] however, rocuronium provides more rapid onset of intubating conditions than vecuronium.[85] As with vecuronium, the duration of action of rocuronium is shorter in younger as compared with older children.[86] The duration of action or rocuronium and vecuronium can be expected to be longer in infants and neonates than in older children.[87] In fact, the duration of action of vecuronium in infants is similar to that of pancuronium.[88] Because these agents are associated with little or no vagolytic activity, bradycardia may result when they are used in combination with high doses of fentanyl or sufentanil.

Depolarizing Agents. Succinylcholine is a short-acting, depolarizing relaxant with a rapid onset of action. These properties make it useful for rapidly securing the airway. Succinylcholine given IV may cause bradycardia or even asystole in the pediatric patient. To attenuate this, atropine (0.1 mg IV) should be given before IV succinylcholine administration. Intramuscular atropine given as part of the premedication will not reliably attenuate succinylcholine dysrhythmias. In the absence of IV access, IM succinylcholine may be used; dysrhythmias are much less common after IM administration. The dose of succinylcholine per kg body weight is highest in infants. 1.0 mg/kg of succinylcholine will provide adequate relaxation for children, whereas for infants, 2.0 mg/kg is required. Likewise, for IM succinylcholine, 2.0 mg/kg will suffice for children, but 4.0 to 5.0 mg/kg is required for infants.

SPECIFIC LESIONS

This section discusses specific lesions and the anesthetic considerations applicable to the lesions. Lesions are not classified as cyanotic or acyanotic because, as elaborated earlier, that often is an artificial distinction.

■ VENTRICULAR SEPTAL DEFECT

Anatomy

An opening in the ventricular septum that permits communication between the right and left ventricles is a ventricular septal defect (VSD). Such communications may exist in one or more locations in the ventricular septum. As illustrated in Figure 6–10, VSDs can be classified by their location in the septum. Subpulmonary or supracristal defects are located in the infundibular septum just below the aortic valve. Subpulmonary lesions may be associated with aortic insufficiency due to a lack of support for the right coronary cusp of the aortic valve. Membranous or perimembranous defects com-

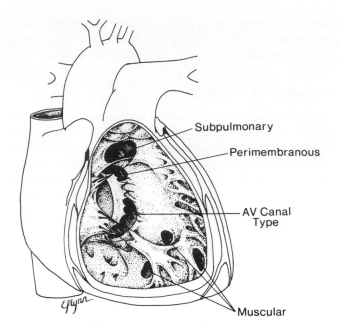

FIGURE 6–10. Location of ventricular septal defects. (AV = atrioventricular.) *(From: Fyler DC, Nadas AS: Congenital heart disease, in Avery ME, Lewis FR (eds):* Pediatric Medicine, *Baltimore, Williams & Wilkins, 1989, p 328.)*

prise approximately 80% of all VSDs and are located in the subaortic region of the membranous septum. Inlet or canal-type defects involve the septum near the atrioventricular (AV) but are different from complete AV canal defects in which there also are abnormalities of the AV valves. Muscular defects are located in the lower trabecular septum and may appear deceptively small on inspection from the right ventricular aspect of the septum. They may be apical, midmuscular, anterior, or posterior.

Physiology

A VSD is an example of a simple shunt. The size of the defect is the critical determinant of the magnitude of shunting. If the defect is small (restrictive shunt), flow through the defect will be limited and there will be a large pressure gradient across the defect. However, as the orifice becomes larger and the pressure gradient across the orifice decreases, the magnitude and direction of shunting becomes more dependent on the relative resistances of the systemic and pulmonary vascular beds. If the defect is large (approximating the size of the aortic valve orifice), there will be little or no pressure gradient across the defect. This is a dependent shunt with shunt magnitude and direction determined only by the relative resistances of the pulmonary and systemic vascular beds.

Because the ratio of PVR to SVR is normally 1:10 to 1:20, VSDs generally result in production of a left-to-right shunt. In some instances, however, the ratio of PVR to SVR may be higher, resulting in near-normal pulmonary blood flow or, in extreme cases, production of a right-to-left shunt.

The infant with a large VSD may have near-normal pulmonary blood flow as a result of high PVR present at birth. By the second week of life, PVR begins to fall to near-normal levels and pulmonary blood flow increases dramatically. Continued decreases in PVR after birth may be delayed by the elevated left atrial pressure that accompanies increased pulmonary blood flow.

Large VSDs predispose the development of PVOD during the first few years of life due to exposure of the pulmonary vasculature to high flows and systemic blood pressures. The increases in PVR that accompany PVOD will ultimately produce bidirectional and right-to-left shunts. Patients with advanced PVOD and markedly increased PVR (Eisenmenger's complex) generally are not candidates for VSD closure, because closure will result in an enormous increase in RV afterload and RV afterload mismatch (*see* Chapter 2). For this reason, large VSDs ($Q_p:Q_s > 2:1$) are corrected early in childhood.

An increase in left atrial volume and pressure parallels the increase in pulmonary blood flow seen with a large VSD. The resultant pulmonary venous congestion increases the work of breathing, decreases pulmonary compliance, and increases airway resistance. All of these factors predispose recurrent pulmonary infections. In VSDs with a large left-to-right shunt, systemic blood flow is maintained at the expense of a large volume load on both the right and left ventricles. This limits the capacity of the patient to meet increased cardiac output demands and may result in pulmonary and systemic congestion at rest. The timing of surgery often is dictated by failure of medical therapy to control this congestion.

Surgical Therapy

VSDs generally are closed with a patch via a variety of approaches, depending on their location. To avoid postoperative compromise of a small ventricle, with its poor compliance and limited capacity for tension development, it is desirable to avoid a ventriculotomy to approach and correct VSDs. Many defects are approachable through the right atrium and tricuspid valve, aorta, or pulmonary artery. However, in some instances, a right ventriculotomy may be the necessary approach. Less commonly, assessment and closure of some muscular defects will require a left ventriculotomy. Because a left ventriculotomy may seriously compromise myocardial function in the infant, palliation with pulmonary artery banding may be preferable to a left ventriculotomy for small infants.

Anesthetic Management

Goals.

1. Maintain heart rate, contractility, and preload to maintain cardiac output. A reduction in cardiac

output will compromise systemic perfusion, despite a relatively high pulmonary blood flow.
2. Avoid decreases in the PVR:SVR ratio. The increase in pulmonary blood flow that accompanies a reduced PVR:SVR ratio necessitates an increase in cardiac output to maintain systemic blood flow.
3. Avoid large increases in the PVR:SVR ratio. An increase may result in production of a right-to-left shunt.
4. In instances in which a right-to-left shunt exists, ventilatory measures to decrease PVR should be used. In addition, SVR must be maintained or increased. These measures will reduce the magnitude of the right-to-left shunt.

Induction and Maintenance. As discussed previously, control of ventilation is the most reliable way to manipulate PVR. Clearly, prompt, and reliable control of the airway at induction is important. For infants and children without congestive heart failure (CHF), an inhalational induction will be well tolerated. For neonates and patients with CHF, induction, maintenance, or both with an inhalation agent may result in profound hypotension. In these instances, an IV induction and maintenance with fentanyl or sufentanil will provide better hemodynamic stability. In particular, for patients with reactive pulmonary vasculature, high doses of fentanyl and sufentanil will be useful in blunting increases in PVR associated with surgical stimulation. In the absence of IV access, IM ketamine and atropine may be used for induction, followed by placement of an IV catheter.

Post-Cardiopulmonary Bypass Management

Closure of the VSD will prevent further exposure of the pulmonary vasculature to high flows and pressures. This usually will result in some immediate decrease in pulmonary artery pressures. For patients with small defects and patients with large VSDs in whom PVOD has not yet developed, near-normal pulmonary artery pressures may result. However, pulmonary artery pressures and PVR will remain elevated in patients with underlying PVOD. In addition, the pulmonary vasculature of these patients will remain hyperresponsive to vasoconstricting stimuli due to medial hypertrophy that accompanies PVOD. Therapy to reduce PVR in the post-cardiopulmonary bypass (CPB) period may be necessary for these patients to avoid RV afterload mismatch (*see* Chapter 2).

Separation from CPB may be complicated by a variety of surgical problems. Inadequate closure of the VSD or the presence of an unrecognized VSD may prevent separation from CPB. Assessment of the presence and location of such defects in the operating room can be accomplished with TEE (*see* Chapter 3). In addition, tricuspid valve damage due to a difficult transatrial approach may produce TR. Patch closure of the VSD may create subaortic or subpulmonic obstruction. Again, TEE is useful. Because the AV node is often near the area where the surgeon is working, heart block may occur. In some instances, use of isoproterenol (0.1 to 0.5 μg/kg/min) may improve A-V nodal conduction. In other instances, temporary epicardial A-V sequential pacing may be necessary to terminate CPB. Finally, if there seems to be complete heart block with a slow ventricular escape rate, the surgeon may decide to take down and redo the patch in an effort to prevent development of permanent heart block.

Goals

1. Maintain heart rate (preferably sinus rhythm) at an age-appropriate rate. Cardiac output is likely to be more heart-rate-dependent in the post-CPB period.
2. Reduce PVR through ventilatory interventions.
3. Inotropic support of the right ventricle may be necessary, particularly if PVR is high and the patient has undergone a right ventriculotomy. The left ventricle will no longer contribute to ejection of blood via the pulmonary artery and the right ventricle will face a high afterload. Dobutamine (5 to 10 μg/kg/min) or dopamine (5 to 10 μg/kg/min) is useful in this instance; both agents provide potent inotropic support without increasing PVR.

■ ATRIAL SEPTAL DEFECT

Anatomy

An atrial septal defect (ASD) is a communication between the left and right atria in the atrial septum. ASDs, like VSDs, are classified by their location. Figure 6–11 illustrates the anatomy of ASDs. ASDs 2° (Ostium secundum defects) comprise 80% of ASDs and result from defects in the septum primum, the septum secundum, or both. Sinus venosus defects are located at the top of the atrial septum and frequently are associated with partial anomalous drainage of the right superior pulmonary vein into the SVC. ASDs 1° (Ostium primum defects) tend to be large and are located in the lower portion of the atrial septum. These defects commonly are associated with abnormalities in the mitral valve, most notably a cleft anterior mitral valve leaflet with associated mitral regurgitation.

Physiology

An ASD is a simple shunt. A small, restrictive defect will allow minimal shunt flow. On the other hand, with a

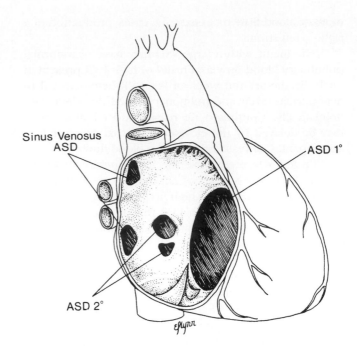

FIGURE 6–11. Location of atrial septal defects (ASDs). *(From: Fyler DC, Nadas AS: Congenital heart disease, in Avery ME, Lewis FR (eds): Pediatric Medicine. Baltimore, Williams & Wilkins, 1989, p 334.)*

large defect (at least 1 cm in diameter), the atria act like a single chamber and shunt magnitude and direction become dependent on the relative resistances of the pulmonary and systemic vascular beds. After the high PVR present after birth declines, a left-to-right shunt occurs because:

1. PVR is 1/10 to 1/20 that of SVR.
2. Increased pulmonary blood flow increases left atrial pressure. This favors flow of blood from the left atrium into the right atrium.
3. RV compliance is greater than LV compliance. This also favors flow of blood from the left to the right atrium.

A large defect will greatly increase pulmonary blood flow but, unlike a VSD, systemic pressures are not transmitted to the pulmonary vasculature. In fact, pulmonary artery pressure may remain normal for many years due to the distensibility of the pulmonary arteries. In contrast to a patient with VSD, the onset of PVOD may not occur until the third or fourth decade of life for a patient with ASD. Finally, a large ASD imposes a large volume load on the right ventricle.

Surgical Therapy

Many ASDs can be sutured closed. The larger defects require a patch closure. Primum ASDs with mitral valve involvement may require mitral valve repair.

Anesthetic Management

Goals

1. Maintain heart rate, contractility, and preload to maintain cardiac output. A reduction in cardiac output will compromise systemic perfusion despite a relatively high pulmonary blood flow.
2. Avoid decreases in the PVR:SVR ratio. The increase in pulmonary blood flow that accompanies a reduced PVR:SVR ratio necessitates an increase in cardiac output to maintain systemic blood flow.
3. Avoid large increases in PVR:SVR ratio. An increase may result in production of a right-to-left shunt.

Induction and Maintenance. Most children with ASDs have excellent cardiac reserve and will handle inhalation induction and maintenance without problems. Good airway management is necessary to allow manipulation of PVR and prevent reversal of left-to-right shunting. The presence of an enlarged atrium may predispose atrial dysrhythmias; these usually are well tolerated.

For children with an isolated ASD and no PVOD, early extubation or extubation in the operating room after repair is possible. An inhalational induction with halothane or sevoflurane followed by placement of an IV and administration of pancuronium 0.1 mg/kg and fentanyl 15 to 20 µg/kg is carried out. Anesthesia is maintained with isoflurane (0.5 to 1.0%) or sevoflurane (1.0 to 2.0%) supplementation. Caudal morphine (70 µg/kg in 5 to 10 mL of preservative-free saline) is administered after induction. A vaporizer on the CPB circuit or propofol 100 µg/kg/min provides anesthesia during CPB.

Post-CPB Management

Separation from CPB usually is not problematic and surgical mortality is less than 1%. In primum defects, the possibility of heart block and residual mitral regurgitation remains. If partial anomalous pulmonary venous drainage (partial pulmonary venous to right atrial drainage) is present and unrecognized, a residual left-to-right shunt may exist after repair. This will increase post-CPB cardiac output requirements and may complicate separation from CPB. Intraoperative TEE can be used to establish this diagnosis before repair.

The pulmonary vasculature is likely to be hyperreactive in the post-CPB period, particularly if PVOD exists. Therefore, it is necessary to use ventilatory measures to reduce post-CPB PVR. These manipulations will prevent right ventricular dysfunction secondary to increased afterload.

Goals

1. Maintain heart rate (preferably sinus rhythm) at an age-appropriate rate. Cardiac output is likely to be more heart-rate-dependent in the post-CPB period.
2. Reduce PVR through ventilatory interventions, particularly for patients with PVOD.
3. Inotropic support of the right ventricle may rarely be necessary when PVR is high and right ventricular dysfunction exists. Dobutamine (5 to 10 µg/kg/min) or dopamine (5 to 10 µg/kg/min) is useful in this instance; both agents provide potent inotropic support without increasing PVR.

■ COMMON ATRIOVENTRICULAR CANAL DEFECTS

Anatomy

Embryologically, there are four endocardial cushions that contribute to the development of the lower ostium primum portion of the atrial septum and the upper inlet portion of the ventricular septum where the AV valves insert. The cushions also contribute to the tissue that forms the septal leaflets of the mitral and tricuspid valves. Therefore, cushion defects, or common atrioventricular canal (CAVC) defects, usually include abnormalities in all these structures. Cushion defects have been classified as types A, B, and C, based on whether the anterior bridging leaflet is divided or undivided and if it is attached or unattached to the septum (*see* Figs. 6–12 and 6–13).

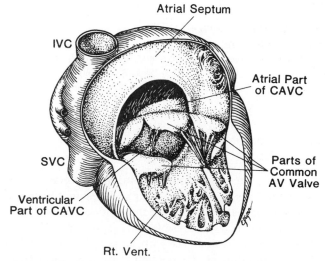

FIGURE 6–12. Right ventricle opened to reveal components of a common atrioventricular canal defect. (AV = atrioventricular; CAVC = common atrioventricular canal; IVC = inferior vena cava; SVC = superior vena cava; Rt Vent = right ventricle.) *(From: Fyler DC, Nadas AS: Congenital heart disease, in Avery ME, Lewis FR (eds): Pediatric Medicine. Baltimore, Williams & Wilkins, 1989, p 341.)*

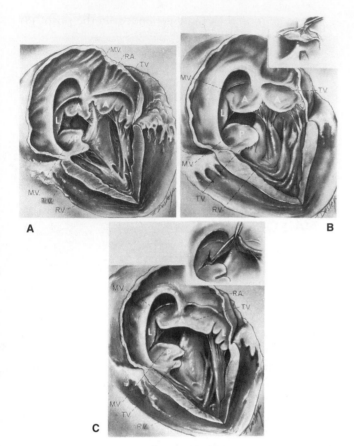

FIGURE 6–13. Types of complete atrioventricular canal. **A.** Type A — the most frequent form of CAVC. The anterior bridging leaflet (A) is divided into mitral and tricuspid portions, both of which are attached to the ventricular septum. The tricuspid portion represents the true anterior tricuspid valve leaflet. In this type of lesion, the VSD does not extend to the aortic valve cusps. **B.** Type B — the least frequent form of CAVC. The anterior bridging leaflet (A) is large, overhangs the ventricular septum and is attached to chordae in the right ventricle. **C.** Type C — the form of CAVC most commonly associated with other major cardiac anomalies. The anterior bridging leaflet (A) is very large, undivided, and unattached to the ventricular septum. The anterior tricuspid leaflet is very hypoplastic and the VSD extends to the aortic valve cusps. (A = anterior bridging leaflet; P = posterior bridging leaflet; L = two lateral leaflets; MV = mitral portions of the leaflets; TV = tricuspid portion of the leaflets; RA = right atrium; RV = right ventricle.) *(From: Feldt RH, et al: Atrial septal defects and atrioventricular canal, in Adams FH, Emmanouilides GG (eds):* Moss' Heart Disease in Infants. *3rd ed. Baltimore, Williams & Wilkins, 1983, p 124.)*

Physiology

These defects result in communication between all four heart chambers as well as abnormalities in the mitral and tricuspid valves. Because the orifice between the four chambers is large, these lesions tend to produce dependent simple shunts. As with large VSDs, this results in (1) production of a large left-to-right shunt; (2) increased pulmonary blood flow; (3) transmission of systemic pressures to the right ventricle and pulmonary arteries; and (4) volume overloading of the right and left ventricles.

As with large VSDs, CAVC defects predispose the early development of PVOD. Advanced PVOD may increase the PVR-SVR ratio such that a bidirectional or right-to-left shunt develops. This is a particular concern for patients with Down's syndrome. CAVC defects are common in these patients, who are particularly prone to early development of PVOD (*see* Chapter 1). In some CAVC defects, the presence of severe mitral insufficiency results in regurgitation of left ventricular blood directly into the right atrium. This increases the left-to-right shunt. In addition, mitral regurgitation increases the volume work of the left ventricle (*see* Chapter 5).

Surgical Therapy

Using one or more pericardial patches, the atrial and ventricular defects are closed. The AV valve apparatus is approximated and resuspended onto the pericardial patch. The surgical approach normally is via a right atriotomy. The mitral valve may need to be repaired (valvuloplasty). If the mitral valve is severely regurgitant, artificial valve replacement may be necessary. This intervention is not without problems. In addition to the obvious problems of anticoagulating small, active children and the need for future valve replacements, placement of an artificial valve may impinge on the left ventricular outflow tract and create subaortic obstruction.

Anesthetic Management

Goals

1. Maintain heart rate, contractility, and preload to maintain cardiac output. A reduction in cardiac output will compromise systemic perfusion despite a relatively high pulmonary blood flow.
2. Avoid decreases in the PVR:SVR ratio. The increase in pulmonary blood flow that accompanies a reduced PVR:SVR ratio necessitates an increase in cardiac output to maintain systemic blood flow.
3. Avoid large increases in PVR:SVR ratio. An increase may result in production of a right-to-left shunt.
4. In instances in which a right-to-left shunt exists, ventilatory measures to decrease PVR should be used. In addition, SVR must be maintained or increased. These measures will reduce the magnitude of the right-to-left shunt.

Induction and Maintenance. Anesthetic management is similar to that for large VSDs. However, the child with CAVC also may have severe mitral regurgitation and a highly reactive pulmonary vasculature. Because control of ventilation is the most reliable way to manipulate PVR, prompt and reliable control of the airway at induction is important. The goal should be to use a reduced FIO_2 and to maintain PCO_2 at 35 to 40 mm Hg. The reduction in FIO_2 tolerated will depend on the individual patient. Inhalational induction and/or maintenance should be reserved for infants and children with small defects, no mitral regurgitation, and no PVOD. Cardiac reserve often is limited or exhausted in patients with large shunts and high PVR. Moreover, the additional volume load imposed on the left ventricle by mitral regurgitation will further limit cardiac reserve. For these reasons, inhalation induction and/or maintenance usually is poorly tolerated in these patients. An IV induction and maintenance with fentanyl or sufentanil will provide better hemodynamic stability. In particular, for patients with reactive pulmonary vasculature, high doses of fentanyl and sufentanil will be useful in blunting increases in PVR associated with surgical stimulation. In addition, high doses of fentanyl or sufentanil will blunt stimulation-induced increases in SVR, which will increase the mitral regurgitant fraction. In the absence of IV access, IM ketamine and atropine may be used for induction, followed by placement of an IV catheter.

Post-CPB Management

Closure of the defects will prevent further exposure of the pulmonary vasculature to high blood flows and pressures. This usually will result in some immediate decrease in pulmonary artery pressures. In patients with small defects and patients with large defects in whom PVOD has not yet developed, near-normal pulmonary artery pressures may result. However, pulmonary artery pressures and PVR will remain elevated in patients with underlying PVOD. In addition, the pulmonary vasculature of these patients (especially patients with Down syndrome) will remain hyperresponsive to vasoconstricting stimuli due to medial hypertrophy that accompanies PVOD. Therapy to reduce PVR in the post-CPB period may be necessary for these patients to avoid RV afterload mismatch (*see* Chapter 2).

Separation from CPB may be complicated by a variety of surgical problems. Inadequate closure of the defects or persistent mitral regurgitation may prevent separation from CPB. Assessment of the presence and location of such defects in the OR can be accomplished with TEE (*see* Chapter 3). The presence of large V waves on the pressure trace obtained from a left atrial catheter may be helpful in assessing the degree of mitral regurgitation, whereas TEE will provide definite information (*see* Chapter 3). Occasionally, patch placement severely reduces the left ventricular chamber size and limits stroke volume. Because the AV node is near the area where the surgeon is working, heart block may occur. In some instances, the use of isoproterenol (0.1 to 0.5 $\mu g/kg/min$) may improve AV nodal conduction. In other

instances, temporary epicardial AV sequential pacing may be necessary to terminate CPB.

Goals

1. Maintain heart rate (preferably sinus rhythm) at an age-appropriate rate. Cardiac output is likely to be more heart rate dependent in the post-CPB period.
2. Reduce PVR through ventilatory interventions.
3. Inotropic support of the right ventricle may be necessary, particularly if PVR is high. The left ventricle will no longer contribute to ejection of blood via the pulmonary artery and the right ventricle will face a high afterload. Dobutamine (5 to 10 $\mu g/kg/min$) or dopamine (5 to 10 $\mu g/kg/min$) is useful in this instance because both agents provide potent inotropic support without increasing PVR.

■ PATENT DUCTUS ARTERIOSUS

Anatomy

The patent ductus ateriosus (PDA) develops from the left sixth aortic arch and connects the main pulmonary trunk with the distal descending aorta distal to the origin of the left subclavian artery (*see* Fig. 6–14). As discussed previously, the duct is a fetal channel that normally closes soon after birth.

Physiology

A PDA is a simple shunt. When the PDA is large, there is little or no pressure gradient across the duct and shunting becomes dependent on the ratio of PVR to SVR.

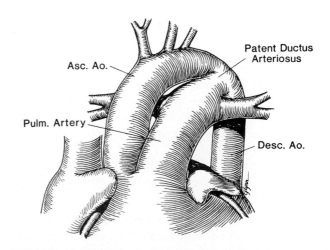

FIGURE 6–14. Patent ductus arteriosus. (Asc Ao = ascending aorta; Desc Ao = descending aorta.) *(From: Fyler DC, Nadas AS: Congenital heart disease, in Avery ME, Lewis FR (eds):* Pediatric Medicine. *Baltimore, Williams & Wilkins, 1989, p 344.)*

Normally, in the postnatal period, this results in a left-to-right shunt and increased pulmonary blood flow. For systemic blood flow to be maintained, left ventricular output must increase and a volume load must be imposed on the left ventricle. The increased pulmonary blood flow increases pulmonary venous return and left atrial pressure. These factors may, in turn, increase PVR and the work of breathing. Finally, runoff of blood from the proximal aorta into the pulmonary artery tends to compromise distal organ perfusion and to decrease aortic diastolic blood pressure, which reduces coronary perfusion pressure.

Fortunately, most patients with PDAs have smaller, restrictive shunts with smaller increases in pulmonary blood flow. Furthermore, the high PVR present after birth tends to limit the shunt magnitude of even the largest PDAs until PVR begins to decrease. However, it is not difficult to see how a PDA could produce CHF and prevent weaning of ventilatory support in an infant.

Surgical Therapy

Closure of the PDA was the first "cardiac" operation, successfully performed by Gross in 1938. The usual surgical approach is via a left thoracotomy. CPB is not used. The ductus is either ligated or ligated and transected. Closure of a PDA currently is being accomplished in some cardiac catheterization laboratories using umbrella devices. An anesthetic often is necessary for this procedure, because catheter insertion is painful and placement of the device may be unsuccessful in an awake, struggling, crying child. Dislodgement of the device downstream into the left pulmonary artery may occur and require surgical intervention.

Anesthetic Management

Goals

1. Maintain heart rate, contractility, and preload to maintain cardiac output. A reduction in cardiac output will compromise systemic perfusion despite a relatively high pulmonary blood flow.
2. Avoid decreases in the PVR:SVR ratio. The increases in pulmonary blood flow that accompany a reduced PVR:SVR ratio necessitate an increase in cardiac output to maintain systemic blood flow.
3. Surgical retraction of the left lung may necessitate high inspired oxygen concentrations to prevent hypoxemia.

Induction and Maintenance. A high proportion of the patients presenting for PDA ligation or embolization are premature infants with respiratory distress syndrome. Age and the likelihood that CHF exists make these patients poor candidates for inhalational anesthesia.

A technique using fentanyl or sufentanil is well tolerated.

For older children with an isolated PDA and no PVOD, early extubation or extubation in the operating room after ligation is possible. An inhalational induction with halothane or sevoflurane followed by placement of an IV and administration of pancuronium 0.1 mg/kg and fentanyl 10 to 15 µg/kg is performed. Anesthesia is maintained with isoflurane (0.5 to 1.0%) or sevoflurane (1.0 to 2.0%) supplementation. Caudal morphine (70 µg/kg in 5 to 10 mL of preservative-free saline) is administered after induction.

■ TETRALOGY OF FALLOT

Anatomy

Tetralogy of Fallot (TOF) (*see* Fig. 6–15) is characterized by a VSD, overriding of the aorta, right ventricular hypertrophy, and pulmonic stenosis (infundibular, valvular, supravalvular, or a combination). The key malformation is underdevelopment of the right ventricular infundibulum and displacement of the infundibular septum resulting in right ventricular outflow tract stenosis. Patients with TOF have displacement of the infundibular septum in an anterior, superior, and leftward direction. The back wall of the right ventricular outflow tract is formed by the infundibular septum and this abnormal displacement results in narrowing of the right ventricular outflow tract. In addition, this displacement of the infundibular septum creates a large malalignment VSD

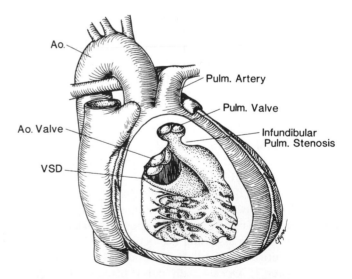

FIGURE 6–15. Anatomy in tetralogy of Fallot (TOF). The following features are notable: malalignment ventricular septal defect (VSD), overriding aorta (Ao), infundibular pulmonic stenosis, small pulmonary arteries. A right-sided aortic arch, as illustrated here, occurs in 25% of patients with TOF. *(From: Fyler DC, Nadas AS: Congenital heart disease, in Avery ME, Lewis FR (eds): Pediatric Medicine. Baltimore, Williams & Wilkins, 1989, p 350.)*

with the aorta overriding the interventricular septum (*see* Fig. 6–16). Abnormalities in the septal and parietal attachments of the outflow tract further exacerbate the infundibular stenosis (*see* Fig. 6–17). The pulmonary annulus usually is hypoplastic and 75% of TOF patients will have both infundibular and valvular stenosis. In addition, varying degrees of main pulmonary artery and branch pulmonary artery hypoplasia may exist as well. A small proportion of patients will have multiple VSDs.

Physiology

TOF is a complex shunt in which a communication (VSD) and a partial obstruction to RV outflow (RV infundibular and valvular stenosis with or without suprapulmonic stenosis) are present. In complex shunts, the resistance to outflow is a combination of the resistance from the obstructive lesions and the vascular resistance. If the resistance from the RV obstructive lesions is high, changes in PVR will have little effect on shunt magnitude and direction. In most patients with TOF, there is a fixed and a dynamic component to RV outflow obstruction. The fixed component is produced by the infundibular, valvular, and supravalvular stenosis. The dynamic component is produced by variations in the caliber of the RV infundibulum.

In patients with TOF, the arterial saturation is a direct reflection of pulmonary blood flow. In the population of patients with TOF, there is a wide variation in the extent of RV outflow obstruction and thus in the amount of pulmonary blood flow. Patients with "Pink Tet" have minimal obstruction to pulmonary blood flow at the right ventricular outflow and pulmonary artery level and may be normally saturated. Some of these patients have a left-to-right shunt with increased pulmonary blood flow. The classic case of TOF includes severe right ventricular outflow obstruction secondary to fixed and variable components. This produces a right-to-left shunt and cyanosis.

Hypoxic or "Tet Spells." The occurrence of hypoxic spells in TOF patients may be life-threatening and should be anticipated in every patient, even those who are not normally cyanotic. The peak frequency of spells is between 2 and 3 months of age; spells occur more frequently in severely cyanotic patients. The onset of spells usually prompts urgent surgical intervention, so it is not unusual for the anesthesiologist to care for an infant who is at great risk for spells during the preoperative period.

The etiology of spells is not completely understood, but infundibular spasm or constriction may play a role. Crying, defecation, feeding, fever, and awakening all can be precipitating events. Paroxysmal hyperpnea is the initial finding. There is an increase in rate and depth of respiration, leading to increasing cyanosis and potential syncope, convulsions, or death. During a spell, the infant will appear pale and limp secondary to poor cardiac output. Hyperpnea has several deleterious effects in maintaining and worsening a hypoxic spell. Hyperpnea increases oxygen consumption through the in-

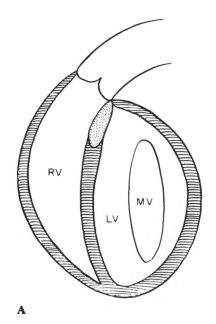

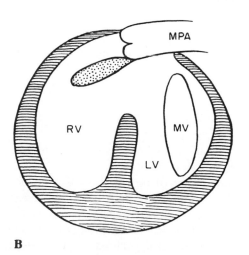

A   **B**

FIGURE 6–16. A. Long-axis view of heart illustrating the normal relationship of the infundibular septum (stippled) and the trabecular septum (striped). **B.** Long-axis view of heart in tetralogy of Fallot. Lack of connection between infundibular and trabecular septum results in malalignment ventricular septal defect. Right ventricular outflow tract is narrowed by upward, anterior tilt of infundibular septum. (RV = right ventricle; LV = left ventricle; MV = mitral valve; MPA = main pulmonary artery.) *(From: Williams RG, Bierman FZ, Sanders SP: Tetrology of Fallot, in* Echocardiographic Diagnosis of Cardiac Malformations. *Boston, Little-Brown, 1986, p 155.)*

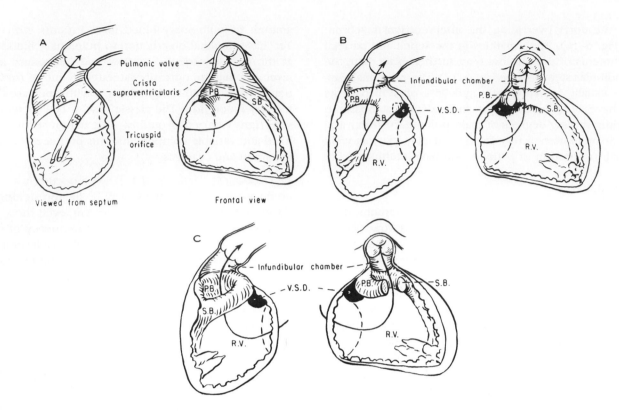

FIGURE 6–17. Spectrum of infundibular stenosis produced by abnormalities in septal and parietal bands of crista supraventricularis. **A.** Normal anatomy of crista supraventricularis. **B.** Moderate infundibular stenosis and creation of an infundibular chamber secondary to hypertrophy and anterior, superior displacement of parietal band. **C.** Severe infundibular stenosis with creation of infundibular chamber secondary to hypertrophy and anterior, superior displacement of both septal and parietal bands. (RV = right ventricle; SB = septal band; PB = parietal band; VSD = ventricular septal defect.) *(From: Guntheroth WG, Kawabori I, Baum D: Tetralogy of Fallot, in Adams FH, Emmanouilides GG (eds): Moss' Heart Disease in Infants. 3rd ed. Baltimore, Williams & Wilkins, 1986, p 216.)*

creased work of breathing. Hypoxia induces a decrease in SVR, which further increases the right-to-left shunt. Hyperpnea also lowers intrathoracic pressure and leads to an increase in systemic venous return. In the face of infundibular obstruction, this results in an increased RV pressure and an increase in the right-to-left shunt. Thus, episodes seem to be associated with events that increase oxygen demand while simultaneous decreases in Po_2 and increases in pH and Pco_2 are occurring.

Treatment of a "Tet spell" includes the following:

1. Administration of 100% oxygen.
2. Placing the patient in a knee–chest position, which transiently increases SVR and reduces the right-to-left shunt.
3. Administration of morphine sulfate, which sedates the patient and may have a depressant effect on respiratory drive and hyperpnea.
4. Administration of 5 to 10 mL/kg of a crystalloid solution. Enhancing preload will increase heart size, which may increase the diameter of the RV outflow tract.
5. Administration of sodium bicarbonate to treat the severe metabolic acidosis that can be seen

during a spell. Correction of the metabolic acidosis will help normalize SVR and reduce hyperpnea. Bicarbonate administration (1 to 2 mEq/kg) in the absence of a blood gas determination is warranted during a spell.

6. Phenylephrine (dose 10 to 20 µg/kg IV or 2 to 5 µg/kg/min as an infusion) can be used to increase SVR and reduce right-to-left shunting. In the presence of severe RV outflow obstruction, phenylephrine-induced increases of PVR will have little or no effect in increasing RV outflow resistance.
7. Beta-adrenergic agonists are absolutely contraindicated. By increasing contractility, they will cause further narrowing of the senotic infundibulum.
8. Administration of propranolol (0.1 mg/kg) or esmolol[89] (0.5 mg/kg followed by an infusion of 50 to 300 µg/kg/min) may reduce infundibular spasm by depressing contractility. In addition, slowing of heart rate may allow for improved diastolic filling (increased preload), increased heart size, and an increase in the diameter of the RV outflow tract (RVOT).

9. Manual compression of the abdominal aorta will increase SVR. This maneuver is particularly effective for the anesthetized patient. After the chest is open, the surgeon can manually compress the ascending aorta to increase impedance to ejection through the LV. This can be effective in terminating a cyanotic episode.

10. TEE is useful in monitoring ventricular dimensions and assessing impending dynamic obstruction of the RVOT.

Surgical Therapy

Palliative Procedures. Palliative procedures to increase pulmonary blood flow are used for patients in whom complicated surgical anatomy precludes definitive repair at the time of presentation. The palliative procedures described below create a systemic-to-pulmonary arterial shunt analogous to a PDA. Ideally, these surgical shunts should be mildly restrictive simple shunts. In the presence of a proximal obstruction to pulmonary blood flow, these shunts produce a left-to-right shunt and an increase in pulmonary blood flow. The volume load imposed on the LV by these shunts parallels the increases in pulmonary flow that they produce.

BLALOCK–TAUSSIG SHUNT. The Blalock–Taussig (BT) shunt (*see* Fig. 6–18A) results from creation of an end-to-side anastomosis of the right or left subclavian artery to the ipsilateral branch pulmonary artery. A modification of this procedure involves interposing a length of Gore-Tex tube graft between the subclavian artery and the branch pulmonary artery. These shunts usually are performed on the side opposite the aortic arch via a thoracotomy without CPB.

WATERSTON SHUNT. This shunt (*see* Fig. 6–18C) results from creation of a side-to-side anastomosis between the ascending aorta and the right pulmonary artery. This procedure is performed via a right thoracotomy without CPB. It often is difficult to size the orifice of this shunt correctly. Too small an orifice will limit pulmonary blood flow, whereas too large an orifice will create pulmonary overperfusion and congestion and predispose development of PVOD in the right lung. In addition, this shunt may produce distortion of the pulmonary artery, making subsequent definitive repair difficult.

POTTS SHUNT. This shunt results from creation of a side-to-side anastomosis between the descending aorta and the left pulmonary artery. This shunt is rarely used today because it is difficult to size properly, may distort the pulmonary artery, and is difficult to take down at the time of the definitive procedure.

CENTRAL SHUNT. This shunt (*see* Fig. 6–18D) is created by placing a synthetic tube graft between the ascending aorta and the main or branch pulmonary artery. This shunt can be performed with or without CPB via a thoracotomy or median sternotomy. It often is used when prior shunt procedures have failed. It is easier to size this shunt than a Waterston or Potts shunt because a tube of known diameter can be placed between the systemic and pulmonary circulations. Use of this shunt has largely replaced use of the Waterston and Potts shunts.

Creation of surgical shunts to increase pulmonary blood flow presents the anesthesiologist with several management problems:

1. When a thoracotomy approach is used, unilateral lung retraction will be required for surgical exposure. The resulting atelectasis may severely compromise oxygenation and CO_2 removal. Intermittent reinflation of the lung may be necessary during the operative procedure. These reinflations should be coordinated with the surgeon. High-frequency jet ventilation (HFJV) has been used with success.

2. For all the shunts described, the main or branch pulmonary artery will have to be partially occluded by a clamp to allow creation of the distal anastomosis. The resulting increase in physiological dead space may compromise oxygenation and CO_2 removal. Efforts to increase pulmonary blood flow by reducing PVR with ventilatory in-

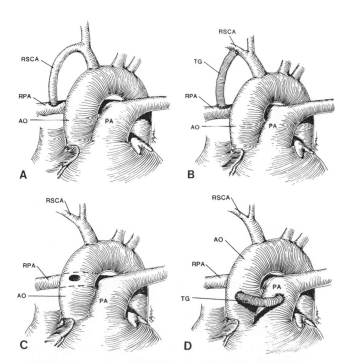

FIGURE 6–18. Surgically created systemic to pulmonary artery shunts. **A.** Blalock–Taussig shunt. **B.** Modified Blalock–Taussig shunt. **C.** Waterston shunt. **D.** Central shunt. (RSCA = right subclavian artery; RPA = right pulmonary artery; AO = aorta; PA = pulmonary artery; TG = tube graft.)

terventions and by increasing left-to-right shunting should be initiated before pulmonary artery occlusion.

3. Partial occlusion of the aorta with a clamp will be necessary during creation of Waterston, Potts, and central shunts. The resulting increase in LV afterload may compromise systolic function. In patients with CHF, inotropic support of the ventricle may be necessary. TEE is useful for monitoring LV function at this point.

4. All of these palliative shunts impose a volume load on the LV. Inotropic support may be necessary to ensure systemic and shunt perfusion after shunt formation.

5. Palliative shunts are mildly restrictive simple shunts. It is important to maintain SVR and reduce PVR to maintain pulmonary blood flow in patients with surgical shunts.

Definitive Procedures. Definitive repair for TOF is being accomplished, even in neonates, if favorable anatomy is present. Surgery is aimed at relieving the outflow obstruction by resection of hypertrophied, obstructing muscle bundles and augmentation and enlargement of the outflow tract with a pericardial patch. Enlargement of the outflow tract may involve extension of the patch across the pulmonary valve annulus and into the main pulmonary artery. If stenosis of the pulmonary artery extends to the bifurcation, the pericardial patch can be extended beyond the bifurcation of the pulmonary arteries. In some cases, a valved conduit from the RV to the PA is placed to prevent the pulmonic insufficiency that develops when a severely stenotic valve is removed. Finally, the VSD(s) is closed.

An important surgical consideration for patients with TOF is the occurrence of coronary artery abnormalities. Approximately 8% of patients have either the left main coronary artery or the left anterior descending artery as a branch of the right coronary artery. In these cases, a right ventriculotomy to enlarge the right ventricular outflow tract will endanger the left coronary artery. In such cases, an extracardiac conduit may be necessary to bypass the outflow tract obstruction and avoid injury to the coronary artery. It is imperative that preoperative evaluation by the cardiologist identifies such an abnormality.

Anesthetic Management

Goals

1. Maintain heart rate, contractility, and preload to maintain cardiac output.
2. Avoid increases in the PVR:SVR ratio. The less severe the RV outflow obstructive lesions, the more important this becomes. Increases in PVR

relative to SVR, and decreases in SVR relative to PVR, will increase right-to-left shunting, reduce pulmonary blood flow, and produce or worsen cyanosis.

3. Use ventilatory measures to reduce PVR.
4. Maintain or increase SVR. This is particularly important when RV outflow obstruction is severe and changes in PVR will have little or no effect on shunt magnitude and direction.
5. Aggressively treat "Tet spells."
6. Maintain contractility. Depression of contractility, particularly in the face of severe RV outflow obstruction, may produce RV afterload mismatch (*see* Chapter 2) and drastically reduce pulmonary blood flow. The exception to this is patients in whom the dynamic component of infundibular obstruction is active. Reducing contractility in these patients may reduce RV outflow obstruction via relaxation of the infundibulum.

Induction and Maintenance. As discussed previously, control of ventilation is the most reliable way to manipulate PVR. Clearly, prompt and reliable control of the airway at induction is important. An inhalational induction will be well tolerated by most infants and children because parallel decreases in PVR and SVR will occur. Nonetheless, systemic hypotension should be avoided or treated promptly. Systemic hypotension is particularly likely to cause or increase right-to-left shunting when RV outflow obstruction is severe and anesthesia-induced decreases in PVR have little effect on decreasing RV outflow resistance.

Ketamine is a useful induction agent in patients with TOF. Ketamine has been shown to cause no significant increase in PVR in these patients. Fentanyl or sufentanil will provide very stable induction and maintenance hemodynamics and will blunt stimulation-induced increases in PVR. Maintenance of anesthesia with fentanyl or sufentanil can be initiated after any of the previously described induction techniques.

Post-CPB Management

After definite repair for TOF, several factors may contribute to depressed RV systolic function:

1. Creation of a right ventriculotomy and placement of the RV outflow patch produces a segment of dyskinetic right ventricle.
2. Protection of the right ventricle from ischemia during aortic cross-clamping is difficult in patients with a hypertrophied right ventricle as occurs in TOF (*see* Chapter 12).
3. Enlargement of the RV outflow tract may create pulmonary regurgitation, which imposes a volume load on the RV.

4. Stenosis or hypoplasia of the distal pulmonary arteries or the inability to completely correct the RV outflow obstruction will impose a pressure load on the RV.
5. A residual VSD will impose a volume load on the RV.

Therefore, despite the relief of RV outflow obstruction, the RV commonly requires inotropic support in the post-CPB period. In instances in which the distal pulmonary arteries are very hypoplastic or surgical correction of RV outflow obstruction is poor, suprasystemic pressures may develop in the RV. In addition, a residual VSD may exist. These problems may not permit separation from CPB. Diagnosis of these surgical problems often can be made efficiently with intraoperative intracardiac saturation and pressure measurements and with intraoperative TEE.

As with all cases involving VSD, closure conduction abnormalities may be a problem (see the VSD discussion earlier in this chapter).

Goals

1. Maintain heart rate (preferably sinus rhythm) at an age-appropriate rate. Cardiac output is likely to be more heart-rate-dependent during the post-CPB period.
2. Reduce PVR through ventilatory interventions.
3. Inotropic support of the right ventricle may be necessary for the reasons addressed. Dobutamine (5 to 10 µg/kg/min) or dopamine (5 to 10 µg/kg/min) are useful in this instance because they provide potent inotropic support without increasing PVR.

■ TETRALOGY OF FALLOT WITH PULMONARY ATRESIA

Anatomy

The anatomy of this lesion is similar to TOF, except that the right ventricular outflow tract is atretic at one or more locations. In addition, the pulmonary arteries tend to be quite hypoplastic. A PDA or systemic–pulmonary collaterals are present as the source of pulmonary blood flow. These collaterals are often numerous, arising from multiple locations off the descending aorta. This anatomy is illustrated in Figure 6–19.

Physiology

TOF with pulmonary atresia is a complex shunt in which a communication (VSD) and total obstruction to RV outflow (pulmonary atresia) are present. This results in obligatory right-to-left shunting across the VSD with

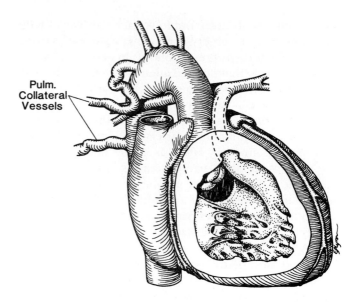

FIGURE 6–19. Anatomy of tetralogy of Fallot with pulmonary atresia. Pulmonary arteries are very small and pulmonary blood flow is supplied via collaterals from descending aorta. *(From: Fyler DC, Nadas AS: Congenital heart disease, in Avery ME, Lewis FR (eds): Pediatric Medicine. Baltimore, Williams & Wilkins, 1989, p 352.)*

complete mixing of systemic and pulmonary venous blood in the LV. Pulmonary blood flow is provided by a downstream simple shunt (PDA or systemic to pulmonary collaterals). For infants, in whom the PDA provides most of the pulmonary blood flow, prostaglandin E_1 infusion (0.05 to 0.1 µg/kg/min) will be necessary to ensure ductal patency.

For patients with TOF and pulmonary atresia, the arterial saturation is dependent on complete mixing. Recall that the arterial saturation in a complete mixing lesion is determined by the systemic venous saturation, pulmonary venous saturation, and $Q_p:Q_s$. In TOF with pulmonary atresia, pulmonary blood flow is greatly reduced and $Q_p:Q_s$ is lower than 1:1. Therefore, as illustrated in Figure 6–5, even with high systemic and pulmonary venous saturations, these patients will be cyanotic.

Surgical Therapy

Palliative Procedures. As with patients with TOF, palliative shunts to increase pulmonary blood flow may be done. For patients with TOF and pulmonary atresia, creation of surgical shunts may be complicated by hypoplastic pulmonary arteries. Hypoplastic pulmonary arteries not only make creation of surgical shunts difficult but their creation may also distort the pulmonary vasculature and make subsequent definitive procedures more difficult. A full discussion of these palliative shunts is covered in the section on tetralogy of Fallot.

Definitive Procedures. The key issue in surgical decision-making in these patients is the location and extent of right ventricular outflow tract atresia. As with correction of TOF, surgery is aimed at relieving the outflow obstruction by resection of hypertrophied, obstructing muscle bundles and augmentation and enlargement of the outflow tract with a pericardial patch. In instances in which the atretic portion is short and close to the pulmonary valve, extension of the RV outflow patch into the pulmonary artery will permit enlargement of the pulmonary artery as it does in patients with TOF and pulmonary artery stenosis. In instances in which the atretic portion is long or distal in the pulmonary artery, creation of a conduit from the RV to the distal pulmonary arteries may be necessary.

Hypoplasia of the distal pulmonary arteries further complicates surgical management. In some instances, the hypoplastic pulmonary arteries are too small to allow creation of the distal anastomosis of a RV to pulmonary artery conduit. These patients are not immediate candidates for an RV-to-PA conduit. A palliative shunt may improve oxygenation and permit growth of the hypoplastic pulmonary arteries so that an RV-to-PA conduit can be constructed at a later date. In other instances, the distal pulmonary arteries are so hypoplastic that they provide significant obstruction to RV outflow, even after correction or bypass of the atretic pulmonary artery segments. For these patients, closure of the VSD is delayed. This allows additional growth of the hypoplastic distal pulmonary arteries while protecting the RV from excessive afterload. VSD closure can be accomplished at a later date when growth of the distal pulmonary arteries reduces RV afterload.

Anesthetic Management

Goals

1. Maintain heart rate, contractility, and preload to maintain cardiac output. Decreases in cardiac output will reduce systemic venous saturation. In a complete mixing lesion, this will reduce arterial saturation.
2. Use ventilatory measures to reduce PVR. This will improve pulmonary blood flow via systemic collaterals.
3. Maintain or increase SVR. This will not affect the magnitude of the obligatory right-to-left shunt but will improve pulmonary perfusion via the PDA, systemic collaterals, or both.
4. Ventilation with 100% oxygen will prevent V/Q abnormalities from decreasing pulmonary venous saturation. A high pulmonary venous saturation will improve arterial saturation in a complete mixing lesion.

Induction and Maintenance. As discussed previously, control of ventilation is the most reliable way to manipulate PVR. Clearly, prompt and reliable control of the airway at induction is important because these patients are hypoxemic. These patients are managed like those with TOF. However, infants who are ductus-dependent for pulmonary blood flow are likely to be hypoxemic and acidotic with little cardiac reserve. These patients are candidates for induction and maintenance with fentanyl or sufentanil.

Post-CPB Management

The same factors that compromise post-CPB RV function in patients with TOF are factors in patients with TOF and pulmonary atresia. In addition, the inability to ligate all of the extensive systemic to pulmonary collaterals may result in a large residual left-to-right shunt after surgical correction. This potentially large left-to-right shunt will impose a volume load on the LV similar to that imposed by a PDA. In some instances, postoperative embolization of these collaterals may be necessary. Conduction abnormalities may be associated with VSD closure.

Goals

1. Maintain heart rate (preferably sinus rhythm) at an age-appropriate rate. Cardiac output is likely to be more heart rate dependent in the post-CPB period.
2. Reduce PVR through ventilatory interventions.
3. Inotropic support of the right ventricle may be necessary for the reasons addressed in the discussion on TOF. Dobutamine (5 to 10 µg/kg/min) or dopamine (5 to 10 µg/kg/min) is useful in this instance because both agents provide potent inotropic support without increasing PVR.

■ TRICUSPID ATRESIA

Anatomy

In tricuspid atresia (TA), there is complete agenesis of the tricuspid valve and no communication between the right atrium and the hypoplastic right ventricle. Anatomic classification is based on the presence or absence of transposition of the great arteries (TGA), the extent of pulmonary atresia, and the size of the VSD. This classification and the frequency of the different lesion types are summarized in Figure 6–20 and Table 6–7. Approximately 70% of patients with TA are type 1 and 30% are type 2.[90] Type 3 lesions are very rare. Fifty percent of all TA patients are type 1B.

Physiology

TA is a complex shunt with complete obstruction to outflow. There is a communication (ASD or patent fora-

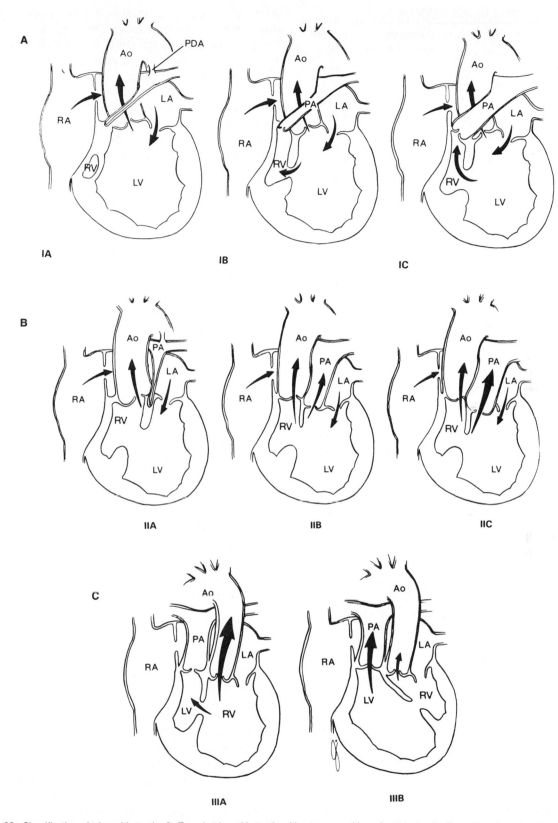

FIGURE 6–20. Classification of tricuspid atresia. **A.** Type 1: tricuspid atresia without transposition of great vessels. Type 1A: pulmonary atresia with pulmonary blood flow via patent ductus arteriosus or bronchial collaterals. Type 1B: small ventricular septal defect and pulmonary stenosis. Type 1C: large ventricular septal defect and no pulmonary stenosis. **B.** Type 2: tricuspid atresia with D-transposition of great vessels. Type 2A: pulmonary atresia with pulmonary blood flow via patent ductus arteriosus or bronchial collaterals. Type 2B: pulmonary stenosis. Type 2C: no pulmonary stenosis. **C.** Type 3: tricuspid atresia with L-transposition of great vessels. Type 3A: subpulmonic stenosis. Type 3B: subaortic stenosis. (Ao = aorta; LA = left atrium; LV = left ventricle; PA = pulmonary artery; PDA = patent ductus arteriosus; RA = right atrium; RV = right ventricle.) *(From: Lake CL: Pediatric Cardiac Anesthesia. Norwalk, CT, Appleton and Lange, 1988, p 301. Used by permission.)*

TABLE 6–7. CLASSIFICATION OF TRICUSPID ATRESIA

	Pulmonary Blood Flow	Frequency (%)
Type 1: No TGV		**70**
A No VSD, with pulmonary atresia	↓	10
B Small VSD, with pulmonary stenosis	↓	50
C Large VSD, no pulmonary stenosis	⇄↑	10
Type 2: D-TGV		**30**
A VSD, with pulmonary atresia	↓	2
B VSD, with pulmonary stenosis	⇄↓	8
C VSD, no pulmonary stenosis	↑↑	20
Type 3: L-TGV		**very rare**
A VSD, with pulmonary or subpulmonary stenosis	↓	
B VSD, with subaortic stenosis	↑	

TGV = transposition of the great vessels; VSD = ventricular septal defect.

men ovale) and a complete obstruction to RA outflow (tricuspid atresia). This results in an obligatory right-to-left shunt at the atrial level with complete mixing of systemic and pulmonary venous blood in the left atrium. When the ASD or foramen ovale is restrictive, there will be a large right atrial to left atrial pressure gradient. This will result in poor decompression of the RA and systemic venous congestion. Pulmonary blood flow is provided by a downstream shunt. This downstream shunt may be simple (VSD without pulmonary stenosis), complex (VSD with pulmonary stenosis), or complex with complete obstruction (pulmonary atresia with or without a VSD). When pulmonary atresia exists (types 1A and 2A), an additional downstream shunt must exist to provide pulmonary blood flow. PDA, bronchial collaterals, or both are the simple downstream shunts that provide all pulmonary blood flow with pulmonary atresia. The amount of pulmonary blood flow associated with each type of TA is summarized in Table 6–7.

Recall that in mixing lesions the degree of cyanosis will be determined largely by $Q_p:Q_s$. Therefore, patients with a $Q_p:Q_s$ less than 1 due to stenotic or atretic pulmonary outflow tracts, restrictive VSDs, or both will be more cyanotic than their counterparts with normal or increased pulmonary blood flow. TA imposes a volume load on the left ventricle, and increased pulmonary blood flow produces an even larger LV volume load. Therefore, patients with TA and increased pulmonary blood flow are likely to present with CHF. Furthermore, patients with increased pulmonary blood flow are at risk to develop PVOD.

Surgical Therapy

Palliative Procedures. The palliative and definitive procedures described here are not applicable solely to patients with TA. They are applicable to any patient with univentricular physiology, that is, patients in whom only one functional ventricle exists. The single ventricle, by necessity, must become the systemic ventricle, regardless of whether it is of right or left ventricular morphology. Systemic and pulmonary blood flow is supplied by the single ventricle in a parallel circulation. Treatment requires creation of a series circulation. To achieve this, the origin of pulmonary blood flow is modified using the palliative and definitive procedures described here. Hypoplastic left heart syndrome is a version of univentricular physiology, which will be described later in this chapter.

PROCEDURES TO INCREASE PULMONARY BLOOD FLOW. More than 70% of patients with tricuspid atresia are severely cyanotic in the neonatal period and require the creation of a systemic-to-pulmonary shunt. Many of these infants will be severely cyanotic and will be dependent on a PDA for pulmonary blood flow. The usual systemic-to-pulmonary shunt is a BT shunt or modified BT shunt. A central shunt also may be used. The Waterston and Potts shunts are associated with a high incidence of excessive pulmonary blood flow and development of PVOD. They are no longer advocated for any patient who may be a candidate for definitive repair for a univentricular heart. For further discussion of these shunts, see the section on TOF.

Aortopulmonary shunts reliably increase pulmonary blood flow, but they have several disadvantages:

- they increase the volume load on the systemic ventricle.
- they potentially distort pulmonary artery anatomy, which makes subsequent definitive repair difficult.
- they potentially expose the pulmonary circulation to higher-than-normal pressures, which can accelerate the development of PVOD, making definitive repair impossible.

To avoid these problems, shunts that divert systemic venous blood directly to the pulmonary circulation have been devised. These shunts reduce ventricular volume to normal. The original such shunt was the Glenn shunt,[91] which involved an end-to-side anastomosis of the cranial end of the transected superior vena cava (SVC) to the distal end of the transected right pulmonary artery (RPA). This procedure is performed through a right thoractomy without CPB. Subsequent modifications have followed. The differences between an aortopulmonary shunt and a shunt that diverts systemic venous blood directly to the pulmonary circulation are summarized in Figure 6–21.

One such modification is a bidirectional Glenn or bidirectional cavopulmonary shunt (*see* Fig. 6–22). This procedure is performed on CPB through a median sternotomy. Previous aortopulmonary shunts are ligated, as

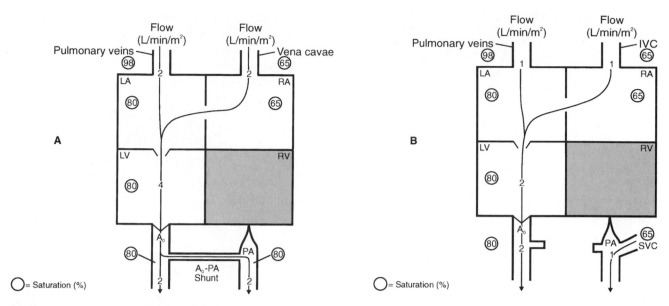

FIGURE 6–21. A. Depiction of saturations and blood flows in tricuspid atresia with a nonrestrictive atrial septal defect (ASD), a hypoplastic right ventricle (RV), and pulmonary atresia palliated with an aortopulmonary shunt. Complete mixing or blending occurs at the atrial level. The left ventricle (LV) is volume overloaded in this parallel circulation to provide pulmonary blood flow. Q_s and Q_p are 2 L/min/m² and the arterial saturation is 80% (Q_p:Q_s = 1:1.) **B.** Depiction of saturations and blood flows in tricuspid atresia with a nonrestrictive ASD, a hypoplastic RV, and pulmonary atresia palliated with a bidirectional cavopulmonary shunt. Complete mixing or blending occurs at the atrial level. The LV is not volume overloaded in this series circulation. Q_s is 2 L/min/m², and Q_p is 1 L/min/m²; Q_p:Q_s = 0.5:1. Nonetheless, cardiac output and arterial saturation are identical in the patient palliated with the aortopulmonary shunt. This is because arterial saturation in a complete mixing lesion is determined by the relative volumes and saturations of systemic and pulmonary venous blood. In this instance, Q_s and the volume of systemic venous blood reaching the right atrium (RA) are not equal because half of Q_s has been diverted to become pulmonary venous blood. As a result, Q_p:Q_s is deceptive here. (Ao = aorta; LA = left atrium; LV = left ventricle; IVC = inferior vena cava; PA = pulmonary artery; RA = right atrium; RV = right ventricle; SVC = superior vena cava.)

is the azygous vein. In this procedure, the SVC is transected at the level of the RPA. The cranial end of the SVC is anatomosed end-to-side to the RPA and the cardiac end of the SVC is oversewn. The main pulmonary artery also may be ligated and oversewn if native pulmonary blood flow is insignificant. Most patients requiring this procedure for univentricular physiology will ultimately undergo a definitive Fontan procedure (see below). To make this transition easier, the hemi-Fontan procedure has been proposed (*see* Fig. 6–23). In one version of this procedure, the bidirectional cavopulmonary shunt is constructed and then the cardiac portion of the SVC is anastomosed end-to-side to the inferior portion of the RPA. The RA–SVC junction is then closed with a patch. The advantage of this procedure is that it makes subsequent dissection for completion of the Fontan easier. Completion of the Fontan procedure then only requires removal of the patch and creation of an intra-atrial baffle to divert the inferior vena cava (IVC) blood up to the SVC orifice. In addition, often during the hemi-Fontan procedure, additional procedures such as enlargement of the atrial septal communication, correction of pulmonary artery stenoses, and AV valve repairs are undertaken.

Because the driving pressure for pulmonary blood flow will be low with cavopulmonary shunts, they are not appropriate for use during the neonatal period, when PVR is very high. After these procedures, the patient's SaO_2 will be no better than that obtained with an aortopulmonary shunt. Desaturated blood from the IVC will continue to mix completely with oxygenated blood from the pulmonary veins and be ejected systemically. SaO_2 will be determined by the factors described for complete mixing lesions.

PROCEDURE TO DECREASE PULMONARY BLOOD FLOW. Patients with TA who have unobstructed pulmonary blood flow have a large volume load imposed on the systemic ventricle, which precipitates CHF. In addition, these patients are at risk of developing PVOD. Pulmonary artery banding is indicated for these patients to reduce pulmonary blood flow and to protect the pulmonary vasculature from pressures. The main pulmonary artery is constricted with a circumferential band. This reduces pulmonary blood flow and distal pulmonary artery pressure by creation of a restrictive lesion. Banding is most effective when pulmonary artery pressure distal to the band is reduced to one-third to one-half of systemic blood pressure. Pulmonary artery banding may cause distortion of the main pulmonary artery. In addition, distortion of branch pulmonary arteries may be caused by migration of the band distally. This

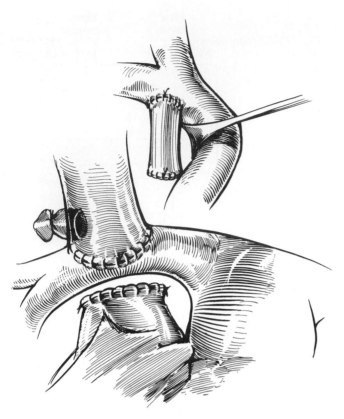

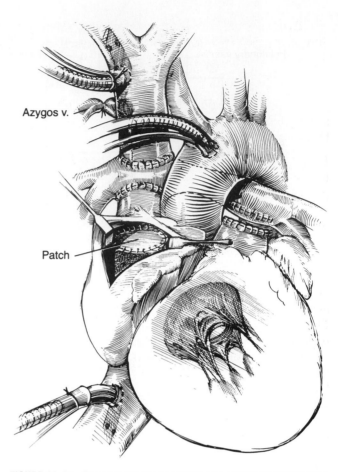

Azygos v.

Patch

FIGURE 6–22. Anatomy of a completed bidirectional cavopulmonary shunt. The cephalad portion of the superior vena cava (SCV) is anastomosed end-to-side to the right pulmonary artery. The right pulmonary artery is in continuity with the left pulmonary artery. A previously modified Blalock–Taussig shunt (right subclavian to right pulmonary artery with interposed Gore-Tex graft) is seen to be ligated and the subclavian artery is being retracted. The azygous vein also is ligated. The cardiac portion of the SVC is oversewn.

FIGURE 61–23. The anatomy of one version of a completed hemi-Fontan. Both the cardiac and cephalic portions of the superior vena cava (SVC) are in continuity with the right pulmonary artery. The right pulmonary artery is in continuity with the left pulmonary artery, and the main pulmonary artery is divided and oversewn. The cardiac portion of the SVC is prevented from supplying blood to the pulmonary arteries due to a patch occluding the right atrium (RA)–SVC junction. Other versions of this procedure do not involve complete transection of the SVC and incorporate patch material to augment pulmonary artery size.

distortion may complicate or preclude definite repair. Pulmonary artery banding is accomplished via a left thoracotomy or a median sternotomy without CPB. An excessively tight pulmonary artery band will severely reduce pulmonary blood flow and expose the pulmonary ventricle to high afterload. Pulse oximetry has proved useful during pulmonary artery banding because arterial desaturation precedes hypotension and bradycardia when banding is excessive.[92] TEE is valuable in assessing RV function during pulmonary artery banding. RV distension may require loosening of the band or initiation of inotropic support. TEE also allows the pressure gradient across the band to be determined (*see* Chapter 3). This will help in determining the tightness of the band.

PROCEDURES TO IMPROVE ATRIAL DECOMPRESSION. The patient with TA must have an atrial communication

to survive. The atrial communication allows an obligatory right-to-left shunt at the atrial level and complete mixing of systemic and pulmonary venous blood in the left atrium. When there is a restrictive ASD or a foramen ovale, the obligatory right-to-left atrial shunt will cause right atrial distension and elevation of right atrial pressure. A high right atrial pressure will result in systemic venous congestion. In the catheterization laboratory, the Rashkind–Miller balloon septostomy enlarges the foramen ovale or ASD and decompresses the right atrium.[93] Older infants and children with a thickened atrial septum may have enlargement accomplished with a blade atrial septostomy in the catheterization laboratory.[94] An enlarged ASD also can be created surgically with the Blalock–Hanlon procedure. The Blalock–Hanlon procedure is a closed procedure performed via a right thoracotomy and does not require CPB.

Placement of the clamps to complete this procedure usually compromises drainage of one or both of the right pulmonary veins. This can produce unilateral pulmonary edema or hemorrhage. TEE will allow the right pulmonary veins to be seen and may guide clamp placement. In addition, TEE will allow assessment of the size of the defect and the pressure gradient across it before leaving the operating room.

Definitive Repair: The Fontan Procedure.

The Fontan procedure was first performed in 1968 and applied to patients with TA.[95] The original operation included a Glenn shunt, which drained the SVC directly into the distal right pulmonary artery. The proximal end of the right pulmonary artery was joined to the right atrial appendage via an aortic valve homograft and a pulmonary valve homograft valve was placed at the IVC-RA junction. The main pulmonary artery was ligated and the ASD was closed. Subsequently, creation of the Glenn shunt and placement of homograft valves at the RA-PA and IVC-RA junctions were eliminated.

Since then, many modifications have been described; some of these are illustrated in Figure 6-24. Despite the modifications, the goal of the procedure is the same: to provide delivery of all systemic venous blood directly to the pulmonary arteries without the benefit of an effective ventricular cavity. In essence, this requires a total cavopulmonary continuity either directly or via the RA. As a result, pulmonary blood flow is essentially nonpulsatile and is dependent on the pressure in the SVC and IVC to be greater than the mean pulmonary artery pressure, which in turn, is greater than the pulmonary venous (usually but not always left) atrial pressure. After completion of the Fontan procedure, the patient will have a normal series circulation and should have a normal SaO_2 barring intrapulmonary shunting.

Appropriate selection is essential to the success of this procedure. Although there is individual variation from institution to institution, certain absolute and relative contraindications can be described:

- Absolute contraindications
  - early infancy
  - PVR > 4 Wood units/m²
  - severe pulmonary artery hypoplasia
  - ejection fraction (EF) < 45%
  - ventricular diastolic pressure > 25 mm Hg
- Relative contraindications
  - age < 1 to 2 years
  - PVR = 2 to 4 Wood units/m²
  - mean pulmonary arterial pressure (PAP) > 15 mm Hg
  - systemic ventricular hypertrophy
  - systemic AV valve regurgitation
  - distorted pulmonary arteries

Recent enthusiasm for the staged Fontan procedure exists because of evidence that survival after the Fontan

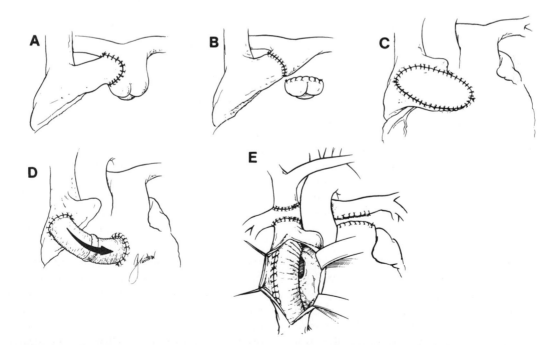

FIGURE 6–24. Modifications of the Fontan procedure. **A.** Direct anastomosis of the right atrial appendage to the main pulmonary artery. **B.** Direct anastomosis of the right atrial appendage to the distal end of the transected main pulmonary artery. **C.** Direct connection of the right atrium to the right ventricle. A pericardial patch is used to create a nonrestrictive orifice. **D.** Connection of the right atrium to the right ventricle via a valved conduit. **E.** Total cavopulmonary connection using an intra-atrial lateral tunnel. The tunnel is prosthetic graft material. A fenestration could be placed in this prosthetic material. Another version not illustrated here would involve connection of the inferior vena cava (IVC) to the pulmonary artery (PA) via a tube graft external to the atrium.

is better in patients undergoing a staged procedure.[96] The staged procedure makes use of a bidirectional cavopulmonary shunt or the hemi-Fontan procedure before the Fontan procedure. The first stage of the procedure has been applied to younger patients (4 to 6 months of age), who are then considered for a Fontan procedure. This allows earlier reduction in the volume overload that accompanies univentricular physiology. There is evidence that these procedures allow systemic ventricular volume load to be reduced to normal and to allow remodeling of the ventricle at lower end-diastolic volume.[97,98]

Acute reduction of systemic ventricular volume in the univentricular heart results in impaired ventricular compliance because wall thickness does not regress as quickly as ventricular volume. The result is impaired ventricular diastolic function and an elevated end-diastolic pressure. This will impede pulmonary venous return, which is a liability in the Fontan procedure, because this will subsequently reduce pulmonary blood flow. A low cardiac output state will result because systemic ventricular output can only equal the quantity of blood that transverses the pulmonary vascular bed.

The staged procedure offers two advantages over the primary Fontan procedure:

1. Impaired ventricular diastolic function, which accompanies acute ventricular volume reduction, has less dire consequences for the patient with a bidirectional cavopulmonary shunt or hemi-Fontan. When there is impairment of pulmonary venous return after one of these procedures, blood from the IVC will continue to provide systemic ventricular filling and cardiac output.
2. The procedures will allow ventricular remodelling such that the Fontan procedure is more likely to succeed when it is performed at a later date.

A risk of the staged procedures is the development of pulmonary arteriovenous malformations, which seem to be the result of diversion of normal hepatic venous blood flow from the pulmonary circulation as occurs in the bidirectional cavopulmonary shunt and hemi-Fontan.[99] An alternative approach to the staged Fontan is the fenestrated Fontan.[100,101] In this procedure, a small hole is left in the connection from the IVC to the pulmonary artery such that systemic venous blood can be shunted to the pulmonary venous atrium when the driving pressure to the lungs becomes high. This provides a "pop-off" valve that allows maintenance of systemic ventricular filling, even if transit of blood across the pulmonary bed is impaired. Therefore, it is halfway between a completed Fontan and a bidirectional cavopulmonary shunt or hemi-Fontan procedure. The fenestration can be closed in the cardiac catheterization laboratory using an umbrella device[100] or, alternatively, it can be closed by tightening a snare purse-string suture around the fenestration left subcutaneously and exposed using local anesthesia.[101]

Anesthetic Management

Goals

1. Maintain heart rate, contractility, and preload to maintain cardiac output. Decreases in cardiac output will reduce systemic venous saturation. In a complete mixing lesion, this will reduce arterial saturation.
2. For patients with pulmonary atresia pulmonary, blood flow may be dependent on ductal patency. A prostaglandin E_1 infusion (0.05 to 0.1 µg/kg/min) will have to be maintained in these patients to maintain ductal patency.
3. For all patients with reduced pulmonary blood flow, efforts should be made to reduce the PVR:SVR ratio. Use of ventilatory interventions to reduce PVR relative to SVR will increase pulmonary blood flow and improve oxygenation.
4. For patients with increased pulmonary blood flow, PVR should be normalized or slightly increased via ventilatory measures to avoid further increases in pulmonary blood flow. Recall that in complete mixing lesions, a Q_p:Q_s higher than 3:1 or 4:1 produces small additional increases in arterial saturation. On the other hand, increases in pulmonary blood flow will necessitate an increase in cardiac output to maintain systemic blood flow. In addition, the increase in LV volume load that accompanies an increased pulmonary blood flow may precipitate CHF.

Induction and Maintenance. Chronic left ventricular volume overload and arterial hypoxemia limit the cardiac reserve of patients with TA. Prompt control of the airway is imperative to avoid accelerating hypoxemia. In patients with increased pulmonary blood flow, CHF may be present. An inhalational induction will be poorly tolerated by neonates and patients with CHF. Use of an inhalation agent to obtain IV access may be tolerated by older patients without CHF. IM ketamine and atropine can be used for neonates and children with CHF to gain IV access. IV induction and maintenance with fentanyl or sufentanil will provide hemodynamic stability without cardiovascular depression. This is important because it is not unusual for TA patients to require inotropic support during palliative procedures.

After the bidirectional cavopulmonary shunt or the hemi-Fontan procedure, all pulmonary blood flow is derived from the SVC. The anatomy of a single ventricle patient is illustrated in Figure 6–21. This figure illustrates that a cavopulmonary shunt can provide the same cardiac output and arterial saturation as an aortopulmonary shunt without volume overloading the systemic ventricle. From a practical point of view, this means that no increase in arterial saturation should be expected in a child who has ligation of an aortopulmonary shunt and creation of a cavopulmonary shunt or hemi-Fontan. Central venous pressure lines placed in the internal jugular vein will no longer measure RA pressure but rather mean upper body systemic venous pressure. The surgeon may choose to place a catheter directly into the RA for pressure monitoring. In the presence of a nonrestrictive ASD, this will also monitor pressure in the pulmonary venous (left) atrium.

Hypoxemia is most commonly the result of low pulmonary blood flow due to elevated PVR. Systemic perfusion will be maintained because IVC blood can provide filling of the systemic ventricle. Arterial saturation will decrease as the amount of desaturated IVC blood in the systemic ventricle increases relative to the amount of saturated pulmonary venous blood.

Efforts to reduce PVR through ventilatory methods should be made. It should be kept in mind that because pulmonary blood flow through the lungs is passive, high airway pressures or mechanical compression of the pulmonary vasculature will impede flow. As a result, hypocarbia ($Paco_2$ = 30 to 35 mm Hg) and an SaO_2 of 75 to 85% should be achieved with relatively large tidal volumes (15 to 20 mL/kg delivered), slow respiratory rates (15 to 20 breaths/min), and short inspiratory times (I:E of 1:3 or 1:4). PEEP should be used with caution.

If arterial saturation is poor after ventilation and acid–base status have been optimized, a restrictive cavopulmonary anastomosis or additional sources of upper extremity blood flow to the heart, such as a persistent left SVC to the coronary sinus, should be ruled out. TEE is very valuable in both instances. Low cardiac output as evidenced by poor perfusion and hypotension requires intervention. This may be the result of hypovolemic, restrictive ASD limiting IVC blood flow to the systemic ventricle, AV valve regurgitation, or systemic ventricular systolic dysfunction. TEE will help sort out the possibilities. If inotropic support is necessary, an agent that does not increase PVR is desirable. Dobutamine 5 to 10 µg/kg/min or amrinone 5 to 10 µg/kg/min after a 3-5 mg/kg loading dose is a reasonable choice.

After the Fontan procedure, all systemic venous blood is directed to the pulmonary arterial system and intracardiac shunting is eliminated. In the presence of normal pulmonary function, this has two important implications:

1. Hypoxemia is much less common than after the bidirectional cavopulmonary shunt or hemi-Fontan because there is no mixing.

2. Low pulmonary blood flow produces low cardiac output. The systemic ventricle can only pump the volume of blood that is delivered to it across the pulmonary vascular bed. This differs from the situation after the bidirectional cavopulmonary shunt or hemi-Fontan because, in these procedures, there is a source of blood supply to the systemic ventricle that does not cross the pulmonary bed.

Management of the patient after the Fontan procedure follows the same principles described for the bidirectional cavopulmonary shunt and hemi-Fontan. However, greater vigilance is needed because detection of the poor perfusion and low cardiac output that are consequences of low pulmonary blood flow is more difficult than the detection of falling arterial saturation. It is an exaggeration, but it is often stated that no child has died after a Fontan due to hypoxemia but many have died of low cardiac output.

A catheter in the internal jugular vein will reflect systemic venous pressure. The surgeon may place a catheter in the common atrial chamber, which functions now as a pulmonary venous (left) atrium. High systemic venous pressures or a high transpulmonary gradient (systemic venous pressure–left atrial pressure) are associated with increased mortality.[102] Generally, a systemic venous pressure less than 20 mm Hg is desirable; higher pressures increase the likelyhood that the repair will have to be taken down.

After ventilation has been optimized and TEE has ruled out systemic ventricular systolic dysfunction, hypovolemia, and anastomotic problems, persistent low output may require fenestration of the Fontan or, in the most extreme cases, takedown and conversion to a hemi-Fontan or bidirectional cavopulmonary shunt.

Spontaneous ventilation is desired postoperatively because it improves the dynamics of nonphasic pulmonary blood flow. However, this advantage can be offset easily by high Pco_2 and elevated catecholamines levels if the child is extubated prematurely. Long-term complications of the Fontan include persistent pleural and pericardial effusions, protein-losing enteropathy, and atrial arrhythmias.

Goals

1. Maintain heart rate (preferably sinus rhythm) at an age-appropriate rate. Cardiac output is likely to be more heart-rate-dependent during the post-CPB period. Atrial systole will augment pulmonary blood flow after the Fontan procedure, although it is not essential to the success of the procedure.
2. Maintain systemic venous pressure of 15 to 20 mm Hg.
3. Reduce PVR through ventilatory interventions.
4. Inotropic support of the systemic ventricle may

be necessary due to ventricular dysfunction induced by chronic volume overload and CPB. Dobutamine (5 to 10 μg/kg/min) or amrinone (5 to 10 μg/kg/min) is useful in this instance because both agents provide potent inotropic support without increasing PVR.

■ TRUNCUS ARTERIOSUS

Anatomy

Truncus arteriosus is characterized by a single great vessel arising from the base of the heart and giving rise to the pulmonary, coronary, and systemic arteries. There is a single semilunar valve, which is usually abnormal, and invariably a large (nonrestrictive) VSD is present. The truncus usually straddles this large VSD. Truncus arteriosus is classified based on the origin of the pulmonary arteries.[103] In type 1, a short pulmonary trunk originates from the truncus and gives rise to both pulmonary arteries. In type 2, both pulmonary arteries arise from a common orifice of the truncus, whereas in type 3, the right and left pulmonary arteries arise separately from the lateral aspect of the truncus. The ventricular septal defect usually is of the infundibular or perimembranous-infundibular type. The truncal valve is tricuspid in most patients, but multiple cusps can be seen and the valve itself may be regurgitant or stenotic. Extracardiac anomalies are seen in approximately 30% of patients.[104]

Physiology

Truncus arteriosus is a simple shunt with a common chamber and complete mixing. The large (nonrestrictive) VSD allows equalization of pressures in the right and left ventricles. As a result, there is bidirectional shunting and complete mixing of systemic and pulmonary venous blood in a functionally common ventricular chamber. This blood is then ejected into the truncal root, which gives rise to the pulmonary, systemic, and coronary circulations. As with all simple shunts, Q_p:Q_s is determined by the ratio of PVR to SVR. However, in truncus arteriosus, the pulmonary and systemic circulations are supplied in parallel from a single vessel, and increases in flow to one circulatory system are likely to produce reductions in flow to the other. Therefore, it is necessary to maintain a delicate balance between PVR and SVR. The physiology has similarities to that described for hypoplastic left heart syndrome (HLHS) (*see* Fig. 6–29).

As with all mixing lesions, a low Q_p:Q_s will reduce arterial saturation, whereas a high Q_p:Q_s will produce CHF without a substantial increase in arterial saturation. Under normal circumstances, the balance of PVR and SVR is such that pulmonary blood flow is high and the patient with truncus arteriosus has symptoms of CHF with mild cyanosis. After cardiac reserve has been ex-

hausted, further decreases in PVR will increase pulmonary blood flow at the expense of systemic and coronary perfusion. This will produce a progressive metabolic acidosis. If PVR increases relative to SVR, systemic blood flow will increase at the expense of pulmonary blood flow and severe hypoxemia will result. This second scenario is particularly likely in patients in whom PVOD has developed in response to high pulmonary blood flow and the transmission of systemic arterial pressures to the pulmonary vasculature. Finally, if truncal valve insufficiency is present, this will obviously impose an additional volume load on the ventricles.

Surgical Therapy

Because of the risk of early development of PVOD, prompt surgical intervention is recommended. Definitive repair of truncus arteriosus requires patch closure of the VSD, detachment of the pulmonary arteries from the truncus, and establishment of right ventricular to pulmonary artery continuity with a valved homograft. The RV-to-PA conduit requires placement of the proximal end of the conduit over a ventriculotomy in the RV free wall. The truncal valves must be assessed at the time of surgery. In some instances, valve repair or replacement is necessary to avoid valvular insufficiency. Considering the problems with valve replacement in a growing child, valvuloplasty is preferred over valve replacement. The valved conduit eventually will require replacement as the child grows.

Anesthetic Management

Goals

1. Maintain heart rate, contractility, and preload to maintain cardiac output. A reduction in cardiac output will compromise systemic perfusion despite relatively high pulmonary blood flow. A decrease in cardiac output will also reduce systemic venous saturation. As with all mixing lesions, a reduction in systemic venous saturation will reduce arterial oxygen saturation.

2. For patients without PVOD, avoid decreases in the PVR:SVR ratio. The increase in pulmonary blood flow that accompanies a reduced PVR:SVR ratio is likely to occur at the expense of systemic and coronary blood flow. Ventilate with a reduced FIO_2 (<40%) and maintain PCO_2 35 to 40 mm Hg. Use of 2 to 4% inspired CO_2 can be used as explained in the section on HLHS.

3. For patients with severe CHF, inotropic support of the ventricles in combination with normocarbia or slight hypercarbia to reduce pulmonary blood flow may be necessary.

4. For patients with PVOD and reduced pulmonary blood flow, ventilatory interventions to reduce

PVR will be necessary. A high PVR will increase systemic and coronary blood flow at the expense of pulmonary blood flow, resulting in hypoxemia.

Induction and Maintenance.   Many of these patients are chronically ill with severe CHF or cyanosis. The neonate with truncus arteriosus often will be intubated and ventilated, requiring inotropic support. Cardiac reserve is so limited that severe hypotension and bradycardia are not uncommon. Ventricular fibrillation can be seen during routine maneuvers, such as opening the pericardium in the prebypass period. Ventilatory control of PVR will help reduce pulmonary blood flow and prevent systemic hypoperfusion. In particular, a high FIo_2 may reduce PVR and increase pulmonary blood flow at the expense of systemic perfusion. Patients with truncus arteriosus are unlikely to tolerate the myocardial depression associated with inhalational anesthetics. Fentanyl or sufentanil in high doses combined with a muscle relaxant will provide hemodynamic stability without myocardial depression.

Post-CPB Management

Post-CPB management may be complicated by ventricular failure. Left ventricular volume overload may occur secondary to truncal valve insufficiency. RV systolic dysfunction may result from RV afterload mismatch (*see* Chapter 2) due to the high pulmonary vascular resistance in patients with PVOD; the right ventriculotomy required for conduit placement; and poor protection of the RV during CPB.

Goals

1. Maintain heart rate (preferably sinus rhythm) at an age-appropriate rate. Cardiac output is likely to be more heart-rate-dependent in the post-CPB period.
2. Reduce PVR when necessary through ventilatory interventions.
3. Inotropic support of the left and right ventricle may be necessary for the reasons addressed previously. Dobutamine (5 to 10 µg/kg/min) or dopamine (5 to 10 µg/kg/min) is useful in this instance because both agents provide potent inotropic support without increasing PVR.

■ TOTAL ANOMALOUS PULMONARY VENOUS RETURN

Anatomy

Total anomalous pulmonary venous return (TAPVR) is present when all of the pulmonary veins drain into the systemic venous system rather than directly into the left atrium. The pulmonary veins join into a single common pulmonary venous structure, which then drains into the systemic venous circulation at the level of the SVC, portal vein, right atrium, or coronary sinus. Often TAPVR is categorized (*see* Fig. 6–25) according to the site of drainage:[105]

- Supracardiac (type 1). In 46% of patients, the pulmonary veins drain into a supracardiac structure. This usually is an anomalous vertical vein that connects the common pulmonary vein with the innominate vein, which then empties into the SVC.
- Intracardiac (type 2). In 24% of patients, drainage is directly into the right atrium or the coronary sinus.

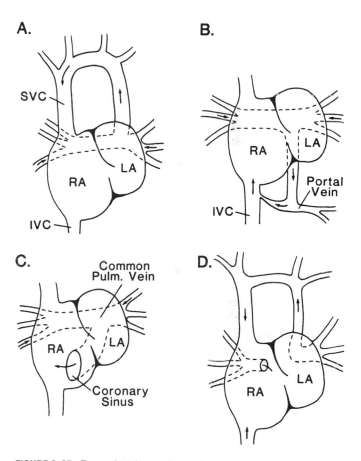

FIGURE 6–25. Types of total anomalous pulmonary venous return (TAPVR). **A.** Supracardiac — pulmonary venous blood returns to common pulmonary vein; the common pulmonary vein drains via a left vertical vein to the innominate vein, the superior vena cava (SVC), and then finally to the right atrium. **B.** Infracardiac — a common pulmonary vein passes through the diaphragm at the esophageal hiatus. The common vein then drains into the portal vein, hepatic vein, or ductus venosus. Obstruction of flow into the inferior vena cava (IVC) and right atrium may be caused by obligatory passage through the liver. **C.** Cardiac — a common pulmonary vein directly enters the right atrium via the coronary sinus. **D.** Mixed — this type involves components of supracardiac, infracardiac, and cardiac drainage. Illustrated here is a combination of cardiac and supracardiac connections. (LA = left atrium; RA = right atrium.) *(From: Fyler DC, Nadas AS: Congenital heart disease, in Avery ME, Lewis FR (eds): Pediatric Medicine. Baltimore, Williams & Wilkins, 1989, p 356.)*

- Infracardiac (type 3). In 22% of patients, drainage is into an infracardiac structure such as the inferior vena cava, portal vein, or hepatic vein. A common pulmonary vein passes through the esophageal hiatus of the diaphragm to reach these infracardiac vessels.
- Mixed (type 4). In 8% of patients, pulmonary venous drainage is a combination of types 1, 2, and 3.

In general, the greater the distance the pulmonary veins travel to empty into the anomalous connection, the greater the likelihood that a stenosis will exist and that there will be pulmonary venous obstruction. For this reason infracardiac drainage commonly is associated with pulmonary venous obstruction.

Physiology

The delivery of all pulmonary venous blood to the right atrium results in a large left-to-right shunt. There is complete mixing of systemic and pulmonary venous blood in the right atrium. There must be a right-to-left shunt if there is to be filling of the left heart and survival outside the uterus. Normally, an ASD or patent foramen ovale exists as the communication with the left heart. The magnitude and direction of shunting across the ASD or foramen ovale is determined by the principles of simple shunting. A small restrictive ASD or foramen ovale will result in a small right-to-left shunt, distended right atrium, reduced systemic blood flow, and increased pulmonary blood flow. This, in turn, will cause volume overload of the right ventricle and systemic venous congestion. A large, nonrestrictive ASD will provide better balance between systemic and pulmonary blood flow because of a larger right-to-left shunt across the atrial communication. Nonetheless, in the absence of PVOD, PVR will be less than SVR in these patients and Q_p will exceed Q_s.

Stenoses in the pulmonary venous drainage system will produce pulmonary venous congestion. This will result in intrauterine and extrauterine development of pulmonary hypertension and PVOD. As a result, patients with pulmonary venous obstruction will have reduced pulmonary blood flow compared with patients without PVOD. In addition, pulmonary venous obstruction will predispose pulmonary edema, much as it does with mitral stenosis. These patients will be hypoxemic because pulmonary edema will reduce pulmonary venous saturation and because, in complete mixing lesions, arterial saturation is largely dependent on a high $Q_p:Q_s$. Efforts to increase pulmonary blood flow in these patients will only worsen the pulmonary edema. Patients with pulmonary venous stenoses present at birth with hypoxemia, poor systemic perfusion, and a metabolic acidosis.

Surgical Therapy

A balloon or blade atrial septostomy at the time of cardiac catheterization may be used to enlarge the ASD or foramen ovale, improve right-to-left shunting, and increase systemic blood flow. Nonetheless, surgical therapy is always necessary for patients with TAPVR. Definitive repair involves (1) reattachment of the pulmonary veins and/or common pulmonary venous trunk to the left atrium and (2) closure of the ASD.

Anesthetic Management

Goals

1. Maintain heart rate, contractility, and preload to maintain cardiac output. Decreases in cardiac output will reduce systemic venous saturation. In a complete mixing lesion, this will reduce arterial saturation.
2. For patients with TAPVR and pulmonary venous obstruction, emergency surgery is necessary. Efforts to increase pulmonary blood flow through ventilatory interventions, pulmonary vasodilators, or ductal patency with prostaglandin E_1 will worsen pulmonary edema.
3. For patients with increased pulmonary blood flow, decreases in the PVR:SVR ratio should be avoided. The increase in pulmonary blood flow that accompanies a reduced PVR:SVR ratio necessitates an increase in cardiac output to maintain systemic blood flow.
4. For patients with increased pulmonary blood flow and right heart failure, ventilatory interventions should be used to increase PVR, reduce pulmonary blood flow, and decrease the volume load on the right ventricle.

Induction and Maintenance. Neonates with pulmonary venous obstruction often arrive in the operating room intubated, ventilated, and on inotropic support. These patients are best anesthetized with a high-dose narcotic technique using fentanyl or sufentanil. Older patients without obstruction and mild CHF may be candidates for an inhalational induction. Alternatively, IM ketamine and atropine may be used to obtain IV access, at which point maintenance with fentanyl or sufentanil can be initiated. Patients with TAPVR, particularly those with venous obstruction, have a highly reactive pulmonary vasculature. High doses of fentanyl and sufentanil will be useful for blunting increases in PVR associated with surgical stimulation.

Post-CPB Management

Residual post-CPB pulmonary venous obstruction may exist because of the small left atrium present in many patients with TAPVR and the technical difficulty of constructing a nonrestrictive surgical anastomosis. RV systolic function may be compromised by labile increases in PVR and the existence of PVOD in patients with preoperative venous obstruction. TEE is valuable in assessing the patency of the pulmonary venous to LA anastomosis and in helping decide whether a revision is necessary.

Goals

1. Maintain heart rate (preferably sinus rhythm) at an age-appropriate rate. Cardiac output is likely to be more heart-rate-dependent in the post-CPB period.
2. In the presence of postoperative pulmonary venous obstruction, efforts to increase pulmonary blood flow may worsen pulmonary edema.
3. For patients with PVOD and reactive pulmonary vasculature, blunting of stress-induced increases in PVR with narcotics is warranted.
4. For patients with PVOD, ventilatory interventions should be used to reduce PVR and improve RV systolic function.
5. Inotropic support of the RV may be necessary, even in the face of a reduced PVR. Dobutamine (5 to 10 µg/kg/min) or dopamine (5 to 10 µg/kg/min) is useful in this instance because both agents provide potent inotropic support without increasing PVR.

■ PULMONARY ATRESIA WITH INTACT VENTRICULAR SEPTUM

Anatomy

There is complete obstruction to RV outflow in pulmonary atresia with intact ventricular septum (PA with IVS). In 80% of patients, the complete outflow obstruction is at the level of the pulmonary valve due to fusion of the valve cusps. The remaining 20% of patients have infundibular and valvular stenosis.[106] It is not unusual to see hypoplasia of the main pulmonary artery trunk and pulmonary artery branches. The RV can be severely hypoplastic (50% of patients) or normal (10% of patients), with the remainder of patients having moderate hypoplasia.[107] Tricuspid valve size generally parallels RV cavity size. Finally, there is an ASD or patent foramen ovale.

Physiology

Pulmonary atresia with IVS is a complex shunt with complete obstruction to outflow. There is a communication (ASD or patent foramen ovale) and a complete obstruction to RV outflow (pulmonary atresia). This results in suprasystemic RV pressures and regurgitation of any blood that reaches the RV back into the RA. Conse-

quently, there is an obligatory right-to-left shunt at the atrial level, with complete mixing of systemic and pulmonary venous blood in the left atrium. When the ASD or foramen ovale is restrictive, there will be a large right atrial to left atrial pressure gradient. This will result in poor decompression of the RA and systemic venous congestion. Pulmonary blood flow is provided by a downstream shunt (PDA). These patients are dependent on ductal patency for pulmonary blood flow and survival. They generally present at birth with profound cyanosis due to reduced pulmonary blood flow. Recall that in complete mixing lesions, arterial saturation will be determined largely by $Q_p:Q_s$. Persistently high RV pressures in the prenatal and neonatal period may result in production of anomalous sinusoidal connections between the right ventricle and the left anterior descending coronary artery.[108] Retrograde coronary blood flow through these ventriculocoronary connections predisposes the LAD coronary circulation to development of proximal obstructive lesions from fibrous myointimal hyperplasia.[109] As a result of these changes, myocardium in the distribution of the distal LAD may be dependent on a high RV pressure to provide retrograde perfusion via ventriculocoronary connections.

Surgical Therapy

Surgical therapy has two objectives: provision of enough pulmonary blood flow to relieve severe hypoxemia, and if possible, relief of RV outflow obstruction such that forward flow through the tricuspid valve, RV, and pulmonary artery is established.[106,107,110] Forward flow through the RV may promote continued growth of the RV. If the RV is large and only pulmonary valvular atresia exists, a pulmonary valvulotomy or a RV outflow patch may be all that is necessary. Because decompression of the RA and RV will occur as long as the ASD or foramen ovale is open, the ASD or foramen ovale cannot be closed unless the RV is capable of providing all of the pulmonary blood flow without failing. If the RV is hypoplastic and the valve is severely atretic, a BT or central shunt (see the TOF section earlier in this chapter) in combination with a RV outflow tract patch may be necessary to provide adequate pulmonary blood flow. If RV growth occurs, the BT shunt may be ligated and the ASD or foramen ovale may be closed at a later date. In cases in which RV growth is inadequate, a Fontan procedure (see the TA section earlier in this chapter) may be necessary at a later date.

Finally, decompression of the RV is contraindicated when significant ventriculocoronary connections and proximal coronary artery lesions exist.[106,107] Myocardial ischemia or infarction distal to coronary lesions may occur when perfusion pressure via ventriculocoronary connections is reduced by RV decompression.[106,107]

Anesthetic Management

Goals

1. Maintain heart rate, contractility, and preload to maintain cardiac output. Decreases in cardiac output will reduce systemic venous saturation. In a complete mixing lesion, this will reduce arterial saturation.
2. Prostaglandin E_1 (0.05 to 0.1 µg/kg/min) infusion will be necessary to ensure ductal patency and pulmonary blood flow. Maintenance of systemic arterial blood pressure will be necessary to ensure adequate pulmonary perfusion pressure via the PDA.
3. Ventilatory interventions to reduce PVR and increase pulmonary blood flow should be used.

Induction and Maintenance. Neonates having PA with IVS often arrive in the operating room intubated, ventilated, and on a prostaglandin E_1 infusion. These patients are best anesthetized with a high-dose narcotic technique using fentanyl or sufentanil. Inotropic support may be necessary to ensure adequate pulmonary perfusion via the PDA.

Post-CPB Management

Patients having PA with IVS who undergo only a pulmonary valvulotomy or RV outflow patching are at high risk for RV systolic dysfunction after CPB, particularly if the RV is hypoplastic. In addition, if the ASD or foramen ovale is left open to allow atrial and ventricular decompression, there may be considerable right-to-left shunting and hypoxemia due to poor RV compliance in these patients. If post-CPB hypoxia is severe, reinstitution of prostaglandin and creation of a systemic to pulmonary artery shunt may have to be considered.

In patients who have undergone a BT or central shunt, pulmonary blood flow will be dependent on a low PVR and maintenance of systemic blood pressure.

Goals

1. Maintain heart rate (preferably sinus rhythm) at an age-appropriate rate. Cardiac output is likely to be more heart-rate-dependent in the post-CPB period.
2. For patients who have undergone only pulmonary valvulotomy or RV outflow tract patching, inotropic support of the RV and maintenance of a low PVR may be necessary. Ventilatory interventions should be used to reduce PVR, whereas dobutamine (5 to 10 µg/kg/min) or dopamine (5 to 10 µg/kg/min) is used for inotropic support.
3. For patients who have received a BT or central shunt, inotropic support may be necessary to maintain systemic and shunt perfusion pressures.

Ventilatory interventions should be used to minimize PVR and increase pulmonary blood flow.

■ COARCTATION OF THE AORTA

Anatomy

Coarctation of the aorta is a congenital narrowing of the descending aorta near the insertion of the ductus arteriosus just distal to the left subclavian artery. Coarctation may involve components that are preductal, postductal, or both. The preductal component usually is caused by segmental tubular hypoplasia of the aortic isthmus or arch. The postductal component usually is caused by a shelf-like invagination of the posterior aortic wall in the region of the ductus arteriosus. Closure of the ductus arteriosus after birth initially occurs at the pulmonary end with constriction of the aortic end normally delayed for several weeks or months. Closure of the aortic end of the ductus arteriosus may abruptly impede flow of blood around an aortic shelf lesion (*see* Fig. 6–26). When coarctation is very severe, distal aortic perfusion may, in part, be supplied with blood from the pulmonary artery via a patent ductus arteriosus (*see* Fig. 6–27). When the development of aortic obstruction is gradual, collateral flow to the distal aorta will be established via the intercostal, internal thoracic, subclavian, and scapular arteries.

Coarctation commonly is associated with cardiac lesions that produce reductions in intrauterine aortic blood flow. The most common lesions associated with coarctation are VSD, hypoplastic left heart syndrome, and abnormalities of the mitral and aortic valves.

Physiology

Coarctation of the aorta produces LV pressure overload and a reduction in lower body perfusion. The physiologic consequences of a coarctation will depend on several factors:

1. The severity of the coarctation.
2. The extent of bypass afforded by the patent or partially patent ductus arteriosus.
3. The extent of collateralization to the distal aorta.
4. The type and severity of associated heart lesions.

Patients presenting in infancy with coarctation are likely to have poor collateralization and to be dependent on patency or partial patency of the ductus arteriosus for distal aortic perfusion. The underlying coarctation usually is severe and the LV is presented with high afterload at birth. This has important consequences:

1. The LV will not have developed the concentric hypertrophy that accompanies a more gradual

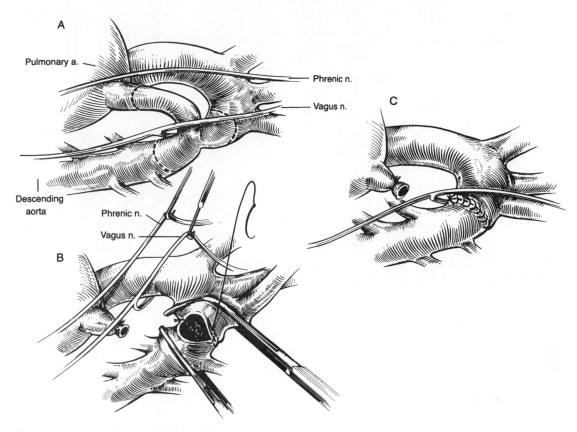

FIGURE 6–26. Anatomy of coarctation of the aorta involving a small patent ductus arteriosus (PDA). Closure of this PDA will create a shelf-like invagination of the posterior aortic wall and increase the severity of the coarctation. The repair shown here (**A** through **C**) is resection of the coarcted segment, ligation of the PDA, and primary end-to-end reanastomosis of the aorta. Clamp placement has compromised flow to the left subclavian artery.

increase in LV afterload (see the section on aortic stenosis in Chapter 5). As a result, LV afterload mismatch (*see* Chapter 2) will occur, resulting initially in distension of the LV and ultimately in reduction of LV output. Distension of the LV will produce LA distension and pulmonary congestion. The reduction in LV output may be so severe that proximal hypertension will not be present.

2. The elevation of LV systolic and diastolic pressures will promote left-to-right shunting via an ASD, VSD, or complete AV canal defect. This, in turn, will dramatically increase pulmonary blood flow at the expense of systemic blood flow and predispose development of PVOD.

3. Descending aortic blood flow will be greatly diminished, which will result in ischemia of distal organs and produce a metabolic acidosis. In many instances, patency of the aortic end of the ductus arteriosus will allow some distal aortic perfusion. When coarctation is severe, distal aortic perfusion will be largely dependent on right-to-left shunt of pulmonary artery blood to the distal aorta via a PDA. This will result in cyanosis

of the abdomen and distal extremities due to their perfusion with systemic venous blood (*see* Fig. 6–27).

Patients presenting in childhood with coarctation will not be ductus dependent and will have well-developed collaterals. In addition, they will have developed the concentric LV hypertrophy that accompanies chronic LV pressure overload lesions. These patients will have proximal aortic hypertension.

Surgical Therapy

Three basic types of repair are used for correction of coarctation of the aorta: subclavian patch angioplasty,[111] synthetic patch angioplasty,[112] and end-to-end anastomosis of the aorta after resection of the coarcted segment.[113] These procedures are performed via a left thoracotomy. It is necessary to cross-clamp the aorta to perform these procedures. For older children, partial CPB or a shunt from proximal to distal aorta may be used if the adequacy of the collateral circulation is in question (*see* Chapter 9).

The advantages and disadvantages of the three techniques are summarized:

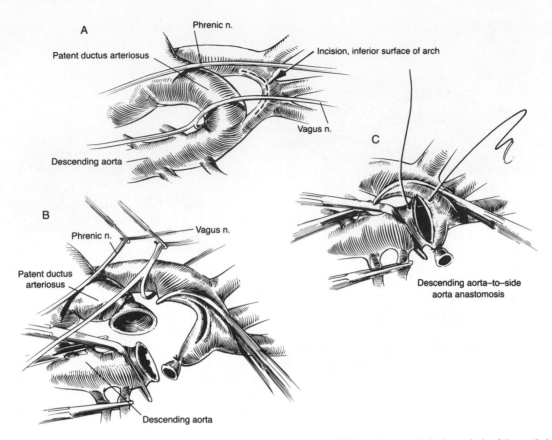

FIGURE 6–27. Anatomy of coarctation of the aorta involving a large patent ductus arteriosus (PDA) and severe tubular hypoplasia of the aortic isthmus (arch). A good portion of the flow to the distal aorta is supplied from R-L shunting through the PDA. The repair shown here (**A** through **C**) is resection of ductal tissue and mobilization of the descending aorta and aortic arch to perform a primary reanastomosis. This increases the caliber of the aortic arch. Clamp placement has compromised flow to the left carotid artery.

1. Subclavian patch — in this technique, the subclavian artery is mobilized, ligated, and divided. The proximal portion of artery is used to repair the coarctation. This technique uses native tissue, puts little pressure on the suture line, and does not create a circumferential scar. It may alter growth potential of the left arm, it may leave ductal tissue behind (predisposing restenosis), and it cannot be used to treat proximal tubular hypoplasia of the isthmus.

2. Patch aortoplasty — in this technique, a synthetic patch is used in place of the subclavian artery tissue. The advantages and disadvantages are similar to those of the subclavian technique.

    Obviously, there is no compromise of left arm perfusion, but there is a documented incidence of subsequent aneurysm formation at the patch site.

3. Resection and end-to-end reanastomosis — in this technique, the ascending and descending aorta is mobilized and the coarcted segment and all ductal tissue are excised. The aortic segments are then reanastomosed together. This technique removes all ductal tissue and can be used to address proximal tubular hypoplasia. It requires extensive dissection, has the potential for suture line tension, and leaves a circumferential scar (which may cause restenosis).

The most devastating complication associated with coarctation repair is the development of paraplegia secondary to spinal cord ischemia. The incidence of paraplegia varies from series to series but is quite low (0.14 to 0.4%). Several factors seem to be associated with an increased risk of developing paraplegia: hyperthermia, prolonged aortic cross-clamp time, elevated cerebral spinal fluid (CSF) pressures, low proximal and distal aortic blood pressures, and poorly developed collaterals to the descending aorta.[114-117]

The major long-term problem associated with coarctation repair in infancy and childhood is recoarctation. It is not clear at this time which of the three techniques provides the best protection from this complication.

Anesthetic Management

Goals

1. Maintain heart rate, contractility, and preload to maintain cardiac output. The high afterload faced by the LV makes it particularly vulnerable to reductions in contractility.
2. For neonates and infants with coarctation, continuation of prostaglandin E_1 (0.05 to 0.1 µg/kg/min) to maintain ductal patency may be necessary to prevent cardiovascular collapse.
3. If there is an associated ASD or VSD, reduction in the PVR:SVR ratio should be avoided. Such reductions will increase pulmonary blood flow and will necessitate an increase in cardiac output to maintain systemic blood flow.
4. Avoid increases in SVR. Increased SVR will worsen LV pressure overload, which may cause large reductions in LV output.
5. Cross-clamping of the aorta may produce impressive proximal hypertension or LV dysfunction. This is less likely in the presence of well-developed collaterals.

Induction and Maintenance.

Neonates and infants presenting for coarctation repair generally are prostaglandin-dependent with compromised distal perfusion and pulmonary congestion. They are not candidates for inhalational anesthesia. Ketamine may worsen the hemodynamic picture by increasing SVR and probably should be avoided. A technique using fentanyl or sufentanil is well tolerated by these patients. In older children with only proximal systemic hypertension, IV or inhalational techniques are well tolerated. Again, ketamine may not be a good choice. Regardless of the technique chosen, it should be appreciated that proximal blood pressure response to stimulation will be exaggerated.

The arterial line should be in the right arm because the other extremities will be unreliable after the clamps have been applied. This is particularly true for the left subclavian patch technique.

The management of proximal systemic hypertension after aortic cross-clamping warrants discussion. Cross-clamping of the thoracic aorta has been shown to produce increases in both proximal aortic blood pressure and CSF pressure and decreases in distal aortic blood pressure.[118-120] Use of sodium nitroprusside to normalize proximal aortic blood pressure results in further increases in CSF pressure and further decreases in distal aortic blood pressure. This combination of increased CSF pressure and reduced aortic blood pressure reduces spinal cord blood perfusion pressure and may place the spinal cord at risk for ischemia. Therefore, vasodilators should be used cautiously to control extreme proximal hypertension and LV dysfunction.

TEE is useful during cross-clamping, particularly for infants with coexisting cardiac lesions. LV function and the extent of intracardiac shunting can be monitored. In some instances of severe coarctation in infants, particularly those with proximal tubular hypoplasia, vasodilator therapy may be insufficient to prevent LV dilatation and inotropic support may be necessary. Inotropic therapy for patients with intracardiac shunts may only serve to increase L-R shunting. Ventilatory control of PVR will be complicated by the fact that the left lung must be retracted for exposure. It is important to know which arch vessels are clamped during the surgical procedure. At least one of the carotid arteries must have maintained flow (*see* Figs. 6–26 and 6–27).

Removal of the cross-clamp will result in reactive hyperemia in distal tissues with subsequent vasodilation. This may produce transient hypotension. In addition, release of lactic acid will increase P_{CO_2} if minute ventilation is not increased. Attention to the surgical procedure will allow these changes to be anticipated. Hyperventilation just before clamp removal is helpful, as is a ready source of intravascular volume expansion. TEE again will help guide therapy. Fortunately, cross-clamp times for these repairs are relatively short (<15 minutes), which reduces the hemodynamic consequences of clamp removal.

Postoperatively, rebound hypertension may occur and persist for up to 1 week. The genesis of this hypertension has not been clearly delineated, but in the early phases, it seems that an altered baroreceptor response resulting in very high circulating levels of catecholamines play a role.[121] In the later phase, the renin–angiotensin system seems to be involved.[122] Beta blockers and vasodilators commonly are necessary to control this hypertension. In the immediate postoperative period, maintenance of anesthesia with additional doses of fentanyl or sufentanil will attenuate the hypertension.

Older children without coexisting diseases are candidates for early extubation using the technique described for PDA ligation.

■ HYPOPLASTIC LEFT HEART SYNDROME

Anatomy

Patients with hypoplastic left heart syndrome (HLHS) have severe stenosis or atresia of all left heart structures. In the most severe form, mitral and aortic atresia with hypoplasia of the left atrium, left ventricle, and aortic arch are present. Distal aortic blood flow occurs via a PDA. Proximal aortic blood flow and coronary blood flow occur by retrograde filling of a tiny ascending aorta via the PDA (*see* Fig. 6–28).

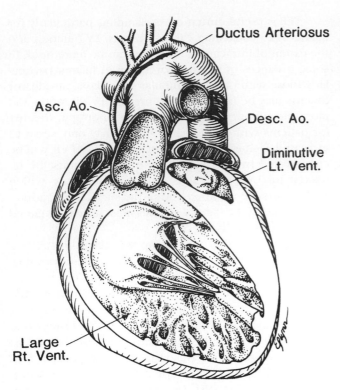

FIGURE 6–28. Anatomy of hypoplastic left heart syndrome (HLHS). Pulmonary and systemic blood flow are both delivered via the right ventricle. Aortic blood flow is provided via a large ductus arteriosus. The proximal aorta and coronary arteries are perfused retrograde via tiny ascending aorta. (Asc. Ao. = ascending aorta; Desc. Ao. = descending aorta; Lt. Vent. = left ventricle; Rt. Vent. = right ventricle.) *(From: Fyler DC, Nadas AS: Congenital heart disease, in Avery ME, Lewis FR (eds): Pediatric Medicine. Baltimore, Williams & Wilkins, 1989, p 370.)*

Physiology

HLHS is a complex shunt with complete obstruction to outflow. There is a communication (ASD or patent foramen ovale) and a complete obstruction to LA outflow (mitral atresia). This results in an obligatory left-to-right shunt at the atrial level with complete mixing of systemic and pulmonary venous blood in the right atrium and ventricle. When the ASD or foramen ovale is restrictive, there will be a large left atrial to right atrial pressure gradient. This will result in poor decompression of the LA and pulmonary venous congestion. Systemic blood flow is provided by a simple downstream shunt (PDA). Closure of the PDA in infants with HLHS drastically reduces coronary and systemic blood flow and results in immediate cardiovascular collapse. Prostaglandin E_1 therapy is lifesaving for these patients.

Because pulmonary and systemic blood flow are supplied by a single ventricle in parallel fashion, it is necessary to maintain a balance between PVR and SVR.[123] An increase in blood flow to one circulation will occur at the expense of flow to the other. If PVR is lowered, pulmonary blood flow will increase, producing a pulmonary steal phenomenon with systemic and coronary hypoperfusion. An increase in the arterial Po_2 and the insidious onset of a metabolic acidosis often heralds impending cardiovascular collapse (*see* Fig. 6–29). Similarly, increases in PVR relative to SVR are likely to improve systemic and coronary perfusion at the expense of pulmonary perfusion. As with all mixing lesions, a reduction in Q_p will produce hypoxemia. If allowed to progress, this too will produce cardiovascular collapse (*see* Fig. 6–29). Obviously, ventilatory control of PVR is imperative in this lesion.

Surgical Therapy

The successful application of the Fontan procedure to a variety of single ventricle lesions prompted Norwood and associates to devise a two-stage treatment plan for patients with HLHS.[124]

Stage 1. The stage 1 procedure is palliative and is designed to allow survival of neonates with HLHS while creating anatomy suitable for a definitive Fontan procedure in stage 2. Palliation is directed toward establishing systemic and pulmonary blood flow without the need for a PDA and toward allowing normal development of the pulmonary vasculature. The stage 1 procedure involves creation of a nonrestrictive ASD to allow complete mixing of systemic and pulmonary venous blood in the right atrium without left atrial distension. To provide adequate systemic blood flow from the right ventricle, the pulmonary artery is transected and the proximal portion used to construct a new ascending aorta (neoaorta). It also may be necessary to use synthetic or homograft material to enlarge the neoaorta. Pulmonary blood flow is provided by either a modified BT or central shunt (see the section on TOF). The anatomy after completion of the stage 1 procedure is illustrated in Figure 6–30.

Stage 2. The stage 2 procedure is the definitive procedure for patients with HLHS. It is basically a modified Fontan procedure, with a total cavopulmonary connection using the lateral atrial tunnel technique shown in Figure 6–24.

As described earlier in the section on the Fontan procedure, there is current enthusiasm for staging of the Fontan procedure. For patients with HLHS, this involves a hemi-Fontan procedure before the Fontan procedure. The hemi-Fontan procedure is performed at approximately 6 to 8 months of age; the definitive Fontan is performed at 1 to 2 years of age. Therefore, stage 2 is divided into two parts. This approach has resulted in better survival of patients with HLHS after stage 1 and better survival after the definitive Fontan procedure.[96,98]

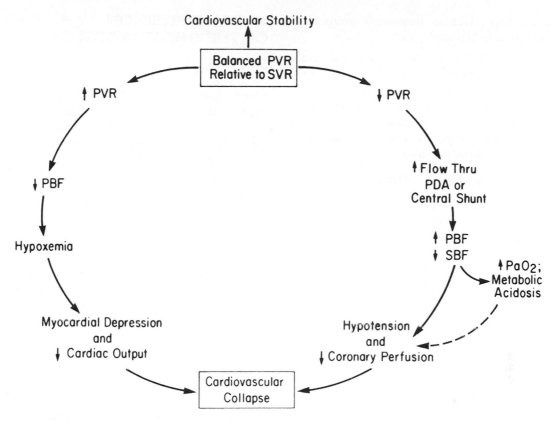

FIGURE 6–29. Consequences of changes in PVR:SVR ratio in patients with hypoplastic left heart syndrome before and after stage 1 palliation. (PVR = pulmonary vascular resistance; SVR = systemic vascular resistance; PBF = pulmonary blood flow; SBF = systemic blood flow; PDA = patent ductus arteriosus.) *(From: Hansen DD, Hickey PR: Anesthesia for hypoplastic left heart syndrome: Use of high-dose fentanyl in 30 neonates. Anesth Analg 1989; 65(2):129.*

Anesthetic Management, Stage 1

Goals

1. Maintain heart rate, contractility, and preload to maintain cardiac output.
2. Maintain ductal patency with prostaglandin E_1 (0.05 to 0.1 µg/kg/min).
3. Maintain a balanced PVR and SVR (*see* Fig. 6-26).
4. Avoid a high FIo_2 unless Po_2 is less than 40 mm Hg or arterial saturation is less than 80%. A high FIo_2, Po_2, or arterial saturation will reduce PVR, which will increase pulmonary blood flow and reduce systemic blood flow. Usually, an FIo_2 of 21% is appropriate for these patients.
5. When pulmonary blood flow increases despite a reduced FIo_2, a gradual increase in arterial saturation and Po_2 will be noted in conjunction with falling arterial blood pressure. It may be necessary to use PEEP and an arterial Pco_2 in the range of 40 to 50 mm Hg to increase PVR. Use of 2 to 4% inspired CO_2 can be used to increase Pao_2 without having to reduce tidal volume and minute ventilation.[125] This will allow maintenance of FRC and a

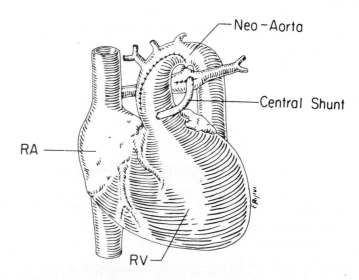

FIGURE 6–30. Anatomy after stage 1 palliation for patients with hypoplastic left heart syndrome. (RA = right atrium; RV = right ventricle.) *(From: Hansen DD, Hickey PR: Anesthesia for hypoplastic left heart syndrome: Use of high-dose fentanyl in 30 neonates. Anesth Analg 1989; 65(2):120.*

satisfactory Paco₂ without pulmonary overperfusion and systemic hypoperfusion.

Induction and Maintenance. These patients usually are extremely ill and may require ongoing resusitation despite the use of prostaglandin. Cardiac reserve is severely limited and control of PVR is imperative. Prompt airway control is necessary and a high-dose fentanyl or sufentanil technique provides the necessary hemodynamic stability for these patients.

Post-CPB Management, Stage 1

After the stage 1 procedure, there is improved perfusion of the proximal aorta and coronary circulation; however, the pulmonary and systemic circulations are still supplied in parallel from a single ventricle. Therefore, as illustrated in Figure 6–29, a balanced PVR relative to SVR is necessary to maintain adequate systemic and pulmonary blood flow. After CPB, it is not uncommon for a high PVR to result in reduced pulmonary blood flow and hypoxemia. As PVR begins to fall later in the post-CPB period, it may be necessary to use ventilatory interventions to reduce pulmonary blood flow.

Goals

1. Maintain heart rate (preferably sinus rhythm) at an age-appropriate rate. Cardiac output is likely to be more heart-rate-dependent during the post-CPB period.
2. When arterial Po₂ is less than 30 mm Hg, aggressive efforts to reduce PVR must be made. A high FIo₂, a Pco₂ of 20 to 25 mm Hg, a pH of 7.50 to 7.60, and low mean airway pressures should be used. In addition, efforts should be made to increase systemic blood pressure to improve pulmonary perfusion pressure via the surgical shunt.
3. Inotropic support of the ventricle may be necessary.
4. Pulmonary overperfusion will have the same consequence as before stage 1, that is, systemic hypoperfusion. Again, use of 2 to 4% CO₂ can be life-saving. If aggressive efforts to balance PVR and SVR fail, the size of the surgical shunt may have to be reduced.

Anesthetic Management, Stage 2

The anesthetic considerations for the stage 2 procedure are identical to those for stage 1, as the pulmonary and systemic circulations are still supplied in parallel from a single ventricle.

Post-CPB Management, Stage 2

The post-CPB management of patients having undergone a hemi-Fontan or Fontan procedure are discussed in detail in the section on tricuspid atresia.

■ TRANSPOSITION OF THE GREAT VESSELS

Anatomy

Ventriculoarterial discordance is the characteristic finding in transposition of the great vessels (TGV) — that is, the great arteries arise from the wrong ventricles (*see* Fig. 6–31). Normally, the aorta arises from the left ventricle posterior and to the left of the pulmonary artery, which arises from the right ventricle. In D-transposition, the aorta arises anterior and to the right of the pulmonary artery. In L-transposition, the aorta arises anterior and to the left of the pulmonary artery. When ventriculoarterial discordance is combined with atrioventricular concordance (right atrium connects to the right ventricle and left atrium connects to the left ventricle), there will be a disruption of the normal series relationship between the systemic and pulmonary circulations (*see* Fig. 6–4). As a result of this arrangement, the pulmonary and systemic circulations will function as two separate parallel circuits. Systemic venous blood will be recirculated through the systemic circulation, whereas pulmonary venous blood will be recirculated through the pulmonary circulation. For survival outside the uterus, there must be a communication between the two circuits.

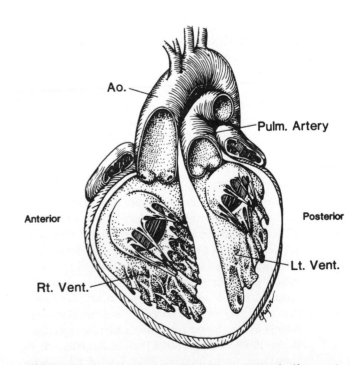

FIGURE 6–31. Anatomy of transposition of the great vessels. (Ao. = aorta; Lt. Vent. = left ventricle; Rt. Vent. = right ventricle.) *(From: Fyler DC, Nadas AS: Congenital heart disease, in Avery ME, Lewis FR (eds): Pediatric Medicine. Baltimore, Williams & Wilkins, 1989, p 370.)*

For patients with complete TGV, the most commonly associated cardiac anomalies are a persistent patent foramen ovale (PFO), PDA, VSD, and subpulmonic stenosis, or left ventricular outflow tract obstruction (LVOTO). Approximately 50% of patients with TGV will present with a PDA before prostaglandin E_1 administration. The foramen ovale is almost always patent, but a true secundum ASD exists in only approximately 5% of patients. Although angiographically detectable VSDs may occur in 30 to 40% of patients, only about one-third of these defects are hemodynamically significant.[126] Therefore, for practical purposes, 75% of patients have an intact ventricular septum (IVS).[127] LVOTO is present in approximately 30% of patients with VSD and most often is due to an extensive subpulmonary fibromuscular ring or mechanical obstruction from malposition of the outlet portion of the ventricular septum.[126] Only 5% of patients with IVS have significant LVOTO. In these patients, there is a dynamic obstruction of the LV outflow tract during systole due to leftward bulging of the ventricular septum and anterior movement of the anterior mitral valve leaflet.[128] Valvular pulmonary stenosis is rare in patients with TGV.[126] Other less commonly seen lesions are functionally important tricuspid or mitral regurgitation (4% each) and coarctation of the aorta (5%).[126]

Bronchopulmonary collateral vessels (aorta to pulmonary artery proximal to the pulmonary capillaries) are visible angiographically in 30% of patients with complete TGV, and the functional patency of these vessels has been demonstrated conclusively.[129]

Physiology

Transposition of the great vessels produces two parallel circulations with recirculation of systemic and pulmonary venous blood. For survival to be possible there must be one or more communications (ASD, VSD, PDA) between the two circuits to allow intercirculatory mixing. This mixing allows oxygenated pulmonary venous blood to be delivered to the systemic circulation and for deoxygenated systemic venous blood to be delivered to the pulmonary circuit. In the steady state, the amount of blood that leaves the systemic circuit to enter the pulmonary circuit must be equal to the amount of blood that leaves the pulmonary circuit to enter the systemic circuit. When intercirculatory mixing occurs, total systemic blood flow is a combination of recirculated systemic venous blood flow and effective systemic blood flow (the amount of saturated pulmonary venous blood that reaches the systemic circulation). Likewise total pulmonary blood flow is a combination of recirculated pulmonary venous blood flow and effective pulmonary blood flow (the amount of desaturated systemic venous blood that reaches the pulmonary circulation). Effective pulmonary blood flow and effective systemic blood flow are always equal, and these flows represent only a small portion of the total blood flow in each circuit (see Fig. 6–4).

Intercirculatory mixing is enhanced by:[130]

1. Large nonrestrictive communications between the pulmonary and systemic circulations (large ASD, VSD, and PDA).
2. High pulmonary blood flow; pulmonary blood flow is increased by a low PVR and by increases in the compliance of the pulmonary ventricle (left ventricle).

The arterial saturation is determined by:[131]

1. The magnitude of intercirculatory mixing.
2. The quantity of systemic venous blood recirculated into the systemic circulation; the less systemic venous blood that is recirculated relative to effective systemic blood flow, the higher the arterial saturation.
3. The saturation of the systemic venous blood; for a given degree of intercirculatory mixing and recirculated systemic blood flow, reductions in systemic venous saturation will reduce arterial saturation. Increases in oxygen consumption, decreases in cardiac output, and decreases in hematocrit all will reduce systemic venous saturation.

It is obvious that patients with a restrictive communication between the two circuits will have poor mixing and hypoxemia. The neonate with TGV and an intact ventricular septum will present with severe, increasing cyanosis as the ductus arteriosus closes. Palliation is directed toward creation of a less restrictive communication to promote better intercirculatory mixing and improve oxygenation as the PDA closes. Prostaglandin E_1 is used to maintain ductal patency and stabilize the neonate while a Rashkind–Miller balloon atrial septostomy is performed in the cardiac catheterization laboratory. After this procedure, the neonate can be brought to the operating room for a definitive procedure.

Patients with pulmonary stenosis will have low pulmonary blood flow and may be hypoxemic despite a relatively large intercirculatory communication. Patients with high pulmonary blood flow, particularly those with a VSD in whom systemic pressures are transmitted to the pulmonary vasculature, are at risk of developing PVOD. In the presence of a good-sized intercirculatory communication, these patients will initially not be hypoxemic. However, the progressive development of PVOD will eventually reduce pulmonary blood flow and produce hypoxemia. Finally, all patients with TGV and increased pulmonary blood flow will have a large volume load imposed on the pulmonary atrium and ventricle (LA and LV).

Surgical Therapy

Intra-Atrial Physiologic Repair: Mustard and Senning Procedures. Both the Mustard and the Senning procedures are atrial switch procedures that surgically create discordant atrioventricular connections in the presence of the preexisting discordant ventriculoarterial connections. Therefore, after repair, systemic venous blood is routed to the LV, which is connected to the pulmonary artery. Likewise, pulmonary venous blood is routed to the RV, which is connected to the aorta. This arrangement results in physiologic but not anatomic correction of TGV. In 1964, Mustard described an operation that redirected venous return via an intra-atrial baffle after excision of the interatrial septum.[132] The baffle, made from pericardium or synthetic material, directed pulmonary venous blood across the tricuspid valve into the right ventricle and out the aorta. Systemic venous blood passed beneath the baffle to the mitral valve, left ventricle, and finally the pulmonary artery (*see* Fig. 6–32). This procedure requires that the right ventricle remain the systemic ventricle and that the tricuspid valve face systemic pressures. There is evidence to suggest that long-term exposure of the right ventricle to systemic pressures results in progressive right ventricular dysfunction.[133,134] Both systemic and pulmonary venous obstruction may occur as the result of this procedure. Finally, the incidence of dysrhythmias after the Mustard procedure is high: 64% of patients have dysrhythmias, 28% of which are serious (bradycardia, sick-sinus syndrome, atrial flutter).[135]

The Senning procedure is an interatrial baffle repair that uses autologous atrial tissue to preserve atrial contractility and optimize atrial growth potential.[136] The Senning procedure is associated with the same long-term problems as the Mustard procedure.

Anatomic Repair or the Arterial (Jatene) Switch Procedure. The arterial switch procedure anatomically corrects the discordant ventriculoarterial connections. After repair, the right ventricle is connected to the pulmonary artery and the left ventricle is connected to the aorta. Clinical success with the Jatene procedure, summarized in Figure 6–33, was achieved in 1975.[137] In brief, the pulmonary artery and the aorta are transected distal to their respective valves. The coronary arteries are initially explanted from the ascending aorta with 3 to 4 mm of surrounding tissue. The explant sites are repaired either with pericardium or synthetic material. The coronary arteries are reimplanted into the proximal pulmonary artery (neoaorta). The great arteries are then switched with the distal pulmonary artery brought anterior (Lecompte maneuver) to be reanastomosed to the old proximal aorta (right ventricular outflow) and the distal aorta reanastomosed to the old proximal pulmonary artery (left ventricular outflow).

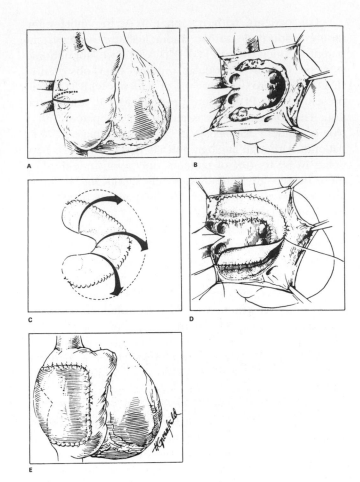

FIGURE 6–32. Details of Mustard operation. **A** through **E.** Creation of atriotomy, enlargement of atrial septal defect, and creation of intra-atrial baffle. Orifice of superior and inferior vena cavae are encircled by distal ends of baffle such that systemic venous blood is directed under baffle across enlarged atrial septal defect into mitral valve, left ventricle, and pulmonary artery. Pulmonary venous blood remains above baffle to be directed across tricuspid valve into right ventricle and aorta. *(From: Lake CL:* Pediatric Cardiac Anesthesia. *Norwalk, CT: Appleton and Lange, 1988, p 234. Used by permission.)*

Most patients with TGV have coronary anatomy, which is suitable for the coronary reimplantation necessary in the arterial switch procedure.[138,139] Patients with certain types of coronary anatomy (inverted coronaries, single right coronary artery) are at risk for postoperative myocardial ischemia and death because reimplantation can result in distortion of the coronary ostia or narrowing of the artery itself.[138] The emergence of two parallel coronary arteries above but in contact with the posterior valve commissure or the intramural origin of the coronaries also presents a technical challenge. These patients may require resuspension of the neopulmonary valve after the coronaries and a surrounding tissue cuff have been excised.[138]

For the arterial switch procedure to be successful, the original pulmonary ventricle (LV) must have suffi-

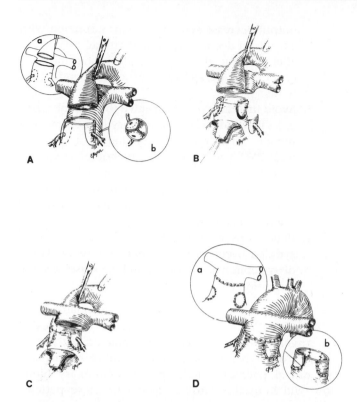

FIGURE 6–33. Details of arterial switch procedure. **A.** Aorta is transected and left and right main coronary arteries are excised using (a) either button of aortic wall or (b) segment of aortic wall extending from rim of aorta. **B.** Equivalent segment of pulmonary arterial wall is excised, and coronary arteries are sutured to pulmonary artery. **C.** Distal pulmonary artery is brought anterior to ascending aorta, and proximal pulmonary artery is anastomosed to distal aorta. **D.** Sites of coronary explantation are repaired using either (a) patch of prosthetic material or (b) segment of percardium. Finally, proximal aorta is sutured to distal pulmonary artery. *(From: Castanda AR, Norwood WI, Jonas RA, et al: Transposition of the great arteries and intact ventricular septum: Anatomical repair in the neonate. Ann Thorac Surg 1984; 38:438–443. Reprinted with permission from the Society of Thoracic Surgeons.)*

cient mass to be capable of becoming the systemic ventricle after the switch. Patient selection and the timing of the surgical procedure are, therefore, important variables in determining the success of this procedure. The Jatene procedure was described originally in patients with TGV and a large VSD or a large PDA.[129] In these patients, the pulmonary ventricle (LV) remains exposed to systemic pressures and the LV mass remains sufficient to support the systemic circulation. For these patients, the arterial switch procedure generally is performed within the first 2 to 3 months of life before intractable CHF or irreversible PVOD intervene.[140]

For patients with TGV and IVS, there is progressive reduction in LV mass as the physiologic pulmonary hypertension present at birth resolves progressively over the first days after birth. Adequate LV mass to support the systemic circulation exists in these patients for only the first 2 or 3 weeks after birth.[141,142] For patients with

TGV and IVS, the arterial switch procedure can be performed primarily or as the second phase of a staged procedure. A successful primary arterial switch procedure generally must be performed within the first 10 days of life. Favorable candidates for the procedure in the neonatal period must have a LV:RV pressure ratio of at least 0.6 by catheterization. Alternatively, two-dimensional echocardiography can be used to noninvasively assess the LV:RV pressure ratio. Three types of ventricular septal geometry have been described. Patients in whom the ventricular septum bulges to the left (type 3), indicating a low pressure in the pulmonary ventricle (LV), are not candidates for a neonatal arterial switch procedure. Patients with septal bulging to the right (type 1), indicating a high pressure in the pulmonary ventricle (LV), and patients with an intermediate septal position (Type 2) are considered good candidates. Most neonates with TGV and IVS who are suitable candidates for an arterial switch procedure have type 2 septal geometry.

The staged arterial switch procedure for TGA with IVS is used for neonates in whom surgery cannot be performed during the first few weeks of life secondary to events such as prematurity, sepsis, low birth weight (<2 kg), or late referral. The LV is prepared to accept the systemic workload by placement of a pulmonary artery band within the first 2 months of life.[143] In addition, an aortopulmonary shunt with entry to the pulmonary artery distal to the band is necessary to prevent hypoxemia. The band must be tight enough to increase pressure in the pulmonary ventricle (LV) to approximately one-half to two-thirds that in the systemic ventricle (RV).[144] This will increase afterload sufficiently to prevent regression of LV mass. However, if the band is too tight, there may be LV decompensation secondary to afterload mismatch. Historically, after 3 to 6 months, the pulmonary artery was debanded, the shunt was taken down, and an arterial switch procedure was performed. Currently, early success has been reported with a rapid two-stage repair in which the arterial switch procedure is performed as early as 1 week after preparatory pulmonary artery banding, often during the same hospitalization.[145,146] This approach is based on the fact that a doubling of LV mass is seen after 1 week of pulmonary artery banding.[145] The staged procedure is complicated by the fact that placement of the pulmonary artery band to the proper tightness is not an easy task and that the pulmonary artery band and systemic to pulmonary artery shunt may result in distortion of the pulmonary artery, making the definite arterial switch procedure difficult.

The arterial switch procedure generally is not performed on patients in whom mechanical LVOTO exists. Correction of the LVOTO is difficult, and without complete correction of the LVOTO, these patients will be left with aortic or subaortic stenosis.[147] On the other hand, patients with dynamic LVOTO have been shown to have no gradient across the LV outflow tract after the arterial switch procedure.[148]

Closure of a VSD preferentially is performed transatrially through the tricuspid valve. It is desirable to avoid approaching a VSD through the RV because an incision in the RV may contribute substantially to postoperative RV dysfunction.

Rastelli Procedure. For patients with TGV, VSD, and severe LVOTO (subpulmonary stenosis), a Rastelli procedure is performed.[149] Closure of the VSD is performed through a right ventriculotomy. The VSD is closed so that LV blood is directed through the aorta. The proximal pulmonary artery is ligated and a valved conduit is placed from the right ventriculotomy to the pulmonary artery, thereby bypassing the subpulmonic stenosis (*see* Fig. 6–34). Subaortic stenosis may result from placement of the VSD patch. Replacement of the valved conduit may be necessary in later years secondary to calcification.

Anesthetic Management

Goals

1. Maintain heart rate, contractility, and preload to maintain cardiac output. Decreases in cardiac output decrease systemic venous saturation with a resultant decrease in arterial saturation.
2. Maintain ductal patency with postaglandin E₁ (0.05 to 0.1 µg/kg/min) in ductal-dependent patients.
3. Avoid increases in PVR relative to SVR. Increases in PVR will decrease pulmonary blood flow and reduce intercirculatory mixing. For patients with PVOD, ventilatory interventions should be used to reduce PVR. For patients with LVOTO that is not severe, ventilatory interventions to reduce PVR increase pulmonary blood flow and intercirculatory mixing.
4. Reductions in SVR relative to PVR should be avoided. Decreased SVR increases recirculation of systemic venous blood and decreases arterial saturation.

Induction and Maintenance. Neonates with TGV and an intact ventricular septum may present for surgery after Rashkind–Miller balloon atrial septostomy or with a prostaglandin E₁ infusion to maintain ductal patency. The increased pulmonary blood flow will limit the cardiac reserve of these patients and the immature myocardium will be sensitive to anesthetic-induced myocardial depression. A high-dose fentanyl or sufentanil technique will provide hemody-

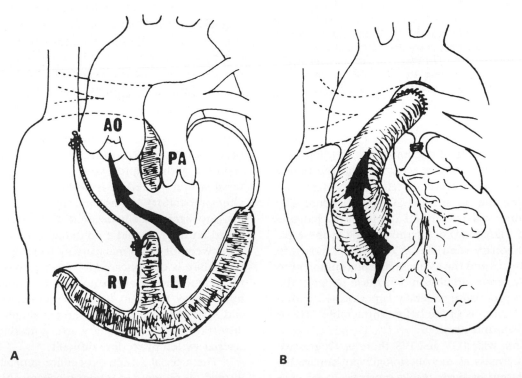

A   **B**

FIGURE 6–34. Schematic of Rastelli procedure for repair of transposition of the great vessels associated with pulmonic stenosis and ventricular septal defect (VSD). **A.** VSD is closed with patch such that left ventricular output is directed across the aortic valve. **B.** Proximal main pulmonary artery is ligated and valved conduit is placed from right ventricle to main pulmonary artery. (AO = aorta; LV = left ventricle; PA = pulmonary artery; RV = right ventricle.) *(From: Lake CL: Pediatric Cardiac Anesthesia. Norwalk, CT, Appleton and Lange, 1988, p 237. Used by permission.)*

namic stability without adversely affecting intercirculatory mixing.

In older children, PVOD may have reduced pulmonary blood flow with resultant hypoxemia. For these patients, prompt airway control and ventilatory interventions to reduce PVR are important. An inhalational induction or a intramuscular ketamine induction followed by placement of an IV and conversion to a high-dose fentanyl or sufentanil technique may be suitable for these patients. A similar approach may be taken for older children with subpulmonic stenosis. A high-dose fentanyl or sufentanil technique is useful in blunting the stress-induced increases in PVR that are so detrimental to these patients.

Post-CPB Management

After atrial baffle repairs, there may be pulmonary and systemic venous obstruction. Systemic venous obstruction will produce systemic venous congestion and a low RA pressure. Pulmonary venous obstruction may result in pulmonary venous and pulmonary arterial hypertension, pulmonary edema, and hypoxemia. Efforts to reduce SVR will reduce the RV afterload and help prevent tricuspid regurgitation. Therapy for atrial dysrhythmias also may be necessary. TEE will prove useful in ruling out pulmonary and systemic venous obstruction. In addition, large baffle leaks that may require surgical revision will be detected.

After the arterial switch procedure, there may be extensive bleeding from the aortic and pulmonary suture lines. Myocardial ischemia may result from technical difficulties in coronary artery reimplantation. Reductions in heart rate, coupled with IV nitroglycerin therapy, may be necessary to treat this ischemia. LV afterload mismatch and distension can occur in patients in which LV systolic function is inadequate and inotropic support of the LV in addition to afterload reduction with vasodilators may be necessary to terminate CPB.

TEE usually allows visualization of the reimplanted coronary arteries and allows patency to be assessed. In addition, TEE will provide on-line assessment of LV function, which may allow early detection of a kinked or compromised coronary anastomosis. Inotropic support of the LV also can be guided by the use of TEE.

Goals

1. Maintain heart rate (preferably sinus rhythm) at an age-appropriate rate. Cardiac output is likely to be more heart-rate-dependent during the post-CPB period. For patients having undergone atrial baffle procedures, antidysrhythmia therapy or pacing may be necessary.
2. Aggressive treatment of myocardial ischemia

(see Chapter 4) is necessary when it occurs after coronary reimplantation.
3. Reductions in aortic and pulmonary artery pressures may be necessary to help prevent suture line bleeding after the arterial switch procedure.
4. Systemic ventricular (RV after atrial baffle procedures and LV after arterial switch procedures) dysfunction may necessitate inotropic and vasodilator therapy to terminate CPB.

■ OBSTRUCTION TO LEFT VENTRICLE FILLING

Anatomy

Several congenital causes of obstruction to LV filling exist:[150]

1. Valvular mitral stenosis. Isolated congenital mitral stenosis is very rare and usually is caused by short, fused chordae tendineae.
2. Parachute mitral valve. In this lesion, two mitral valve leaflets are attached to shortened chordae that insert on the same papillary muscle.
3. Supravalvular mitral stenosis. In this lesion, an obstructive ring of thickened endocardium is found above the mitral valve downstream from the atrial appendage.
4. Cor triatriatum. In this lesion, an obstructive membrane is located upstream of the atrial appendage.

Physiology

All of these lesions have the same physiologic consequences as valvular mitral stenosis: obstruction to LV diastolic filling and pulmonary venous congestion. The physiology of mitral stenosis is discussed in detail in Chapter 5.

Surgical Therapy

Resection of a supravalvular ring or a cortriatum membrane normally results in a satisfactory result. Repair of the mitral valve is a superior alternative to mitral valve replacement because placement of artificial valves in infants and children is fraught with difficulties. A low-profile valve must be used to prevent LV outflow tract obstruction. A mechanical valve generally is chosen over a porcine or homograft valve because of the short in-situ half-life of these valves. Mechanical valves require long-term anticoagulation, which may be problematic for growing, active children.

The anesthetic and post-CPB management of patients with mitral stenosis is discussed in detail in Chapter 5.

■ LEFT VENTRICLE OUTFLOW TRACT OBSTRUCTION

Anatomy

Several categories of congenital LV outflow tract obstruction exist:[151]

1. Valvular aortic stenosis, most commonly caused by a bicuspid aortic valve. Most of these patients will remain asymptomatic until the fourth or fifth decade of life. In infants presenting with valvular aortic stenosis, the LV may be small. These patients may represent a milder form of hypoplastic left heart syndrome.

2. Subaortic stenosis, which may occur secondary to a discrete membranous ring located 1 to 2 cm below the aortic valve or to a fibromuscular overgrowth of the LV outflow tract that produces a tunnel-like stenosis.

3. Supravalvular stenosis, which may occur as the result of a discrete membrane, hourglass narrowing of the ascending aorta just above the sinus of Valsalva, or diffuse hypoplasia of the ascending aorta.

Physiology

The physiologic consequences of aortic stenosis are discussed in detail in Chapter 5. Infants with severe aortic stenosis warrant additional discussion, however. Infants with aortic stenosis tend to have a small LV and varying degrees of endocardial fibroelastosis secondary to prolonged subendocardial ischemia. When aortic stenosis is severe in the neonatal period, systemic blood flow and survival may be dependent on right-to-left shunting across a patent ductus arteriosus. This will result in perfusion of the periphery with systemic venous blood and will produce cyanosis. The coronary arteries will be perfused with desaturated blood at a low perfusion pressure. This, combined with the high LVEDP that accompanies aortic stenosis, will exacerbate myocardial ischemia.

Surgical Therapy

These lesions usually are approached by transecting or opening the ascending aorta. Subaortic lesions are then approached across the aortic valve. Resection of discrete subvalvular or supravalvular membranes is relatively straightforward. Treatment of fibromuscular tunnel-like stenosis is difficult. Resection of the fibromuscular tissue is limited by potential damage to surrounding structures such as the conduction system, mitral valve and the septum. In some instances, repair of a tunnel-like stenosis may require widening of the LV outflow tract with a patch and an aortic valve replacement.[152] Hourglass deformities of the ascending aorta may be repaired by widening the root with a patch. Diffuse hypoplasia of the ascending aorta may require replacement of the aortic root with graft material and reimplantation of the coronary arteries. In some cases of complex multilevel obstruction, an LV apex to descending aorta conduit may be necessary.[153]

Postrepair TEE can be used to detect residual gradients and to rule out damage to the mitral valve and ventricular septum. In particular, the presence of a small VSD should be ruled out.

The anesthetic and post-CPB management of patients with aortic stenosis is discussed in detail in Chapter 5.

■ REFERENCES

1. Hickey PR, Hansen DD, Norwood WI, Castenada AR: Anesthetic complications in surgery for congenital heart disease. *Anesth Analg* 1984; **63**:657-664.

2. Flyer D: Report on the New England Regional Infant Cardiac Program. *Pediatrics* 1980; **65**:375-461.

3. Hecker JF: *The Sheep as an Experimental Animal.* Orlando, Academic Press, 1983, pp 1-17.

4. Kirkpatrick SE, Corell JW, Friedman WF: A new technique for the continuous assessment of fetal and neonatal cardiac performance. *Am J Obstet Gynecol* 1973; **116**:963-972.

5. Assali NS, Brinkman CR, Nuwayhid B: Comparison of maternal and fetal cardiovascular functions in acute and chronic experiments in the sheep. *Am J Obstet Gynecol* 1974; **120**:411-425.

6. Assin S, Tyler TL, Wallis R: The effect of prostaglandin E₁ on fetal pulmonary vascular resistance. *Proc Soc Exp Biol Med* 1975; **148**:584-587.

7. Smith RW, Morris JA, Assali NS: Effects of chemical mediators on the pulmonary and ductus arteriosus circulation in the fetal lamb. *Am J Obstet Gynecol* 1964; **89**:252-260.

8. Friedman WF, Hirschlau MJ, Pitlick PT, Kirkpatrick SE: Pharmacologic closure of patent ductus arteriosus in the premature infant. *N Engl J Med* 1976; **295**:526-529.

9. Lynch JJ, Schuchard GH, Gross CM, Wann LS: Prevalance of right-to-left atrial shunting in a healthy population: Detection by Valsalva maneuver contrast echocardiography. *Am J Cardiol* 1984; **53**:1478-1480.

10. Dubourg O, Bourdarias JP, Farcot JC, et al: Contrast echocardiographic visualization of cough-induced right to left shunt through a patent foramen ovale. *J Am Coll Cardiol* 1984; **4**: 587-594.

11. Cassin S, Dawes GS, Mott JC, et al: The vascular resistance of the foetal and newly ventilated lung of the lamb. *J Physiol* 1964; **171**:61-79.

12. Reynolds SRM: The fetal and neonatal pulmonary vasculature in the guinea pig in relation to hemodynamic changes at birth. *Am J Anat* 1958; **98**:97-127.

13. Rudolph AM, Heymann MA: Fetal and neonatal circulation and respiration. *Annu Rev Physiol* 1974; **36**:187-207.

14. Adams FH: Fetal and neonatal circulations, in Adams FH, Emmanoulides GC (eds): *Heart Disease in Infants, Children and Adolescents.* Baltimore, Williams & Wilkins, 1983, pp 11-17.

15. Berman W, Musselman J: Myocardial performance in the newborn lamb. *Am J Physiol* 1979; **237**:H66-H70.

16. Friedman WF: Intrinsic physiological properties of the developing heart. *Prog Cardiovasc Dis* 1972; **15**:87-111.

17. Romero T, Corell J, Friedman WF: A comparison of pressure-volume relations of the fetal, newborn and adult heart. *Am J Physiol* 1972; **222:**1285–1290.

18. McGoon DC, Mair DD: On the unmuddling of shunting, mixing, and streaming. *J Thorac Cardiovasc Surg* 1990; **100:**77–82.

19. Hickey PR, Wessel DL: Anesthesia for treatment of congenital heart disease, in Kaplan JA (ed): *Cardiac Anesthesia*. 2nd ed, vol 2. New York, Grune & Stratton, 1987, pp 635–723.

20. Hoffman JIE, Rudolph AM, Heymann MA: Pulmonary vascular disease with congenital heart lesions: Pathologic features and causes. *Circulation* 1981; **64:**873–877.

21. Rabinovitch M, Haworth SG, Castaneda AR, et al: Lung biopsy in congenital heart disease: A morphometric approach to pulmonary vascular disease. *Circulation* 1978; **58:**1107–1122.

22. Fishman A: Hypoxia on the pulmonary circulation: How and where it acts. *Circ Res* 1976; **38:**221–231.

23. Rudolph AM, Yuan S: Response of the pulmonary vasculature to hypoxia and H+ ion concentration changes. *J Clin Invest* 1966; **45:**399–411.

24. Abman SH, Wolfe RR, Accurso FJ: Pulmonary vascular response to oxygen in infants with severe bronchopulmonary dysplasia. *Pediatrics* 1985; **75:**80–84.

25. Malik AB, Kidd BSL: Independent effects of changes in H+ and CO_2 concentration on hypoxic pulmonary vasoconstriction. *J Appl Physiol* 1973; **34:**318–323.

26. Schreiber MD, Heyman MA, Soifer SJ: Increased arterial pH, not decreased $PaCO_2$, attenuates hypoxia-induced pulmonary vasconstriction in newborn lambs. *Pediatr Res* 1986; **20:**113–117.

27. Drummond WH, Gregory GA, Heyman MA: The independent effect of hyperventilation, tolazoline and dopamine on infants with persistent pulmonary hypertension. *J Pediatr* 1981; **98:**603–611.

28. Wessel DL, Hickey PR, Hansen DD: Pulmonary and systemic hemodynamic effects of hyperventilation in infants after repair of congenital heart disease. *Anesthesiology* 1987; **67:**A526.

29. Morray JP, Lynn AM, Mansfield PB: Effect of pH and PCO_2 on pulmonary and systemic hemodynamics after surgery in children with congenital heart disease and pulmonary hypertension. *J Pediatr* 1988; **113:**474–479.

30. West JB: *Respiratory Physiology: The Essentials.* Baltimore, Williams & Wilkins, 1974.

31. Johns RA: EDRF/nitric oxide: The endogenous nitrovasodilator and a new cellular messenger. *Anesthesiology* 1991; **75:**927–931.

32. Furchgott RF, Zawadzki JV: The obligatory role of endothelial cells in relaxation of arterial smooth muscle by acetylcholine. *Nature* 1980; **288:**373–376.

33. Palmer RMJ, Ferrige AG, Monacada SA: Nitric oxide release accounts for the biological activity of endothelium-derived relaxing factor. *Nature* 1987; **327:**524.

34. Ignarro LJ, Lippton H, Edwards JC, et al: Mechanism of vascular smooth muscle relaxation by organic nitrates, nitrites, nitroprusside and nitric oxide: Evidence for the involvement of S-nitrosothiols as active intermediates. *J Pharmacol Exp Ther* 1981; **218:**739–749.

35. Moncada S, Palmer RMJ, Higgs EA: Nitric oxide: Physiology, pathophysiology, and pharmacology. *Pharmacol Rev* 1991; **43:**109–143.

36. Johns RA: Endothelium-derived relaxing factor: Basic review and clinical implications. *J Cardiothorac Vasc Anesth* 1991; **5:**69–79.

37. Body SC, Hartigan PM, Shernan SK, et al: Nitric oxide: Delivery, measurement, and clinical applications. *J Cardiothorac Vasc Anesth* 1995; **9:**748–763.

38. Miller OI, Celermajer DS, Deanfield JE, et al: Very-low-dose inhaled nitric oxide: A selective pulmonary vasodilator after operations for congenital heart disease. *J Thorac Cardiovasc Surg* 1994; **108:**487–494.

39. Wessel DL, Adatia I, Giglia TM, et al: Use of inhaled nitric oxide and acetycholine in the evaluation of pulmonary hypertension and endothelial function after cardiopulmonary bypass. *Circulation* 1993; **88:**2128–2138.

40. Girard C, Neidecker J, Laroux MC, et al: Inhaled nitric oxide in pulmonary hypertension after total repair of total anomalous pulmonary venous return. *J Thorac Cardiovasc Surg* 1993; **106:**369.

41. Okamoto K, Sato T, Kurose M, et al: Successful use of inhaled nitric oxide for treatment of severe hypoxemia in an infant with total anomalous pulmonary venous return. *Anesthesiology* 1994; **81:**256–259.

42. Morris GN, Lowson SM, Rich GF: Transient effects of inhaled nitric oxide for prolonged postoperative treatment of hypoxemia after surgical correction of total anomalous pulmonary venous return. *J Cardiothorac Vasc Anesth* 1995; **9:**713–716.

43. Sellden H, Winberg P, Gustafsson LE, et al: Inhalation of nitric oxide reduced pulmonary hypertension after cardiac surgery in a 3.2-kg infant. *Anesthesiology* 1993; **78:**577–580.

44. Journois D, Pouard P, Mauriat P, et al: Inhaled nitric oxide as a therapy for pulmonary hypertension after operations for congenital heart defects. *J Thorac Cardiovasc Surg* 1994; **107:**1129–1135.

45. Roberts JD, Polander DM, Lang P, et al: Inhaled nitric oxide in persistent pulmonary hypertension of the newborn. *Lancet* 1992; **340:**818–819.

46. Kinsella JP, Neish SR, Sheffer E, et al: Low-dose inhalational nitric oxide in persistent pulmonary hypertension of the newborn. *Lancet* 1992; **340:**819–820.

47. Zwissler B, Rank N, Jaenicke U, et al: Selective pulmonary vasodilatation by inhaled prostacyclin in a newborn with congenital heart disease and cardiopulmonary bypass. *Anesthesiology* 1995; **82:**1512–1516.

48. Pappert D, Busch T, Gerlach H, et al: Aerosolized prostacyclin versus inhaled nitric oxide in children with severe respiratory distress syndrome. *Anesthesiology* 1995; **82:**1507–1511.

49. Hickey PR, Hansen DD, Wessel D: Blunting of the stress response in the pulmonary circulation of infants by fentanyl. *Anesth Analg* 1985; **64:**1137–1142.

50. Greenwood RD, Rosenthal A, Parisi L, et al: Extracardiac abnormalities in infants with congenital heart disease. *Pediatrics* 1975; **55:**485–492.

51. Alswang M, Friesen RH, Bangert P: Effect of preanesthetic medication on carbon dioxide tension in children with congenital heart disease. *J Cardiothorac Vasc Anesth* 1994; **8:**415–419.

52. Laishley RS, Burrows FA, Lerman J, Roy WL: Effect of anesthetic induction regimes on oxygen saturation in cyanotic congenital heart disease. *Anesthesiology* 1986; **65:**673–677.

53. Greeley WJ, Bushman GA, Davis DP, Reves JG: Comparative effects of halothane and ketamine on systemic arterial oxygen saturation in children with cyanotic heart disease. *Anesthesiology* 1986; **65:**666–668.

54. Hensley FA, Larach DR, Martin DE, et al: The effect of halothane/nitrous oxide/oxygen mask induction on arterial hemoglobin saturation in cyanotic heart disease. *J Cardiothorac Anesth* 1987; **1:**289–296.

55. Hickey PR, Hansen DD, Cramolini GM, et al: Pulmonary and systemic hemodynamic responses to ketamine in infants with normal and elevated pulmonary vascular resistance. *Anesthesiology* 1985; **62:**287–293.

56. Bini M, Reves JG, Berry D, et al: Ejection fraction during ketamine anesthesia in congenital heart disease. *Anesth Analg* 1984; **63:**S186.

57. Faithfull NS, Haider R: Ketamine for cardiac catheterization: An evaluation of its use in children. *Anaesthesia* 1971; **26:**318–323.

58. Coppel DL, Dundee JW: Ketamine anesthesia for cardiac catheterization. *Anaesthesia* 1972; **27:**25–31.

59. Hickey PR, Hansen DD, Wessel DL: Pulmonary and systemic responses to fentanyl in infants. *Anesth Analg* 1985; **64:**483–486.

60. Moore RA, Yang SS, McNicholas KW, et al: Hemodynamic and anesthetic effects of sufentanil as the sole anesthetic for pediatric cardiovascular surgery. *Anesthesiology* 1985; **62:**725-731.

61. Davis PJ, Cook DR, Stiller RL, Davin-Robinson KA: Pharmacodynamics and pharmacokinetics of high-dose sufentanil in infants and children undergoing cardiac surgery. *Anesth Analg* 1987; **66:**203-208.

62. Hickey PR, Hansen DD: Fentanyl- and sufentanil-oxygen-pancuronium anesthesia for cardiac surgery in infants. *Anesth Analg* 1984; **63:**117-124.

63. Anand KJS, Hickey PR: Halothane-morphine compared with high dose sufentanil for anesthesia and postoperative analgesia in neonatal cardiac surgery. *N Engl J Med* 1992; **326:**1-9.

64. Schulte Sasse U, Hess W, Tarnow J: Pulmonary vascular responses to nitrous oxide in patients with normal and high pulmonary vascular resistance. *Anesthesiology* 1985; **57:**9-13.

65. Hickey PR, Hansen DD, Strafford M, et al: Pulmonary and systemic effects of nitrous oxide in infants with normal and elevated pulmonary vascular resistance. *Anesthesiology* 1986; **65:**374-378.

66. Barash PG, Glanz S, Katz JD, et al: Ventricular function in children during halothane anesthesia: An echocardiographic evaluation. *Anesthesiology* 1978; **49:**79-85.

67. Wolf WJ, Neal MB, Peterson MD: The hemodynamic and cardiovascular effects of isoflurane and halothane anesthesia in children. *Anesthesiology* 1986; **64:**328-333.

68. Glenski JA, Friesen RH, Berglund NL, et al: Comparison of the hemodynamic and echocardiographic effects of sufentanil, fentanyl, isoflurane, and halothane for pediatric cardiovascular surgery. *J Cardiothorac Anesth* 1988; **2:**147-155.

69. Wear R, Robinson S, Gregory GA: The effect of halothane on the baroresponse of adult and baby rabbits. *Anesthesiology* 1982; **56:**188-196.

70. Lerman J, Robinson S, Willis MM, Gregory GA: Anesthetic requirement for halothane in young children 0-1 month and 1-6 months of age. *Anesthesiology* 1983; **59:**421-424.

71. Friesen RH, Lichtor JL: Cardiovascular depression during halothane anesthesia in infants: A study of three induction techniques. *Anesth Analg* 1982; **61:**42-45.

72. Friesen RH, Lichtor JL: Cardiovascular effects of inhalation induction with isoflurane in infants. *Anesth Analg* 1983; **62:**411-414.

73. Friesen RH, Henry DB: Cardiovascular changes in preterm neonates receiving isoflurane, halothane, fentanyl, and ketamine. *Anesthesiology* 1986; **64:**238-242.

74. Murat I, Lapeyre G, Saint-Maurice C: Isoflurane attenuates baroreflex control of heart rate in human neonates. *Anesthesiology* 1989; **70:**395-400.

75. Rao CC, Boyer MS, Krishna G, Paradise RR: Increased sensitivity of the isometric contraction of the neonatal isolated rat atrial to halothane, isoflurane, and enflurane. *Anesthesiology* 1986; **64:**13-18.

76. Fisher DM, Robinson S, Brett CM, et al: Comparison of enflurane, halothane, and isoflurane for diagnostic and therapeutic procedures in children with malignancies. *Anesthesiology* 1985; **63:**647-650.

77. Morgan P, Lynn AM, Parrot C, Morray JP: Hemodynamic and metabolic effects of two anesthetic techniques in children undergoing surgical repair of acyanotic congenital heart disease. *Anesth Analg* 1987; **66:**1028-1030.

78. Smiley RM: An overview of induction and emergence characteristics of desflurane in pediatric, adult, and geriatric patients. *Anesth Analg* 1992; **75:**S38-S46.

79. Warltier DC, Pagel PS: Cardiovascular and respiratory actions of desflurane: Is desflurane different from isoflurane? *Anesth Analg* 1992; **75:**S17-S31.

80. Ebert TJ, Harkin CP, Muzi M: Cardiovascular responses to sevoflurane: A review. *Anesth Analg* 1995; **81:**S11-S22.

81. Lerman J: Sevoflurane in pediatric anesthesia. *Anesth Analg* 1995; **81:**S4-S10.

82. Holzman RS, van der Velde ME, Kaus SJ, et al: Sevoflurane depresses myocardial contractility less than halothane during induction of anesthesia in children. *Anesthesiology* 1996; **85:**1260-1267.

83. Cabal LA, Siassa B, Artal R: Cardiovascular and catecholamine changes after administration of pancuronium in distressed neonates. *Pediatrics* 1985; **75:**284-287.

84. Woelfel SK, Brandom BW, Cook R, et al: Effects of bolus administration of ORG-9426 in children during nitrous oxide-halothane anesthesia. *Anesthesiology* 1992; **76:**939-942.

85. Scheiber G, Ribeiro FC, Marichal A, et al: Intubating conditions and onset of action after rocuronium, vecuronium, and atracurium in young children. *Anesth Analg* 1996; **83:**320-324.

86. Vuksanaj D, Fisher DM: Pharmacokinetics of rocuronium in children aged 4-11 years. *Anesthesiology* 1995; **82:**1104-1110.

87. Goudsouzian NG, Ryan JF, Savarese JJ: The neuromuscular effects of pancuronium in infants and children. *Anesthesiology* 1974; **41:**95-98.

88. Fisher DM, Miller RD: Neuromuscular effects of vecuronium (ORG NC45) in infants and children during N_2O, halothane anesthesia. *Anesthesiology* 1983; **58:**519-523.

89. Nussbaum J, Zane EA, Thys DM: Esmolol for treatment of hypercyanotic spells in infants with tetralogy of Fallot. *J Cardiothorac Anesth* 1989; **3:**200-202.

90. Vlad P: Tricuspid atresia, in Keith JD, Rowe RD, Vlad P (eds): *Heart Disease in Infancy and Childhood.* 3rd ed. New York, Macmillan, 1978, pp 518-541.

91. Glenn WWL, Ordway NK, Talner NS, Call BP: Circulatory bypass of the right side of the heart: VI. Shunt between superior vena cava and distal right pulmonary artery. Report of clinical application to 38 cases. *Circulation* 1965; **31:**172-189.

92. Casthely PA, Redko V, Dluzneski J, et al: Pulse oximetry during pulmonary artery banding. *J Cardiothorac Anesth* 1987; **1:**297-299.

93. Rashkind WJ, Miller WW: Creation of an atrial septal defect with thoracotomy: A palliative approach to complete transposition of the great vessels. *JAMA* 1966; **196:**991-992.

94. Park SC, Neches WH, Zuberbuhler JR, et al: Clinical use of blade atrial septostomy. *Circulation* 1978; **58:**600-608.

95. Fontan F, Baudet E: Surgical repair of tricuspid atresia. *Thorax* 1971; **26:**240-248.

96. Norwood WI, Jacobs ML, Murphy JD: Fontan procedure for hypoplastic left heart syndrome. *Ann Thorac Surg* 1992; **54:**1025-1030.

97. Chang AC, Hanley FL, Wernovsky G, et al: Early bidirectional cavopulmonary shunt in young infants. Postoperative course and early results. *Circulation* 1993; **88:**149-158.

98. Jacobs ML, Rychik J, Rome JJ, et al: Early reduction of the volume work of the single ventricle: The hemi-Fontan procedure. *Ann Thorac Surg* 1996; **62:**456-462.

99. Srivastava D, Preminger T, Lock JE, et al: Hepatic venous blood and the development of pulmonary arteriovenous malformations in congenital heart disease. *Circulation* 1995; **92:**1217-1222.

100. Bridges ND, Lock JE, Castenada AR: Baffle fenestration with subsequent transcatheter closure. Modification of the Fontan operation for patients at increased risk. *Circulation* 1990; **82:**1681-1689.

101. Laks H, Pearl JM, Haas GS, et al: Partial Fontan: Advantages of an adjustable intertrial communication. *Ann Thorac Surg* 1991; **52:**1084-1095.

102. Knott-Craig CJ, Schaff H, Puga FJ, et al: Therapeutic implications of intraoperative pressure measurements after the Fontan operation. *Ann Thorac Surg* 1994; **57:**937-940.

103. Collett RW, Edwards JE: Persistent truncus arteriosus: A classification according to anatomic types. *Surg Clin North Am* 1949; **29:**1245-1270.

104. Calder L, Van Praagh R, Van Praagh S, et al: Truncus arteriosus communis: Clinical, angiographic and pathologic findings in 100 patients. *Am Heart J* 1976; **92:**23-38.

105. Hawkins JA, Clark EB, Doty DB: Total anomalous pulmonary venous connection. *Ann Thorac Surg* 1983; **36:**548-560.

106. Rowe RD, Freedom RM, Mehrizi A, Bloom KB: *The Neonate with Congenital Heart Disease.* 3rd ed. Philadelphia, WB Saunders, 1981, pp 328-349.

107. Van Praagh R, Ando M, Van Praagh S, Senno A: Pulmonary atresia: Anatomic considerations, in Kidd BS, Rowe RD (eds): *The Child with Congenital Heart Disease after Surgery.* Mt. Kisko, NY, Futura, 1976, pp 103-134.

108. O'Connor WN, Cottrill CM, Johnson GL, et al: Pulmonary atresia with intact ventricular septum and ventriculocoronary communications: Surgical significance. *Circulation* 1982; **65:**805-809.

109. Coles JG, Freedom RM, Lightfoot NE, et al: Long-term results in neonates with pulmonary atresia and intact ventricular septum. *Ann Thorac Surg* 1989; **47:**213-217.

110. Lewis AB, Wells W, Lindesmith GC: Evaluation and treatment of pulmonary atresia with intact ventricular septum in infancy. *Circulation* 1983; **67:**1318-1323.

111. Zeimer G, Jonas RA, Perry SB, et al: Surgery for coarctation of the aorta in the neonate. *Circulation* 1986; **74**(suppl 1):25-31.

112. Del Nido PJ, Williams WG, Wilson GJ, et al: Synthetic patch angioplasty for repair of coarctation of the aorta: Experience with aneurysm formation. *Circulation* 1986; **74**(suppl 1):31-36.

113. Gross RE: Coarctation of the aorta. Surgical treatment of 100 cases. *Circulation* 1950; **1:**41-55.

114. Symbas PN, Pfaender LM, Drucker MH: Cross-clamping of the descending aorta. *J Thorac Cardiovasc Surg* 1983; **85:**300-305.

115. Brewer LA, Fusberg RG, Mulder GA: Spinal cord complications following surgery for coarctation of the aorta. A study of 66 cases. *J Thorac Cardiovasc Surg* 1972; **64:**368-381.

116. Krieger KH, Spence FC: Is paraplegia after repair of coarctation of the aorta due principally to distal hypoperfusion during aortic cross-clamping? *Surgery* 1985; **97:**2-6.

117. Crawford FA, Sade RM: Spinal cord injury associated with hyperthermia during coarctation repair. *J Thorac Cardiovasc Surg* 1984; **87:**616-618.

118. Hantler CB, Knight PR: Intracranial hypertension following cross-clamping of the thoracic aorta. *Anesthesiology* 1982; **56:**146-147.

119. D'Ambra MN, Dewhurst W, Jacobs M, et al: Cross-clamping the thoracic aorta. Effect on intracranial pressure. *Circulation* 1988; **78**(suppl 3):198-202.

120. Nugent M, Kaye MP, McGoon DC: Effects of nitroprusside on aortic and intraspinal pressures during thoracic aortic crossclamping. *Anesthesiology* 1984; **61:**A68.

121. Benedict CR, Graham-Smith DG, Fisher A: Changes in plasma catecholamines and dopamine beta hydroxylase after corrective surgery for coarctation of the aorta. *Circulation* 1977; **57:**598-602.

122. Rocchini AP, Rosenthal A, Barger AC, et al: Pathogenesis of paradoxical hypertension after coarctation resection. *Circulation* 1976; **54:**382-387.

123. Hansen DD, Hickey PR: Anesthesia for hypoplastic left heart syndrome: Use of high dose fentanyl in 30 neonates. *Anesth Analg* 1986; **65:**127-132.

124. Norwood WI, Lang P, Hansen DD: Physiologic repair of aortic atresia-hypoplastic left heart syndrome. *N Engl J Med* 1983; **308:**23-26.

125. Jobes DR, Nicoloson SC, Steven JM, et al: Carbon dioxide prevents pulmonary overcirculation in hypoplastic left heart syndrome. *Ann Thorac Surg* 1992; **54:**150-151.

126. Paul MH: Complete transposition of the great arteries, in Adams FH, Emmanoulides GC, Riemenschneider TA (eds): *Moss' Heart Disease in Infants, Children, and Adolescents.* Baltimore, Williams & Wilkins, 1989, pp 371-423.

127. Castaneda AR, Mayer JE: Neonatal repair of transposition of the great arteries, in Long WA (ed): *Fetal and Neonatal Cardiology.* Philadelphia, WB Saunders, 1990, pp 789-795.

128. Aziz KU, Paul MH, Idriss FS, et al: Clinical manifestations of dynamic left ventricular outflow tract stenosis with D-transposition of the great arteries with intact ventricular septum. *Am J Cardiol* 1979; **44:**290-297.

129. Aziz KL, Paul MH, Rowe RD: Bronchopulmonary circulation in D-transposition of the great arteries: Possible role in genesis of accelerated pulmonary vascular disease. *Am J Cardiol* 1977; **39:**432-438.

130. Mair DG, Ritter DD: Factors influencing intercirculatory mixing in patients with complete transposition of the great arteries. *Am J Cardiol* 1972; **30:**653-658.

131. Mair DD, Ritter DG: Factors influencing systemic arterial oxygen saturation in complete transposition of the great arteries. *Am J Cardiol* 1973; **31:**742-748.

132. Mustard WT: Two stage correction of transposition of the great vessels. *Surgery* 1964; **55:**469-472.

133. Okuda H, Nakazama M, Imai Y: Comparison of ventricular function after Senning and Jantene procedures for complete transposition of the great arteries. *Am J Cardiol* 1985; **55:**530-534.

134. Peterson RJ, Franch RH, Fajman WA, Jones RH. Comparison of cardiac function in surgically corrected and congenitally corrected transposition of the great arteries. *J Thorac Cardiovasc Surg* 1988; **96:**227-236.

135. Bink-Boelkens MTE, Velvis H, Homan vander Heide JJ: Dysrhythmias after atrial surgery in children. *Am Heart J* 1983; **106:**125-130.

136. Senning A: Surgical correction of transposition of the great vessels. *Surgery* 1959; **45:**966-980.

137. Jatene AD, Fontes VF, Paulista PP, et al: Anatomic correction of transposition of the great vessels. *J Thorac Cardiovasc Surg* 1976; **72:**364-370.

138. Yacoub MH, Radley-Smith R: Anatomy of the coronary arteries in transposition of the great arteries and methods for their transfer in anatomical correction. *Thorax* 1978; **33:**418-424.

139. Mayer JE, Sanders SP, Jonas RA, et al: Coronary artery pattern and outcome of the arterial switch operation for transposition of the great arteries. *Circulation* 1990; **82**(suppl 5):139-145.

140. Bove EL, Beekman RH, Snider AR, et al: Arterial repair for transposition of the great arteries and large ventricular septal defect in early infancy. *Circulation* 1988; **78**(suppl 3):26-31.

141. Bano-Rodrigo A, Quero-Jimenez M, Moreno-Granado F, Gamallo-Amat C: Wall thickness of ventricular chambers in transposition of the great arteries: Surgical implications. *J Thorac Cardiovasc Surg* 1980; **79:**592-597.

142. Danford D, Huhta J, Gutgesell H: Left ventricular wall stress and thickness in complete transposition of the great arteries: Implications for surgical intervention. *J Thorac Cardiovasc Surg* 1985; **89:**610-615.

143. Yacoub MH, Radley-Smith R, MacLaurin R: Two-stage operation for anatomical correction of transposition of the great arteries with intact ventricular septum. *Lancet* 1977; **1:**1275-1278.

144. Ilbawi MN, Idriss FS, DeLeon SY, et al: Preparation of the left ventricle for anatomical correction in patients with simple transposition of the great arteries. *J Thorac Cardiovasc Surg* 1987; **94:**87-94.

145. Boutin C, Wernosky G, Sanders S, et al: Rapid two-stage arterial switch operation. Evaluation of left ventricular systolic mechanics late after an acute pressure overload stimulus in infancy. *Circulation* 1994; **90:**1294-1303.

146. Boutin C, Jonas RA, Sanders SP, et al: Rapid two-staged arterial switch operation. Acquisition of left ventricular mass after pulmonary artery banding in infants with transposition of the great arteries. *Circulation* 1994; **90:**1304–1309.

147. Idriss FS, DeLeon SY, Nikaidoh H, et al: Resection of left ventricular outflow obstruction in d-transposition of the great arteries. *J Thorac Cardiovasc Surg* 1977; **74:**343–351.

148. Yacoub MH, Arensman FW, Keck E, Radley-Smith R: Fate of dynamic left ventricular arteries. *Circulation* 1983; **68**(suppl 2): 56–62.

149. Rastelli GC, McGoon DC, Wallace RB: Anatomic correction of transposition of the great arteries with ventricular septal defect and subpulmonary stenosis. *J Thorac Cardiovasc Surg* 1969; **58:**545–552.

150. Ruckman RN, Van Praagh R: Anatomic types of congenital mitral stenosis: Report of 49 autopsy cases with diagnostic and surgical implications. *Am J Cardiol* 1978; **42:**592–601.

151. Ho SY, Anderson RH: The morphology of the aortic valve with regard to congenital malformations, in Dunn JM (ed): *Cardiac Valve Disease in Children.* New York, Elsevier, 1988, pp 3–21.

152. Konno S, Imai Y, Iida Y, et al: New method for prosthetic valve replacement in congenital aortic stenosis associated with hypoplasia of the aortic valve ring. *J Thorac Cardiovasc Surg* 1975; **70:**909–917.

153. Brown JW, Girod DA, Hurwitz RA, Caldwell RL: Apicoaortic conduits for complex left ventricular outflow obstruction in children, in Dunn JM (ed): *Cardiac Valve Disease in Children.* New York, Elsevier, 1988, pp 60–77.

7

Anesthesia for Heart, Heart–Lung, and Lung Transplantation

James A. DiNardo

■ HEART TRANSPLANTATION

Cardiac transplantation can be considered for patients with end-stage cardiac dysfunction that is unresponsive to maximal medical therapy for which no surgical options exist except cardiac replacement. Most adult patients are New York Heart Association (NYHA) functional class IV (symptoms at rest). These patients have an expected 1-year survival of approximately 50 to 60% with optimal medical therapy.[1] A subgroup of ambulatory NYHA functional class III patients (symptoms with limited exertion) with an impairment of exercise tolerance (VO_2max < 14 mL/kg/min) predictive of reduced 1-year survival also can be considered for transplantation.[2]

For infants and children, the natural history of end-stage cardiac dysfunction is not as well delineated; 6-year survival ranges from 20 to 84%.[1] In addition, end-stage cardiac dysfunction is more difficult to define. Growth failure secondary to severe cardiac dysfunction is useful in identifying end-stage disease. Progressive pulmonary hypertension, which could preclude transplantation at a later date, also is considered an important indication for transplantation.

Ninety percent of adult patients presenting for cardiac transplantation have either a dilated cardiomyopathy (DCM) or an ischemic cardiomyopathy.[3] Less commonly, patients with end-stage valvular heart disease or with intractable, life-threatening arrhythmias not amenable to medical therapy or insertion of an im-

planted cardioverter defibrillator (ICD) are transplanted. Cardiac transplantation also has been used for unresectable cardiac tumors,[4] sarcoidosis, amyloidosis, active myocarditis, hypertrophic cardiomyopathies, and refractory angina not amenable to angioplasty or surgical revascularization. Enthusiasm regarding heart transplantation for patients with amyloidosis and sarcoidosis is tempered by evidence that systemic progression of these diseases may limit the long-term effectiveness of heart transplantation.[5,6] Enthusiasm regarding heart transplantation for patients with acute myocarditis is tempered by evidence that mortality and rejection rates may be higher in these patients.[7]

DCM and complex congenital heart disease represent the two major indications for heart transplantation for pediatric patients.[1] In patients younger than 1 year of age, 78% of transplants are for congenital heart disease, primarily hypoplastic left heart syndrome (HLHS). In patients between 1 and 5 years of age, the indications for heart transplantation are divided equally between congenital heart disease and DCM. Most children requiring transplantation for congenital lesions in this age group have had at least one palliative or definite prior cardiac surgical procedure. In patients between 6 and 18 years of age, the primary indication (63%) for heart transplantation is DCM.

Contraindications to heart transplantation are outlined in Table 7–1. They represent medical conditions that have been demonstrated to or are suspected to re-

TABLE 7–1. RECIPIENT SELECTION CRITERIA FOR HEART AND LUNG TRANSPLANTATION[30]

Absolute contraindications

1. History of emotional instability, medical noncompliance, or active substance abuse
2. Fixed pulmonary hypertension (only for cardiac transplantation, not for heart–lung or lung transplantation)
3. Significant cerebral vascular disease
4. Active malignancy or life-limiting coexistent disease

Relative contraindications

1. Physiological age older than 60 years
2. Significant peripheral vascular disease
3. Active peptic ulcer or diverticular disease
4. Severe bronchitis or chronic obstructive pulmonary disease (only for cardiac transplantation, not for heart–lung or lung transplantation)
5. Morbid obesity
6. Disease likely to recur in allograft (such as sarcoid or amyloid for cardiac allografts)
7. Irreversible hepatic or renal dysfunction
8. Recent pulmonary embolus associated with pulmonary infarction (only for cardiac transplantation, not for heart–lung or lung transplantation)
9. Immunologic sensitization to donor antigens
10. Severe osteoporosis
11. Active infection
12. Diabetes with end-organ dysfunction

duce long-term functional recovery or survival. Severe osteoporosis, active peptic ulcer or diverticular disease, active infection, and morbid obesity all are conditions that are likely to be worsened by the necessity of a lifelong immunosuppressive regiment including steroids. Corticosteroids also complicate the management of blood sugars for patients with diabetes, who are at increased risk of survival-reducing vascular complications.[8] Nonetheless, carefully selected patients with diabetes without end-organ dysfunction have been shown to have 2- to 4-year survival similar to nondiabetics.[9] Chronic lung disease identified as a FEV < 50% predicted, a $FEV_1 < 1$ L, and a FEV_1:FVC ratio < 1 is believed to predispose postoperative respiratory failure, reduced survival from lung disease alone, and an increased risk of infection on immunosuppression.[1] Survival is favorable for elderly patients (> 55 years of age), but careful selection is necessary, particularly for patients older than 65 years of age, because they are at increased risk for infectious and steroid complications.[10]

■ DILATED CARDIOMYOPATHY

Dilated cardiomyopathies (DCMs) commonly are classified as either idiopathic or secondary. In secondary dilated cardiomyopathies, a variety of etiological factors, both acquired and hereditary, seem to cause or at least predispose development of a cardiomyopathy.[11] Some secondary DCMs are potentially reversible. Toxins (including alcohol and cocaine), pregnancy, infectious agents (including CMV and toxoplasmosis), and metabolic abnormalities (including thiamine deficiency and hypo- and hyperthyroidism) all have been identified as potentially reversible forms of secondary DCM.[12] Idiopathic cardiomyopathy is not reversible because no clear etiological factors have been identified. Familial and genetic factors, viral and other cyotoxic insults, immune abnormalities, and metabolic, energetic, and contraction abnormalities all have been investigated to determine the pathogenesis of idiopathic DCM. It is likely that several factors interact to cause disease in susceptible patients. This topic is discussed in depth elsewhere.[11,12]

Ischemic cardiomyopathy is considered a separate entity from DCM. However, histologically and functionally, an ischemic cardiomyopathy is indistinguishable from the various forms of DCM, except for the presence of atheromatous disease and areas of previous infarction seen in ischemic cardiomyopathies. For the sake of discussion here, all three entities (idiopathic, secondary, and ischemic) will be considered as DCM.

Management of adults and children with DCM presenting for heart transplantation will be covered in this chapter. Management of children with HLHS and other congenital lesions presenting for heart transplantation is discussed in Chapter 6.

Pathophysiology and Adaptation

Regardless of the initiating cause, the alterations in ventricular function in DCM are remarkably consistent (see Fig. 7–1). Biventricular dysfunction is common in idiopathic and secondary DCM. In ischemic cardiomyopathy, dysfunction may be limited to the left ventricle. Loss of myocardial tissue, as occurs with infarction or from direct myocardial damage, results in overload and subsequent hypertrophy of the remaining active myocardium.[13] For the postinfarction patient, this process has come to be known as ventricular remodeling.[14,15] Hypertrophy of active myocardium serves to reduce wall stress and energy consumption. However, the process of hypertrophy results in changes that adversely affect myocardial energy balance and ultimately produces progressive myocardial dysfunction. Increases in capillary density do not keep pace with replication of sarcomeres, and the distance between capillaries increases, resulting in poor substrate delivery to hypertrophied myocardium. In addition, the process of hypertrophy increases the cellular ratio of myofibrils to mitochondria, creating the potential for oxygen imbalance at the cellular level. Eventually, myocardial necrosis results in replacement of myocardium with connective tissue. This produces progressive impairment of contractility, which in turn, stimulates further

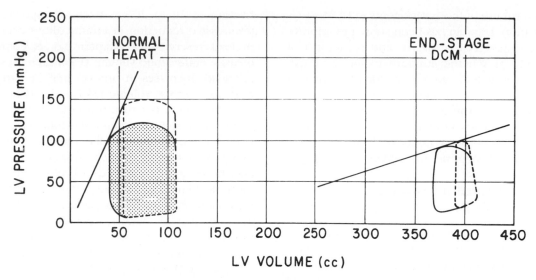

FIGURE 7–1. Pressure–volume (PV) loops from a normal heart and a dilated cardiomyopathy (DCM) heart. The DCM heart is dilated, has depressed systolic function, has reduced stroke volume at rest, and is prone to afterload mismatch. Stroke volume at rest for each heart is represented by the solid PV loop. Stroke volume after an increase in afterload with preload and contractility held constant is represented by the dotted PV loop. Note the marked decrease in stroke volume in the DCM as compared with the normal heart with comparable increases in afterload.

hypertrophy and progression of myocardial necrosis. Ventricular dilatation occurs as the result of this progressive replacement of myocardium with connective tissue and as a result of the eccentric hypertrophy (*see* Chapter 5) in the surviving myocardium.

Metabolic down-regulation and uncoupling of cardiac beta receptors is a common feature in DCM. Norepinephrine (NE) secretion is enhanced in patients with low-output cardiac failure with the degree of elevation paralleling the severity of the failure.[16] Serum NE levels may be two to three times normal due to enhanced release and reduced reuptake of NE by adrenergic terminals. There are reduced concentrations of NE in the atrial and ventricular tissue of failing hearts with the degree of depletion paralleling the reduction in ejection fraction.[16] The consequence of prolonged elevation of NE is gradual down-regulation (reduction in receptor density) of cardiac $beta_1$ receptors and partial uncoupling of cardiac $beta_1$ receptors from adenylate cyclase.[17,18] Again, the extent of down-regulation and uncoupling parallels the degree of contractile impairment. Interestingly, there is a greater decrease in the density of $beta_1$-adrenergic receptors in patients with idiopathic cardiomyopathy as compared with ischemic cardiomyopathy. This may be due to long-term adrenergic overstimulation or anti-beta-receptor antibodies in idiopathic cardiomyopathy.[18]

Uncoupling of $beta_1$ adrenoreceptors from the effector enzyme adenylate cyclase involves phosphorylation of the receptors by beta-adrenergic receptor kinase.[17] Progressive cardiac dysfunction also produces an increases in the ratio of the inhibitory guanine nu-

cleotide regulatory protein (G_i) to the stimulatory guanine nucleotide regulatory protein (G_s).[19] G_i inhibits and G_s stimulates adenylate cyclase. Uncoupling of $beta_1$ adrenoreceptors and an increased ratio of G_i: G_s both result in reduced levels of cyclic adenosine monophosphate (cAMP) and reduced movement of calcium into myocytes.

The consequence of down regulation of $beta_1$ receptors, uncoupling of $beta_1$ receptors, and an increased G_i:G_s ratio is an impaired ability of DCM hearts to produce cAMP. Therefore, the contractile response of the DCM heart to beta-adrenegeric receptor agonists (epinephrine, dopamine, dobutamine, isoproterenol, and norepinephrine) and phosphodiesterase inhibitors (amrinone, milrinone) is markedly impaired. The contractile response to raising intracellular calcium and to cardiac glycosides (digoxin) is retained. In addition, although the depletion of myocardial norepinephrine stores does not affect the intrinsic contractile function of the myocardium, it does result in an impaired contractile response to indirect-acting beta-adrenergic agonists such as ephedrine.

Considering that excessive sympathetic stimulation is a major pathophysiological factor in DCM, the use of beta-blocking agents in treatment is being investigated. Treatment with metoprolol has been demonstrated to improve quality of life and ventricular function but not survival in the only large multicenter trial to date.[20] Treatment with metoprolol also results in upregulation of beta receptors and improved contractile response to catecholamines.[21] Nonetheless, beta blockers remain an investigational drug for patients with DCM.

The long-term use of inotropic agents in DCM also is under investigation. Digoxin has been shown to improve ejection fraction, exercise capacity, and symptoms of heart failure in DCM. Whether it improves survival is currently being investigated. Long-term administration of other oral and intravenous inotropic agents has not proved as promising. Amrinone, milrinone, and enoxmone have not been shown to improve exercise capacity or symptoms and have been associated with increased cardiovascular mortality (primarily sudden death).[11,22]

Ventricular Diastolic Function and the Atrial Transport Mechanism

Impairment of ventricular relaxation (see Chapter 2) is seen in DCM. However, the marked reduction in chamber compliance that accompanies ventricular dilatation masks this pattern. Instead, the rapid equilibration of left atrial and ventricular end-diastolic pressures produces a restrictive mitral inflow pattern with abrupt premature closure of the mitral valve (see Chapter 3).[23] Progressive ventricular dilatation produces atrial enlargement due to the longstanding increase in atrial afterload produced by an elevated ventricular end-diastolic pressure. In many instances, the atria will be dilated, hypokinetic, and filled with spontaneous contrast on echocardiographic examination. In these patients, the contribution of atrial systole to ventricular filling will be minimal. As a consequence of these changes, patients with DCM require high mean atrial pressures to ensure adequate ventricular filling.

Myocardial Oxygen Balance

Obviously, in patients with an ischemic cardiomyopathy, myocardial oxygen balance will be altered for reasons discussed in detail in Chapter 4. However, myocardial blood flow abnormalities also are present in patients with DCM despite the presence of angiography normal coronary arteries. It has been proposed that functional small-vessel abnormalities due to either increased vascular tone or endothelial abnormalities account for decreased global baseline myocardial blood flow and impaired coronary reserve in DCM.[24] Regional perfusion defects also are seen in 45% of DCM hearts without demonstrable coronary lesions. Furthermore, myocardial ischemia (angina and ST segment depressions) has been detected in patients with DCM who are subjected to pacing-induced tachycardia and to coronary vasodilation from dipyridamole infusion.[24]

Left Ventricular Systolic Function

The hallmark of DCM is impaired contractile function with an ejection fraction < 45% required for diagnosis. When a patient presents for transplantation, an ejection fraction of 10 to 20% is likely. Compensation for the progressive reduction in contractility occurs by use of preload reserve (see Chapter 2). As contractility decreases, end-systolic volume (ESV) increases for a given afterload. Increases in preload initially can be used to normalize stroke volume (SV) under these conditions. Preload reserve is exhausted when the sacromeres are stretched to their maximum diastolic length. When this occurs, there will be no further augmentation of the velocity of shortening by increasing diastolic fiber length, and the ventricle behaves as if preload were fixed. For a given level of contractility, after preload reserve has been exhausted, additional increases in afterload will be accompanied by parallel decreases in stroke volume. This is defined as a state of afterload mismatch. Patients with end-stage DCM will have exhausted preload reserve and will exhibit afterload mismatch (see Fig. 7-1). In addition, patients with DCM have a fixed SV due to exhaustion of preload reserve and an inability to decrease ESV by increasing contractility.

Unfortunately, the result of this compensation process is progressive ventricular dilatation. Dilatation of the ventricle has several important consequences. As described in Chapter 5, ventricular dilatation can produce mitral insufficiency secondary to dilation and deformation of the valve annulus. This type of functional mitral insufficiency is common in DCM. Dilatation of the ventricle also results in elevated wall stress (wall stress = $[P \times r]/2h$) at the conclusion of isovolemic contraction. Because wall stress is synonymous with afterload (see Chapter 2), ventricular dilatation further compromises systolic function by producing increased afterload at a given systolic blood pressure.

Right Ventricular Function and the Pulmonary Vasculature

In instances in which DCM produces biventricular dysfunction, the right ventricle will exhibit the same alterations in systolic function, afterload sensitivity, and diastolic dysfunction described for the left ventricle. In addition, the prolonged elevations of left atrial pressure (LAP) seen in progressive DCM have profound effects on the pulmonary vasculature and right ventricular function. Early in the disease, elevated LAP is transmitted to the pulmonary venous system and there is reversible passive elevation of the pulmonary artery pressures while pulmonary vascular resistance (PVR) remains normal (see Fig. 5-7). Right ventricular function remains unchanged. As the disease progresses, reactive changes occur in the pulmonary vasculature. Prolonged perivascular edema results in arterial intima fibroelastosis and nonreversible elevations in PVR due to obliterative changes in the distal pulmonary vasculature known as pulmonary vascular occlusive disease

(PVOD). Progression of this process presents an large increase in right ventricular afterload similar to that seen in severe mitral stenosis (*see* Fig. 5–7). Similar changes occur in infants and children, who develop PVOD for reasons examined in detail in Chapter 6.

The RV is poorly adapted to generate pressures that approach systemic. As a result, afterload mismatch occurs, the RV invariably fails, and RV output falls. Peripheral edema and hepatic congestion ensue. Right ventricular failure and dilation also may lead to functional tricuspid regurgitation and worsening symptoms of right heart failure. In the steady state, RV output and LV output must be equal. Therefore, LV output also is limited by RV failure.

Increased, fixed PVR remains an absolute contraindication to heart transplantation (Table 7-1). When the postischemic donor right ventricle is acutely exposed to the elevated PVR of the recipient, severe right heart failure develops secondary to afterload mismatch. PVR in excess of 5 Wood units (mean peak [PAP] – mean [PAOP])/cardiac output) and transpulmonary gradient (mean PAP – mean PAOP) in excess of 15 mm Hg both have been clearly associated with increased postoperative mortality in adults.[25,26] In children, a PVRI in excess of 6 to 7 Wood units/m² and a transpulmonary gradient > 15 mm Hg have been associated with increased postoperative mortality.[25,27-29] Patients with a PVR > 4 Wood units or a pulmonary vascular resistance index (PVRI) > 6 Wood units/m² usually are evaluated for a reversible component.[30] It has been demonstrated that adults in whom PVR can be reduced using nitroprusside or prostaglandin E₁ to < 2.5 Wood units while maintaining a systolic blood pressure > 85 mm Hg have a postoperative mortality similar to patients with a resting PVR < 2.5 Wood units.[31] Most adult transplant centers believe that a PVR < 5 Wood units after drug therapy presents an acceptable risk.[32] In infants and children, the threshold is less clear. Some centers consider a PVRI < 4 to 6 Wood units/m² and a transpulmonary gradient < 15 mm Hg with inotropes, oxygen, nitroprusside, or prostaglandin E₁ testing a necessity,[28,29] whereas others will accept a PVRI of 7 to 8 Wood units/m².[33]

Effect of Heart-Rate Alterations on Hemodynamics

Patients with DCM have a fixed SV and, as a result, are dependent on maintenance of their baseline heart rate to maintain cardiac output. With exhausted preload reserve, reductions in heart rate will not be accompanied by increases in SV as seen in the normal heart. Therefore, reductions in heart rate will be accompanied by cardiac output decreases. Heart-rate increases will reduce diastolic filling time and will reduce end-diastolic volume (EDV) and SV. Heart-rate increases generally will

result in no change in cardiac output because the reduction in SV will be offset by the increase in heart rate. Elevations in right and left atrial pressures by volume infusion to compensate for reduced diastolic filling time are not practical because they will increase systemic and pulmonary venous congestion. For patients with an ischemic DCM, heart-rate increases may exacerbate myocardial ischemia (*see* Chapter 4).

Effect of Afterload Alterations on Hemodynamics

As discussed in Chapter 2, reduced contractility is represented by a linear left ventricular pressure–volume relationship that is shifted downward and to the right and that has a less positive slope. As the result of impaired contractile function patients with DCM have enhanced sensitivity to afterload (*see* Fig. 7–1). Small increases in afterload result in comparatively large increases in ESV. For a given EDV, this results in a large reduction in SV. Conversely, afterload reduction with maintenance of EDV will produce concomitant increases in SV. This partly explains the unequivocal success of vasodilator therapy (the angiotensin-converting enzyme (ACE) inhibitor enalapril) in improving NYHA functional class and reducing mortality in patients with end-stage DCM.[34-36] Aggressive perioperative afterload reduction is difficult considering the low systolic blood pressure of most patients with DCM.

■ THE DONOR

The following guidelines are used to select donors after the diagnosis of irreversible brain death has been made. The diagnosis of brain death and preoperative management of the donor is discussed in detail elsewhere.[1]

1. Age less than 40 years — most centers will not accept female donors older than 45 years of age or male donors older than 40 years of age. Exceptions are made.
2. Absence of significant cardiac disease or trauma — donors with known cardiac disease or severe myocardial contusion from trauma are not acceptable. Severe myocardial contusion usually is identified by a history of blunt chest trauma, CPK MB elevations, and echocardiographic evidence of severe ventricular dysfunction. Patients who have suffered cardiac arrest are not necessarily excluded from consideration but are considered with reservations pending subsequent evaluation of function both clinically and echocardiographically. Generally, a desirable donor heart is maintained with less than 10 μg/kg/min of dopamine.

3. Low probability of coronary artery disease — coronary angiography is not commonly employed in evaluation of donors. However, as the age of acceptable donors increases, it may become more common.
4. No active severe infection or malignancy with the possibility of metastases — most extracranial malignancies disqualify a donor.
5. Negative serologies for human immunodeficiency virus or hepatitis B.
6. ABO compatibility and human lymphocyte antigen (HLA) screen — the donor and recipient must be ABO blood type compatible. HLA typing for cardiac transplantation is not routine. The recipient's blood is tested against a standard panel of blood cells containing a diverse human lymphocyte sample. This screen is called the percent reactive antibody (PRA) screen. If the PRA has 5 to 15% reactivity, most centers will proceed with transplantation based on ABO compatibility. If the PRA is greater than 15%, then a lymphocyte cross-match between donor and recipient blood must be performed. This is a time-consuming process because donor blood must be transported to the transplant center.
7. Appropriate donor size — for adult patients, the donor's body weight should be between 80 and 120% of the recipient's body weight. For adults, use of undersized hearts (donor/recipient weight ratio < 0.75) may be associated with increased mortality for patients receiving preoperative inotropes or with ventricular assist devices (VADs).[37] At the other extreme, use of oversized donor hearts (donor/recipient weight ratio > 1.25) may be associated with increased mortality.[38]

Size constraints for infants and children differ from adults. For infants, the weight of the donor should be no more than 2.5 times the weight of the recipient.[39] For recipient's older than 18 months of age, the body weight of the donor should not be more than 25 to 50% of the recipient's weight. Hearts transplanted into infants and children demonstrate normal cardiac chamber dimensional growth.[40,41]

Most centers prefer donors at the upper limits of size for their adult and pediatric patients with pulmonary hypertension, although data to support this practice are lacking.

■ ANESTHETIC MANAGEMENT

Goals

1. Avoid increases in afterload; afterload reduction can be attempted with caution, but EDV must be maintained.

2. Maintain preload.
3. Maintain or enhance contractility.
4. Maintain heart rate.
5. Avoid hypercarbia, hypoxemia, and acidemia, which tend to cause pulmonary hypertension and may result in acute RV decompensation.

Preoperative Evaluation

Preoperative evaluation is covered in detail in Chapters 1 and 6. Cardiac transplant patients typically undergo extensive medical evaluation. A summary of this evaluation is readily available to the anesthesiologist through the transplant coordinator. An example of a summary sheet is shown in Figure 7–2. Several unique management problems are common in patients with DCM. Use of aprotinin (*see* Chapter 10) should be considered for patients at risk for postoperative bleeding.

Ventricular Arrhythmias. More than 70% of DCM patients have asymptomatic, nonsustained ventricular tachycardia seen on ambulatory monitoring.[42] Antiarrhythmic therapy is problematic for these patients considering the negative inotropic and arrhythmogenic effects of many of the agents, the altered drug pharmacokinetics in heart failure, and the low efficacy of these agents for patients with severe LV dysfunction. In addition, although therapy can reduce ventricular arrhythmias and improve exercise tolerance and ventricular function, reduction in the incidence of sudden death is unproven.[11] An implanted cardioverter defibrillator (ICD) may be necessary for patients with symptomatic ventricular arrhythmias if medical therapy is not effective or cannot be tolerated.

Thromboembolic Phenomena. Patients with an ejection fraction less than 30% and patients with atrial fibrillation are particularly at risk for the formation of atrial and ventricular mural thrombi and subsequent systemic or pulmonary embolization.[43,44] In addition, patients with left ventricular aneurysms as the result of extensive prior infarction are also at higher risk for mural thrombus formation. Long-term oral anticoagulation, primarily with coumadin, is common for patients with DCM. This will complicate the management of hemostasis after termination of CPB.

Preoperative Mechanical Ventricular Support and the Total Artificial Heart. At present, the limiting factor in the number of patients who can be offered a heart transplant is the availability of donor hearts.[45] In the United States, it is estimated that although 40,000 patients per year could benefit from a heart transplant, only approximately 2,200 heart transplants are being performed per year. Furthermore, 20% of suitable transplant candidates die before a donor heart can be found.[46] As a result, mechanical assist de-

ORTHOTOPIC HEART TRANSPLANT EVALUATION REPORT
♥♥ THE UNIVERSITY OF ARIZONA HEALTH SCIENCES CENTER, TUCSON, AZ ♥♥

```
NAME:                    UMC HOSNUM:        AGE: 62   RACE: ---   FROM: Kern/Slepian      NYHA: Class IV

BLOOD TYPE: A-   AB: neg  DAT: neg  WT: 81.1 kg  HT: 182.0 cm  BP: 160/107  AP: 104  PREGNANCIES:  0  TRANSFUSIONS:  0

DIAGNOSIS: Coronary Artery Disease (Ischemic)              Coordinator:    Wild        S.S.:  798-78-86UM
HLA: A1 1  A2 3  B1 8  B2 35 BW1 -- BW2 -- DR1 -- DR2 --  CYTO SCREEN: 01-10-96 NEG
```

HX: A 61 year old male with ischemic cardiomyopathy, MI 7/95 (silent ischemia).

Sestamibi 10/95=Large perfusion defect apex and inferolateral, inferior and posterior septal walls. No evidence of stress-related myocardial ischemia.
Thallium 1/96=Significant perfusion to the anterolateral wall w/o evidence of significant redistribution.

```
MEDS: DYAZIDE     37.500/25/ PO SPIMURAN    200.000 PO QD
      LISINOPRIL  10.000 PO BID  MYCOSTATIN     5.000 PO TID
      NEORAL (Ge 125/100/ PO SPLITPREDNISONE  10/5/ PO SPLIT M
      RIOPAN      30.000 PO QID  ZANTAC       150.000 PO BID
```

CARD BX: Date: ------- RESULT: ---

CATH: Date: 08-04-95 RA: 7 RV: 55/ 7 PA: 53/ 20/ 30
  LV: ---/--- AO: ---/---/--- PCW: 20 CO: 4.75
  CI: --- SVR: --- PVR: 2.11 EF: --- CORONARIES: Abnormal
  Circ 100% occluded, LAD 73% after takeoff of first diagonal.

CHEST AND ABDOMEN CT SCAN: Date: 01-11-96
  Minimal bibasilar pleural thickening and minimal right basilar dependent atelectasis or edema. Minimal amount of ascities. Left renal cyst.

CHEST X-RAY: Date: 01-01-96 RESULT: Negative
  Cardiomegaly
DENTAL PANOREX/CONSULT: Date: 01-10-96 RESULT: Normal
  No infectious process. Some tempromandibular degenerative changes.
2D ECHO: Date: 01-03-96
  LVEF 10-20% mod dilated ischemic LV with motion defects Severe alteration of LVDP. Trace MR, TR and 1+ pulmonic insufficiency. RVEF 30-40%. Mild LA enlargement.

EKG: Date: 01-11-96 HR: 77 RHYTHM: NSR
  BLOCK: 1st Degree   ARRHYTHMIAS: None
  Anterolateral infarct

HOLTER: Date: 12-11-95 PVC's/HR: 147   PAC's/HR: ---
  MIN HR: 53 MAX HR: 112 MEAN HR: 70
  total 3285 VPB
MUGA SCAN: Date: 01-10-96 LVEF: 15%   RVEF: 17%

TREADMILL: Date: 01-11-96 EX: 5.09 min.sec METS: 3.00
  MVO2= 8.5 ml/kg/min.

VASCULAR STUDIES: Date: 01-11-96
  Minimal disease noted in the left prox. ICA.

HEMATOLOGY		
WBC	14.0	10-06-96
HGB	10.7	10-06-96
HCT	31.6	10-06-96
SEGS	84.0	10-06-96
BANDS	8.0	10-06-96
LYMPHS	6.0	10-06-96
MONOS	2.0	10-06-96
EOS	0.0	10-06-96
BASOS	0.0	10-06-96
PLT	184.0	10-02-96
RETIC	1.1	10-02-96

RENAL		
NA	142.0	10-06-96
K	3.5	10-06-96
CL	103.0	10-06-96
CO2	27.0	10-06-96
GLUC	102.0	10-06-96
BUN	18.0	10-06-96
CR	0.8	10-06-96
CA++	9.7	09-27-96
DIG	0.7	09-28-96
UR ACI	6.7	09-27-96
NOREPI	-----	--------

SKIN TESTS		
COCCI: 48hr --- 72hr ---	PPD : 48hr ---- 72hr ---	
MUMPS: 48hr --- 72hr ---	HIST: 48hr ---- 72hr ---	

LFT'S		
T. BILI	0.3	10-06-96
D. BILI	-----	--------
SGOT	34.0	10-06-96
SGPT	20.0	10-06-96
ALK PHOS	34.0	10-06-96
LDH	134.0	09-27-96
CK	1391.0	10-03-9
MB	122.9	10-03-96
CHOLEST	189.0	09-27-96
TRIGLY	148.0	09-27-96
HDL	49.0	08-28-96
LDL	139.0	06-05-96
ALBUMIN	4.0	09-27-96
T PROTE	7.7	09-27-96
AG RATIO	-----	--------

ABG'S 06-06-96	
%O2	21.00
PO2	73.00
SAT	94.60
PCO2	36.10
PH	7.46
HCO3	26.00

PFT'S 06-06-96		
FVC	2.60/	0.86%
PREDICTED	3.03	
FEV1	2.32/	0.92%
PREDICTED	2.50	

COAG'S		
PT	13.5	10-02-96
C PT	-----	--------
PTT	27.8	10-02-96
FSP	-----	--------
FIBRINO	-----	--------
ANTITH III	-----	--------
FACTOR X	-----	--------

URINE		
24HR CR CL	-----	--------
VOL	1908.0	06-06-9

UA		
PH	5.0	10-02-96
SP GR	1.0	10-02-96
PROTEIN	[<10]	10-02-96
GLUC	[NEG]	10-02-96
WBC'S	0.0	10-02-96
RBC'S	0.0	10-02-96
CAST	NONE	10-02-96

SEROLOGY		
HIV	06-05-96	NEG
AMYA	10-02-96	
ANA	10-02-96	[NEG],NOT DETECTED,TEST PERFORMED AT ARUP (ASSOCIATED REGIONAL,AND UNIVERSITY PATHLOGISTS,INC.);,DIRECTOR: RONALD L. WEISS,M.D.
CMV	10-02-96	REACTIVE BY ENZYME IMMUNOASSAY.,DONOR'S SERUM,TRANFUSION STATUS UNKNOWN
COCCI	10-02-96	
HEP BS	06-05-96	[NRE],NONREACTIVE BY ENZYME IMMUNOASSAY
HEP C	06-05-96	[NRE],NONREACTIVE BY ENZYME IMMUNOASSAY
HTLV1	06-05-96	SERUM
RUBELL	06-05-96	0.36

CULTURES		
BLOOD	10-02-96	FINAL 100796
RSP/AS	10-03-96	2+ MIXED FLORA
URINE	06-05-96	NO GROWTH 1 DAY
```

SOCIAL SERVICE:_____  PSYCH EVAL:_____  INSURANCE:_____
COMMENTS/ADDITIONAL CONSULTATIONS:_____

ACCEPT/REFUSE:_____

**FIGURE 7–2.** A typical transplant evaluation sheet for a patient awaiting heart transplantation. This patient has an ischemic cardiomyopathy. Similar data sheets exist for patients awaiting heart–lung and lung transplantation.
```

vices and the total artificial heart are being used as a bridge to cardiac transplantation until suitable donor hearts are found.[47-49] Management of patients with mechanical assist devices or total artificial heart presenting for transplantation will be discussed in Chapter 11.

Previous Cardiac Surgical Procedures. All patients who have undergone previous cardiac surgical procedures are likely to have prolonged dissection times and are at risk for bleeding. Adequate intravenous access is a necessity. All blood products must be cytomegalovirus (CMU) compatible and transfused through leukocyte filters.

Many patients with ischemic DCM will have undergone prior coronary artery bypass surgery. In addition, nicking or cutting of the existing extracardiac conduits (internal mammary arteries and reverse saphenous veins) can severely compromise myocardial perfusion. Likewise, surgical manipulation of these conduits may result in embolization of atherosclerotic plaques into the distal coronary vascular bed with subsequent transmural myocardial ischemia.[50,51] A determination of how much myocardium is supplied by the conduits that are patent can be made from the most recent catheterization report. Other patients will have undergone placement of an ICD via a sternotomy or thoracotomy.

Many children with congenital heart disease will have undergone prior procedures. Physical examination should include an evaluation of the limitations to vascular access and monitoring sites imposed by previous surgery and catheterizations. A child who has undergone a palliative shunt procedure may have a diminished pulse or an unobtainable blood pressure in the arm in which the subclavian artery has been incorporated into the shunt. Children who have undergone multiple palliative procedures may have poor peripheral venous access and previous surgical cutdown sites may exist. Children having multiple cardiac catheterizations may have absent or compromised femoral arterial and venous access. Such findings have obvious implications regarding arterial and venous catheter placement, sphyingomonometric blood pressure monitoring, the use of pulse oximetry, and the mode of induction.

Premedication

Most patients will have been called into the hospital on short notice and many will have eaten solid food in the previous 6 to 8 hours. In addition, patients will have taken their initial doses of oral immunosupressive drugs, usually cyclosporine and azathioprine or mycophenolate moftil. Cyclosporine usually is administered with 10 to 20 mL of liquid. It is important to verify that these medications have been taken. To reduce the risk of aspiration in adults and older children, a nonparticulate antacid such as bicitra (30 mL) should

be given in addition to intravenous metaclopromide 10 mg and an H_2 receptor blocker such as ranitidine 50 mg. For infants and smaller children, a period of 2 to 3 hours of NPO status is sufficient and usually transpires before induction.

Premedication for adults and children is most safely and effectively titrated by the anesthesiologist before induction and while lines are placed and the history and physical examination are completed. Midazolam 0.03 to 0.05 mg/kg in divided doses works well to reduce anxiety. Supplemental oxygen should be administered, because hypoxemia will exacerbate existing pulmonary hypertension. For neonates and infants, premedication is not necessary.

Preinduction

Some transplant patients will be receiving intravenous inotropic and vasodilator therapy when they arrive for surgery. These agents should be continued via a reliable intravenous route. Sterility is of the utmost importance because the patients will be immunosuppressed.

Adults. All patients should have two large-bore peripheral intravenous lines (14 gauge). Electrocardiogram (ECG) monitoring should allow assessment of V_5, I, II, III, aVR, aVL, and aVF. Baseline recording of all seven leads should be obtained for comparative purposes. Normally two leads (II and V_5) are monitored simultaneously intraoperatively. A radial artery catheter is placed with local anesthesia before induction of anesthesia.

We do not normally place a pulmonary artery catheter in patients for heart transplantation. The advantages of a pulmonary artery catheter are discussed in Chapter 3. The disadvantages as they apply to cardiac transplant patients are:

- technical difficulty in advancing the catheter in patients with a dilated right ventricle and low cardiac output
- risk of atrial and ventricular ectopy leading to hemodynamic compromise
- increased risk of infection
- catheter must be withdrawn into the sterile sheath during excision of the recipient's heart
- catheter must be readvanced across new suture lines into the donor heart as cardiopulmonary bypass (CPB) is terminated

A triple-lumen catheter is placed in the left internal jugular vein after induction of anesthesia. The distal lumen is continuously transduced to measure central venous pressure (CVP). The proximal lumen is used for injection and infusion of drugs. The middle lumen is flushed and left for later use as a route for nutrition if necessary. The right internal jugular vein is not used because it is the preferred route to obtain the endomyocardial biopsies that are used to monitor rejection postoperatively. In addition to the triple-lumen catheter, placement of an introducer sheath in the left internal jugular vein for use as reliable site of rapid fluid administration is warranted if peripheral access is poor. We use biplane or multiplane transesophageal echocardiography (TEE) (see Chapter 3) to help manage the patient pre- and post-CPB. After transplantation TEE is used to assess left and right ventricular function, measure pulmonary artery pressures (using a tricuspid regurgitation jet), and guide management of pulmonary artery hypertension and RV dysfunction if necessary.

INFANTS AND CHILDREN.   An inhalational induction, particularly with halothane, is likely to be poorly tolerated by children with DCM. Placement of an intravenous catheter before induction is optimal. EMLA cream can be used if necessary in older children. ECG monitoring should allow assessment of V5, I, II, III, aVR, aVL, and aVF. Baseline recording of all seven leads should be obtained for comparative purposes. Normally, two leads (II and V5) are monitored simultaneously intraoperatively. A radial artery catheter is placed after induction of anesthesia. The technique and catheter size is discussed in detail in Chapter 6. An appropriately sized double-lumen central venous line (see Chapter 6) is placed in the left internal jugular vein after induction. We use a pediatric biplane TEE probe in children weighing less than 15 to 20 kg and the adult multiplane TEE probe in children weighing more than 20 to 30 kg to help manage the patient pre- and post-CPB.

Induction and Maintenance

Generally, 50 to 75 µg/kg of fentanyl or 10 to 15 µg/kg of sufentanil is used as the primary anesthetic for induction and maintenance before CPB. These agents have no effect on myocardial contractility and cause a reduction in peripheral vascular resistance only through a diminution in central sympathetic tone.[52-55] An inhalation-based technique will be poorly tolerated by patients with DCM due to limited contractile reserve, dependence on preload, and limited ability to respond to decreases in afterload. A benzodiazepine should be included as a part of the premedication or should be administered intraoperatively to prevent awareness. Alternatively, administration of small, supplemental doses of an inhalational agent can be used to prevent awareness.

A traditional rapid-sequence induction will be poorly tolerated by patients with DCM, considering the abrupt hemodynamic changes that usually occur. If the risk of aspiration is deemed to be high, the following induction sequence is performed with the patient in a slightly head-up position and cricoid pressure is applied from commencement of induction until the trachea is intubated. After several minutes of denitrogenation and with the patient breathing 100% oxygen, induction begins with an infusion of fentanyl 500 µg/min or sufentanil 100 µg/min over 5 to 10 minutes. Vasodilator infusions such as nitroprusside should be tapered down or off at this time. A system of graded stimulation is used to assess anesthetic depth. After loss of consciousness, the hemodynamic response to insertion of an oral airway, followed by insertion of a urinary catheter, is used to gauge the need for additional narcotic to blunt the hemodynamic response to tracheal intubation. Larngoscopy is performed carefully and should not be prolonged. If an upward trend in heart rate or blood pressure is noted as laryngoscopy commences, laryngoscopy should be terminated and additional narcotic should be titrated. If there is poor visualization of the trachea, laryngoscopy should be terminated and intubating conditions should be improved by changing head position, using a stylet, or changing blades. This approach will help prevent long, stimulating larnygoscopies that compromise hemodynamics. If the entire narcotic dose is not used for induction, the remainder is infused slowly in anticipation of the skin incision.

Vecuronium or pancuronium 0.02 mg/kg or cis-atracurium 0.04 mg/kg is administered approximately 1 to 2 minutes before starting the narcotic infusion. Pancuronium is a better choice for infants and smaller children because the vagolytic and sympathometic effects of pancuronium can be used to counteract the vagotonic effects of high doses of fentanyl or sufentanil. As the patient loses consciousness, the remainder of the total dose of vecuronium or pancuronium 0.1 mg/kg or cis-atracurium 0.2 mg/kg is administered and controlled ventilation with 100% O_2 is initiated. This regimen minimizes the risk of narcotic-induced rigidity without undue stress to the patient.

When prompt control of the airway is desirable, etomidate 0.15 to 0.3 mg/kg may be used to hasten loss of consciousness during narcotic infusion. Etomidate produces minimal cardiovascular effects at this dosage when administered in conjunction with narcotics.[56] Alternatively, sufentanil 5 µg/kg and succinylcholine 1.0 to 1.5 mg/kg or etomidate 0.15 to 0.30 mg/kg and 10 µg/kg or sufentanil 1 µg/kg can be used in a rapid-sequence technique.[57]

If bradycardia with hemodynamic compromise occurs, it must be treated promptly. A small dose of pancuronium (0.015 to 0.05 mg/kg) often is effective if vecuronium or cis-atracurium has been used. Atropine should be used cautiously. Atropine administration may initiate tachycardia, and atropine, unlike beta₁-adrenergic agents, increases heart rate without any reduction in the duration of systole. Therefore, for equal increases in heart rate, atropine will cause a greater reduction in the duration of diastole and will compromise subendocardial perfusion to a greater degree than a beta$_1$-adrenergic agent. Ephedrine (a direct- and indirect-acting beta and alpha agonist) 0.03 to 0.07 mg/kg is a reliable agent to increase heart rate without compromising diastole. In addition, the augmentation in diastolic blood pressure obtained is beneficial when hypotension accompanies bradycardia.

Tachycardia is detrimental for patients with ischemic DCM and should be treated to avoid subendocardial ischemia and hemodynamic compromise. The first strategy should be to terminate noxious stimuli and then increase the depth of anesthesia as necessary. The use of a short- or long-acting beta blockers is not recommended considering the severely depressed systolic function present.

If hypotension due to reduced SVR occurs during the narcotic infusion, small doses of phenylephrine (0.5 to 1.5 µg/kg) and volume infusion (5 mL/kg) to increase preload to preinduction levels usually will correct the problem. A dose of phenylephrine very reliably causes an increase in systemic vascular resistance (SVR). Caution must be exercised when alpha agonists are administered to patients with severe systolic dysfunction. The goal should be to normalize SVR. Overzealous use of phenylephrine will increase afterload, induce afterload mismatch, and severely reduce SV. If the patient fails to respond with a prompt increase in aortic blood pressure, an inotropic agent should be started to avoid a downward spiral of ventricular dilatation, increased wall stress, reduced SV, and further hypotension. Dobutamine 5 to 10 µg/kg/min is a reasonable choice because it is potent inotrope that does not increase afterload. Using noxious stimulation such as larnygoscopy and intubation to treat hypotension in the lightly anesthetized patient with DCM must be avoided. These stimuli will produce a sudden, dramatic increase in afterload. The subsequent afterload mismatch will produce ventricular dilatation and may produce an additional reduction in blood pressure.

When surgical stimulation (skin incision, sternotomy, sternal spreading, and aortic manipulation) produces hypertension, additional doses of sufentanil (1 to 5 µg/kg) or fentanyl (5 to 25 µg/kg) traditionally have been used. Recent data do not support this practice. After a patient has received high doses of sufentanil (10 to 30 µg/kg) or fentanyl (50 to 100 µg/kg), administration of an additional agent as an infusion or a bolus will not reliably blunt the hemodynamic response to noxious stimuli.[58] Control of hypertension may require the use of vasodilator agents or adjuvant anesthetic agents. Sodium nitroprusside is a ready titratable, potent arteriolar dilator and can be used effectively to treat hypertension. An infusion can be started at 0.25 µg/kg/min and titrated upward. However, because sodium nitroprusside is a potent arteriolar dilator, it has the potential to induce a coronary steal in the presence of the appropriate anatomy.[59] This will be of concern for patients with ischemic DCM.

Nitroglycerin dilates large coronary vessels and does not dilate arterioles; therefore, it is not implicated in the steal phenomena. Systemically, nitroglycerin has it greatest dilating capacity on the venous beds and arterial dilation occurs only at higher doses. Despite this, when used in appropriate doses, nitroglycerin and nitroprusside have been shown to be equally effective in treatment of hypertension associated with coronary artery bypass surgery.[60,61] For treatment of hypertension, nitroglycerin is started at 0.5 µg/kg/min and may have to be increased up to 20 µg/kg/min.

The following adjuvant anesthetic agents also are useful:

1. Benzodiazepines — diazepam, midazolam, and lorazepam administered in conjunction with fentanyl or sufentanil have been implicated in causing decreases in peripheral vascular resistance with subsequent hypotension.[62-64] Therefore, they must be titrated with caution. Diazepam in increments of 0.03 to 0.07 mg/kg, midazolam in increments of 0.015 to 0.03 mg/kg, or lorazepam in increments of 0.007 to 0.015 mg/kg are reasonable.

2. Inhalational anesthetics — N$_2$O is not a good choice as an adjuvant agent; it has a weak myocardial depressant effect that normally is counteracted by the sympathetic outflow it produces. In patients with DCM and elevated catecholamine levels, down-regulated beta receptors; and reduced myocardial norepinephrine stores, the myocardial depressant effects will predominate. In addition, N$_2$O combined with high-dose opiates does elevate pulmonary vascular resistance, particularly in the presence of preexisting pulmonary hypertension.[65] Isoflurane, sevoflurane, or desflurane can be used in low concentrations (<0.75 MAC) to supplement a narcotic anesthetic. These agents will produce a small decrease in SVR with minimal myocardial depression. This makes them a better choice than enflurane or halothane.

■ POST-CARDIOPULMONARY BYPASS MANAGEMENT

Management of the patient with a transplanted heart is founded on a solid understanding of the surgical procedure and the physiology of the transplanted heart as outlined here.

Surgical Technique

The technique for **orthotopic heart transplantation** that has been used almost exclusively for the last 25 years is that described by Lower and Shumway (*see* Figs. 7–3 through 7–5).[66] Most heart transplants performed in the world are orthotopic. In this procedure, the recipient's heart is excised and replaced entirely with a donor heart. The procedure is performed through a median sternotomy with hypothermic CPB, bicaval cannulation, and aortic cross-clamping. After commencement of CPB, the recipient's heart is excised to just above the atrioventricular groove, leaving:

- a large cuff of left atrium containing all four pulmonary veins

- a large cuff of right atrium containing the superior vena cava (SVC) and inferior vena cava (IVC)
- the ascending aorta just distal to the aortic valve
- the main pulmonary artery just distal to the pulmonic valve

The donor left and right atria are anastomosed to the cuffs of the recipient left and right atria while the donor and recipient aorta and pulmonary artery are anastomosed. This technique creates large atrial cavities with abnormal geometry. This results in a less than optimal contribution of atrial systole to ventricular filling. In

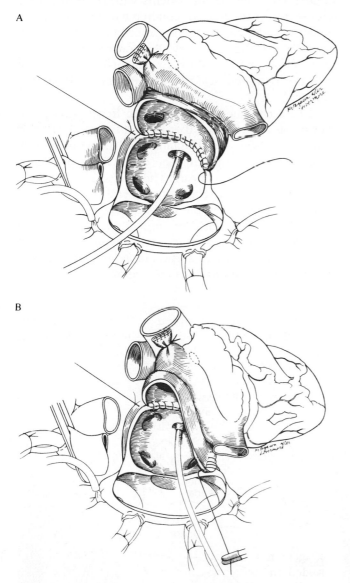

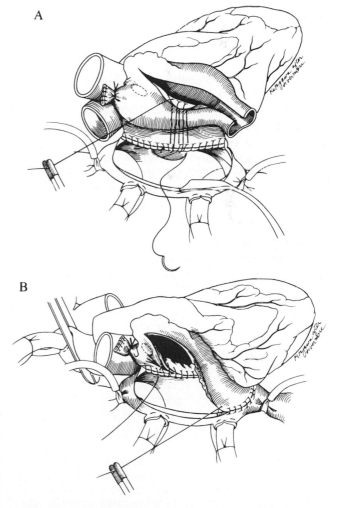

FIGURE 7–3. Operative technique for orthotopic heart transplantation. **A.** The recipient heart has been excised leaving a cuff of right atrium containing the superior vena cava (SVC) and inferior vena cava (IVC) and a cuff of left atrium containing all four pulmonary veins. The beginning of the left atrial anastomosis is depicted. The sinoatrial (SA) node of the donor heart is depicted by the dashed oval in the right atrium. The donor SVC is ligated. **B.** Details of the anastomosis between the recipient and donor left atria.

FIGURE 7–4. A. The left atrial anastomosis is complete and the new intra-atrial septum is being completed. **B.** The right atrial anastomosis is being completed using a portion of the donor IVC.

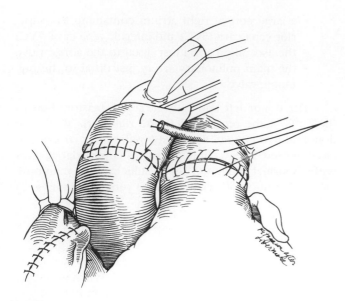

FIGURE 7–5. Details of the completed aortic and pulmonary artery anastomoses. The aortic cannula and cross-clamp are depicted. In an effort to reduce the ischemic interval, the surgeon may release the aortic cross-clamp after completion of the atrial and aortic suture lines and complete the pulmonary artery anastomosis while the heart is being reperfused.

addition, the distorted anatomy contributes to the development of functional mitral and tricuspid regurgitation. It also is associated with the development of atrial septal aneurysms, atrial thrombus, and sinus node injury.[67-69] These problems have led to application of a more anatomical orthotopic technique in which the recipient's atria are completely excised, leaving the SVC, the IVC, and a small cuff of left atrium containing all four pulmonary veins.[70] Early results are encouraging.

Compared with the biatrial technique, patients demonstrate a reduction in right and left atrial size, a reduction in right atrial pressure and a reduction in mortality from right ventricular failure (presumably as a result of improved right atrial function), a lower incidence of atrial arrhythmias, a lower incidence of sinus node dysfunction, a lower incidence of atrial thrombus formation, and a lower incidence of tricuspid regurgitation.[71,72] It remains to be seen whether this new technique will result in long-term outcome improvement.

For children with congenital heart lesions, the technical aspects of the surgical procedure are more challenging. For example, for patients with HLHS, the aorta must be reconstructed. For children having undergone a Fontan or bidirectional Glenn procedure, a caval reconstruction may be necessary. Pulmonary artery reconstruction may be necessary for patients with pulmonic atresia or right ventricle (RV) to pulmonary artery (PA) conduits.

The technique for **heterotopic heart transplantation** was described by Barnard and Losman in 1975.[73] Heterotopic heart transplantation is a rarely used technique that involves placing the donor heart parallel to the recipient's native heart. The donor heart can be placed parallel to the recipient's left and right ventricles or in parallel with just the left ventricle, depending on the technique chosen. The procedure is performed through a median sternotomy with hypothermic CPB, bicaval cannulation, and aortic cross-clamping. The surgical technique and options are summarized as follows (*see* Fig. 7–6):

- an anastomosis between the donor and recipient left atria. The anastomotic site in the donor left

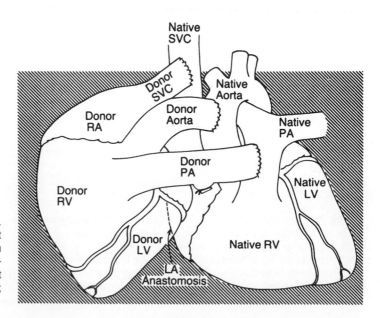

FIGURE 7–6. Operative technique for heterotopic heart transplantation. In this representation, the donor heart is in parallel with both the recipient LV and RV. The donor right pulmonary artery in continuity with the main pulmonary artery provides the added length necessary to reach the recipient pulmonary artery without use of a conduit. (LA = left atrium; LV = left ventricle; PA = pulmonary artery; RA = right atrium; RV = right ventricle; SVC = superior vena cava.)

atrium incorporates the entry sites of the left pulmonary veins, whereas the orifices of the right pulmonary veins are ligated.

- an end-to-side anastomosis between the donor SVC and the recipient SVC.
- an end-to-side anastomosis of the donor aorta to the ascending aorta of the recipient
- an end-to-side anastomosis of the donor pulmonary artery to the main pulmonary artery of the recipient. This requires an interposed piece of conduit to extent the length of the donor pulmonary artery. Alternatively, the donor right pulmonary artery in continuity with the main pulmonary artery can provide the added length without use of a conduit. When only LV support is desired, the donor pulmonary artery can be anastomosed to the free wall of the recipient right atrium. This places the donor heart in parallel only with the recipient LV.
- paced linkage of the donor and recipient heart produces functional improvement in both hearts.[74] With paced linkage, there is sensing of the donor atrium and pacing of the recipient atrium to produce recipient systole during diastole of the donor heart.

Indications for heterotopic heart transplantation have evolved since its initial description. At present, heterotopic heart transplantation is indicated for:

1. Patients with severe LV dysfunction with markedly elevated PVR and preserved RV function. In this setting, only LV support is needed.
2. Patients in whom the procured cardiac allograft is either small or has been subjected to a severe ischemic insult such that it is unlikely to be successful in the orthotopic position.
3. As a biological ventricular assist device (*see* Chapter 11).
4. As an adjuvant to other procedures (coronary revascularization, ventricular aneurysmectomy) for management of end-stage ischemic heart disease.[75]

The potential disadvantages of heterotopic heart transplantation are:

1. A reduced survival rate when compared with orthotopic transplantation.[76] There also seems to be increased morbidity for heterotopic heart transplantation when comparing patients receiving a smaller donor heart in the orthotopic position with patients receiving a similiarly undersized donor heart in the heterotopic position.[77]
2. The native heart may serve as a source of thromboembolism.

3. The native heart continues to require management of the underlying disease process.
4. Positioning of the donor heart in the right hemithorax may compromise pulmonary function.

Physiology of the Transplanted Heart

The functional and anatomic characteristics of the transplanted heart are summarized:

Autonomic Nervous System. Regardless of the surgical technique used, the orthotopically transplanted heart is devoid of sympathetic and parasympathetic innervation.[78] The most important consequence of this is an altered baroreceptor response. Normally, vagal afferent fibers from the atria and ventricles produce tonic inhibition of central sympathetic outflow. When atrial and ventricular volumes are reduced, vagal afferent outflow is reduced and central sympathetic outflow increases. In addition, activation of carotid and aortic baroreceptors by hypotension increases central sympathetic outflow. The result is direct sympathetic stimulation of the heart and generation of circulating catccholamines.

In the transplanted heart, no direct sympathetic stimulation of the heart is possible. Response to activation of barorectors in the patient with a transplanted heart is dependent on generation of circulating catecholamines for inotropic and chronotropic response. It normally takes several minutes to generate appropriate levels of circulating catecholamines. Although systemic catecholamine generation in response to arterial hypotension is enhanced,[79] reflex systemic catecholamine release in response to reduced atrial and ventricular volumes is impaired due to atrial and ventricular vagal deafferentation.[80] As a result of these changes, abrupt decreases in blood pressure will not be compensated for as quickly as normal in heart transplant patients.

The response of baroreceptors to endogenous and exogenous vasopressors in heart transplant patients is normal, but feedback to the donor heart is absent.[81] Therefore, increases in blood pressure will be accompanied by a reflex decrease in recipient atrial rate but not in donor atrial rate. As a result, there will be no reflex decrease in the transplanted heart rate in response to phenylephrine or norepinephrine-induced hypertension.

Early in exercise, increases in cardiac output are acquired by increases in SV, with EDV increasing and ESV remaining unchanged.[82] As exercise progresses, cardiac output increases as the result of systemic catecholamine-induced increases in heart rate with maintenance of SV.[83]

Cardiac denervation produces presynaptic supersensitivity due to denervation-associated loss of neuronal catecholamine uptake. As a result, there is increased sensitivity to catecholamines that are taken up by adrenergic nerve terminals (epinephrine, norepinephrine) with no increase in sensitivity to catecholamines that are not taken up (isoproteronol).[84,85] Evidence exists to suggest that reinnervation of the left ventricle with efferent sympathetic fibers occurs after 1 year or more.[86-88] Stimulation of these reinnervating sympathetic efferents produces a chronotropic response,[89] a subnormal increase in dP/dT, and a decrease in coronary blood flow. The ability of some transplant patients to experience angina suggests reinnervation with sympathetic afferents.[90,91] On the other hand, it seems that reinnervation of cardiac vagal afferents is unlikely.[92] In summary, sympathetic efferent and afferent reinnervation may occur in some patients during the years after cardiac transplantation. When reinnervation occurs, it has some physiologic importance.

Heart Rate. Long-term follow-up has demonstrated that the resting atrial rate of the transplanted human heart is approximately 90 to 110 bpm. This is significantly greater than the resting atrial rate of the innervated human heart and demonstrates that the predominant effect on sinus rate in man is a slowing effect of the parasympathetic system. Heart-rate increases with exercise in heart-transplant patients are achieved through stimulation of cardic beta$_2$ receptors by circulating catecholamines.[93] The increases in heart rate do not occur until after several minutes of exercise and they parallel the increase in serum catecholamines.[94] Despite this, the heart-rate response with exercise in transplanted hearts is attenuated relative to that seen in normal hearts[95,96] due to the lack of efferent innervation of the SA node.[97]

LV Systolic Function. The left ventricle of the transplanted heart exhibits normal contractile function and also exhibits reserve in response to an afterload challenge.[98] LVEDV and LVESV have been found to be reduced, whereas SV and EF remain normal or low normal due to the parallel reductions in EDV and ESV.[95,98,99] LV mass is increased due to concentric hypertrophy as the result of the arterial hypertension, which accompanies cyclosporine immunosuppression.[100,101]

RV Systolic Function. The right ventricle exhibits normal systolic function. RVEDV and RVESV are larger than normal, and RV wall thickness is increased. This is probably secondary to the persistent tricuspid regurgitation present in most patients.[30] In patients with preoperative pulmonary hypertension, persistence of RV dilatation and tricuspid regurgitation is the result of remodeling of the donor RV in response to recipient pulmonary circulation.[102] The dilation and tricuspid regurgitation persist despite resolution of pulmonary hypertension.[102]

Atrial Function. Following the biatrial technique, both right and left atrial areas are larger than normal.[103]

These patients have reduced right and left atrial emptying compared with normal subjects; the portion of total atrial emptying contributed by the recipient atrium is much less than that contributed by the donor atrium.[104-106] In addition, the asynchronous contraction of donor and recipient atrium results in wide variations in diastolic flow.[106] Following the bicaval technique, patients have right atrial emptying comparable to normal subjects and left atrial emptying, although reduced compared with normal subjects, is better than that seen in biatrial technique patients.[105] In addition, the left and right dimensions are smaller in patients with the bicaval as compared with the biatrial technique.[105]

Diastolic Function. LV diastolic dysfunction has been noted immediately after orthotopic cardiac replacement[107,108] and is related to the postischemic state.[109] This dysfunction is characterized by a restrictive ventricular filling pattern (*see* Chapter 3) that improves during the first several months after transplantation.[107] At that time, the restrictive pattern is occult until unmasked by volume loading.[108] This restrictive pattern may manifest clinically as reduced preload reserve in response to exercise and afterload increases.[95,99,110,111] The etiology of this continued dysfunction is unclear. It may be inherent to the small allograft LVEDV. Whether patients who receive hearts from donors smaller than themselves may be at particular risk for reduced preload reserve is debatable.[112,113] Rejection episodes are known to impair diastolic function,[114] but it is unclear whether recurring rejection episodes produce progressive LV and RV diastolic dysfunction in the form of a restrictive-constrictive pattern.[115-117]

There also is deficient acceleration of LV relaxation during exercise, which along with restrictive inflow, contributes to the elevations in LVEDP and LAP seen during exercise.[118] This impairment of relaxation may be due to loss of adrenergic tone due to denervation, ischemic injury at the time of harvest, or cyclosporine-induced arterial hypertension.

Based on the above discussion, the important characteristics of the transplanted heart in the immediate postoperative period can be summarized as follows.

Impaired Systolic Function. Systolic dysfunction in the donor heart may occur for a variety of reasons.[119,120]

ISCHEMIA-REPERFUSION INJURY. This is the most common cause of allograft systolic dysfunction post-CPB. Preservation of the donor heart standardly involves application of the aortic cross-clamp and delivery of cold cardioplegia to induce arrest in diastole, followed by cold storage at 4°C. The ischemic interval, the time from when the aortic cross-clamp is applied in the donor until the aortic cross-clamp is removed after implantation of the heart in the recipient is extremely important. The longer this ischemic interval, the more likely there is to be biventricular systolic dysfunction secondary to myocardial fibrosis.[121] Because there is an incremental increase in mortality with ischemic times > 3.5 hours, it is desirable to keep the interval less than 4 hours.[122] In an effort to reduce the ischemic interval, the surgeon may release the aortic cross-clamp after completion of the atrial and aortic suture lines and complete the pulmonary artery anastomosis while the heart is being reperfused. Prolonged and excessive inotropic support of the donor heart before cross-clamping also is undesirable because it contributes to post-transplant ischemic dysfunction.

BRAIN DEATH.   Donors who experience brain death as the result of a sudden rise in intracranial pressure (ICP) exhibit a hyperdynamic cardiovascular response, massive increases in plasma epinephrine, and histological evidence of severe myocardial ischemia.[123] Slower increases in ICP produce less of a hyperdynamic response, smaller increases in plasma epinephrine, and mild ischemic myocardial damage. The right ventricle seems to be more vulnerable to the effects of brain death than the left ventricle.[124] In addition, the altered geometry of the RV after biatrial implantation may contribute to dysfunction during the immediate postoperative period.[124]

HYPERACUTE REJECTION.   This rare event is caused by ABO blood group incompatibility or cytotoxic recipient antibodies against donor lymphocytes. It presents as cyanosis and mottling of the allograft in conjunction with profoundly impaired systolic function. It is impossible to separate these patients from CPB for any extended period of time. The only therapy available is excision of the allograft with placement of a total artificial heart (*see* Chapter 11). The time necessary (several hours to weeks) to screen potential donors for reactive antigens makes continued support on CPB impractical. This type of rejection is preventable by careful donor and recipient ABO typing and screening for percent reactive antibody (PRA).

MYOCARDIAL CONTUSION.   Patients with severe myocardial contusions are excluded as donors. Patients with lesser degrees of dysfunction from blunt trauma may exhibit impaired systolic function in the post-CPB period.

MYOCARDIAL INFARCTION.   Considering the careful screening of donors that is performed routinely, this is a very rare cause of immediate allograft dysfunction. It has been reported[125] in a 62-year-old donor with a normal coronary arteriogram who was found subsequently to have a 75% LAD stenosis at autopsy. With an increase in the acceptable age for donors, this is likely to become a more common problem.

RV Afterload Mismatch.   Impaired right ventricular performance is a particular risk in the presence of recipient pulmonary hypertension. RV afterload mismatch may occur as the result of severely depressed RV systolic function and normal PAP and PVR or, more commonly, as the result of less severely depressed RV systolic function and elevated PAP and PVR. This may result in acute allograft RV dysfunction severe enough to prevent termination of CPB. Therapy in this setting will need to be directed toward inotropic support of the RV and selective reduction of PVR.

Sinus and AV Node Dysfunction.   Ischemic injury to the sinus and AV node may produce bradycardia, nodal rhythmn, or heart block. SA node dysfunction is much more common; approximately 20% of patients need permanent atrial pacing.[126,127] In some instances, an appropriate sinus rate can be obtained with isoproterenol. In other instances, atrial or AV sequential pacing may be necessary.

Impaired Diastolic Function.   The postischemic state of the transplanted heart is characterized by increased ventricular stiffness and limited preload reserve resulting in a fixed stroke volume.[128] Increases in heart rate obtained with pacing will reduce diastolic filling time (*see* Fig. 4–3). This, in turn, will produce reductions in EDV and SV for a given ESV. The net result will be little or no change in cardiac output.[128] Atrial or AV sequential pacing is likely to be superior to ventricular pacing due to the presence of an appropriately timed atrial systole. For a given right or left atrial pressure, atrial pacing or atrioventricular (AV) sequential pacing will provide a higher ventricular EDV than ventricular pacing.

Inotropic support is useful for patients with limited preload reserve in both sinus and paced rhythms because SV can be augmented at a given afterload by reducing ESV. Inotropic agents allow SV to be maintained as heart rate increases, thereby producing increases in cardiac output. This occurs because the reductions in EDV produced by reduced diastolic filling time are offset by the reductions in ESV produced by enhanced contractility. Optimal heart rate is 100 to 110 bpm for adults and older children, whereas 130 to 150 bpm is optimal for neonates and infants. Higher heart rates result in progressive reductions in SV such that cardiac output remains constant or falls.

Preparations for terminating CPB are discussed in Chapter 10. Particular attention must be paid to deairing the heart. Severe ventricular dysfunction may follow ejection of air down the coronary arteries. The right ventricle is particularly at risk because of the anterior location of the right coronary ostia. TEE is valuable in guiding the deairing process.

A dose of methylprednisolone (usually 10 mg/kg in children and 500 mg in adults) will be given after aortic cross-clamp removal. In some institutions, the dose will be given after termination of CPB.

Historically, isoproterenol, which is a potent chronotrope, dromotrope, inotrope, and vasodilator, has been used to enhance cardiac output during the immediate post-CPB period.[128] Isoproterenol works well for patients in whom minimal inotropic support of the RV and LV is necessary. This is most likely when the donor heart requires minimal inotropic support before cross-clamping, the ischemic interval is short, and recipient pulmonary artery pressure is low or mildly elevated. Generally, isoproterenol is infused at 0.01 to 0.05 μg/kg/min (adults) or 0.05 to 0.25 μg/kg/min (children). At these doses, heart rate is maintained in an age-appropriate range, inotropic support of the RV and LV is provided, and PVR and SVR are reduced. Higher doses of isoproterenol increase the incidence of hemodynamic changes that are unfavorable to the myocardial energetics of the postischemic heart. Isoproterenol increases MVO_2, reduces aortic diastolic blood pressure, is arrhythmogenic, and increases heart rate. All of these variables tend to exacerbate myocardial ischemia. Furthermore, as the doses of isoproterenol increase, it may be difficult to maintain systemic blood pressure due to prohibitive decreases in SVR. Due to these side effects, doses in excess of 0.01 to 0.05 μg/kg/min (adults) or 0.05 to 0.25 μg/kg/min (children) are rarely useful as a means of providing additional inotropic support or as a method of increasing heart rate.

When isoproternol is ineffective in producing the desired heart rate, atrial or AV sequential pacing should be initiated. This combination will allow maintenance of SV as heart rate is increased. When isoproterenol is ineffective in producing the desired inotropic effect, alternative inotropic agents should be initiated. The need for additional inotropic support can be determined with either TEE or a pulmonary artery catheter. TEE will reveal ventricular dilatation and global hypokinesis. Regional wall motion abnormalities are also possible, but the ischemic insult usually is diffuse. Atrial enlargement and dilation of the mitral or tricuspid valve annulus with subsequent mitral or tricuspid regurgitation also is possible. Pressure monitoring will reveal an elevated CVP (>15 mm Hg), elevated PCWP (>20 mm Hg), or both. Cardiac output will be reduced (<2.0 l/min/m²). The advantage of the pulmonary artery catheter is that it allows measurement of PAP and calculation of PVR and SVR. PAP can be estimated with TEE using a tricuspid regurgitation jet and the CVP measurement (*see* Chapter 3).

The properties of the various inotropic agents are reviewed in detail in Chapter 4. The choice of agent should be tailored to the clinical picture. Epinephrine 0.01 to 0.1 μg/kg/min (adults) or 0.05 to 0.5 μg/kg/min (children) is a better choice than dobutamine, amirinone, or milrinone when SVR and systemic blood pressure are low. Dobutamine 5 to 10 μg/kg/min, amrinone 5 to 10 μg/kg/min after a 1.5-mg/kg loading dose, or milrinone 0.5 to 0.75 μg/kg/min after a 50-μg/kg loading dose are better choices when PAP and PVR are elevated.

When RV afterload mismatch exists with preserved LV systolic function, there will be low cardiac output, low systemic blood pressure, elevated CVP, elevated PAP, and low PCWP. TEE will reveal a dilated right atrium and ventricle with an underfilled, hyperkinetic left ventricle. Tricuspid regurgitation will be likely.

Therapy involves inotropic support and pulmonary vasodilatation. Pulmonary vasodilatation with intravenous agents is problematic because simultaneous reduction of SVR occurs. Simultaneous reduction of a normal SVR may compromise RV and systemic organ perfusion. Isoproterenol has historically been used during the post-cardiac transplant setting. Although isoproterenol is a potent inotrope and a pulmonary vasodilator, it is not a selective pulmonary vasodilator. Its beta₂ effects cause parallel reductions in PVR and SVR.[129] Other intravenous pulmonary vasodilators have been evaluated in heart transplant patients. Prostaglandin E_1 (PGE_1), prostacyclin (PGI_2), sodium nitroprusside (SNP), and nitroglycerin (NTG) are pulmonary vasodilators.[130-132] Unfortunately, they are not selective pulmonary vasodilators because they cause reductions in SVR as well. In theory, PGE_1 should be a selective pulmonary vasodilator because it experiences a pronounced first-pass elimination in the lungs while PGI_2, SNP, and TNG are metabolized in one circulation time. In reality, all four drugs reduce PVR while causing a decrease in SVR such that the ratio of PVR:SVR is unchanged or, in the case of PGI_2, slightly increased.[129,131] Efforts to reduce PVR with PGE_1, PGI_2, SNP, and TNG may require simultaneous use of inotropes and vasoconstrictors to maintain systemic blood pressure.[125,133] The simultaneous use of inotropic support is of benefit to the afterload-mismatched RV as well. Use of PGI_2 to reduce PVR seems to result in better maintenance of stroke volume and cardic output than PGE_1, TNG, and SNP due to less of a venodilating effect.[129,131]

The use of the inhaled pulmonary vasodilators nitric oxide (NO) and aerosolized PGI_2 is more promising. These agents are selective for the pulmonary circulation. NO delivered at 20 ppm has been shown to selectively reduce PVR by 35% in all heart transplant recipients.[131] In the subset of patients with a PVR > 3 Woods units, NO reduces PVR by 50%.[131] Evidence suggests that the peak effect in reducing PVR occurs at 20 ppm.[131,134] NO has been used to successfully reduce PVR in heart transplant patients in whom SNP and PGI_2 have failed.[135] Unfortunately, NO is not currently (1996) approved by the Food & Drug Administration (FDA). Recently, aerosolized PGI_2 (2 to 50 ng/kg/min) has proved useful in selectively lowering PVR after cardiac surgery[136] and is comparable to

NO in acute respiratory distress syndrome (ARDS).[137] It is not FDA approved either.

In summary, inhaled NO (20 ppm) is a reliable, selective pulmonary vasodilator but is not widely available. Aerosolized PGI_2 (2 to 50 ng/kg/min) also may prove useful. Intravenous PGI_2 5 to 20 ng/kg/min may be superior to PGE_1 0.05 to 0.2 µg/kg/min or SNP 0.5 to 1.0 µg/kg/min in reducing PAP and PVR while maintaining cardiac output and systemic blood pressure.

In addition to pharmacologic methods, efforts to reduce PVR with ventilatory interventions are essential. This topic is reviewed in detail in Chapter 6. A combination of a high inspired FiO_2, an arterial $PO_2 > 60$ mm Hg, an arterial PCO_2 of 20 to 30 mm Hg, a pH of 7.50 to 7.60, and low inspiratory pressures without high levels of PEEP will produce reliable reductions in PVR.

It is important to rule out a mechanical cause of increased impedance to RV ejection when RV dysfunction exists in the presence of low pulmonary artery pressures. Kinking of the pulmonary artery anastomosis has been observed to cause mechanical obstruction of the RV.[138,139] Kinking may be observed directly by the surgeon. Alternatively, it may be detected by TEE. It also is diagnosed readily by direct measurement of a pressure gradient between the RV and PA.

When univentricular or biventricular failure is severe and refractory to inotropic and vasodilator agents, a ventricular assist or circulatory assist device may be necessary to support circulation until the ventricles can recover (*see* Chapter 11).

Goals

1. Maintain sinus rhythm at 100 to 120 bpm in adults and older children and at 130 to 150 bpm in neonates and infants. Atrial or AV sequential pacing may be required.
2. Avoid pulmonary artery hypertension by treating hypercarbia, hypoxemia, and acidemia.
3. Aggressively treat pulmonary artery hypertension with vasodilator therapy to avoid RV failure. If RV failure does occur, inotropic support of the RV and pulmonary vasodilation may be necessary.
4. Maintain RAP and LAP to optimize SV in the setting of increased ventricular stiffness.
5. Inotropic support of the LV may be necessary if the ischemic interval is long.

■ SURGERY FOR CARDIAC TRANSPLANT PATIENTS

The success of heart transplantation makes it likely that anesthesiologists will encounter patients with transplanted hearts for a variety of noncardiac surgical proce-

dures. Some of the surgical procedures are purely elective, whereas others are likely to be urgent or emergent. Most surgical procedures are the direct result of complications of triple-drug (cyclosporine, azathioprine, prednisone) immunosuppressive therapy. These complications are listed in Table 7–2. The incidence of complications requiring general surgical consultation in heart transplant patients is 35 to 40%.[140-143] Many of these complications require operative intervention. Progression of atherosclerotic vascular disease also results in surgical intervention for aortic and peripheral vascular surgery.[144] Finally, heart transplant patients undergo all types of elective surgery, including cosmetic surgery.

Cardiac transplant patients have a unique set of management issues, in addition to those associated with the denervated heart. They are outlined as follows.

Cardiac Allograft Vasculopathy. This is currently the survival limiting factor after heart transplantation. It accounts for one-third of the late deaths after transplantation as the result of myocardial infarction, congestive heart failure, and sudden death. The incidence of angiographic coronary artery disease (CAD) in cardiac transplant patients is 10% per year posttransplantation. Similar incidence and outcome exist in the pediatric heart transplant population (including neonates) as well.[145,146] Angiographic CAD is associated with a greater than 3-fold increase in the risk of a cardiac event.[147] When the more sensitive method of intravascular ultrasound is used, intimal thickening is found to be universal in transplant coronary arteries at 1 year.[148] The prognostic significance of early intimal thickening has not yet been delineated clearly.

The pathogenesis of cardiac allograft vasculopathy is complex, multifactorial, and incompletely understood. It is believed that immunologic mechanisms in conjunction with nonimmunologic risk factors produce endothelial injury with subsequent myointimal hyperplasia.[149] It differs from atherosclerotic CAD in a number of ways. Atherosclerotic lesions are eccentric, focal, proximal lesions of large epicardial vessels that contain calcium, disrupt the internal elastic media, and develop over years. Cardiac allograft vasculopathy is associated with concentric, diffuse lesions that do not disrupt the elastic lamina

---

TABLE 7–2. COMPLICATIONS OF IMMUNOSUPPRESSION

Gingivigval hyperplasia related to cyclosporine[279]

Pancreatitis related to azathioprine and prednisone[280]

Cholelithiasis and cholecystitis related to cyclosporine[281,282]

Malignancies related to immunosuppression[283,284]

Complications of steroid use: cataracts, retinal detachment, aseptic hip necrosis, perforated viscus, gastrointestinal hemorrhage[285]

Complications of infection: abscess drainage in a variety of organs

and that progress rapidly. Focal, traditional atherosclerotic plaques also are seen in cardiac allografts.[150]

An immunologic mechanism is supported by the association of cardiac graft vasculopathy with histologic vascular rejection and its association with HLA antibodies.[149] Nonetheless, the direct association of cardiac allograft vasculopathy with histologic rejection and with leukocyte histocompatability remains a controversial subject.

A role for cytomegalovirus (CMV) has been proposed in the development of cardiac allograft vasculopathy. Both active CMV infection[151,152] and recipient pretransplantation (CMV) seropositivity have been identified as risk factors for development of cardiac allograft vasculopathy.[153] Direct CMV endothelial damage and CMV enhanced expression of other inflammatory mediators is the proposed mechanism.

Hyperlipidemia, specifically hypercholesterolemia, hypertriglyceridemia, and increased low-density lipoprotein (LDL) are common after heart transplantation, obesity, steroids, and cyclosporine all are implicated as causes.[149] It remains to be seen whether treatment of hyperlipidemia will have an effect on regression of cardiac allograft vasculopathy.

Older age at the time of transplantation also is a risk factor for development of cardiac allograft vasculopathy.[149] It has been suggested that male recipients of female allografts are at higher risk of developing cardiac allograft vasulopathy due to a higher degree of intimal hyperplasia by intravascular ultrasound detected at 1 year.[154] Finally, the presence of preexisting donor (CAD) does not accelerate the progression of cardiac allograft vasculopathy.[155]

Surveillance is difficult for a number of reasons. Patients with heart transplants may not experience angina or typical ECG changes with myocardial ischemia and infarction due to afferent sympathetic denervation.[156] Some patients who do experience angina with ischemia have been demonstrated to have evidence of functional sympathetic reinnervation.[90] Noninvasive tests for ischemia, specifically echocardiography, rest/exercisegated radionuclide wall motion, dipyridamole thallium scintigraphy, exercise thallium scintigraphy, and ambulatory ECG, have low sensitivity and predictive value for detecting CAD after transplantation.[157-159] Recently, use of dobutamine stress echocardiography has shown promise as a noninvasive technique for detection of CAD in heart transplant patients.[160,161] Considering these limitations, transplant centers currently use yearly coronary angiography as a screen for CAD. More frequent angiograms may be indicated to monitor progression in individual patients.

Therapeutic options are limited. Recent studies demonstrate that therapy with calcium entry blockers (diltiazem, nifedipine, and verapamil) or angiotensin-converting enzyme (ACE) inhibitors (enalapril, lisinopril, captopril) limits progression of cardiac allograft vasculopathy.[162,163] More invasive approaches involve angioplasty[164] and directional arthrectomy.[165] Only discrete proximal vessel disease is amenable to angioplasty and atherectomy. With angioplasty, short-term morbidity and success is similar to that seen in atherosclerotic disease, but the restenosis rate is high and long-term prognosis remains poor.[164] Finally, in the most severe cases, coronary artery bypass surgery[166] and retransplantation have been used. The diffuse nature of the coronary lesions makes bypass surgery an option only in selected cases. The survival rates for retransplantation are significantly less than for initial transplantation and the incidence of malignancy is twice that of first transplants.[167]

Post-transplantation Arterial Hypertension. This problem occurs in 75% of transplant patients at long-term follow-up.[168] It is not related to the conventional risk factors associated with hypertension and is multifactorial.[100]

CYCLOSPORINE. Cyclosporine immunosuppression has been implicated because virtually all patients receiving cyclosporine develop hypertension.[169] This is the result of cyclosporine-induced renal afferent arteriolar vasoconstriction and nephrotoxicity.[170] Because cyclosporine causes enhanced secretion of creatinine, the creatinine clearance overestimates the glomerular filtration rate (GFR).

CORTICOSTEROIDS. Corticosteroids have been implicated secondary to their mineralocorticoid effects. Corticosteroids also promote weight gain and the development of obesity.

The resultant hypertension produces LV hypertrophy. As SVR increases, there are parallel reductions in ejection fraction. In obese patients, there also is development of eccentric hypertrophy and further reduction in ejection fraction.[171] Therapy is necessary to prevent severe LV hypertrophy and impaired ventricular function.[101] This usually requires treatment with multiple classes of antihypertensive agents.[100] Calcium entry blockers (CEBs) and ACE inhibitors often are used as first-line agents because of their ability to slow the progression of cardiac allograft vasculopathy. In addition, CEBs provide additive immunosuppression to conventional therapy.[172] Diltiazem has the added advantage of reducing cyclosporine clearance, thereby allowing the cyclosporine dosage to be reduced by approximately one-third.[173]

Atrial and Ventricular Arrhythmias. The incidence of atrial and ventricular arrhythmias during initial hospitalization after transplantation is 55% and 79%, respectively.[174,175] At late follow-up, the incidence of atrial arrhythmias is 40 to 50%, whereas the incidence of ventricular arrhythmias is 43%.[175] An increased incidence of atrial arrhythmias during rejection has been reported in some[169] but not all series.[175] In general, atrial arrhythmias during the initial hospitalization are benign, except for atrial fibrillation. Development of atrial fibrillation is associated with a 3-fold increase in the risk of death. The risk of death is particularly high in patients who develop atrial fibrillation more than 2 weeks after transplantation.[175]

Permanent atrial pacing is required in approximately 10 to 20% of both pediatric[176] and adult recipients with symptomatic and assymptomatic bradycardia. Development of bradycardia seems to be related to a longer ischemic interval for the donor heart.[126,127]

SBE Prophylaxis. Bacterial endocarditis is a rare complication in heart transplant patients. Nonetheless, because of the extent of the suture lines and the immunosuppressed status of the patient, it is recommended the American Heart Association (AHA) guidelines for SBE prophylaxis be followed.[30]

Rejection. Most patients have at least one acute rejection episode despite adequate immunosuppression. Most rejection episodes occur within the first 3 months after transplantation with decreasing incidence thereafter.[177] Late episodes of acute rejection are more common in patients with more than two episodes of rejection in the first year and is most likely to occur within a month after an acute infection. Surveillance during the first year is accomplished with endomyocardial biopsies of the right ventricle via the right internal jugular vein every week for the first 4 to 8 weeks. Biopsies are not performed routinely in children younger than 6 months old or less than 5 kg but are performed selectively to confirm suspected rejection. Biopsies are graded from 0 to 4 based on histologic criteria. No rejection is 0, mild rejection is 1, and severe rejection is 4. After the first year, an annual biopsy is performed in most institutions. In some institutions, no biopsies are performed after the first year considering the low incidence of late rejection episodes and the invasive nature of the procedure.[178] Obviously, if clinical evidence of rejection exists, more frequent biopsies may be indicated to document rejection and to assess regression of histologic changes with treatment.

Noninvasive methods of rejection surveillance have been investigated, including serologic, electrocardiographic, echocardiographic, and nonechocardiographic imaging. Echocardiography is the most promising but has some important limitations. Rejection episodes are associated with development of a restrictive mitral inflow pattern as assessed by Doppler analysis. Specifically, there is a shortening of both the isovolumic relaxation time and the pressure half-time associated with an increase in the velocity of passive, early ventricular filling.[114] Unfortunately, the dependence of these indices on loading conditions and the presence of preexisting diastolic abnormalities limits the sensitivity and specificity of this type of analysis in detecting moderate rejection.[114,179,180] Echocardiographic indices of systolic function remain unaltered in mild to moderate rejection, whereas severe rejection is characterized by global systolic dysfunction.

Mild rejection frequently resolves spontaneously and is not treated. Mild rejection by biopsy usually is not associated with clinical evidence of allograft dysfunction such as hypotension, elevated jugular venous pressure, rales, sinus rate > 110, atrial fibrillation, bradycardia, or systolic dysfunction by echo.[181] Moderate or more severe rejection is accompanied by evidence of allograft dysfunction and is treated. Although normal allografts have maintained coronary vasodilator reserve,[182] moderate allograft rejection is associated with impaired reserve.[183,184] Normal reserve returns after treatment of rejection. Rejection also is accompanied by an attenuated coronary vasodilatory response to nitroglycerin.[185]

First-line therapy for moderate rejection is oral or intavenous pulsed steroids. In the approximately 10% of cases in which mild rejection by biopsy is associated with allograft dysfunction, pulsed steroid therapy is necessary. Severe rejection usually is treated with steroids and, in some institutions, a lympholytic agent such as polyclonal antithymocyte globulin (ATG) or murine monoclonal antibody (OKT3) is added.

Response to Drugs. The response to various drugs is altered in heart transplant patients secondary to the denervated state of the allograft:

1. Digoxin — digoxin prolongs AV node conduction in a biphasic manner. The initial effect is mediated vagally and is absent in the transplanted heart. The chronic effect is mediated directly and is present in the transplanted heart. The inotropic properties also are directly mediated and present.

2. Muscarinic antagonists — atropine, glycopyrrolate, and scopolamine produce competitive inhibition of acetylcholine at the muscarinic receptors of postgangionic cholinergic nerves such as the vagus. As a result, these drugs will not increase heart rate in the transplanted heart.[186] The effects of these drugs on other organs with cholinergic innervation will remain.

3. Acetylcholinesterase inhibitors — the contention that agents such as neostigmine and edrophonium have no cardiac effects while they continue to have systemic effects has been challenged recently. Bradycardia after administration of neostigmine, which was reversed

with atropine, has been demonstrated in a heart transplant patient.[187] In addition, sinus arrest after administration of neostigmine and glycopyrrolate for reversal of neuromuscular blockade reversal has been reported in two heart transplant patients.[188] It has been demonstrated that neostigmine produces direct stimulation of cholinergic receptors on cardiac ganglion cells with subsequent release of acetylcholine.[189] In addition, allograft denervation hypersensitivity of both the postganglionic neurons and the muscarinic myocardial receptors has been demonstrated.[190] These factors, combined with intrinsic allograft sinoatrial (SA) node dysfunction may produce severe SA node dysfunction or sinus arrest after acetylcholinesterase inhibitor administration in heart transplant patients.

4. Beta-adrenergic agonists — as discussed previously, there is increased sensitivity to catecholamines that are taken up by adrenergic nerve terminals (epinephrine, norepinephrine) with no increase in sensitivity to catecholamines that are not taken up (isoproterenol).[84,85] Improvements in systolic function with beta-adrenergic agents are obtainable during acute rejection episodes.[191]

5. Beta-adrenergic antagonists — these agents retain their usual activity. The sinus rate of both the donor and recipient slow equally, demonstrating that the predominant effect is caused by blockade of circulating catecholamines. There also will be a normal increase in the refractoriness of the AV node.[192]

6. Calcium entry blockers — these agents directly suppress the sinus and AV nodes and, thus, should have normal activity. Nonetheless, the negative chronotropic and dromotropic effects of verapamil have been demonstrated to be more pronounced in the transplanted heart.[193] There will be no reflex tachycardia from agents with strong vasodilator properties such as nifedipine.

7. Vagolytic and vagotonic agents — drugs with vagolytic activity (pancuronium, demerol) will not increase heart rate, whereas drugs with vagotonic activity (fentanyl, sufentanil) will not decrease heart rate.

8. Adenosine — the magnitude and duration of adenosine's negative chronotropic and dromotropic effects is 3 to 5 times greater in the transplanted heart.[194]

9. Ephedrine — cardiac drugs that are both direct and indirect acting will have a diminished effect because only the direct effect will be present.

Anesthetic Considerations

A variety of regional and general anesthetic techniques have been used safely and successfully in the anesthetic management of patients with heart transplants.[195-197] In patients without evidence of allograft dysfunction, the following principles are useful:

1. Aseptic technique is essential.
2. Appreciate that compensation for acute alterations in preload, afterload, and contractility are incomplete and delayed; postural effects are magnified.
3. Heart-rate and blood-pressure increases due to inadequate anesthesia will be delayed until circulating catecholamine levels increase.
4. Bradycardia will compromise cardiac output secondary to the reduced baseline stroke volume and the delayed ability to increase stroke volume in compensation; atropine is not useful, whereas isoproterenol and ephedrine are useful.
5. Acetylcholinesterase inhibitors (neostigmine, edrophonium) for reversal of neuromuscular blockade may have cardiac effects. Anticholingeric agents (atropine, glycopyrrolate) must be given to block the peripheral muscarinic effects of these agents and to attenuate cardiac effects.
6. Central venous pressure monitoring, when indicated, should be obtained via a route other than the right internal jugular vein.
7. Reflex bradycardia will not accompany administration of vasopressor agents (phenylephrine), nor will directly induced bradycardia accompany administration of agents with vagotonic activity.
8. Reflex tachycardia will not accompany administration of vasodilator agents (sodium nitroprusside, nifedipine, hydralazine), nor will directly induced tachycardia accompany administration of agents with vagolytic activity.
9. Stress-dose steroid coverage should be administered to patients receiving steroids as part of their immunosuppression.

For patients with moderate to severe rejection, systolic function will be compromised and inotropic support before induction may be warranted. Emphasis should be placed on providing an anesthetic that allows gradual adaptation of a heart with diminished reserve.

■ HEART–LUNG TRANSPLANTATION

Heart–lung transplantation (HLT) can be considered for patients with end-stage cardiopulmonary disease unresponsive to maximal medical therapy for which no surgical options exist except combined heart–lung replacement. Increasingly, in an effort to make maximum use of donated organs, double lung transplantation (DLT) and single lung transplantation (SLT) are being used for patients with pulmonary disease without secondary severe cardiac dysfunction. The number of heart–lung transplants peaked in 1989 and has continued to decline as the result of this increase of the use of DLT and SLT.[3]

For adults, the primary indications for HLT, based on 1995 Registry data,[3] are primary pulmonary hypertension (PPH) (30%), Eisenmenger's syndrome secondary to congenital heart disease (28%), and septic lung disease such as cystic fibrosis and bronchiectasis (15%). Other indications include emphysema, alpha$_1$ antitrypsin deficiency, and interstitial pulmonary fibrosis. For children, the primary indications are congenital heart disease (40%), primary pulmonary hypertension (24%), and cystic fibrosis (16%). Most pediatric heart–lung transplantations are in children aged 6 to 18 years old; the remainder are in the 1- to 5-year-old range.[3]

■ SINGLE LUNG TRANSPLANTATION

Single lung transplantation (SLT) can be considered for patients with end-stage lung disease without significant cardiac dysfunction. Generally, patients with an LV ejection fraction (EF) > 35% and a RVEF > 25% are considered suitable. 1995 Registry data[3] indicate that, for adults, SLT is used primarily for patients with obstructive lung disease from emphysema (42%) and alpha$_1$ antitrypsin deficiency (16%). It also is used for patients with idiopathic pulmonary fibrosis (17%).

Increasingly, SLT is being used for patients with pulmonary hypertension from PPH (9%) and Eisenmenger's syndrome (2%) in whom there is no coexistent severe cardiac dysfunction.

For children, most lung transplantations are performed in the 6- to 18-year-old age group. SLT is used much less frequently than in adults and is used for patients with Eisenmenger's syndrome in conjunction with repair of intracardiac lesions.[198-201]

■ DOUBLE LUNG TRANSPLANTATION

Double lung transplantation (DLT) is also considered for patients with end-stage pulmonary disease without significant cardiac dysfunction. Two approaches to double lung transplantation exist: bilateral sequential single lung transplantation (BSSLT) and en-bloc double lung transplantation. Again, patients with an LVEF > 35% and a RVEF > 25% are considered suitable. The trend has been to reserve double lung transplantation for patients in whom SLT is not an option. Based on 1995 Registry

data,[3] the primary indications for DLT in adults are cystic fibrosis (36%), emphysema (17%), alpha$_1$ antitrypsin deficiency (13%), and PPH (10%). In addition, DLT has been used in conjunction with cardiac repair in adults with Eisenmenger's syndrome.[202]

In children, the primary indications are cystic fibrosis (38%), PPH (19%), and Eisenmenger's syndrome in conjunction with a repair of intracardiac lesions (10%).

Contraindications to HLT, SLT, and DLT are similar to those for heart transplantation and are outlined in Table 7–1.

■ SPECIFIC DISEASE STATES

Obstructive Lung Disease. The most common indication for lung transplantation is obstructive lung disease secondary to emphysema or alpha$_1$ antitrypsin deficiency. Patients considered for transplantation generally have an FEV$_1$ < 1 L, a requirement for supplemental O$_2$ at rest, and CO$_2$ retention. Pulmonary hypertension is uncommon in these patients. Concomitant CAD must be ruled out because many of these patients have long histories of smoking.

Both SLT and BSSLT have been used for these patients. SLT is relatively contraindicated in two subsets of emphysema patients: those with severe bullous disease and those with bronchiectasis. Severe bullous disease may result in preferential ventilation of the nontransplanted lung. Bronchiectasis introduces the risk of leaving an infected lung in communication with the transplanted lung in an immunocompromised patient. These subsets of patients usually are considered for BSSLT.

In other patients, both SLT and BSSLT provide good early functional results. BSSLT provides better long-term functional results but is associated with a higher operative mortality.[203] Therefore, some centers consider BSSLT in younger emphysema patients.

Pulmonary Fibrosis. These patients have restrictive pulmonary physiology. Patients considered for transplantation generally have a FVC < 1.5 L and a FEV$_1$ < 1.2 L, a requirement for supplemental O$_2$ at rest, and CO$_2$ retention. Moderate to severe pulmonary hypertension is common in these patients.

SLT provides good function results in these patients as the transplant lung is preferentially ventilated and perfused. Preferential ventilation of the transplant lung occurs because it is more compliant than the native lung. Preferential perfusion of the transplant lung occurs because PVR is higher in the native lung.

Primary Pulmonary Hypertension (PPH). Patients in whom the cause of pulmonary hypertension is unexplained are said to have PPH. For the diagnosis of

PPH to be made, the secondary causes of pulmonary hypertension must be ruled out. Common causes of secondary pulmonary hypertension include mitral stenosis, congenital heart disease, pulmonary embolism, and pulmonary venous obstruction. Seventy-three percent of PPH patients are female; the mean age at presentation is 34 years and the 5-year survival rate is 20%.[204]

Survival is enhanced by coumadin anticoagulation therapy, presumably because the presence of low cardiac output and pulmonary vascular endothelial injury places these patients at risk for pulmonary thrombosis and worsening pulmonary hypertesion.[205] High-dose calcium channel blockers also improve survival, but only in the subgroup of patients who experience a greater than 25% decrease in PVR and pulmonary artery pressure.[206] Continuous PGI_2 infusion improves survival and functional status. However, it usually is reserved for patients with NYHA functional class III–IV.[207-209]

All patients with PPH have RV dysfunction. PPH produces RV afterload mismatch and subsequent RV hypertrophy. Chronic exposure to the loading conditions that produce hypertrophy results in progressive ventricular dysfunction as the result of progressive fibrosis and cell death.[13] RV dilatation with dilation of the tricuspid valve annulus and TR are common.

Opinion regarding the best procedure for patients with PPH is evolving. Heart–lung transplantation is the procedure of choice in PPH patients with severe end-stage RV dysfunction or severe biventricular dysfunction. At present, the trend is to offer all other PPH patients SLT or BSSLT.[210-216]

This strategy has evolved because: (1) except in cases of end-stage RV systolic dysfunction, substantial recovery of the right ventricle is possible with the normalization of pulmonary artery pressures, which occurs after SLT and DLT,[217,218] and (2) use of SLT and BSSLT makes better use of the limited organ supply.

At present, there is conflicting opinion regarding whether SLT is the optimal procedure for patients with PPH. In the experience of one large center, short-term survival, long-term survival, and functional status of patients with pulmonary hypertension after SLT is comparable to patients without pulmonary hypertension undergoing SLT.[210,212,213] Another large center reports significantly increased mortality, prolonged intensive care unit stay, and less symptomatic improvement in SLT patients with pulmonary hypertension as compared with SLT patients with normal pulmonary artery pressures.[202,212] Furthermore, patients with pulmonary hypertension undergoing SLT have significant long-term ventilation/perfusion mismatch due to preferential perfusion of the transplanted lung and preferential ventilation of the native lung.[201,211] In addition, these patients are at risk for development of acute postoperative pulmonary edema secondary to overperfusion of the allograft. As a result, some centers prefer BSSLT or HLT for patients with PPH.[201,219-221]

Eisenmenger Syndrome. This term is used to describe patients with congenital heart disease and pulmonary hypertension severe enough to cause reversal of left-to-right shunts. Eisenmenger's syndrome evolves in patients with intracardiac or great vessel left-to-right shunts. Initially, the left-to-right shunt produces increased pulmonary blood flow and eccentric hypertrophy of the cardiac chambers involved. With a ventricular septal defect (VSD), there will be hypertrophy of the left and right ventricle; with an atrial septal defect (ASD), there will be enlargement of the right atrium, left atrium, and right ventricle. Prolonged exposure of the pulmonary vasculature to increased pulmonary blood flow and pressure leads to development of pulmonary hypertension and pulmonary vascular occlusive disease (PVOD). This process is described in detail in Chapter 6. PVOD produces right ventricular concentric hypertrophy. As PVOD advances and pulmonary vascular resistance approaches and then exceeds systemic vascular resistance, intracardiac shunting becomes bidirectional and then right to left.

In the short term, the processes of eccentric and concentric hypertrophy provide appropriate adaptation. However, chronic exposure to the loading conditions that produce hypertrophy results in progressive ventricular dysfunction as the result of progressive fibrosis and cell death.[13] As a result, these patients usually have severe biventricular dysfunction and generally are not candidates for SLT and BSSLT. When LV function is preserved, repair of the congenital cardiac defect can be performed in conjunction with SLT and BSSLT procedures. As with PPH, there is debate regarding whether SLT is the appropriate operation for patients with pulmonary hypertension secondary to Eisenmenger's syndrome.

Cystic Fibrosis. Cystic fibrosis is a multisystem disease and is the most common fatal inherited disease among Caucasians.[222] Its pathophysiology is reviewed extensively elsewhere.[223] Pulmonary involvement is inevitable, and 95% of affected adults die of respiratory complications. Airway obstruction secondary to viscous secretions, edema, and reactive airways leads to air trapping and an increase in FRC, RV, and total lung capacity. FEV_1 and FVC are reduced. In addition, lung damage occurs as the result of bacterial infections. Most patients with cystic fibrosis eventually are colonized by *Pseudomonas aeruginosa.* This pathogen is responsible for producing extensive tissue damage both directly and by antigenic stimulation of the immune system. Because *Pseudomonas* cannot be eradicated effectively, recurrent infections and remissions are the norm. Recently, aerosol administration of recombinant human DNase (rhDNase) has been shown to reduce the risk of infectious exacerbations requiring parenteral antibiotics and to improve pulmonary function.[224] rhDNase reduces the viscoelasticity, reduces the adhesiveness, and improves the mucociliary transportability of cystic fibrosis sputum.

The chronic hypoxemia, acidosis, and physical loss of pulmonary vessels and lung tissue that occur as the result of these pulmonary changes eventually produce pulmonary hypertension and the development of cor pulmonale. Right ventricular hypertrophy and dilatation develop. Chronic exposure to the loading conditions that produce hypertrophy results in progressive ventricular dysfunction as the result of progressive fibrosis and cell death.[13]

In cases in which severe right ventricular dysfunction exists, HLT is the procedure of choice. In cases in which right ventricular function is normal or slightly impaired, BSSLT is used by some centers in place of HLT. SLT is not an option for patients with cystic fibrosis because the transplanted lung will quickly become contaminated and infected by secretions from the remaining lung. SLT with contralateral pneumonectomy has been used but has not been widely accepted.[225]

Additional management problems are presented by the presence of pancreatic insufficiency. Eighty-five percent of patients with cystic fibrosis have pancreatic insufficiency severe enough to cause steatorrhoea and malabsorption.[226] Insufficient caloric absorption and the anorexia of chronic disease combined with the increased caloric demands of chronic infection may result in malnutrition. Enteral and parenteral feeding may be necessary. Vitamin K deficiency may result in prolongation of the prothrombin time.[227] Glucose intolerance is common (40% of adults); frank diabetes mellitus occurs in 25% of adult patients.[228]

Subclinical liver disease and hepatomegly secondary to fatty infiltration are common.[229] Only rarely is liver dysfunction severe enough to cause hepatocellular dysfunction and hypersplenism. As a result, thrombocytopenia and coagulation factor deficiencies are rare.

■ THE DONOR

Only 5 to 20% of all solid organ donors are suitable lung donors. This occurs as the result of blunt thoracic trauma, the potential for aspiration during resuscitation, overaggressive fluid resuscitation, and neurogenic pulmonary edema. The guidelines used to select donors for lung transplantation are summarized below:

1. Age younger than 55 years
2. Adequate gas exchange — the donor should have a $PaO_2 > 300$ mm Hg on $FiO_2 = 1.0$ and PEEP = 5 cm H_2O or $PaO_2 > 100$ mm Hg on $FiO_2 = 0.4$ and PEEP = 5 cm H_2O. Pulmonary compli-

ance should be normal with static pressure < 20 mm Hg and peak pressure < 30 mm Hg at a tidal volume of 15 mL/kg.
3. Normal bronchoscopic examination
4. Normal serial chest radiographs
5. No history of pulmonary disease. A smoking history is acceptable in some centers.
6. Appropriate donor size — some programs compare donor and recipient lung size using chest radiograph measurements. A growing practice is comparison of donor and recipient total lung capacity from nomograms based on age, height, and sex. In patients with obstructive lung disease, an allograft with 15 to 20% greater volume than that predicted for the recipient can be used. These patients have huge pleural cavities.
7. No active severe infection or malignancy with the possibility of metastases
8. Negative serologies for human immunodeficiency virus (HIV) or hepatitis B
9. ABO compatibility and human lymphocyte antigen screen

The guidelines used to select donors for HLT are the combination of those for heart transplantation and those for lung transplantation.

Harvest of the lungs usually is accomplished in conjunction with harvest of the heart. PGE_1 500 μg is given in the pulmonary artery just before circulatory arrest and harvest. The vena cavae are transected, an incision is made in the left atrial appendage, and the aorta is cross-clamped and cold cardioplegia is given. At this point, the pulmonary artery is infused with 3 L of cold Euro-Collins or University of Wisconsin solution, which is vented out the incision in the left atrial appendage. Ventilation is discontinued and the lungs are allowed to partially deflate. The trachea is stapled and divided. The heart–lung block is then removed. When the heart and lungs are to be used for separate recipients, adequate portions of pulmonary artery and left atrial-pulmonary vein cuff must be allocated to each recipient. With the trachea or bronchi stapled, the lungs are immersed in a cold crystalloid solution at 4° C and transported partially inflated. Although the maximum ischemic time is 6 to 8 hours, the optimal ischemic time should not exceed 5 to 6 hours because short- and intermediate-term patient survival is reduced.[230,231]

■ OPERATIVE PROCEDURE AND PATIENT POSITIONING

HLT is performed through a median sternotomy with hypothermic CPB, bicaval cannulation, and aortic cross-clamping. The recipient undergoes resection of the heart–lung block, leaving only a right atrial cuff in continuity with the IVC and SVC, the cut end of the distal trachea, and the cut end of the proximal ascending aorta. The donor heart–lung block is implanted with anastomoses of the right atrium, distal trachea, and ascending aorta.

SLT is performed through a standard thoracotomy with the patient in the lateral thoracotomy position. The donor lung block contains a cuff of left atrium with two pulmonary veins, the bronchus, and the branch pulmonary artery. The other donor lung and the donor heart can be used for two other recipients.[232] One lung ventilation (OLV) is established and a pneumonectomy is performed, followed by implantation of the donor lung with anastomoses at the left atrium, bronchus, and branch pulmonary artery. This procedure often can be performed without CPB.

Two very different surgical procedures are used for DLT. The en-bloc procedure[233] is performed on CPB with hypothermia, bicaval cannulation, aortic cross-clamping, and cardioplegic arrest of the recipient heart. A median sternotomy is used. The donor double lung block consists of the two lungs, the distal trachea, the main pulmonary artery, and a large left atrial cuff with all four pulmonary veins. The donor heart can be used for another recipient. The block is implanted with anastomoses at the trachea, posterior left atrium, and main pulmonary artery after bilateral recipient pneumonectomies. This procedure has been plagued by poor healing of the tracheal anastomosis and reduced long-term survival compared with BSSLT.[234]

BSSLT is the other approach to DLT.[233] This procedure often can be performed without CPB, which is considerably more challenging for the anesthesiologist. This procedure is performed with the patient supine through a sternal bithoracotomy. Proper positioning is necessary to provide adequate exposure for the thoracotomy portion of the incision. One approach is to position the patient's arms suspended over the head. This is cumbersome and consumptive of the small amount of space available at the head of the table. In addition, it exposes the patient to an increased risk of brachial

plexus injuries. With proper positioning of two rolls, one on either side of the patient's spine extending from the cervical to the lumbar region, the arms can be remained tucked at the patient's side. Each donor lung block contains a cuff of left atrium with two pulmonary veins, the bronchus, and the branch pulmonary artery. The donor heart can be used for another recipient. OLV is established and a pneumonectomy is performed, followed by implantation of the donor lung with anastomoses at the left atrium, bronchus, and branch pulmonary artery. The procedure is then repeated for the next donor lung.

Use of CPB

The indications for use of CPB are summarized in Table 7–3.

HLT and En-bloc DLT. HLT and en-bloc DLT both require hypothermic CPB with aortic cross-clamping as described previously.

SLT and BSSLT. Elective CPB is used for SLT and BSSLT for the following subsets of patients:

- infants and small children[235-237]
- patients with pulmonary hypertension
- patients undergoing lung transplantation and simultaneous repair of intracardiac defects.

For all other patients with SLT and BSSLT, CPB is initiated only when hemodynamic, gas exchange, or technical difficulties are encountered in the course of the procedure. The most recent experience demonstrates that most SLT and BSSLT patients without pulmonary hypertension can be managed without CPB.[238-240] One group's experience suggests a higher incidence of need for CPB in patients with restrictive lung disease. Criteria have been established to predict which patients with restrictive lung disease undergoing SLT will need CPB. Preoperative criteria include RVEF < 27% during exercise, SaO_2 < 85% during exercise, and an exercise duration of <3 minutes. Intraoperative criteria include an SaO_2 < 90% with an FiO_2 of 1.0, baseline mean

TABLE 7–3. INDICATIONS FOR CPB AND OLV IN LUNG TRANSPLANTATION

Type of Transplant	CPB	OLV
HLT	full hypothermic, aortic X-clamp	no
En-block double-lung transplantation	full hypothermic, aortic X-clamp, cardioplegic arrest	no
SLT, BSSLT		
infants/small children	full normothermic	no
intracardiac defect repair	full hypothermic, aortic X-clamp, cardioplegic arrest	no
pulmonary hypertension	partial normothermic	yes
all others	partial normothermic if necessary	yes

BSSLT, bilateral sequential single-lung transplantation; CPB, cardiopulmonary bypass; HLT, heart–lung transplantation; OLV, one-lung ventilation; SLT, single-lung transplantation.

PA pressure > 40 mm Hg, mean PA pressure > 50 mm Hg with the pulmonary artery clamped, severe systemic hypotension, and a cardiac index < 2.0 L/min/m².[241]

The incentive to avoid CPB when possible is the evidence that use of CPB contributes to postoperative graft dysfunction in the form of an increased arterial/alveolar oxygen ratio, increased severity of radiographic pulmonary injury, and prolonged postoperative intubation.[242]

Full CPB is used for infants and small children[243] and for all patients undergoing simultaneous repair of an intracardiac lesion. Aortic cross-clamping and cardioplegic arrest are only necessary when intracardiac defects are repaired. Normothermic partial CPB is used for all other cases of SLT and BSSLT. Cannulation of the ascending aorta and the right atrium is used for bilateral SLT and right SLT. For patients undergoing left SLT, descending aorta and pulmonary artery cannulations have been used. Alternatively, femoral vein and artery cannulation can be used.

■ ANESTHETIC MANAGEMENT

Goals

1. Patients with obstructive lung disease may exhibit auto-PEEP, stacking of breaths, and hemodynamic compromise with positive pressure ventilation. Ventilatory interventions will be necessary.
2. Preexisting LV or RV dysfunction requires that contractility be maintained or enhanced.
3. Avoid hypercarbia, hypoxemia, and acidemia, which will exacerbate pulmonary hypertension and may result in acute RV decompensation.
4. Avoid increase in the PVR:SVR ratio in patients with Eisenmenger's syndrome. This will increase right-to-left shunting and worsen hypoxemia.

Preoperative Evaluation

Preoperative evaluation is covered in detail in Chapters 1 and 6. Lung transplant patients typically undergo extensive medical evaluation. A summary of this evaluation is readily available to the anesthesiologist through the transplant coordinator. An example of a summary sheet is shown in Figure 7–2.

Premedication

Most patients will have been called into the hospital on short notice and many will have eaten solid food in the previous 6 to 8 hours. In addition, patients will have taken their initial doses of oral immunosuppressive drugs, usually cyclosporine and azathioprine or mycophenolate moftil. Cyclosporine usually is administered with 10 to 20 mL of liquid. It is important to verify that these medications have been taken. To reduce the risk of aspiration in adults and older children, a nonparticulate antacid such as bicitra 30 mL should be given in addition to intravenous metaclopromide 10 mg and an intravenous H_2 receptor blocker such as ranitidine 50 mg. For infants and smaller children a period of 2 to 3 hours of NPO status is sufficient and usually transpires before induction.

Premedication for adults and children is most safely and effectively titrated by the anesthesiologist before induction and while lines are placed and the history and physical examination are completed. Midazolam 0.03 to 0.05 mg/kg in divided doses works well to reduce anxiety. Supplemental oxygen should be administered because hypoxemia will exacerbate existing pulmonary hypertension.

Preinduction

Some transplant patients will be receiving intravenous inotopic and vasodilator therapy when they arrive for surgery. These agents should be continued via a reliable intravenous route. Sterility is of the utmost importance because the patients will be immunosuppressed. Patients with bronchospastic disease should receive bronchodilator therapy before induction. Likewise, patients with cystic fibrosis should receive nebulized acetylcysteine or rhDNase to help break up tenacious secretions.

Adults. All patients should have two large-bore peripheral intravenous lines (14 gauge). If the patient's arms are suspended over the head, venous access in or below the antecubital fossa is not practical because flow will be impaired. Placement of one or more introducer sheaths in the internal jugular vein for use as reliable sites of rapid fluid administration is warranted if peripheral access is poor or the arms are to be suspended over the head. ECG monitoring should allow assessment of V_5, I, II, III, aVR, aVL, and aVF. Baseline recording of all seven leads should be obtained for comparative purposes. Normally, two leads (II and V_5) are monitored simultaneously intraoperatively. If a left thoractomy incision is used, V_5 is not an option because the lead will be in the operative field. A radial or femoral artery catheter is placed with local anesthesia before induction of anesthesia. When a femoral artery catheter is used, it should be placed in femoral artery contralateral to the one that will be used if femoral artery contralateral to the one that will be used if femoral artery cannulation for CPB is used.

We place a pulmonary artery catheter in adults for SLT and BSSLT. We place the catheter after induction in patients who are unable to lie flat or to cooperate. Some centers use PA catheters that allow continous cardiac output and mixed venous O_2 saturation (SVO_2) monitoring (*see* Chapter 3). The PA catheter is an important tool in managing the patient during pneumonectomy and clamping of the pulmonary artery. In addition, information obtained from the PA catheter is used to determine whether completion of the procedure without CPB is feasible. We do not make an effort to direct the pulmonary artery catheter into the contralateral pulmonary artery in patients undergoing SLT. We pull the catheter back into the main pulmonary artery before pulmonary artery clamping and then advance the catheter into the contralateral pulmonary artery.

For HLT and en-bloc DLT, we do not place a PA catheter for the same reasons we do place one in heart transplant patients. A triple-lumen catheter is placed in the internal jugular vein after induction of anesthesia in HLT patients. The right internal jugular vein can be used because endomyocardial biopsies are not routinely used to monitor myocardial rejection postoperatively. In patients with en-bloc DLT, the right internal jugular can be used because endomyocardial biopsies are not necessary.

We use biplane or multiplane TEE (*see* Chapter 3) to help manage the patient pre- and post-CPB. After transplantation, TEE is used to assess left and right ventricular function, measure pulmonary artery pressures (using a tricuspid regurgitation jet), and guide management of pulmonary artery hypertension and RV dysfunction if necessary. In addition, TEE is used to assess the pulmonary arterial and pulmonary venous anastomoses after lung transplantation.[244,245] TEE also has proved useful in detection and treatment of dynamic, infundibular RV outflow tract obstruction after lung transplantation.[246] Patients with RV hypertrophy may have apposition of the walls of the infundibulum in systole, when RV afterload is reduced after donor lung implantation. Hypovolemia and inotrope use tend to exacerbate this problem.

A thoracic or lumbar epidural is used for postoperative pain management in SLT and BSSLT patients. The catheter is placed preoperatively in those patients who are unlikely to require CPB. This generally can be accomplished before induction but can be accomplished after induction and intubation. For patients requiring CPB, the epidural catheter is placed postoperatively after reversal of heparinization and correction of coagulation deficiencies. The catheter generally can be placed before leaving the operating room. In thoracic catheters, we infuse 0.25% bupivacaine and fentanyl 5 µg/mL at 4 to 8 mL/hr. In lumbar catheters, we use preservative-free morphine 0.05 mg/mL at 5 to 10 mL/hr.

Children.　Placement of an intravenous catheter before induction is optimal. EMLA cream can be used if necessary for older children. ECG monitoring should allow assessment of V_5, I, II, III, aVR, aVL, and aVF. Baseline recording of all seven leads should be obtained for

comparative purposes. Normally, two leads (II and V_5) are monitored simultaneously intraoperatively. If a left thoracotomy incision is used, V_5 is not an option because the lead will be in the operative field. A radial or femoral artery catheter is placed after induction of anesthesia. The technique and catheter size is discussed in detail in Chapter 6. Central venous pressure monitoring is placed after induction. For older children undergoing SLT or BSSLT without CPB or with partial CPB, a PA catheter is placed. For all other children, an appropriately sized double-lumen central venous line (*see* Chapter 6) is placed. The right internal jugular vein is the preferred site. We use a pediatric biplane TEE probe for children weighing less than 15 to 20 kg and the adult multiplane TEE probe for children weighing more than 20 to 30 kg to help manage the patient pre- and post-CPB as described previously for adult patients.

For older children undergoing SLT and BSSLT, a lumbar or thoracic epidural catheter is placed for postoperative pain management. The same guidelines outlined for adults are followed, except that the catheter is never placed before induction and intubation.

Management of OLV

The indications for use of OLV are summarized in Table 7–3. In procedures performed with full CPB, lung isolation and OLV are not necessary. These procedure can be managed with a standard single-lumen endotracheal tube. The anesthetic plan for SLT and BSSLT in adults and older children must include a method of lung isolation and OLV because these procedures are being performed increasingly without CPB or with partial CPB. When partial CPB is used, OLV to the perfused, nonoperative lung is necessary (*see* Chapter 10). Four methods of lung isolation and OLV are available:

Endobronchial Intubation.　A standard endotracheal tube (ETT) is used and then a bronchoscope is used to direct the ETT down the main stem bronchus of the lung that is to be ventilated.

ADVANTAGES
- applicable to any size patient with use of an appropriate-sized ETT.
- placement is easy with the appropriate-sized fiberoptic bronchoscope. When the right main stem bronchus is intubated, visualization of the right upper lobe (RUL) bronchus is possible with the bronchoscope. This helps prevent occlusion of the RUL bronchus by the balloon of the ETT.
- suctioning of secretions via the ETT before endobronchial intubation is easy because a large suction catheter or fiberoptic bronchoscope can be used.

- when the procedure is completed, the ETT does not have to be replaced.

DISADVANTAGES

- some deflation of the nonventilated lung will occur passively, but most will occur by absorption of gas. For patients with emphysema, this will result in slow, poor lung deflation and poor operating conditions.
- suctioning of the nonventilated lung and application of CPAP to the nonventilated lung is impossible.
- in taller patients, a standard ETT may not be long enough to extend far enough into the main stem bronchus to provide isolation.

Single-lumen Endotracheal Tube Plus a Bronchial Blocker. This technique involves use of a Fogarty catheter and a standard ETT.[247] Laryngoscopy is performed and the Fogarty catheter is placed in the trachea, followed by placement of the endotracheal tube. A fiberoptic bronchoscope is used to guide the catheter down the bronchus, which is to be blocked and not ventilated while the ETT remains in the trachea.

ADVANTAGES

- is applicable to any size patient with use of an appropriate-sized ETT and bronchial blocker. Fogarty catheters with balloon sizes from 0.5 to 3 mL are available.
- placement is easy with the appropriate-sized fiberoptic bronchoscope.
- suctioning of secretions via the ETT before placement of the blocker is easy because a large suction catheter or fiberoptic bronchoscope can be used.
- when the procedure is completed, the ETT does not have to be replaced and the Fogarty catheter can be removed.

DISADVANTAGES

- deflation of the blocked lung must occur by absorption of gas. For patients with emphysema, this will result in slow, poor lung delfation and poor operating conditions.
- suctioning of the nonventilated lung and application of continuous positive airway pressure (CPAP) to the nonventilated lung is impossible.
- maintaining the position of the blocker in the main stem bronchus during surgical manipulation may be difficult or impossible. In patients with cystic fibrosis undergoing BSSLT, this introduces the risk of contamination of the first lung transplanted with secretions from the remaining diseased lung.

- visualization of the RUL bronchus with a fiberoptic bronchoscope is impossible with the blocker in the right main stem bronchus. As a result, occlusion of the RUL bronchus by the balloon of the blocker may occur due to the high takeoff of the RUL bronchus. This makes surgical excision of the right lung and the subsequent transplant bronchial anastomosis technically difficult.
- the bronchial blocker balloon is a high-pressure balloon that may compromise bronchial mucosal blood flow.

Univent Tube. This is a standard endotracheal tube with a 3-mm outer diameter bronchial blocker, which passes through a 4-mm channel incorporated within the lumen of the endotracheal tube. The bronchial blocker has a 2-mm internal diameter lumen. These tubes are available with internal diameters from 6.0 to 9.0 mm in 0.5-mm increments. Because of the presence of the enclosed bronchial blocker, the external diameter of these tubes is considerably larger. The external diameter of the 8-mm Univent tube is 13 mm.[248] Optimal placement of the bronchial blocker requires use of a fiberoptic bronchoscope.

ADVANTAGES

- the arrangement of the blocker as an integral part of the ETT provides better stability of the blocker within the main stem bronchus during surgical manipulation.
- the internal lumen of the blocker will allow some decompression of the nonventilated lung and will allow the application of CPAP.
- when the procedure is completed, the Univent tube does not have to be replaced with a standard ETT. The bronchial blocker can be withdrawn into the internal channel and the Univent tube can be left in place.

DISADVANTAGES

- due to the large external diameter, these tubes are useful only for patients of normal adult size.
- the internal lumen of the blocker is too small to allow adequate suctioning of secretions.
- as with a standard bronchial blocker, occlusion of the RUL bronchus by the balloon of the blocker may occur.
- the bronchial blocker balloon is a high-pressure balloon that may compromise bronchial mucosal blood flow.

Double-lumen Endotracheal Tube. DLTs are available in sizes from 26 to 43 French. The outer diameter of a 26-French DLT is 5.5 mm.[249] Both right- and left-sided tubes are available. Right-sided tubes have a side lumen in the bronchial tube that must be positioned over the RUL bronchus so that the balloon of the bronchial lumen does not occlude the RUL bronchus. Fiberoptic bronchoscopy is necessary to ensure proper positioning of both right- and left-sided DLTs.

ADVANTAGES

- deflation and suctioning of the nonventilated lung is easily accomplished.
- application of CPAP to the nonventilated lung is easy.
- the endobronchial tube is not dislodged easily with surgical manipulation.
- visualization of the RUL bronchus with the DL tube in place is accomplished easily with a fiberoptic bronchoscope.

DISADVANTAGES

- alignment of the RUL lumen of a right-sided DLT tube with the patient's RUL can be difficult, particularly in the presence of thick secretions.
- the smallest available DLT tube is appropriate for children aged 7 to 8 years.
- suctioning tenacious secretions through the small lumens of the DL tube is more difficult than through the lumen of a standard ETT.
- when the procedure is completed, the DLT must be exchanged for a standard ETT.

A left-sided DLT is the method of choice for lung isolation in adult and pediatric patients undergoing SLT and BSSLT at our institution. On balance, it provides the greatest versatility and ease of placement. A left-sided DLT, when properly placed, with use of a fiberoptic bronchoscope does not compromise surgical exposure for the left pneumonectomy and the subsequent transplant bronchial anastomosis. For children who are too small for a 26-French DLT, a single-lumen ETT and full CPB are used.

Induction and Maintenance

Generally, 50 to 75 µg/kg of fentanyl or 10 to 15 µg/kg of sufentanil is used as the primary anesthetic for induction and maintenance. A benzodiazepine should be included as a part of the premedication or be administered intraoperatively to prevent awareness. Alternatively, administration of small, supplemental doses of an inhalational agent can be used to prevent awareness.

Many patients with end-stage pulmonary disease will be unable to lie flat due to severe dyspnea. These patients are induced in the sitting position and, as they lose consciousness, they are slowly placed supine. For patients in whom the risk of aspiration is deemed to be high, induction is performed with the patient in a slightly head up position and cricoid pressure is applied from commencement of induction until the trachea is intubated.

After several minutes of denitrogenation and with the patient breathing 100% oxygen, induction begins with an infusion of fentanyl 500 µg/min or sufentanil 100 µg/min over 5 to 10 minutes. A system of graded stimulation is used to assess anesthetic depth. After loss of consciousness, the hemodynamic response to insertion of an oral airway followed by insertion of a urinary catheter is used to gauge the need for additional narcotic to blunt the hemodynamic response to tracheal intubation. Larnygoscopy is performed carefully and should not be prolonged. If an upward trend in heart rate or blood pressure is noted as laryngoscopy commences, laryngoscopy should be terminated and additional narcotic should be titrated. If there is poor visualization of the trachea laryngoscopy should be terminated and intubating conditions improved by changing head position, using a stylet or changing blades. This approach will help prevent long stimulating laryngoscopies that compromise hemodynamics. If the entire narcotic dose is not used for induction, the remainder is infused slowly in anticipation of the skin incision.

Vecuronium or pancuronium 0.02 mg/kg or cisatracurium 0.04 mg/kg is administered approximately 1 to 2 minutes before starting the narcotic infusion. Pancuronium is a better choice for infants and smaller children because the vagolytic and sympathomimetic effects of pancuronium can be used to counteract the vagotonic effects of high doses of fentanyl or sufentanil. As the patient loses consciousness, the remainder of the total dose of vecuronium or pancuronium 0.1 mg/kg or cis-atracurium 0.02 mg/kg is administered and controlled ventilation with 100% O_2 initiated. This regimen minimizes the risk of narcotic-induced rigidity without undue stress to the patient.

Narcotic-induced rigidity with subsequent difficulty ventilating can have disastrous consequences for these patients. Therefore, when more prompt control of the airway is desirable, etomidate 0.15 to 0.3 mg/kg and succinylcholine 1.0 to 1.5 mg/kg in conjunction with fentanyl 5 to 10 µg/kg or sufentanil 1 µg/kg may be used. Etomidate produces minimal cardiovascular effects at this dosage when administered in conjunction with narcotics.[56]

When a left-sided DLT is needed, placement is accomplished as follows:

1. The trachea is intubated such that the tracheal cuff is just below the vocal cords and the tube is rotated 90° to the left. The trachea cuff is inflated and the patient is ventilated. The bronchial lumen will be located just above the carina in most normal-sized patients.
2. An appropriate-sized fiberoptic bronchoscope is introduced down the bronchial lumen and the right and left main stem bronchi are identified.

In some instances, it may be necessary to pull the DLT back slightly if the tip of the bronchial lumen is past the carina. For patients with cystic fibrosis or bronchiectasis, thick secretions may make identification difficult. A suction catheter and saline irrigation may have to be introduced down the bronchial lumen to clear secretions. Suctioning through the bronchoscope is difficult considering the small caliber scopes that can fit down the DLT. Alternatively, aggressive cleanout with an SLT and a large bronchoscope can be accomplished before placement of the DLT.

3. The bronchoscope is advanced down the left main stem bronchus and the left upper lobe bronchus is identified.

4. While the operator keeps the tip of the bronchoscope above the left upper lobe bronchus orifice, the tracheal balloon is deflated and the DLT is advanced into the left main stem bronchus over the bronchoscope. The tip of the bronchial lumen should be confirmed to be above the left upper lobe bronchus. The tracheal balloon is reinflated and ventilation continues.

5. The bronchoscope is now placed down the tracheal lumen. Ideally, the tracheal lumen should be positioned just above the right main stem bronchus with the bronchial balloon below the rim of the orifice of the left main stem bronchus. If the DLT has been advanced too far down the left main stem bronchus, the tracheal lumen may lie within the left main stem bronchus. This is unlikely if the tip of the bronchial lumen lies above the left upper lobe bronchus.

6. If the tracheal lumen is within the left main stem bronchus, the tracheal balloon is deflated and the DLT is pulled back until the tracheal lumen provides unobstructed access to the right main stem bronchus. The bronchial balloon should remain at or below the rim of the left main stem bronchus orifice. The tracheal balloon is reinflated.

7. After proper positioning is confirmed, the bronchial balloon is inflated while the bronchoscope remains in the tracheal lumen. The bronchial balloon should not herniate out the left main stem bronchus when the balloon is inflated. If the balloon herniates out of the left main stem bronchus, the DLT must be advanced slightly into the left main stem bronchus.

8. Positioning of the DLT should be rechecked with the bronchoscope after the patient has been moved into final position. DLT placement may change after movement of the patient into the lateral decubitus position.

For patients with obstructive lung disease (emphysema, alpha$_1$ antitrypsin deficiency, cystic fibrosis) induction and positive pressure ventilation may produce profound hypotension. This cardiovascular compromise is secondary to air trapping or auto-PEEP.[250-252] This auto-PEEP reduces SV and cardiac output through the following:

- reductions in venous return to the RV resulting in a decrease in RVEDV
- increased impedance to RV ejection by mechanical compression of the pulmonary arterial system resulting in an increase in RVESV
- shift of the interventricular septum into the LV, which increases LV stiffness and reduces LVEDV.

This combination is particularly detrimental for patients with compromised RV systolic function and RV afterload mismatch. Treatment requires volume administration to (10 to 15 ml/kg of a balanced salt solution) to normalize RVEDV and intropic support to improve RV systolic function and normalize RVESV. Dobutamine 5 to 10 µg/kg/min and epinephrine 0.01 to 0.1 µg/kg/min (adults) or 0.05 to 0.5 µg/kg/min (children) are both effective. In addition, ventilation with a rapid initial inflation followed by an inspiratory hold or pause and a long expiration time is necessary (low I/E). This may require hand ventilation, although pressure-control ventilation with a Siemens 900 ventilator works well. PEEP should not be used. TEE is extremely valuable in assessing ventricular filling and contractile function in this setting because filling pressures will not provide an accurate measure of ventricular volumes.

In the most severe instances, intermittent periods of apnea may be necessary. This apneic oxygenation may exacerbate preexisting pulmonary hypertension, CO_2 retention, and hypoxemia. Evaluation of pulmonary artery pressures and cardiac output with a PA catheter, RV and LV function with TEE, and arterial saturation with pulse oximetry are necessary to determine the extent of hypoventilation that can be tolerated. With appropriate monitoring marked acidemia (pH of 6.94) and hypercarbia (PaCO$_2$ of 150 mm Hg) can be tolerated during lung transplantation.[253] In rare cases, initiation of CPB may be necessary.

Blood loss may be impressive during dissection for pneumonectomy in HLT, SLT, and double lung transplantation patients with dense adhesions from previous thoracic surgery or for patients with cystic fibrosis[254] or bronchiectasis. A rapid transfusion device may be necessary in some cases. Some centers use aprotinin (*see* Chapter 10) in both children and adults when CPB is used or when there are dense adhesions regardless of whether CPB is used or not.[255,256] In addition to red cells, component therapy with FFP and platelets often is necessary, particularly when CPB is used.[253] Manipulation of the lungs in patients with cystic fibrosis or bronchiectasis may result in release of endotoxins with subsequent decrease in SVR, hyperpyrexia, and increased metabolic rate. Management of the recipient without use of CPB under these conditions is extremely difficult.[257]

After one or both of the lungs have been implanted and perfused, most centers administer methylprednisolone (usually 10 mg/khg for children and 500 mg for adults). After lung implantation has been completed, 5 to 10 cm H_2O PEEP is applied and the FiO_2 selected is the lowest necessary to obtain a PaO_2 of 90 to 100 mm Hg. This is done because the postischemic lung is vulnerable to oxygen-free radial toxicity. At the termination of the procedure, patients with DLTs have the DLT replaced with a large single-lumen ETT. The large tube size allows easy access for postoperative fiberoptic bronchoscopy.

Special Considerations for SLT and BSSLT

Management of OLV and pulmonary artery clamping for recipient pneumonectomy and allograft implantation in SLT and BSSLT patients without CPB is a challenge. The task is made easier for patients undergoing SLT if the lung with the poorest ventilation and perfusion is removed and replaced. For patients undergoing BSSLT, the lung with the poorest ventilation and perfusion should be removed and replaced first.

Maintenance of body temperature is a challenge when CPB is not used.[258] A warming blanket under the patient, an actively humidified breathing circuit, a fluid/blood warmer, and a forced warm air blanket over the patient all are necessary.

OLV. Collapse of the operative lung and OLV is likely to exacerbate air trapping and the subsequent hemodynamic compromise and CO_2 retention. Treatment with volume administration, inotropes, and ventilatory interventions is warranted as described previously. Marked hypercarbia with acidemia is likely and generally is well tolerated. Aggressive suctioning may be necessary to failiitate collapse of the operative lung. PaO_2 also is likely to decrease, due to intrapulmonary shunting, until the ipsilateral pulmonary artery is clamped. Administration of CPAP to the nonventilated lung, insufflation of O_2 to the nonventilated lung, or high-frequency jet ventilation (HFJV) of the nonventilated lung may improve oxygenation.

Clamping of the PA. Recipient pneumonectomy requires clamping of the ipsilateral pulmonary artery. Before clamping of the pulmonary artery, the pulmonary artery catheter is withdrawn into the main pulmonary artery. Palpation by the surgeon will confirm its position proximal to the proposed cross-clamp site. Af-

ter the ipsilateral pulmonary artery has been clamped, the catheter is advanced into the contralateral pulmonary artery. Clamping of the pulmonary artery may compromise RV function due to afterload mismatch. This is most likely in patients with mild to moderate preexisting pulmonary hypertension and in those with impaired RV function. This is the primary reason why patients with severe pulmonary hypertension require elective CPB. If there is any doubt regarding the ability of the patient to tolerate pulmonary artery clamping, a trial of clamping is recommended. TEE is used to assess RV function. In addition, increased PAP and CVP, falling cardiac index, and SVO_2 may occur.

Allograft Implantation. Immediately after allograft implantation and washout of Euro-Collins solution and prostaglandin, there may be profound, transient systemic hypotension. Treatment requires fluid administration and alpha-adrenergic support. After implantation of the donor lung, there usually is an immediate reduction in PA pressures and an improvement in pulmonary compliance and gas exchange. This period may be followed by allograft dysfunction characterized by deteriorating gas exchange, decreasing pulmonary compliance, and elevated PA pressures. This is the result of noncardiogenic, reperfusion pulmonary edema. Two factors predispose this process:

1. preexisting pulmonary hypertension, which results in overperfusion of the donor lung.
2. a long ischemic interval, which enhances capillary permeability.

PEEP (5 to 15 cm H_2O) usually is necessary to maintain adequate gas exchange when allograft dysfunction occurs. Increased capillary permeability and the lack of pulmonary lymphatic drainage in the allograft requires that crystalloid administration be judicious. Excessively large tidal volumes should be avoided because over inflation of the allograft will contribute to elevated PA pressures through mechanical compression of the pulmonary vasculature.

If allograft dysfunction is severe, implantation of the second lung in BSSLT patients may require CPB. If CPB is not used, implantation of the second lung is managed as described for the first lung.

Indications for CPB. The decision to use CPB is individualized for each patient. The use of CPB may become necessary at any of the following points during SLT or BSSLT:

- following induction of anesthesia
- following initiation of OLV
- following PA clamping
- following OLV and PA clamping on the contralateral side after allograft implantation

CPB is not necessary for increased pulmonary artery pressures unless there is evidence of deteriorating RV function. TEE assessment of RV function is supplemented by use of CVP determinations. Increasing CVP, RV distension, worsening global hypokinesis, and new or worsening TR despite inotropic support with epinephrine and dobutamine and intravenous pulmonary vasodilation with nitroglycerin 0.5 to 5 µg/kg/min, PGE_1 0.05 to 0.2 µg/kg/min, or PGI_2 5 to 20 ng/kg/min are indications for use of CPB. Inhaled NO has been used both intraoperatively and postoperatively to treat pulmonary hypertension from graft dysfunction.[259,260] When it becomes readily available, it will undoubtedly prove useful.

TEE is used to monitor LV function as well. TEE assessment of LV function is supplemented by use of PCWP determinations. Hypoxemia, hypercarbia, and reduced systemic blood pressure can all contribute to LV dysfunction. Progressive deterioration in LV function (new wall motion abnormalities, LV distension, new or worsening MR) despite aggressive pharmacologic and ventilatory interventions is an indication for CPB.

In addition, cardiac index <2 L/min/m^2, SVO_2 < 60%, mean arterial pressure (MAP) < 50 to 60 mm Hg, SaO_2 < 85 to 90%, and pH < 7.00 despite aggressive ventilatory and pharmacologic interventions are all indications for use of CPB. A metabolic acidosis is difficult to treat because sodium bicarbonate administration will produce CO_2, which must be eliminated by increased alveolar ventilation. Obviously, increasing alveolar ventilation often is not possible.

■ POST-CARDIOPULMONARY BYPASS MANAGEMENT

Preparations for terminating CPB are discussed in Chapter 10. Particular attention must be paid to deairing the heart. Severe ventricular dysfunction may follow ejection of air through the coronary arteries. The right ventricle is particularly at risk due to the anterior location of the right coronary ostia. TEE is valuable in guiding the deairing process.

Patients undergoing HLT have a denervated heart and are managed in the post-CPB period in the same manner as that described for heart transplant patients.

RV function usually improves dramatically after lung implantation due to the immediate reduction in pulmonary artery pressures. Despite this, patients with en-bloc DLT,[261] BSSLT, or SLT may require inotropic support. Patients requiring aortic cross-clamping and cardioplegic arrest are at particular risk for post-CPB right and left ventricular dysfunction. In addition, the presence of lung allograft dysfunction may contribute to post-CPB RV dysfunction as the result of elevated PA pressures.

■ POSTOPERATIVE CARE

In rare instances, extracorporeal membrane oxygenation and independent lung ventilation may be necessary after SLT in patients with pulmonary hypertension secondary to reperfusion pulmonary edema.[262] Postoperative independent lung ventilation with a DLT has been used for patients with SLT to minimize preferential ventilation and air trapping in the native lung in patients with obstructive lung disease.[250-252] For these patients, the native lung has high compliance and air trapping can result in hyperinflation with subsequent displacement of the mediastinum and compression of the donor lung. Differential ventilation with hypoventilation of the native lung has been used successfully to avoid this problem. Preferential perfusion of the donor lung occurs after SLT, especially for patients with pulmonary hypertension. In cases of severe V/Q mismatch, selective hypoventilation of the native lung combined with positioning the patient in the lateral position with the donor lung in the nondependent position may be necessary in the postoperative period. This will minimize overventilation of the native lung and overperfusion of the donor lung. In patients with SLT with a fibrotic native lung, positioning the patient with the donor lung dependent may help equalize ventilation to the both lungs.

■ SURGERY IN LUNG TRANSPLANT PATIENTS

As with heart transplant patients, lung transplant, and HLT patients may require surgical procedures. Some are purely elective, whereas others are likely to be urgent or emergent. Most surgical procedures are the direct result of complications of triple-drug (cyclosporine, azathioprine, prednisone) immunosuppressive therapy. These complications are listed Table 7-2. The incidence of complications requiring general surgical consultation and intervention in lung transplant patients is 16%.[263] In addition, lung transplant patients suffer airway and vascular anastomotic complications that require operative intervention.[264,265] The incidence of airway complications in SLT and BSSLT is 12 to 17% per anastomosis with an associated mortality rate of 2 to 3%.[266] Nine percent of nonlethal airway complications require operative intervention.[266] Similar statistics exist in pediatric patients.[237,243] The most common intervention required is for treatment of bronchial stenosis. This usually involves flexible and rigid bronchoscopy for laser excision of granulation tissue, stent placement, or balloon dilatation.

Lung transplant and HLT patients present a unique set of management issues. They are outlined here:

1. Loss of cough reflex due to transection of vagal fibers — this makes the patient with a transplanted lung prone to retention of secretions and at risk for pulmonary infections. The risk of aspiration should not be significantly increased as the innervation of the larynx, epiglottis, and proximal trachea remain normal. However, laryngeal nerve injury during dissection can result in loss of protective airway reflexes.

2. Reduction in lung volumes — mild proportional reductions in all lung volumes are seen long term in patients after HLT, DLT, and SLT.[267] These reductions are not due to reduced elastic properties of the transplanted lung but are secondary to the volume constraints of the recipient chest cavity and to the strength and efficiency of the thoracic musculature.[268] In fact, the improvement in elastic recoil and the reduced chest wall distention that follow SLT for emphysema substantially reduce the work of breathing and dyspnea.[269]

3. Ventilatory response to CO_2 — HLT and DLT patients have total vagal denervation, whereas SLT patients retain vagal innervation to the native lung. HLT, BSSLT, and SLT patients all increase minute ventilation in response to CO_2 rebreathing-induced hypercapnia. However, while SLT patients increase both tidal volume and respiratory rate, HLT and BSSLT patients exhibit an increase in tidal volume with little or no respiratory rate response.[270-272]

4. Ventilatory response to hypoxia — lung transplant patients have an increase in tidal volume and respiratory rate comparable to normal patients in response to hypoxia.[272]

5. Rejection — acute rejection of the transplanted lungs can be diagnosed both clinically and with transbronchial biopsies via a flexible bronchoscope. In the absence of clinical evidence of rejection (dyspnea, fever, diffuse perihilar infiltrate on chest radiograph) biopsies are performed at regular intervals postoperatively. Obviously, if clinical evidence of rejection exists, more frequent biopsies may be indicated to document rejection and to assess regression of histologic changes with treatment. Biopsies are graded from 0 to 4 based on histologic criteria.[273] No rejection is 0 with mild rejection 1 and severe rejection 4.

   Acute rejection of the lungs is very common; 98% of patients experience an acute rejection episode in the first month post-transplantation. In fact, it is not uncommon for patients to experience two or three acute rejection episodes during the first several months post-transplanta-

tion. Rejection of the heart in HLT patients, on the other hand, is uncommon. Because rejection of the heart and lungs is not synchronous, heart biopsies are performed in HLT patients only if there is clinical evidence of heart rejection. Rejection is treated with oral or intravenous pulsed steroids. Persistent rejection unresponsive to steroids usually is treated with a lympholytic agent such as polyclonal antithymocyte globulin (ATG) or murine monoclonal antibody (OKT3).

6. Bronchiolitis obliterans syndrome (BOS) and bronchiolitis obliterans (BO) — BOS is a clinical entity characterized by declining FEV_1, FEF_{25-75}, and FEF_{50}/FVC. BOS is graded based on the reduction in FEV_1 compared with the best baseline value. (O: FEV_1 80 to 100%; 1: FEV_1 65 to 80%; 2: FEV_1 50 to 65%; 3: FEV_1 less than 50%). BO is a pathologic diagnosis based on histologic evidence of fibrous scarring of membraneous and respiratory bronchioles with partial or complete obliteration of the lumen.

   BOS and BO are the main sources of morbidity and mortality after lung transplantation. The prevalence of BOS and BO for HLT, SLT, and BSSLT patients is 50 to 60% at 3 years and 80% at 10 years in large series.[274-277] The mortality rate for patients with BOS and BO is 50% in these same series.

   Once established, BOS and BO follow a progressive downhill course. Patients with BOS and BO ultimately develop severe obstructive pulmonary disease and progressive hypoxemia. Recently, augmented immunosuppression has been shown to attenuate this downhill course and improve survival.[274] In severe progressive cases, retransplantation is the only option. However, the results are not encouraging, with a 1-year survival of 35%, as BOS and BO usually reoccur within a short time.[278]

   The etiology is multifactorial with rejection and CMV infection both implicated. It is believed that an alloimmune injury occurs with subsequent release of immunologic mediators and production of growth factors that lead to luminal obliteration and scarring of small airway.[274] Monitoring for BO is accomplished with transbronchial biopsies.

7. Response to drugs — HLT patients have a denervated heart and have drug responses identical to those described for heart transplant patients.

8. HLT patients — these patients will have all of the cardiac problems outlined previously for heart transplant patients.

Anesthetic Considerations

1. Sterile technique is essential.
2. Patients with stenotic airways and patients with BOS and BO may exhibit airtrapping and auto PEEP.
3. Diminished cough reflex makes clearing of secretions difficult. Laryngeal damage will predispose aspiration.
4. Lymphatic interruption necessitates careful fluid administration to avoid interstitial pulmonary fluid accumulation.
5. Placement of ETTs must take into account the position of the tracheal or bronchial anastomoses.
6. Patients will preoperative CO_2 retention may exhibit CO_2 retention for 2 to 3 weeks postoperatively as the central chemoreceptors reset.
7. HLT patients will present the same cardiac challenges as heart transplant patients.
8. Stress-dose steroid coverage should be administered to patients receiving steroids as part of immunosuppression.

■ REFERENCES

1. O'Connell JB, Bourge RC, Costanzio-Nordin MR, et al: Cardiac transplantation: Recipient selection, donor procurement, and medical followup. *Circulation* 1992; **86**:1061–1079.
2. Mancini DM, Eisen H, Kussmaul W, et al: Value of peak exercise oxygen consumption for optimal timing of cardiac transplantation in ambulatory patients with heart failure. *Circulation* 1991; **83**:778–786.
3. Hosenpud JD, Novick RJ, Breen TJ, et al: The registry of the International Society for Heart and Lung Transplantation: Twelfth offical report, 1995. *J Heart Lung Transplant* 1995; **14**:805–815.
4. Goldstein DJ, Oz MC, Rose EA, et al: Experience with heart transplantation for cardiac tumors. *J Heart Lung Transplant* 1995; **14**:382–386.
5. Hosenpud JD, DeMarco T, Frazier H, et al: Progression of systemic disease and reduced long-term survival in patients with cardiac amyloidosis undergoing heart transplantation. Follow-up results of a multicenter survey. *Circulation* 1991; **84**(suppl 3):III-338–III-343.
6. Oni AA, Hershberger RE, Norman DJ, et al: Recurrence of sarcoidosis in a cardiac allograft: Control with augmented corticosteroids. *J Heart Lung Transplant* 1992; **11**:367–369.
7. O'Connell JB, Dec GW, Goldenberg IF, et al: Results of heart transplantation for active lymphocytic myocarditis. *J Heart Transplant* 1990; **9**:351–360.
8. Munoz E, Lonquist J, Radovancevic B, et al: Long-term results in diabetic patients undergoing cardiac transplantation. *J Heart Transplant* 1991; **10**:189–190.
9. Rhenman MJ, Rhenman B, Icenogle T, et al: Diabetes and heart transplantation. *J Heart Transplant* 1988; **7**:356–358.
10. Heroux AL, Costanzo-Nordin MR, O'Sullivan JE, et al: Heart transplantation as a treatment option for end-stage heart disease in patients older than 65 years of age. *J Heart Lung Transplant* 1993; **12**:573–579.
11. Dec GW, Fuster V: Idiopathic dilated cardiomyopathy. *N Engl J Med* 1994; **331**:1564–1575.
12. Johnson RA, Palacois I: Dilated cardiomyopathies of the adult. *N Engl J Med* 1982; **307**:1051–1058, 1119–1125.
13. Katz AM: Cardiomyopathy of overload: A major determinant of prognosis in congestive heart failure. *N Engl J Med* 1990; **322**:100–110.
14. Pfeffer MA, Braunwald E: Ventricular remodeling after myocardial infarction. Experimental observations and clinical implications. *Circulation* 1990; **81**:1161–1172.
15. Pfeffer MA: Left ventricular remodeling after acute myocardial infarction. *Annu Rev Med* 1995; **46**:455–466.
16. Thomas JA, Marks BH: Plasma norepinephrine in congestive heart failure. *Am J Cardiol* 1978; **41**:233–243.
17. Ungerer M, Bohm M, Elce JS, et al: Altered expression of β-adrenergic receptor kinase and $β_1$-adrenergic receptors in the failing human heart. *Circulation* 1993; **87**:454–463.
18. Bristow MR, Anderson FL, Port JD, et al: Differences in β-adrenergic neuroeffector mechanisms in ischemic versus idiopathic dilated cardiomyopathy. *Circulation* 1991; **84**:1024–1039.
19. Neumann J, Schmitz W, Scholz H, et al: Increase in myocardial G_1 proteins in heart failure. *Lancet* 1988; **22**:936.
20. Waagstein F, Bristow MR, Swedberg K et al: Beneficial effects of metroprolol in idiopathic dilated cardiomyopathy. *Lancet* 1993; **342**:1441–1446.
21. Heilbrunn SM, Shah P, Bristow MR, et al: Increased beta receptor density and improved hemodynamic response to catecholamine stimulation during long-term metroprolol therapy in heart failure from dilated cardiomyopathy. *Circulation* 1989; **79**:483.
22. Packer M, Carver JR, Rodeheffer RJ, et al: Effect of oral milrinone on mortality in severe chronic heart failure. *N Engl J Med* 1991; **325**:1468–1475.
23. Appleton CP, Hatle LK, Popp RL: Relation of transmitral flow velocity patterns to left ventricular diastolic function: New insights from a combined hemodynamic and Doppler echocardiographic study. *J Am Coll Cardiol* 1988; **12**:426–444.
24. Neglia D, Parodi O, Gallopin M, et al: Myocardial blood flow response to pacing tachycardia and to dipyridamole infusion in patients with dilated cardiomyopathy without overt heart failure. A quantitative assessment by positron emission tomography. *Circulation* 1995; **92**:796–804.
25. Kirklin JK, Naftel DC, Kirlin JW, et al: Pulmonary vascular resistance and the risk of heart transplantation. *J Heart Transplant* 1988; **7**:331–336.
26. Murali S, Kormos RL, Uretsky BF, et al: Preoperative pulmonary hemodynamics and early mortality after orthotopic cardiac transplantation: The Pittsburgh experience. *Am Heart J* 1993; **126**:896–904.
27. Addonizio LJ, Gersony WM, Robbins RC, et al: Elevated pulmonary vascular resistance and cardiac transplantation. *Circulation* 1987; **76**(suppl V):V-52–V-56.
28. Webber SA, Fricker FJ, Michael M, et al: Orthotopic heart transplantation in children with congenital heart disease. *Ann Thorac Surg* 1994; **58**:1664–1669.
29. Bando K, Konnishi H, Komatsu K, et al: Improved survival following pediatric cardiac transplantation in high-risk patients. *Circulation* 1993; **88**:218–223.
30. Taylor AJ, Bergin JD: Cardiac transplantation for the cardiologist not trained in transplantation. *Am Heart J* 1995; **129**:578–592.
31. Costard-Jackle A, Fowler MB: Influence of preoperative pulmonary artery pressure on mortality after heart transplantation: Testing of potential reversibility of pulmonary hypertension with nitroprusside is useful in defining a high risk group. *J Am Coll Cardiol* 1992; **19**:48–54.
32. Miller LW, Kubo SH, Young JB, et al: Report of the Consensus Conference on Candidate Selection for Heart Transplantation, 1993. *J Heart Lung Transplant* 1995; **14**:562–571.
33. Sarris GE, Smith JA, Bernstein D, et al: Pediatric cardiac transplan-

tation. The Stanford experience. *Circulation* 1994; **90**(part 2):II-51–II-55.

34. The SOLVD Investigators: Effect of enalapril on survival in patients with reduced left-ventricular ejection fractions and congestive heart failure. *N Engl J Med* 1991; **325**:293–302.

35. The CONSENSUS Trial Study Group: Effects of enalapril on mortality in severe congestive heart failure: results of the Cooperative North Scandinavian Enalapril Survival Study (CONSENSUS). *N Engl J Med* 1987; **316**:1429–1435.

36. Cohn JN, Johnson G, Ziesche S, et al: A comparison of enalapril with hydralazine-isosorbide dinitrate in the treatment of chronic congestive heart failure. *N Engl J Med* 1991; **325**:303–310.

37. Blackbourne LH, Tribble CG, Langenburg SE, et al: Successful use of undersized donor

38. Costanzo-Nordin MR, Liao Y, Grusk BB, et al: Oversizing of donor hearts: Beneficial or detrimental? *J Heart Lung Transplant* 1991; **10**:717–730.

39. Turrentine MW, Kesler KA, Caldwell R, et al: Cardiac transplantation in infants and children. *Ann Thorac Surg* 1994; **57**:546–554.

40. Bernstein D, Kolla S, Miner M, et al: Cardiac growth after pediatric heart transplantation. *Circulation* 1992; **85**:1433–1439.

41. Addonizio LJ, Gersony WM: The transplanted heart in the pediatric patient. Growth or adaptation. *Circulation* 1992; **85**:1624–1626.

42. Costanzo-Nordin MR, O'Connell JB, Engelmeier RS, et al: Dilated cardiomyopathy: Functional status, hemodynamics, arrhythmias, and prognosis. *Cathet Cardiovasc Diag* 1985; **11**:445–453.

43. Falk RH, Foster E, Coats MH: Ventricular thrombi and thromboembolism in dilated cardiomyopathy: A prospective follow-up study. *Am Heart J* 1992; **123**:136–142.

44. Dunkman WB, Johnson GR, Carson PE, et al: Incidence of thromboembolic events in congestive heart failure. *Circulation* 1993; **87**(suppl VI):VI-94–VI-101.

45. Evans RW, Manninen DL, Garrison LP, Maier AM. Donor availability as the primary determinant of the future of heart transplantation. *JAMA* 1986; **255**:1892–1898.

46. Copeland JG, Emery RW, Levinson MM, Copeland J, McAleer MJ, Riley JE: The role of mechanical support and transplantation in treatment of patients with end stage cardiomyopathy. *Circulation* 1985; **72**(suppl 2):II-7–II-12.

47. McCarthy PM, Portner PM, Tobler HG, et al: Clinical experience with the Novacor ventricular assist system. Bridge to transplantation and the transition to permanent application. *J Thorac Cardiovasc Surg* 1991; **102**:578–587.

48. Joyce LD, Johnson KE, Toninato CJ, et al: Results of the first 100 patients who received Symbion Total Artificial Hearts as a bridge to cardiac transplantation. *Circulation* 1989; **80**(suppl III): III-192–III-201.

49. Copeland JG, Smith R, Icenogle T, et al: Orthotopic total artificial heart bridge to transplantation: Preliminary results. *J Heart Transplant* 1989; **8**:124–138.

50. Keon WJ, Heggtveit HA, Leduc J: Perioperative myocardial infarction caused by atheroembolism. *J Thorac Cardiovasc Surg* 1982; **84**:849–855.

51. Grondin CM, Pomar JL, Herbert Y: Re-operation in patients with patent atherosclerotic coronary vein grafts. *J Thorac Cardiovasc Surg* 1984; **87**:379–385.

52. Rosow CE, Philbin DM, Keegan CR, Moss J: Hemodynamics and histamine release during induction with sufentanil or fentanyl. *Anesthesiology* 1984; **60**:489–491.

53. Stanley TH, Webster LR: Anesthesia requirements and cardiovascular effects of fentanyl-oxygen and fentanyl-diazepam-oxygen anesthesia in man. *Anesth Analg* 1978; **57**:411–426.

54. Sebel PS, Bovil JG: Cardiovascular effects of sufentanil anesthesia. *Anesth Analg* 1982; **61**:115–119.

55. Howie MB, McSweeney TD, Lingam Maschke SP: A comparison of fentanyl-O$_2$ and sufentanil-O$_2$ for cardiac anesthesia. *Anesth Analg* 1985; **64**:877–887.

56. Waterman PM, Bjerke R: Rapid sequence induction in patients with severe ventricular dysfunction. *J Cardiothorac Anesth* 1988; **2**:602–606.

57. Butterworth JF, Bean E, Royster RL: Sufentanil is preferable to etomidate during rapid-sequence anesthesia induction for aorto-coronary bypass surgery. *J Cardiothorac Anesth* 1989; **3**:396–400.

58. Philbin DM, Roscow CE, Schneider RC, et al: Fentanyl and sufentanil anesthesia revisited: How much is enough? *Anesthesiology* 1990; **73**:5–11.

59. Mann T, Cohn PF, Holman BL, et al: Effect of nitroprusside on regional myocardial blood flow in coronary artery disease. Results in 25 patients and comparison with nitroglycerin. *Circulation* 1978; **57**:732–737.

60. Flaherty JT, Magee PA, Gardner TL, et al: Comparison of intravenous nitroglycerin and sodium nitroprusside for treatment of acute hypertension developing after coronary artery bypass surgery. *Circulation* 1982; **65**:1072–1077.

61. Kaplan JA, Jones EL: Vasodilator therapy during coronary artery surgery. Comparison of nitroglycerin and nitroprusside. *J Thorac Cardiovasc Surg* 1977; **77**:301–309.

62. Tomicheck RC, Rosow CE, Philbin DA, et al: Diazepam-fentanyl interaction — hemodynamic and hormonal effects in coronary artery surgery. *Anesth Analg* 1983; **62**:881–884.

63. Heikkila H, Jalonen J, Arola M: Midazolam as adjunct to high-dose fentanyl anesthesia for coronary artery bypass grafting operation. *Acta Anaesthesiol Scand* 1984; **28**:683–689.

64. Heikkila H, Jalonen J, Laaksonen V: Lorazepam and high-dose fentanyl anaesthesia: Effects on hemodynamics and oxygen transportation in patients undergoing coronary revascularization. *Acta Anaesthesiol Scand* 1984; **28**:357–361.

65. Schulte-Sasse U, Hess W, Tarnow J: Pulmonary vascular response to nitrous oxide in patients with normal and high pulmonary vascular resistance. *Anesthesiology* 1982; **57**:9–13.

66. Lower RR, Stofen RR, Shumway NE: Homovital transplantation of the heart. *J Thorac Cardiovasc Surg* 1961; **41**:196.

67. Angermann CE, Spes CH, Tammen A, et al: Anatomic characteristics and valvular function of the transplanted heart: Transthoracic versus transesophageal echocardiographic findings. *J Heart Lung Transplant* 1990; **9**:331–339.

68. Kaye DM, Anderson ST, Federman J: Electrocardiographic and echocardiographic features of left atrial size after orthotopic cardiac transplantation. *Am J Cardiol* 1992; **70**:1096–1099.

69. Fernandez AL, Llorens R, Herreros JM, et al: Intracardiac thrombi after orthotopic heart transplantation: Clinical significance and etiological factors. *J Heart Lung Transplant* 1994; **13**:236–240.

70. Saram MA, Campbell CS, Yonan NA, et al: An alternative surgical technique in orthotopic cardiac transplantation. *J Cardiovasc Surg* 1993; **8**:344–349.

71. El Gamel A, Yonan NA, Grant S, et al: Orthotopic cardiac transplantation: A comparison of standard and bicaval Wythenshawe techniques. *J Cardiovasc Thorac Surg* 1995; **109**:721–730.

72. Deleuze PH, Benvenuti C, Mazzucotelli JP, et al: Orthotopic cardiac transplantation with direct caval anastomosis: Is it the optimal procedure? *J Cardiovasc Thorac Surg* 1995; **109**:731–737.

73. Barnard CN, Losman JG: Left ventricular bypass. *S Afr Med* 1975; **49**:303–312.

74. Morris-Thurgood J, Cowell R, Paul V, et al: Hemodynamic and metabolic effects of paced linkage following heterotopic cardiac transplantation. *Circulation* 1994; **90**:2342–2347.

75. Ridley PD, Khaghani A, Musumeci F, et al: Heterotopic heart transplantation and recipient heart operation in ischemic heart disease. *Ann Thorac Surg* 1992; **54**:333–337.

76. Kriett JM, Kaye MP: The registry of the International Society for

Heart and Lung Transplantation: Eighth official report, 1991. *J Heart Lung Transplant* 1991; **10**:491-498.

77. Kawaguchi AT, Gandjbakhch I, Desruennes M, et al: Orthotopic vs heterotopic heart transplantation in donor/recipient size mismatch. *Transplant Proc* 1995; **27**:1277-1281.

78. Kent KM, Cooper T: The denervated heart. A model for studying autonomic control of the heart. *N Engl J Med* 1974; **291**:1017-1021.

79. Altered cardiovascular and neurohumoral responses to head-up tilt after heart-lung transplantation. *Circulation* 1990; **82**:863-871.

80. Mohanty PK, Thames MD, Arrowood JA, et al: Impairment of cardiopulmonary baroreflex after cardiac transplantation in humans. *Circulation* 1987; **75**:914-921.

81. Ellenbogen KA, Mohanty PK, Szentpetery S, et al: Arterial baroreflex abnormalities in heart failure. Reversal after orthotopic cardiac transplantation. *Circulation* 1989; **79**:51-58.

82. Hsu DT, Garofano RP, Douglas JM, et al: Exercise performance after pediatric heart transplantation. *Circulation* 1993; **88**:II-238-II-242.

83. Pope SE, Stinson EB, Daughter GT, et al: Exercise response of the denervated heart in long-term cardiac transplant recipients. *Am J Cardiol* 1980; **46**:213-218.

84. Gilbert EM, Eiswirth CC, Mealey PC, et al: β-adrenergeric supersensitivity of the transplanted human heart is presynaptic in origin. *Circulation* 1989; **79**:344-349.

85. von Scheidt W, Bohm M, Schneider B, et al: Isolated presynaptic inotropic β-adrenergic supersensitivity of the transplantation denervated human heart in vivo. *Circulation* 1992; **85**:1056-1063.

86. Wilson RF, Christensen BV, Olivari MT, et al: Evidence for structural sympathetic reinnervation after orthotopic cardiac transplantation in humans. *Circulation* 1991; **83**:1210-1220.

87. Burke MN, McGinn AL, Homans DL, et al: Evidence for functional sympathetic reinnervation of left ventricle and coronary arteries after orthotopic cardiac transplantation in humans. *Circulation* 1995; **91**:72-78.

88. Lord S, Holt N, Brady S, et al: Hemodynamic effects of sympathetic efferent reinnervation after orthotopic cardiac transplantation. *Circulation* 1995; **91**:3023-3024.

89. Lord S, Holt N, Brady S, et al: Hemodynamic effects of sympathetic efferent reinnervation after orthotopic cardiac transplantation. *Circulation* 1995; **91**:3023-3024.

90. Stark RP, McGinn AL, Wilson RF: Chest pain in cardiac-transplant recipients. Evidence of sensory reinnervation after cardiac transplantation. *N Engl J Med* 1991; **324**:1791-1794.

91. Schroeder JS, Hunt SA: Chest pain in cardiac-transplant recipients. *N Engl J Med* 1991; **324**:1805-1807.

92. Arrowood JA, Goudreau E, Minisi A, et al: Evidence against reinnervation of cardiac vagal afferents after human orthotopic cardiac transplantation. *Circulation* 1995; **92**:402-408.

93. Leenen FHH, Davies RA, Fourney A: Role of cardiac β$_2$ receptors in cardiac responses to exercise in cardiac transplant patients. *Circulation* 1995; **91**:685-690.

94. Pope SE, Stinson EB, Daughters GT, et al: Exercise response of the denervated heart in long-term cardiac transplant recipients. *Am J Cardiol* 1980; **46**:213-218.

95. Pflugfelder PW, Purves PD, McKenzie FN, et al: Cardiac dynamics during supine exercise in cyclosporine-treated heart transplant recipients: Assessment by radionuclide angiography. *J Am Coll Cardiol* 1987; **10**:336-341.

96. Mandak JS, Aaronson KD, Mancini DM: Serial assessment of exercise capacity after heart transplantation. *J Heart Lung Transplant* 1995; **14**:468-478.

97. Quigg RJ, Rocco MB, Gauthier DF, et al: Mechanism of the attenuated heart rate response to exercise after orthotopic cardiac transplantation. *J Am Coll Cardiol* 1989; **14**:338-344.

98. Borow KM, Neumann A, Arensman FW, et al: Left ventricular contractility and contractile reserve in humans after cardiac transplantation. *Circulation* 1985; **71**:866-872.

99. Kao AC, Trigt PV, Shaeffer-McCall GS, et al: Allograft diastolic dysfunction and chromtropic incompetence limit cardiac output response to exercise two to six years after heart transplantation. *J Heart Lung Transplant* 1995; **14**:11-22.

100. Starling RC, Cody RJ: Cardiac transplant hypertension. *Am J Cardiol* 1990; **65**:106-111.

101. Farge D, Julien J, Amrein C, et al: Effect of systemic hypertension on renal function and left ventricular hypertrophy in heart transplant recipients. *J Am Coll Cardiol* 1990; **15**:1095-1101.

102. Bhatia SJS, Kirshenbaum JM, Shemin RJ, et al: Time course of resolution of pulmonary hypertension and right ventricular remodeling after orthotopic cardiac transplantation. *Circulation* 1987; **76**:819-826.

103. Gorcsan J, Snow FR, Paulsen W, et al: Echocardiographic profile of the transplanted human heart in clinically well recipients. *J Heart Lung Transplant* 1992; **11**:80-89.

104. Cresci S, Goldstein JA, Cardona H, et al: Impaired left atrial function after heart transplantation: Disparate contribution of donor and recipient atrial components studied on-line with quantitative echocardiography. *J Heart Lung Transplant* 1995; **14**:647-653.

105. Freimark D, Silverman JM, Aleksic I, et al: Atrial emptying with orthotopic heart transplantation using bicaval and pulmonary venous anastomoses: A magnetic resonance imaging study. *J Am Coll Cardiol* 1995; **25**:932-936.

106. Triposkidis F, Starling R, Haas GJ, et al: Timing of recipient atrial contraction: A major determinant of transmitral diastolic flow in orthotopic cardiac transplantation. *Am Heart* 1993; **126**:1175-1181.

107. St. Goar FG, Gibbons R, Schnittger I, et al: Left ventricular diastolic function. Doppler echocardiographic changes soon after cardiac transplantation. *Circulation* 1990; **82**:872-878.

108. Young JB, Leon CA, Short D, et al: Evolution of hemodynamics after orthotopic heart and heart-lung transplantation: Early restrictive patterns persisting in occult fashion. *J Heart Transplant* 1987; **6**:34-43.

109. Davies RA, Koshal A, Walley V, et al: Temporary diastolic noncompliance with perserved systolic function after heart transplantation. *Transplant Proc* 1987; **19**:3444-3447.

110. Schulman DS, Herman BA, Edwards TD, et al: Diastolic dysfunction in cardiac transplant recipients: An important role in the response to increased afterload. *Am Heart J* 1993; **125**:435-442.

111. Paulus WJ, Bronzwaer JGF, Felice H, et al: Deficient acceleration of left ventricular relaxation during exercise after heart transplantation. *Circulation* 86:1175-1185.

112. Hosenpud JD, Morton MJ, Wilson RA, et al: Abnormal exercise hemodynamics in cardiac allograft recipients 1 year after cardiac transplantation. Relation to preload reserve. *Circulation* 1989; **80**:525-532.

113. Hosenpud JD, Pantely GA, Morton MJ, et al: Relationship between recipient:donor body size matching and hemodynamics 3 months following cardiac transplantation. *J Heart Lung Transplant* 1989; **8**:241-244.

114. Valantine HA, Yeon T, Gibbons R, et al: Sensitivity and specificity of diastolic indexes for rejection surveillance: Temporal correlation with endomyocardial biopsy. *J Heart Lung Transplant* 1991; **10**:757-756.

115. Hosenpud JD, Pantely GA, Morton MJ, et al: Lack of progressive "restrictive" physiology after heart transplantation despite intervening episodes of allograft rejection: Comparison of serial rest and exercise hemodynamics one and two years after transplantation. *J Heart Lung Transplant* 1990; **9**:119-123.

116. Skowronski EW, Epstein M, Ota D, et al: Right and left ventricular function after cardiac transplantation. Changes during and after rejection. *Circulation* 1991; **84**:2409-2417.

117. Valantine HA, Appleton CP, Hatle LK, et al: A hemodynamic and Doppler echocardiographic study of ventricular function in long-term cardiac allograft recipients. Etiology and prognosis of restrictive-constrictive physiology. *Circulation* 1989; **79**:66–75.

118. Paulus WJ, Bronzwaer JGF, Felice H, et al: Deficient acceleration of left ventricular relaxation during exercise after heart transplantation. *Circulation* 1991; **86**:1175–1185.

119. Hauptman PJ, Aranki S, Mudge GH, Jr, et al: Early cardiac allograft failure after orthotopic heart transplantation. *Am Heart J* 1994; **127**:179–186.

120. Walley VM, Masters RG, Boone SA, et al: Analysis of deaths after heart transplantation: The University of Ottawa Heart Institute experience. *J Heart Lung Transplant* 1993; **12**:790–801.

121. Pickering JG, Boughner DR: Fibrosis in the transplanted heart and it relation to donor ischemic time. *Circulation* 1990; **81**:949–958.

122. Hosenpud JD, Novick RJ, Breen TJ, et al: The registry of the International Society for Heart and Lung Transplantation: Eleventh official report, 1994. *J Heart Lung Transplant* 1994; **13**:561–570.

123. Shivalkar B, Van Loon J, Wieland W, et al: Variable effects of explosive or gradual increase of intracranial pressure on myocardial structure and function. *Circulation* 1993; **87**:230–239.

124. Van Trigt P, Bittner HB, Kendal SW, et al: Mechanisms of transplant right ventricular dysfunction. *Ann Surg* 1995; **221**:666–676.

125. Turnage WS, Rosenfeld LE: Intraoperative acute myocardial failure after orthotopic heart transplantation. *J Cardiothorac Vasc Anesth* 1995; **9**:598–602.

126. Payne ME, Murray KD, Watson KM, et al: Permanent pacing in heart transplant recipients: Underlying causes and long-term results. *J Heart Lung Transplant* 1991; **10**:738–742.

127. Miyamoto Y, Curtiss EI, Kormos RL, et al: Bradyarrhythmia after heart transplantation: Incidence, time course, and outcome. *Circulation* 1990; **82**:313–317.

128. Stinson EB, Caves PK, Griepp RB, et al: Hemodynamic observations in the early period after human heart transplantation. *J Thorac Cardiovasc Surg* 1975; **69**:264–270.

129. Prielipp RC, McLean R, Rosenthal MH, et al: Hemodynamic profiles of prostaglandin E$_1$, isoproteronol, prostacyclin, and nifedipine in vasoconstrictor pulmonary hypertension in sheep. *Anesth Analg* 1988; **67**:722–729.

130. Armitage JM, Hardesty RL, Griffith BG: Prostaglandin E$_1$: An effective treatment of right heart failure after orthotopic heart transplantation. *J Heart Transplant* 1987; **6**:348–351.

131. Kieler-Jensen N, Lundin S, Ricksten S-E: Vasodilator therapy after heart transplantation: Effects of inhaled nitric oxide and intravenous prostacyclin, prostaglandin E$_1$, and sodium nitroprusside. *J Heart Lung Transplant* 1995; **14**:436–443.

132. Kieler-Jensen N, Milocco I, Rickstein S-E: Pulmonary vasodilatation after heart transplantation: A comparison among prostacycline, sodium nitroprusside and nitroglycerin on right ventricular function and pulmonary selectivity. *J Heart Lung Transplant* 1992; **12**:179–184.

133. D'Ambra MN, LaRaia PJ, Philbin DM, et al: Prostaglandin E$_1$: A new therapy for refractory right heart failure and pulmonary hypertension after mitral valve replacement. *J Thorac Cardiovasc Surg* 1985; **89**:567–572.

134. Kieler-Jensen N, Rickstein S-E, Stenquist O, et al: Inhaled nitric oxide in the evaluation of heart transplant candidates with elevated pulmonary vascular resistance. *J Heart Lung Transplant* 1994; **13**:366–375.

135. Williams TJ, Salamonsen RF, Snell G, et al: Preliminary experience with inhaled nitric oxide for acute pulmonary hypertension after heart transplantation. *J Heart Lung Transplant* 1995; **14**:419–423.

136. Zwissler B, Rank N, Jaenicke U, et al: Selective pulmonary vasodilatation by inhaled prostacyclin in a newborn with congenital

137. heart disease and cardiopulmonary bypass. *Anesthesiology* 1995; **82**:1512–1516.

137. Pappert D, Busch T, Gerlach H, et al: Aerosolized prostacyclin versus inhaled nitric oxide in children with severe respiratory distress syndrome. *Anesthesiology* 1995; **82**:1507–1511.

138. Dreyfus G, Jebara V, Couetil J, et al: Kinking of the pulmonary artery: a treatable cause of acute right ventricular failure after heart transplantation. *J Heart Transplant* 1990; **9**:575–576.

139. Gieraerts R, Schertz C, Ghignone M: Right ventricular failure after heart transplantation caused by a kink in the pulmonary artery anastomosis. *J Cardiothorac Anesth* 1989; **3**:470–472.

140. Parascandola SA, Wisman CB, Burg JE, et al: Extracardiac surgical complications in heart transplant recipients. *J Heart Transplant* 1989; **8**:400–406.

141. Steed DL, Brown B, Reilly JJ, et al: General surgical complications in heart and heart-lung transplantation. *Surgery* 1985; **98**:739–744.

142. Colon R, Frazier OH, Kahan BD, et al: Complications in cardiac transplant patients requiring general surgery. *Surgery* 1988; **103**:32–38.

143. Merrel SW, Ames SA, Nelson EW, et al: Major abdominal complications following cardiac transplantation. *Arch Surg* 1989; **124**:889–894.

144. Bull DA, Hunter GC, Copeland JG, et al: Peripheral vascular disease in heart transplant recipients. *J Vasc Surg* 1992; **16**:546–554.

145. Pahl E, Zales VR, Fricker J, et al: Posttransplant coronary artery disease in children. A multicenter national survey. *Circulation* 1994; **90**(part 2):II-56–II-60.

146. Addonizio LJ, Hsu DT, Douglas JF, et al: Decreasing incidence of coronary artery disease in pediatric cardiac transplant recipients using increased immunosupression. *Circulation* 1993; **88**(part II):II-224–II-229.

147. Uretsky BF, Kormos RL, Zerbe TR, et al: Cardiac events after heart transplantation: Incidence and predictive value of coronary arteriography. *J Heart Lung Transplant* 1992; **11**:S45–51.

148. St. Goar FG, Pinto FJ, Alderman EL, et al: Intracoronary ultrasound in cardiac transplant recipients. In vivo evidence of "angiographically silent" intimal thickening. *Circulation* 1992; **85**:979–987.

149. Ventura HO, Mehra MR, Smart FW, et al: Cardiac allograft vasculopathy: Current concepts. *Am Heart J* 1995; **129**:791–779.

150. Johnson DE, Gao SZ, Schroeder JS, et al: The spectrum of coronary artery pathologic findings in human cardiac allografts. *J Heart Transplant* 1989; **8**:349–359.

151. Loebe M, Schuler S, Zais O, et al: Role of cytomegalovirus infection in the development of coronary artery disease in the transplanted heart. *J Heart Transplant* 1990; **9**:707–721.

152. Grattan MT, Moreno-Cabral CE, Starnes VA, et al: Cytomegalovirus infection is associated with cardiac allograft rejection and atherosclerosis. *JAMA* 1989; **261**:3561–3566.

153. McGiffin DC, Savunen T, Kirlin JK, et al: Cardiac transplant coronary artery disease. A multivariate analysis of pretransplant risk factors for disease development and morbid events. *J Thorac Cardiovasc Surg* 1995; **109**:1081–1089.

154. Mehra MR, Stapleton DD, Ventura HO, et al: Influence of donor and recipient gender on cardiac allograft vasculopathy. An intravascular study. *Circulation* 1994; **90**(part II):II-78–II-82.

155. Botas J, Pinto FJ, Chenzbraun A, et al: Influence or preexistent donor coronary artery disease on the progression of transplant vasculopathy. An intravascular ultrasound study. *Circulation* 1995; **92**:1126–1132.

156. Gao SZ, Schroeder JS, Hunt SA, et al: Acute myocardial infarction in cardiac transplant recipients. *Am J Cardiol* 1989; **64**:1093–1096.

157. Smart FW, Ballantyne CM, Cocanougher B, et al: Insensitivity of noninvasive tests to detect coronary artery vasculopathy after heart transplant. *Am J Cardiol* 1991; **67**:243–247.

158. Smart FW, Grinstead WC, Cocanougher B, et al: Detection of transplant arterioplasty: Does exercise thallium scintigraphy im-

prove noninvasive diagnostic capabilities? *Transplant Proc* 1991; **23**:1189–1192.

159. Mairesse GH, Marwick TH, Melin JA, et al: Use of exercise electrocardiography, technetium-99m-MIBI perfusion tomography, and two-dimensional echocardiography for coronary disease surveillance in a low-prevalence population of heart transplant patients. *J Heart Lung Transplant* 1995; **14**:222–229.

160. Akosah KO, Mohanty PK, Funai JT, et al: Noninvasive detection of transplant coronary artery disease by dobutamine stress echocardiography. *J Heart Lung Transplant* 1994; **13**:1024–1038.

161. Derumeaux G, Redonnet M, Mouton-Schleifer D, et al: Dobutamine stress echocardiography in orthotopic heart transplant recipients. *J Am Coll Cardiol* 1995; **25**:1665–1672.

162. Mehra MR, Ventura HO, Smart FW, et al: An intravascular ultrasound study of the influence of angiotensin-converting enzyme inhibitors and calcium entry blockers on the development of cardiac allograft vasculopathy. *Am J Cardiol* 1995; **75**:853–854.

163. Schroeder JS, Gao S-H, Alderman EL, et al: A preliminary study of diltiazem in the prevention of cpronary artery disease in heart-transplant recipients. *N Engl J Med* 1993; **328**:164–170.

164. Halle AA, Wilson RF, Massin EK, et al: Coronary angioplasty in cardiac transplant patients. Results of a multicenter study. *Circulation* 1992; **86**:458–462.

165. Strikwerda S, Umans V, van der Linden MM, et al: Percutaneous directional atherectomy for discrete lesions in cardiac transplant patients. *Am Heart J* 1992; **6**:1686–1690.

166. Copeland JC, Butman SM, Sethi G: Successful coronary artcry bypass grafting for high-risk left main coronary artery atherosclerosis after cardiac transplantation. *Ann Thorac Surg* 1990; **49**:106–110.

167. Ensley RD, Hunt S, Renlund DG, et al: Predictors of survival after repeat heart transplantation: The registry of the International Society for Heart and Lung Transplantation, and Contributing Investigators. *J Heart Lung Transplant* 1992; **11**:S142–158.

168. Ozdogan E, Banner N, Fitzgerald M, et al: Factors influencing the development of hypertension after heart transplantation. *J Heart Lung Transplant* 1990; **9**:548–553.

169. Scherrer U, Vissing SF, Morgan BJ et al: Cyclosporine-induced sympathetic activation and hypertension after heart transplantation. *N Engl J Med* 1990; **323**:693–699.

170. Luke RG: Mechanism of cyclosporine-induced hypertension. *Am J Hypertens* 1991; **4**:468–471.

171. Ventura HO, Johnson MR, Grusk B, et al: Cardiac adaptation to obesity and hypertension after heart transplantation. *J Am Coll Cardiol* 1992; **19**:55–59.

172. Weir MR: Theraputic benefits of calcium channel blockers in cyclosporine-treated organ transplant recipients: Blood pressure control and immunosuppression. *Am J Med* 1991; **5A**:32S–36S.

173. Macdonald P, Connell J, Harvison A, et al: Diltiazem co-administration reduces cyclosporine toxicity after heart transplantation: A prospective randomized trial. *Transplant Proc* 1992; **24**:2259–2262.

174. Little RE, Kay GN, Epstein AE, et al: Arrhythmias after orthotopic cardiac transplantation. Prevalence and determinants during initial hospitalization and late follow-up. *Circulation* 1989; **80**(suppl 3):140–146.

175. Pavri BB, O'Nunain SS, Newell JB, et al: Prevalence and prognostic significance of atrial arrhythmias after orthotopic cardiac transplantation. *J Am Coll Cardiol* 1995; **25**:1673–1680.

176. Baum D, Bernstein D, Starnes VA, et al: Pediatric heart transplantation at Stanford: Results of a 15 year experience. *Pediatrics* 1991; **88**:203–214.

177. Kirklin JK, Naftel DC, Bourge RC, et al: Rejection after cardiac transplantation: A time-related risk factor analysis. *Circulation* 1992; **86**:236–241.

178. Sethi GK, Rosado LJ, McCarthy M, et al: Futility of yearly heart

biopsies in patients undergoing heart transplantation. *J Thorac Cardiovasc Surg* 1992; **104**:90–93.

179. Paulsen W, Magid N, Sagar K, et al: Left ventricular function of heart allografts during acute rejection: An echocardiographic assessment. *Heart Transplant* 1985; **5**:525–528.

180. Amende I, Simon R, Seegers A, et al: Diastolic dysfunction during acute cardiac allograft rejection. *Circulation* 1990; **81**(suppl 3):66–70.

181. Yeoh T-K, Frist WH, Eastburn TE, et al: Clinical significance of mild rejection of the cardiac allograft. *Circulation* 1992; **86**(suppl 2):II-267–II-271.

182. McGinn AL, Wilson RF, Olivari MT, et al: Coronary vasodilator reserve after human orthotopic cardiac transplantation. *Circulation* 1988; **78**:1200–1209.

183. Nitenberg A, Tavolaro O, Benvenuti C, et al: Recovery of a normal coronary vascular reserve after rejection therapy in acute human cardiac allograft rejection. *Circulation* 1990; **81**:1312–1318.

184. Chan SY, Kobashigawa J, Stevenson LW, et al: Myocardial blood flow at rest and during pharmacological vasodilation in cardiac transplants during and after successful treatment of rejection. *Circulation* 1994; **90**:204–212.

185. Pinto FJ, St. Goar FG, Fischell TA, et al: Nitroglycerin-induced coronary vasodilatation in cardiac transplant recipients. Evaluation with in vivo intracoronary ultrasound. *Circulation* 1992; **85**:69–77.

186. Cannon DS, Graham AF, Harrison DC: Electrophysiological studies in the denervated transplanted human heart. Response to atropine and pacing. *Circ Res* 1973; **23**:268–278.

187. Backman SB, Ralley FE, Fox GS: Neostigmine produces bradycardia in a heart transplant patient. *Anesthesiology* 1993; **78**:777–779.

188. Beebe DS, Shumway SJ, Maddock R: Sinus arrest after intravenous neostigmine in two heart transplant recipients. *Anesth Analg* 1994; **78**:779–782.

189. Backman SB, Bachoo M, Polosa C: Mechanisms involved in the bradycardia produced by neostigmine. *Can J Anaesth* 1991; **38**:A125.

190. Priola DV, Spurgeon HA: Cholinergic sensitivity of the denervated heart. *Circ Res* 1977; **41**:600–606.

191. DeBroux E, Lagace G, Dumont L, et al: Efficacy of dobutamine in the failing transplanted heart. *J Heart Lung Transplant* 1992; **11**:1133–1139.

192. Cannon DS, Rider AK, Stinson EB, et al: Electrophysiological studies in the denervated transplanted human heart. II. Response to norepinephrine, isoproteronol and propranolol. *Am J Cardiol* 1975; **36**:859–866.

193. Qi A, Tuna IC, Gornick CC, et al: Potentiation of cardiac electrophysiologic effects of verapamil after autonomic blockade or cardiac transplantation. *Circulation* 1987; **75**:888–893.

194. Ellenbogen KA, Thames MD, DiMarco JP, et al: Electrophysiological effects of adenosine in the transplanted human heart. Evidence of supersensitivity. *Circulation* 1990; **81**:821–828.

195. Kanter SF, Samuels SI: Anesthesia for major operations on patients who have transplanted hearts. A review of 29 cases. *Anesthesiology* 1977; **46**:65–68.

196. Bricker SRW, Sugden JC: Anaesthesia for surgery in a patient with a transplanted heart. *Br J Anaesth* 1985; 634–637.

197. Melendez JA, Delphin E, Lamb J, et al: Noncardiac surgery in heart transplant recipients in the cyclosporine era. *J Cardiothorac Vasc Anesth* 1991; **5**:218–220.

198. Lupinetti FM, Bolling SF, Bove EL, et al: Selective lung or heart-lung transplantation for pulmonary hypertension associated with congenital cardiac anomalies. *Ann Thorac Surg* 1994; **57**:1545–1548.

199. Spray TL, Mallory GB, Canter CE, et al: Pediatric lung transplantation for pulmonary hypertension and congenital heart disease. *Ann Thorac Surg* 1992; **54**:216–223.

200. Bridges ND, Mallory GB, Huddleston CB, et al: Lung transplanta-

tion in children and young adults with cardiovascular disease. *Ann Thorac Surg* 1995; **59**:813-821.

201. Bando K, Armitage JM, Paradis IL, et al: Indications for and results of single, bilateral, and heart-lung transplantation for pulmonary hypertension. *J Thorac Cardiovasc Surg* 1994; **108**:1056-1065.

202. Aeba R, Griffith BP, Hardesty RL, et al: Isolated lung transplantation for patients with Eisenmenger's Syndrome. *Circulation* 1993; **88**:452-455.

203. Patterson GA, Cooper JD: Lung transplantation, in Pearson FG, Deslauriers J, Ginsberg RJ, et al (eds): *Thoracic Surgery.* New York, Churchill Livingstone, 1995, pp 931-959.

204. Fuster V, Steele PM, Edwards WD, et al: Primary pulmonary hypertension: Natural history and the importance of thrombosis. *Circulation* 1984; **70**:580-587.

205. Butt AY, Higenbottam T: New therapies for primary pulmonary hypertension. *Chest* 1994; **105**:21S-25S.

206. Rich S: Medical treatment of primary pulmonary hypertension: A bridge to transplantation? *Am J Cardiol* 1995; **75**:63A-66A.

207. Nootens M, Freels S, Kaufmann E, et al: Timing of single lung transplantation for primary pulmonary hypertension. *J Heart Lung Transplant* 1994; **13**:276-281.

208. Brenot F: Primary pulmonary hypertension. Case series from France. *Chest* 1994; **105**(suppl 2):33S-36S.

209. Palevsky HI, Fishman AP: The management of primary pulmonary hypertension. *JAMA* 1991; **265**:1014-1020.

210. Pasque MK, Trulock EP, Cooper JD, et al: Single lung transplantation for pulmonary hypertension. Single institution experience in 34 patients. *Circulation* 1995; **92**:2252-2258.

211. Bando K, Keenan RJ, Paradis IL, et al: Impact of pulmonary hypertension on outcome after single-lung transplantation. *Ann Thorac Surg* 1994; **58**:1336-1342.

212. Davis RD Jr, Trulock EP, Manley J, et al: Differences in early results after single-lung transplantation. *Ann Thorac Surg* 1994; **58**:1327-1334.

213. Cooper JD, Patterson GA, Trulock EP: Results of single and bilateral lung transplantation in 131 consecutive recipients. *J Thorac Cardiovasc Surg* 1994; **107**:460-470.

214. Pasque MK, Trulock EP, Kaiser LR, et al: Single-lung transplantation for pulmonary hypertension. Three-month hemodynamic follow-up. *Circulation* 1991; **84**:2275-2279.

215. Frist WH, Carmicheal LC, Loyd JE, et al: Transplantation for pulmonary hypertension. *Transplant Proc* 1993; **25**:1159-1161.

216. Pasque MK, Kaiser LR, Dresler CM, et al: Single lung transplantation for pulmonary hypertension. Technical aspects and immediate hemodynamic results. *J Thorac Cardiovasc Surg* 1992; **103**:475-481.

217. Kramer MR, Valantine HA, Marshall SE, et al: Recovery of the right ventricle after single-lung transplantation in pulmonary hypertension. *Am J Cardiol* 1994; **73**:494-500.

218. Ritchie M, Waggoner AD, Davila-Roman VG, et al: Echocardiographic characterization of the improvement in right ventricular function in patients with severe pulmonary hypertension after single-lung transplantation. *J Am Coll Cardiol* 1993; **22**:1170-1174.

219. Dromer C, Velly JF, Jougon J, et al: Long-term functional results after bilateral lung transplantation. *Ann Thorac Surg* 1993; **56**:68-72.

220. Chapelier A, Vouch P, Macchiarini P, et al: Comparative outcome of heart-lung and lung transplantation for pulmonary hypertension. *J Thorac Cardiovasc Surg* 1993; **106**:299-307.

221. Parquin F, Cerrina J, Le Roy Ladurie F, et al: Comparison of hemodynamic outcome of patients with pulmonary hypertension after double-lung or heart-lung transplantation. *Transplant Proc* 1993; **25**:1157-1158.

222. Davis PB, Di Sant' Agnese PA: Diagnosis and treatment of cystic fibrosis. *Chest* 1984; **85**:802-809.

223. Walsh TS, Young CH: Anaesthesia and cystic fibrosis. *Anaesthesia* 1995; **50**:614-622.

224. Shak S: Aerosolized recombinant human DNase I for the treatment of cystic fibrosis. *Chest* 1995; **107**(suppl 2):65S-70S.

225. Shennib H, Massard G, Gauthier R, et al: Single lung transplantation for cystic fibrosis: is it an option? Cystic Fibrosis Transplant Study Group. *J Heart Lung Transplant* 1993; **12**:288-293.

226. Kopelman H: Cystic fibrosis: Gastrointestinal and nutritional aspects. *Thorax* 1991; **46**:261-267.

227. Durie PR: Vitamin K and the management of patients with cystic fibrosis. *Can Med Assoc J* 1994; **151**:933-936.

228. Webb AK, David TJ: Clinical management of children and adults with cystic fibrosis. *BMJ* 1994; **308**:459-462.

229. Tanner MS, Taylor CJ: Liver disease in cystic fibrosis. *Arch Dis Childhood* 1995; **72**:281-284.

230. Kshettry VR, Kroshus TJ, Burdine J, et al: Does donor organ ischemia over four hours affect long-term survival after lung transplantation? *J Heart Lung Transplant* 1995; **16**:169-174.

231. Snell GI, Rabinov M, Griffiths A, et al: Pulmonary allograft ischemic time: An important predictor of survival after lung transplantation. *J Heart Lung Transplant* 1995; **15**:160-168.

232. Haydock DA, Low DE, Trulock EP, et al: Pulmonary "twinning" procedure: Use of lungs from one donor for single-lung transplantation in two recipients. *Ann Thorac Surg* 1992; **54**:1189-1192.

233. Patterson GA, Cooper JD, Geldman B, et al: Technique of successful clinical double-lung transplantation. *Ann Thorac Surg* 1988; **45**:626-633.

234. Bisson A, Bonnette P: A new technique for double lung transplantation. "Bilateral single lung transplantation." *J Thorac Cardiovasc Surg* 1992; **103**:40-46.

235. Bridges ND, Mallory GB Jr, Huddleston CB, et al: Lung transplantation in children and young adults with cardiovascular disease. *Ann Thorac Surg* 1995; **59**:813-820.

236. Armitage JM, Kurland G, Michaels M, et al: Critical issues in pediatric lung transplantation. *J Thorac Cardiovasc Surg* 1995; **109**:60-65.

237. Metras D, Kreitmann B, Riberi A, et al: Bilateral single-lung transplantation in children. *Ann Thorac Surg* 1995; **60**:S578-S581.

238. Triantafillou AN, Pasque MK, Huddleston CB, et al: Predictors, frequency, and indications for cardiopulmonary bypass during lung transplantation in adults. *Ann Thorac Surg* 1994; **57**:1248-1251.

239. Girard C, Mornex JF, Gamondes JP, et al: Single lung transplantation for primary pulmonary hypertension without cardiopulmonary bypass. *Chest* 1992; **102**:967-968.

240. Raffin L, Michel-Cherqui M, Sperandio M, et al: Anesthesia for bilateral lung transplantation without cardiopulmonary bypass: Initial experience and review of intraoperative problems. *J Cardiothorac Vasc Anesth* 1992; **6**:409-417.

241. deHoyos A, Demajo W, Snell G, et al: Preoperative prediction for the use of cardiopulmonary bypass in lung transplantation. *J Thorac Cardiovasc Surg* 1993; **106**:787-796.

242. Aeba R, Griffith BP, Kormos RL, et al: Effect of cardiopulmonary bypass on early graft dysfunction in clinical lung transplantation. *Ann Thorac Surg* 1994; **57**:715-722.

243. Spray TL, Mallory BB, Canter CB, et al: Pediatric lung transplantation. Indications, techniques, and early results. *J Thorac Cardiovasc Surg* 1994; **107**:990-1000.

244. Ross DJ, Vassolo M, Kass R, et al: Transesophageal echocardiographic assessment of pulmonary venous flow after single lung transplantation. *J Heart Lung Transplant* 1993; **12**:689-694.

245. Hausmann D, Daniel WG, Mugge A, et al: Imaging of pulmonary artery and vein anastomoses by transesophageal echocardiography after lung transplantation. *Circulation* 1992; **86**(suppl 2):II-251-II-258.

246. Gorcsan J 3d, Reddy SC, Armitage JM, et al: Acquired right ven-

tricular outflow tract obstruction after lung transplantation: Diagnosis by transesophageal echocardiography. *J Am Soc Echocardiol* 1993; **6**:324-326.

247. Soberman MS, Kraenzler EJ, Licina M, et al: Airway management during bilateral sequential lung transplantation for cystic fibrosis. *Ann Thorac Surg* 1994; **58**:892-894.

248. Scheller MS, Kriett JM, Smith CM, et al: Airway management during anesthesia for double-lung transplantation using a single-lumen endotracheal tube with an enclosed bronchial blocker. *J Cardiothorac Vasc Anesth* 1992; **6**:204-207.

249. Rowe R, Andropoulos D, Heard M, et al: Anesthetic management of pediatric patients undergoing thoracoscopy. *J Cardiothorac Vasc Anesth* 1994; **8**:563-566.

250. Smiley RM, Navedo AT, Kirby T, Schulman LL: Postoperative independent lung ventilation in a single-lung transplant recipient. *Anesthesiology* 1991; **74**:1144-1148.

251. Thomas BJ, Siegel LC: Anesthetic and postoperative management of single-lung transplantation. *J Cardiothorac Vasc Anesth* 1991; **5**:266-267.

252. Heerdt PM, Triantafillou A: Perioperative management of patients receiving a lung transplant. *Anesthesiology* 1991; **75**:922-923.

253. Quinlan JJ, Buffington CW: Deliberate hypoventilation in a patient with air trapping during lung transplantation. *Anesthesiology* 1993; **78**:1177-1181.

254. Peterson KL, DeCampli WM, Feeley TW, et al: Blood loss and transfusion requirements in cystic fibrosis patients undergoing heart-lung or lung transplantation. *J Cardiothorac Vasc Anesth* 1995; **9**:59-62.

255. Jaquiss RDB, Huddleston CB, Spray TL: Use of aprotinin in pediatric lung transplantation. *J Heart Lung Transplant* 1995; **14**:302-307.

256. Kesten S, de Hoyas A, Chaparro C, et al: Aprotinin reduces blood loss in lung transplant recipients. *Ann Thorac Surg* 1995; **59**:877-879.

257. Chaney MA: Hypermetabolism during bilateral single-lung transplantation requiring cardiopulmonary bypass. *J Cardiothorac Vasc Anesth* 1995; **9**:565-570.

258. Lee BS, Sarnquist FH, Starnes VA: Anesthesia for bilateral single-lung transplantation. *J Cardiothorac Vasc Anesth* 1992; **6**:201-203.

259. Myles PS, Venema HR: Avoidance of cardiopulmonary bypass during bilateral sequential lung transplantation using inhaled nitric oxide. *J Cardiothorac Vasc Anesth* 1995; **9**:571-574.

260. Adatia I, Lillehei C, Arnold JH, et al: Inhaled nitric oxide in the treatment of postoperative graft dysfunction after lung transplantation. *Ann Thorac Surg* 1994; **57**:1311-1318.

261. Gayes JM, Giron L, Nissen MD, Plut D: Anesthetic considerations for patients undergoing double-lung transplantation. *J Cardiothorac Vasc Anesth* 1990; **4**:486-498.

262. Badesch DB, Zamora MR, Jones S, et al: Independent ventilation and ECMO for severe unilateral pulmonary edema after SLT for primary pulmonary hypertension. *Chest* 1995; **107**:1766-1770.

263. Smith PC, Slaughter MS, Petty MC, et al: Abdominal complications after lung transplantation. *J Heart Lung Transplant* 1995; **14**:44-51.

264. Griffith BP, Magee MJ, Gonzalez IF, et al: Anastomotic pitfalls in lung transplantation. *J Thorac Cardiovas Surg* 1994; **107**:743-753.

265. Higano ST, Gaffney M, Nishimura RA, et al: Intravascular ultrasound to assess anastomotic patency after lung transplantation. *Ann Thorac Surg* 1995; **60**:442-444.

266. Shennib H, Massard G: Airway complications in lung transplantation. *Ann Thorac Surg* 1994; **57**:506-511.

267. Williams TJ, Grossman RF, Maurer JR: Long-term functional follow-up of lung transplant recipients. *Clin Chest Med* 1990; **11**:347-358.

268. Glanville AR, Theodore J, Harvey J, et al: Elastic behavior of the transplanted lung. Exponential analysis of static pressure-volume relationships. *Am Rev Respir Dis* 1988; **137**:308-312.

269. Scott JP, Gillespie DJ, Peters SG, et al: Reduced work of breathing after single lung transplantation for emphysema. *J Heart Lung Transplant* 1995; **14**:39-43.

270. Trachiotis GD, Knight SR, Hann M, et al: Respiratory responses to CO_2 rebreathing in lung transplant recipients. *Ann Thorac Surg* 1994; **58**:1709-1717.

271. Trachiotis GD, Knight SR, Pohl MS, et al: Tidal volume and respiratory rate changes during CO_2 rebreathing after lung transplantation. *Ann Thorac Surg* 1994; **58**:1718-1720.

272. Sanders MH, Owens GR, Sciurba FC, et al: Ventilation and breathing pattern during progressive hypercapnia and hypoxia after human heart-lung transplantation. *Am Rev Respir Dis* 1989; **140**:38-44.

273. Yousem SA, Berry GJ, Cagle PT, et al: Revision of the 1990 working formulation for the classification of pulmonary allograft rejection: Lung rejection study group. *J Heart Lung Transplant* 1996; **15**:1-15.

274. Reichenspurner H, Girgis RE, Robbins RC, et al: Obliterative bronchiolitis after lung and heart-lung transplantation. *Ann Thorac Surg* 1995; **60**:1845-1853.

275. Sundaresna S, Trulock EP, Mohanakumar T, et al: Prevelance and outcome of bronchiolitis obliterans syndrome after lung transplantation. *Ann Thorac Surg* 1995; **60**:1341-1347.

276. Keller CA, Cagle PT, Brown RW, et al: Bronchiolitis obliterans in recipients of single, double, and heart-lung transplantation. *Chest* 1995; **107**:973-980.

277. Nathan SD, Ross DJ, Belman MJ, et al: Bronchiolitis obliterans in single-lung transplant recipients. *Chest* 1995; **107**:967-972.

278. Novick RJ, Kaye MP, Patterson GA, et al: Redo lung transplantation: A North American-European experience. *J Heart Lung Transplant* 1993; **12**:5-16.

279. Raleitshak-Plus EM, Hefti A, Lortsher R: Initial observation that cyclosporine A induces gingival enlargement in man. *J Clin Periodontol* 1983; **10**:237-246.

280. Mallory A, Kern F: Drug-induced pancreatitis: A critical review. *Gastroenterology* 1980; **78**:813-820.

281. Spes CH, Angerman CE, Beyer RW, et al: Increased incidence of cholelithiasis in heart transplant recipients receiving cyclosporine therapy. *J Heart Transplant* 1990; **9**:404-407.

282. Girardet RE, Rosenbloom P, DeWeese BM, et al: Significance of asymptomatic biliary tract disease in heart transplant recipients. *J Heart Transplant* 1989; **8**:391-399.

283. Penn I: The changing pattern of posttransplant malignancies. *Transplant Proc* 1991; **23**:1101-1103.

284. Bernstein D, Baum D, Berry G, et al: Neoplastic disorders after pediatric heart transplantation. *Circulation* 1993; **88**(part 2):II-230-II-237.

285. Augustine SM, Yeo CJ, Buchman TG, et al: Gastrointestinal complications in heart and in heart-lung transplant patients. *J Heart Lung Transplant* 1991; **10**:547-556.

Anesthesia for Pericardial Disease

James A. DiNardo

Effective anesthesia for patients with pericardial disease depends on a thorough understanding of the physiologic alterations that the diseased pericardium imposes on the heart. This physiologic insight must be considered with other aspects of a patient's underlying disease that may complicate the anesthetic management. This chapter reviews the normal physiology of the pericardium, followed by a discussion of the physiologic derangements caused by a pericardial effusion or a constricting pericardium. Diseases that can cause pericardial dysfunction will be discussed, including aspects of illnesses that affect anesthetic management, independent of the state of the pericardium. Finally, the anesthetic management of generic patients with pericardial tamponade and constrictive pericarditis will be reviewed. It must be understood that many patients will manifest a combined picture of a pericardial effusion, either acute or chronic, together with some degree of constrictive physiology.

The normal pericardium is a dual envelope that surrounds the heart and separates the chambers from the bordering chest wall anteriorly, pleura laterally, and great vessels posteriorly. The pericardium contains approximately 25 mL of an ultrafiltrate of plasma, which layers within the atrial-ventricular groove. The oblique sinus lies behind the posterior wall of the left atrium, where the pericardium is tightly adherent to the vena cava and pulmonary veins. This defines an area of the pericardial space in which an effusion does not collect

unless it is very large or under pressure.[1] The parietal layer of the pericardium is composed of fibrous and elastic fibers that are responsible for its stiffness. The low compliance of the normal pericardium is responsible for the fundamental pathophysiologic mechanism seen in pericardial tamponade, and accounts for the difference in presentation between an acutely developing effusion and a much larger, but more slowly accumulating, collection of fluid.

The presenting symptoms of pericardial diseases are, in part, referable to the innervation of the pericardium and the location of adjacent structures. A large pericardial effusion may present as dyspnea, dysphagia, cough, hiccups, or hoarseness due to compression of adjacent lung, esophagus, diaphragm, or recurrent laryngeal nerve.[2] Afferents from the pericardium travel via the phrenic nerve, entering the spinal cord at C4 to C6, and pericardial pain often is symptomatically indistinguishable from a diaphragmatic source. The phrenic nerves travel along the lateral aspects of the pericardium, where they are subject to mechanical or cold-induced injury, especially from maneuvers to keep the heart cold during cardiac surgery.[3]

The function of the normal pericardium is not well established. Although it has been invoked as a barrier to the spread of infection or malignancy, this has been difficult to demonstrate unequivocally. More frequently mentioned, and the subject of much investigation, is the role of the pericardium in limiting acute cardiac dilatation and in the coupling of diastolic filling of the right and left ventricles so that stroke volumes are similar.[2,4] Although there is clear echocardiographic evidence that increases in right ventricular diastolic dimensions are accompanied by a posterior shift of the interventricular septum and diminished left ventricular diastolic volume,[5] there are two lines of evidence that raise question regarding the hemodynamic significance of these findings in healthy patients with normal ventricular filling volumes. First, patients with a congenitally absent pericardium often come to medical attention because of an abnormal chest x-ray, not because of a physiologic derangement or symptom.[4,6] Second, right and left ventricular function has been demonstrated to be the same whether the pericardium is intact or opened.[7,8] In contrast, the physiologic function of the pericardium is seen clearly in situations of increased intrapericardial volume, as in patients with pericardial tamponade.

The pericardium can be involved in a variety of disease states, either as the primary lesion or secondarily. There are two principle physiologic expressions of pericardial disease: (1) effusion, with or without tamponade physiology resulting; and (2) constriction. It is essential to realize that both pericardial tamponade and constrictive pericarditis produce ventricular diastolic dysfunction. The principal physiologic lesion in either case is inadequate filling of the ventricles during diastole. However, there are differences in diastolic dysfunction resulting from a pericardial effusion and that due to constrictive pericarditis, and the diagnosis is predicated on these differences. An understanding of the physiology of these diastolic limitations will provide the anesthesiologist with the tools to safely anesthetize these patients, partly independent of the specific etiology of their pericardial disease.

Normally, venous return to the right side of the heart is accelerated during ventricular systole. This is due, in part, to a reduction in total intrapericardial volume (cardiac structures plus pericardial contents), which generates a pressure gradient from the vena cava to the right atrium. This increased rate of venous flow is represented in the right atrial waveform by the X descent (*see* Fig. 8-1). The second surge in venous return occurs during the latter phase of atrial systole, when the tricuspid valve opens. This is visualized as the Y descent in the right atrial waveform (*see* Fig. 8-1). Analysis of the right atrial (or central venous) pressure waveform and right ventricular pressure tracing, and measurement of the pulmonary capillary wedge pressure in the catheterization laboratory, usually differentiates pericardial tamponade from constrictive pericarditis. Although there are situations in which the pathophysiology is that of a combined lesion, this conceptual separation allows a clearer understanding of the relevant physiology.

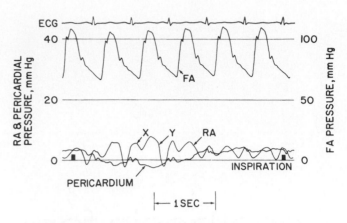

FIGURE 8–1. Right atrial pressure (RA) waveform with simultaneous electrocardiogram and femoral arterial pressure waveform (FA). RA tracing demonstrates timing of X and Y descents relative to cardiac cycle. Recordings were taken from a patient with pericardial tamponade after pericardiocentesis. Also shown is simultaneous intrapericardial pressure (pericardium) and respiratory cycle (inspiration). *(From: Lorell BH, Grossman W: Profiles in constrictive pericarditis, restrictive cardiomyopathy, and cardiac tamponade, in Grossman W (ed):* Cardiac Catheterization and Angiography. *3rd ed. Philadelphia, Lea & Febiger, 1986.)* (See Chapter 3 for detailed descriptions of atrial waveforms.)

■ PERICARDIAL EFFUSION (TAMPONADE)

Pericardial tamponade is one consequence of a pericardial effusion. The clinical manifestations and hemodynamic consequences of blood or other fluid in the pericardial space are determined primarily by the rate of accumulation of the effusion, if the pericardium is of normal compliance. A slowly accumulating effusion allows time for the pericardium to stretch; this increased compliance allows very large effusions to be asymptomatic. Conversely, left ventricular perforation leading to only a few hundred milliliters of blood in the pericardial space will cause fatal tamponade very quickly. The compliance curve of the normal pericardium is such that there is little change in intrapericardial pressure until a critical volume is reached, after which further incremental increases in volume cause large increases in intrapericardial pressure (*see* Fig. 8-2). When intrapericardial fluid accumulates rapidly, there is little distension of the normally stiff pericardium. This generates a sharp elevation in intrapericardial pressure for a relatively small volume of fluid, which produces a constraining or limiting force to filling of the ventricular chambers.

The pathophysiology of pericardial tamponade is best seen in acute, hemorrhagic pericardial tamponade. This typically occurs in penetrating cardiac injuries, such as knife wounds or chamber puncture injuries sustained in the catheterization laboratory, or during blind pericardiocentesis. Claude Beck's classic description of the physical findings in acute pericardial tamponade is seen primarily in this setting: hypotension, elevated venous

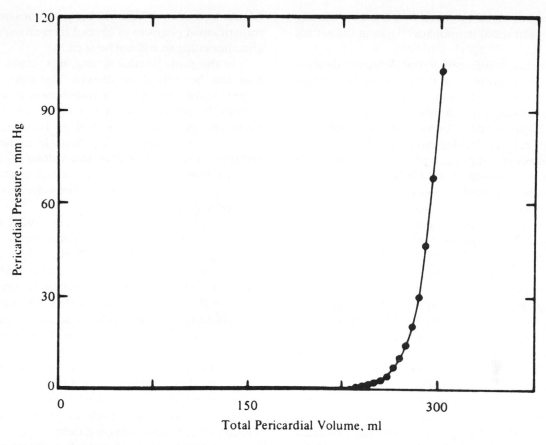

FIGURE 8–2. Total intrapericardial pressure as a function of changing intrapericardial volume. Until a critical volume is reached, there is little rise in pressure. After that "knee" has been reached, however, small additional increments in volume result in large changes in intrapericardial pressure. In pericardial tamponade, it is necessary to remove only enough fluid to be below the "knee" of the curve to temporarily reverse the tamponade physiology. *(From: Holt JP: The normal pericardium. Am J Cardiol 1970;* **26:***455–465.)*

pressure, and a small "quiet" heart.[9] Hypotension is due to a markedly reduced stroke volume caused by the compression of cardiac chambers by the effusion, especially on the right side.[10] An elevation in the central venous pressure also reflects the restriction to cardiac filling imposed by the tense pericardium. The central venous pressure waveform will demonstrate a prominent X descent, reflecting the accelerated venous return associated with ventricular systole and with the elevation of central venous pressure. Ventricular systole reduces total interpericardial volume by a quantity equal to the stroke volume, thereby allowing enhanced atrial filling. In addition, the right atrial waveform will demonstrate the absence of the Y descent, reflecting the increased ventricular end-diastolic pressure due to reduced distensibility induced by the tense intrapericardial effusion (*see* Fig. 8–3).

The diagnosis of pericardial tamponade should be entertained, even in the absence of an elevated central venous pressure if there is reason to believe that a sig-

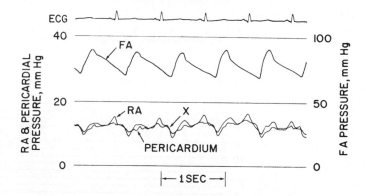

FIGURE 8–3. Simultaneous femoral arterial (FA), right atrial (RA), and intrapericardial pressure waveforms from patient with pericardial tamponade. Note exaggerated X descent, absent Y descent, equilibration of right atrial and intrapericardial pressures, and systemic hypotension. Patient subsequently had 1800 mL of effusion removed (Fig. 8–1 is same patient after removal of 300 mL). *(From: Lorell BH, Grossman W: Profiles in constrictive pericarditis, restrictive cardiomyopathy, and cardiac tamponade, in Grossman W (ed): Cardiac Catheterization and Angiography. 3rd ed. Philadelphia, Lea & Febiger, 1986.)*

nificant volume of blood has been lost from the circulation ("occult pericardial tamponade"[11]), as in the setting of trauma.

Cardiac echocardiography is the definitive diagnostic technique for documenting the presence and magnitude of a pericardial effusion. It can be performed rapidly at the bedside with no morbidity and is the most sensitive technique available for locating an effusion.[12] In addition, there are echocardiographic correlates that allow the diagnosis of tamponade physiology to be established.[12] This is especially helpful when hemodynamic compromise due to a rapidly accumulating effusion does not allow time for formal cardiac catheterization.

The echocardiographic magnitude of a pericardial effusion is graded as "large, moderate, or small."[13] In the supine patient, effusions layer initially along the dependent surfaces of the heart. As the volume of the effusion increases, it appears apically, laterally, and then anteriorly.[12] The typical echocardiographic features suggesting tamponade physiology resulting from an effusion are: right atrial collapse, which occurs just before ventricular systole; right ventricular collapse in early diastole; and a reduction in right ventricular dimensions during end-diastole.[14] The interventricular septum is displaced posteriorly during early diastole as a consequence of the increase in right ventricular size.[15,16] The echocardiographic demonstration of right atrial and right ventricular collapse in the presence of an effusion can be highly predictive of tamponade physiology, except in situations in which right ventricular compliance is already low, as in preexisting pulmonary hypertension or a right ventricular infarction. When wall stiffness does not allow intrapericardial pressure to exceed intracavitary pressure, chamber collapse will not be seen.[17]

In the postoperative setting, this "classic" presentation may be difficult to discern. The formation of intrapericardial clot alters the distribution of an effusion, as does the presence of anterior adhesions between the heart and pericardium, as well as between the pericardium and anterior mediastinum. In addition, in the setting of a reduced intravascular volume — as in hypovolemia from bleeding — patients will manifest a low central venous pressure despite hemodynamically significant pericardial tamponade.[11]

The definitive method of documenting tamponade physiology has been cardiac catheterization. In patients with straightforward tamponade, right atrial catheterization reveals an accentuated X descent and absent Y descent, as well as an elevated central venous pressure. There will be equalization (within ~5 torr) of right atrial, right ventricular end-diastolic, and pulmonary capillary wedge or left atrial pressures. These pressures will equal intrapericardial pressure, when measured during pericardiocentesis (*see* Fig. 8–4). It must be remembered that these findings apply only to patients who do not have an underlying condition that alters right or left ventricular compliance, such as prior infarction, pulmonary hypertension, ongoing ischemia, or left ventricular hypertrophy from chronic hypertension or aortic stenosis. Any of these situations will result in ventricular end-diastolic pressures that will remain elevated after drainage of the effusion.

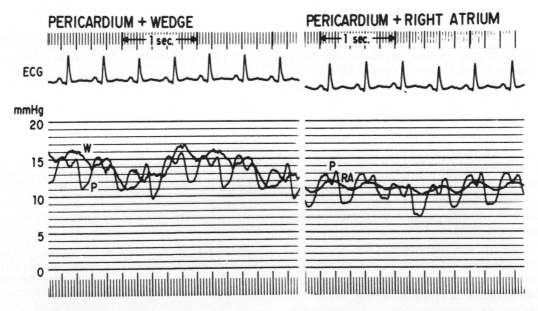

FIGURE 8–4. Pressure waveforms obtained from patient with pericardial tamponade, demonstrating elevation and equilibration of right and left heart filling pressures (P = intrapericardial pressure; W = pulmonary capillary wedge pressure; RA = right atrial pressure). Prominent X and absent Y descents are also present. (*From: Shabetai R: Diseases of the pericardium, in Wyngaarden JB, Smith LH (eds):* Cecil Textbook of Medicine. *18th ed. Philadelphia, WB Saunders, 1988.*)

A physical finding often seen in pericardial tamponade (but neither always nor exclusively) is pulsus paradoxus, which is an exaggeration of the normal 5-torr decrease in systolic blood pressure associated with inspiration. Pulsus paradoxus is the difference in torr between the point when the systolic systemic pressure is first auscultated during inspiration and when it is heard consistently throughout the respiratory cycle. A pulsus paradoxus is present when this difference exceeds 10 torr. It can also be measured easily from the waveform of an intra-arterial catheter (*see* Fig. 8–5). Although a number of mechanisms for pulsus paradoxus have been postulated, recent echocardiographic studies have provided a coherent explanation.[15,16,18] During inspiration, the negative pressure gradient between the periphery and the intrathoracic veins is increased. This increase in negative intrathoracic pressure is transmitted to the intrapericardial structures, accelerating the rate of venous return to the right-sided chambers of the heart. The resultant increase in right ventricular dimensions causes a shift of the interventricular septum to the left, diminishing left ventricular diastolic filling and reducing left ventricular stroke volume and subsequent systolic arterial pressure.[15,16,18] This mechanism has been confirmed by pulse wave Doppler echocardiography. Normally, there is a small increase (<25%) in early tricuspid blood flow velocity and a concomitant small decrease (<10%) in early mitral blood flow velocity with inspiration as compared with expiration. This pattern is exaggerated in the presence of tamponade with early tricuspid flow velocity increasing by as much as 130% and early mitral flow

velocity decreasing by as much as 50% with inspiration as compared with expiration.[19]

Although detection of pulsus paradoxus in a hypotensive patient who has an elevated central venous pressure and a known etiology for a pericardial effusion supports the diagnosis of pericardial tamponade, it must be remembered that pulsus paradoxus can be found in patients with disorders unrelated to pericardial tamponade. These include severe chronic obstructive pulmonary disease, asthma, and pulmonary embolism. Further, pulsus paradoxus may be absent in patients with pericardial tamponade who have coexistent cardiac pathology. Any condition that allows equalization of venous return between the right and left sides of the heart, such as an atrial septal defect, will prevent expression of a pulsus paradoxus. In addition, pulsus paradoxus will not be demonstrable whenever the interventricular shift that accompanies inspiration is prevented by conditions that reduce left ventricular compliance and distensibility, such as left ventricular hypertrophy, left ventricular failure, infarction, ischemia, or aortic valve incompetence. Further, pulsus paradoxus may not be demonstrable in patients with elevated right ventricular end-diastolic pressure due to pulmonary hypertension or pulmonary outflow obstruction.[17,20]

The therapy for hemodynamic compromise due to pericardial tamponade is drainage. The recommended approach for removal of the effusion will depend on the severity of hemodynamic compromise, which in turn, is partially dependent on the rate of accumulation of the effusion. Rapid intrapericardial bleeding from a cardiac puncture wound, for example, will quickly limit ventricular diastolic filling to a point incompatible with life. In this setting, when the diagnosis is readily apparent and the patient presents in impending shock, percutaneous pericardiocentesis under ultrasound and local anesthesia will be life-saving. Due to the steep portion of the pericardial compliance curve (*see* Fig. 8–2), removal of only a few hundred milliliters will be sufficient to restore an adequate stroke volume. This will allow time for more definitive diagnostic evaluation, such as cardiac catheterization, if indicated, or more definitive surgical therapy, such as formal open pericardiostomy or pericardiectomy.

Blind pericardiocentesis is associated with an unacceptably high rate of complications, including pneumothorax, coronary artery or internal mammary artery laceration, or ventricular chamber perforation.[21] These complications are even more likely if there are pericardial adhesions between the pericardium and anterior mediastinum, as in postoperative cardiac surgical patients, or between the pericardium and epicardium, as in patients who have received chest irradiation or had an illness associated with pericarditis. The success of pericardiocentesis is partly a function of the etiology of the effusion. Pericardiocentesis under fluoroscopic or

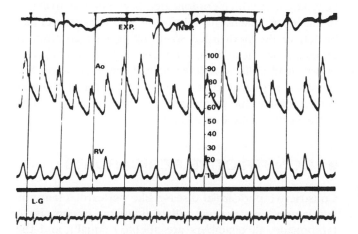

FIGURE 8–5. Pulsus paradoxus is demonstrated by 25 torr decrease in systolic arterial pressure (A$_o$ = aortic pressure) associated with inspiration (insp) compared with expiration (exp). Also demonstrated is inspiratory increase in right ventricular pressure (RV). Patient had pericardial tamponade and hypovolemia from ruptured aortic aneurysm. *(From: Shabetai R, Fowler NO, Guntheroth WG: The hemodynamics of cardiac tamponade and constrictive pericarditis. Am J Cardiol 1970; **26**:480–489.)*

echocardiographic control is very successful for large malignant or uremic effusions, whereas pericardiocentesis for a postoperative effusion, even under fluoroscopic guidance, is only successful in 50% of cases.[21]

Pericardiocentesis at our institution is carried out in the catheterization laboratory, under full fluoroscopic and echocardiographic control, except when patients are in extremis.[2] The patient is placed in a semireclining position, which allows anterior and inferior pooling of the effusion. A subxiphoid approach is used to avoid such vital structures as the pleura and coronary and internal mammary arteries (see Fig. 8–6). A short-beveled needle containing local anesthesia and connected to equipotent electrocardiographic leads is advanced, with constant aspiration, until fluid is obtained, ventricular disrhythmias is induced, or an injury current is demonstrated. If there is any question of intraventricular puncture, a few milliliters of contrast is injected, which quickly identifies the location of the needle tip. Usually, biventricular catheterization is performed simultaneously, to document the hemodynamic significance of the effusion, with tamponade demonstrated by equalization of right atrial, right ventricular end-diastolic, pulmonary capillary wedge, or left ventricular end-diastolic, and intrapericardial pressures. Biventricular catheterization also allows identification of any coexistent abnormalities, such as vena caval compression syndrome, pulmonary hypertension, or pulmonary outflow tract obstruction, or altered ventricular end-diastolic pressure. In addition, the hemodynamic efficacy of pericardiocentesis can be documented by restoration of the Y descent on the right atrial waveform. Therapeutically, a soft

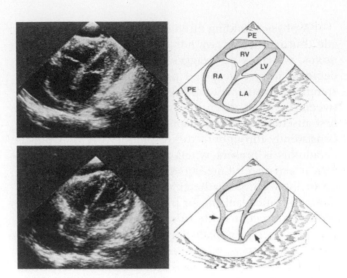

FIGURE 8–7. Subcostal four-chamber echocardiographic view from a patient with a large pericardial effusion and tamponade. The top image is during end-ventricular systole; the atria are full and not compressed. The bottom image is during late ventricular diastole/early ventricular systole. There is collapse of both the right and left atria. Collapse of the left atria with tamponade is unusual due to the tethering effect of the pulmonary veins.

catheter can be inserted into the pericardial space to allow continuous drainage of the effusion. This is especially helpful in those situations in which the effusion is accumulating rapidly, and the risk of subsequent tamponade is high, as in a right ventricular puncture during cardiac catheterization. We have had recent experience with this situation, where, to conserve blood, the drained pericardial blood was reinfused into the patient before transport to the operating room.[22] While hemodynamically successful, the reinfusion led to a systemic coagulopathy, which complicated perioperative management. In the absence of reinfusion, a sterile catheter can be left in the pericardial space to provide continuous drainage for a few days, if necessary. If impending cardiovascular collapse makes formal catheterization impossible, pericardiocentesis can be performed under echocardiographic guidance, using an injection of saline as the contrast agent (see Fig. 8–7).

■ CONSTRICTIVE PERICARDITIS

Constrictive pericardial disease, like pericardial tamponade, causes a restriction to diastolic filling. In contrast to tamponade, all chambers are affected equally, and the pattern of restriction to filling is distinctly different. The clinical manifestations of constrictive pericarditis may be quite subtle and easily mistaken for a restrictive cardiomyopathy.

Pulse wave Doppler echocardiography can be used to differentiate a restrictive cardiomyopathy from con-

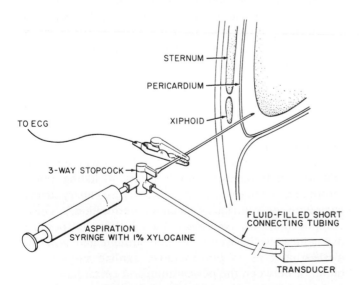

FIGURE 8–6. Technique of pericardiocentesis. *(From: Lorell BH, Grossman W: Profiles in constrictive pericarditis, restrictive cardiomyopathy, and cardiac tamponade, in Grossman W (ed): Cardiac Catheterization and Angiography. 3rd ed. Philadelphia, Lea & Febiger, 1986.)*

strictive pericarditis. The reciprocal changes in early tricuspid and mitral flow velocities seen with inspiration as compared with expiration in tamponade also are seen to a lesser degree in constriction. No such respiratory changes are seen in patients with restrictive cardiomyopathy.

The underlying pathologic process in constrictive pericarditis is a thickened, fibrotic, scarred, and densely adherent pericardium, with the visceral and parietal layers often fused and occasionally calcified (*see* Fig. 8–8). The antecedent illness may be subclinical pericarditis, with fibrin deposition and subclinical effusion formation, a pericardial effusion with incomplete resorption or drainage, or an infiltrative or reactive process.

The physiologic manifestation of constrictive pericarditis is equal impairment of late diastolic filling of all chambers of the heart. Over time, this results in symptoms compatible with biventricular failure. Early in the course of the patient's illness, fluid retention partially compensates for the restriction in diastolic filling by

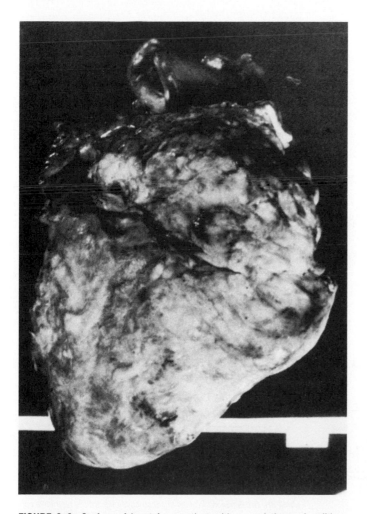

FIGURE 8–8. Surface of heart from patient with constrictive pericarditis, tuberculous in origin. *(Used courtesy of Stuart Schnitt, MD, Department of Pathology, Beth Israel Hospital, Boston.)*

maintaining an elevated central venous volume. This results in a clinical picture similar to right-sided congestive heart failure, with ascites, pleural effusions, and occasionally peripheral edema. As a further compensation, reflex tachycardia serves to maintain stroke volume and cardiac output. Although myocardial systolic function usually is intact, epicardial compression of coronary arteries with resultant ischemia can occur.[23] As stroke volume becomes limiting due to inadequate preload, symptoms of chronic low cardiac output prevail, including weight loss, fatigue, muscle wasting, and cachexia.

In the catheterization laboratory, the stiff, unyielding pericardium is revealed by characteristic findings. Chamber filling is initially very rapid, due to the elevation in venous pressure. This is seen as prominent X and Y descents, imparting a characteristic "M" or "W" shape to the atrial pressure waveform (*see* Fig. 8–9). There is early diastolic equilibration of pressure within all four chambers, revealed by the equalization of pressures in diastole between the atrium and ventricle. Ventricular filling is initially rapid, due to the increased venous pressure, which is revealed as a sharp dip in intraventricular pressure. After the limit to filling imposed by the stiff, unyielding pericardium has been reached, further diastolic filling is halted abruptly. Graphically, this appears as a "square root sign" or "dip and plateau," characteristic of constrictive pericarditis (*see* Fig. 8–10). An additional finding in constrictive pericarditis is Kussmaul's sign, the apparently paradoxical rise in central venous pressure with inspiration. In pericardial tamponade, the increase in negative intrathoracic pressure associated with inspiration is transmitted to the heart, resulting in a transient decrease in central venous pressure, stroke volume, and systolic pressure (pulsus paradoxus). In contrast, the thickened unyielding pericardium in constrictive pericarditis prevents the changes in intrathoracic pressure

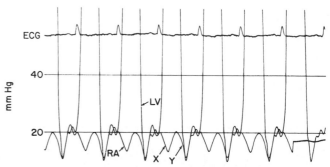

FIGURE 8–9. Right atrial (RA) and left ventricular (LV) pressure waveforms obtained from patient with constrictive pericarditis. Prominent X and Y descents give characteristic "M" and "W" appearance to the right atrial pressure waveform. Note also that right and left heart pressures are elevated and equal throughout diastole. *(From: Lorell BH, Grossman W: Profiles in constrictive pericarditis, restrictive cardiomyopathy, and cardiac tamponade, in Grossman W (ed): Cardiac Catheterization and Angiography. 3rd ed. Philadelphia, Lea & Febiger, 1986.)*

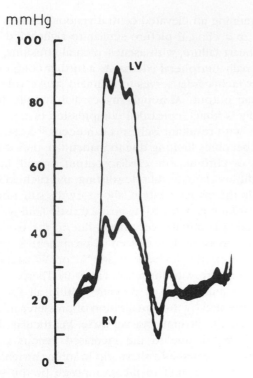

FIGURE 8–10. Right (RV) and left ventricular (LV) pressure tracings from a patient with constrictive pericarditis, demonstrating the rapid early diastolic filling, followed by the abrupt cessation of filling once the limit imposed by the pericardium has been reached. This has been described as a "dip and plateau" or "square root" sign. Note also the equilibration throughout diastole of right and left ventricular pressures. *(From: Shabetai R: The Pericardium. New York, Grune & Stratton, 1981, p 161.)*

associated with ventilation from being transmitted to the heart. This results in either no change or an increase in central venous pressure at the time of inspiration (*see* Fig. 8–11). This difference in the effect of ventilation has important clinical implications for the anesthetic management of these two groups of patients.

Table 8-1 summarizes the differences between pericardial and constrictive pericarditis.

■ ETIOLOGIES OF PERICARDIAL DISEASE

Although the underlying hemodynamic alterations caused by constrictive or effusive pericarditis have a major effect on the anesthetic management of these patients, the underlying illness must be given equal or even greater weight in the considerations necessary for a safe anesthetic. This section will review the anesthetic implications of those disease states that may require pericardial surgical intervention (either pericardial drainage or pericardiectomy) as part of their treatment. Pericardial derangements in these illnesses may be subclinical or may present a combination of effusive and constrictive patterns.

Uremia

Pericardial effusions may be seen in as many as 20% of patients with renal failure who are maintained with hemodialysis and may be associated with a 10 to 20% mortality rate despite hemodialysis.[24,25] Initiation or intensification of hemodialysis will resolve a hemodynamically significant effusion in two-thirds of patients.[25] Operative drainage for uremic pericardial effusions should be reserved for patients who have not responded to augmentation for their dialysis regimen. The effusion itself may be hemorrhagic, and if left untreated, may evolve into constrictive pericarditis. Although asymptomatic effusions are common in patients with chronic renal failure, the presence of echocardiographic findings associated with tamponade physiology suggests the need for cardiac catheterization and surgical drainage.

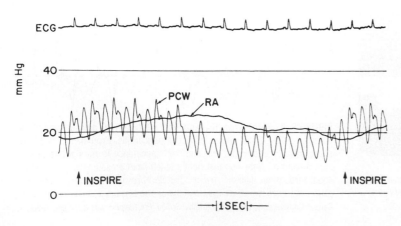

FIGURE 8–11. Right atrial (RA) and pulmonary capillary wedge (PCW) pressure waveforms from a patient with constrictive pericarditis, demonstrating the rise in central venous pressure associated with inspiration (arrow marks onset of inspiration). *(From: Lorell BH, Grossman W: Profiles in constrictive pericarditis, restrictive cardiomyopathy, and cardiac tamponade, in Grossman W (ed): Cardiac Catheterization and Angiography. 3rd ed. Philadelphia, Lea & Febiger, 1986.)*

TABLE 8–1. COMPARISON BETWEEN PERICARDIAL TAMPONADE AND CONSTRICTIVE PERICARDITIS

	Tamponade	Constriction
Duration of symptoms	hours to days	months to years
Chest pain and/or friction rub	usually	infrequently
Pulsus paradoxus	prominent	absent or minimal
Kussmaul's sign	absent	often present
Radiographic heart size	usually enlarged	usually normal
Pericardial calcification	absent	often present
Atrial fibrillation, abnormal P waves	absent	often present
Pericardial effusion	always	absent
Y descent on RA waveform	absent	deep
"Dip and plateau" on RV, LV trace	absent	present, diagnostic
Positive pressure ventilation	to be avoided	not harmful
Full pericardiectomy	occasionally	usually

(LV = left ventricle; RA = right atrial; RV = right ventricle.) (Used by permission of B. Lorell. Modified from: Lorell B: Pericardial disease, in Braunwald E (ed): Heart Disease. 3rd ed. Philadelphia, WB Saunders, 1988.)

Renal failure alters the anesthetic management of patients with a pericardial effusion or constrictive pericarditis in a number of ways. The preoperative evaluation must include close scrutiny of the patient's coagulation capability, due to the impairment of platelet function associated with uremia. A refractory coagulopathy argues for drainage of an effusion under direct vision, rather than percutaneously. Efforts to correct a coagulopathy should be undertaken before surgical intervention for constrictive pericarditis, because surgical hemostasis of raw, bleeding surfaces will be most difficult to achieve in the presence of a bleeding disorder. A prolonged bleeding time might be corrected by the administration of desmopressin (DDAVP), 0.3 to 0.4 µg/kg.[26,27] Fortunately, most patients with pericardial disease as a consequence of renal failure develop an effusion rather than constrictive disease.

The presence of renal failure will alter the metabolic fate of anesthetic agents, especially nondepolarizing muscle relaxants. Atracurium or perhaps vecuronium are preferred nondepolarizing muscle relaxants, because of their independence from renal function for metabolic clearance.[28] Although patients with chronic renal failure are adapted to a higher than normal baseline plasma potassium concentration and succinylcholine does not seem to cause greater than normal increases in plasma potassium, it should be avoided, if possible, to prevent the possibility of further hyperkalemia.[29]

Infectious Pericarditis

Tuberculosis. Although tuberculosis advanced enough to involve the pericardium is uncommon in industrialized countries, the recent increase in the number of immunosuppressed patients, whether iatrogenically for transplants or secondary to HIV infection (AIDS), may result in an increase in tuberculous pericarditis in the near future. Pericardial involvement can be due to hematogenous spread of the tubercle bacillus or from contiguous infection from adjacent lung or mediastinum. Among all causes of acute pericarditis, tuberculosis seems to account for approximately 4%.[30] The presentation is quite varied; most patients will have a fever, pericardial friction rub, and pleural and pericardial effusions, with fully 40% demonstrating tamponade physiology. Clinical presentation includes symptoms related primarily to systemic tuberculosis (fever, weight loss, night sweats), pericardial tamponade, or acute pericarditis. In most patients, tuberculous pericarditis is self-limiting and clinically seems to be idiopathic in origin until other evidence of tuberculosis is discovered. Many patients with pericardial effusions will require pericardiectomy to treat a reaccumulation of fluid, in spite of initial pericardiocentesis. In one prospective series, one-half of patients with acute tuberculous pericarditis developed constrictive pericarditis requiring pericardiectomy 2 to 4 months after presentation. This was despite treatment with isoniazid, ethambutol, and rifampin.[30] Additional treatment with steroids seems to have no influence on the subsequent development of constrictive pericarditis. The diagnosis of tuberculous pericarditis may be delayed for weeks after presentation, even when it is consistently searched for. Sputum culture is the most frequent positive diagnostic test in those patients who present with acute pericarditis. Acid-fast staining of pericardial fluid is infrequently positive, unlike culture results. Pathologic examination of pericardial biopsy specimens is occasionally positive. Untreated tuberculous pericarditis has a high mortality, in the range of 30 to 40%. Some authors recommend early surgery for a pericardial window, to prevent effusion reaccumulation, and possibly the development of late constriction, with early full pericardiectomy indicated if a thickened pericardium is found at that time.[31-33] However, study of a very large series of patients with acute tuberculous pericarditis who were treated with a triple antituberculous drug regimen revealed that, compared with percutaneous pericardiocentesis, open surgical drainage was useful only in eliminating the need for subsequent pericardiocentesis, but not in altering the overall course.[34] In contrast to other studies, oral steroid therapy did improve survival, reduce the need for subsequent pericardiocentesis and pericardiectomy, and perhaps reduce the incidence of subsequent constrictive pericarditis.

Viral Infections. Viral pericarditis can be due to a variety of agents, including Coxsackie B, Echoviruses, varicella, mumps, hepatitis B, or cytomegalovirus, especially when the patient is immunosuppressed.

Bacterial Infections. Etiologic agents usually are staphylococcus, pneumococcus, or meningococcus. Infection spreads from adjacent sites and occurs in association with hematogenously seeded bacterial endocarditis or from extension of a subdiaphragmatic abscess.[2] Although acute bacterial pericarditis is unusual in the antibiotic era, purulent pericarditis occurs most often in immunosuppressed patients (malignancy, AIDS, iatrogenic, burns) or in the setting of a preexisting effusion (such as with uremia). Constriction may be a late consequence of incomplete drainage of a purulent effusion.

Fungal Infections. Histoplasmosis is the most common etiology, in those areas in which the fungus is endemic. As with other infectious agents, pericardial involvement is most likely in those patients who are immunosuppressed. If the patient has received amphotericin B, consideration must be given to the possibility of impaired renal function and, less frequently, hemolysis or hypokalemia.

Idiopathic Pericarditis

This is the most common cause of acute pericarditis in many series (40% of cases) and certainly includes many cases of viral pericarditis in which the virus is not identified.

Post-Myocardial Infarction Pericarditis

Pericarditis within a few days to a week after myocardial infarction occurs in 5 to 10% of patients. The typical presentation is new chest pain, associated with an evanescent pericardial friction rub. New chest pain after a myocardial infarction must be differentiated from other, more serious complications of an infarction. New chest pain of peri-infarction pericarditis must be distinguished from that of unstable angina, an extension of

the original infarction, or an additional infarction, using serial electrocardiograms and cardiac-specific creatine phosphokinase isoenzyme concentrations. New chest pain associated with a murmur may herald a postinfarction ventricular septal defect (VSD) or postinfarction mitral regurgitation, due to papillary muscle rupture or ischemia. The latter conditions usually are associated with hemodynamic compromise, whereas pericarditis after an acute infarction is not. If there is serious question of differentiating the more benign pericarditis from the other two conditions, echocardiography will resolve the issue quickly. If a patient with postinfarction pericarditis requires surgical intervention, appropriate anesthetic management will be determined primarily by the presence and severity of underlying myocardial ischemia as well as residual myocardial systolic function (*see* Chapter 4).

Connective Tissue Disorders

Systemic Lupus Erythematosus. The systemic manifestations of lupus erythematosus are protean. Pericarditis is the most frequent cardiac manifestation, with tamponade occurring infrequently and constrictive pericarditis occurring rarely. Myocardial involvement may lead to conduction abnormalities or, infrequently, contractile dysfunction with direct impairment of systolic function.[35,36] There may be direct involvement of cardiac valves in 20% of patients with lupus. In some, valvular dysfunction may be severe enough to be clinically significant. In an unselected series of patients with lupus, valvular abnormalities, either the verrucae of Libman-Sacks endocarditis, or valvular insufficiency, were seen echocardiographically in 15 to 20% and usually were clinically silent.[37] These lesions, or more commonly, distorted or perforated valves, typically left sided, may require surgical replacement in a small percentage of lupus patients. Rarely, an arteritis can result in clinically significant coronary artery disease. In addition, accelerated atherosclerosis in patients with lupus, in part a consequence of prolonged corticosteroid use, increases the risk of myocardial ischemia and infarction. Patients with lupus severe enough to necessitate operative intervention for effusive, pericardial, or valvular disease usually are receiving systemic steroid therapy and will need prophylactic corticosteroid therapy to protect them from a chronically suppressed pituitary-adrenal axis.

Nonsteroidal anti-inflammatory agents may interfere with platelet thromboxanes, resulting in a coagulation defect. However, fewer than 10% of patients with lupus will have a significant thrombocytopenia. Lupus patients may have a circulating anticoagulant, which presents as an otherwise unexplained prolonged partial thromboplastin time (aPTT). The lupus anticoagulant is a test-tube anticoagulant only, interfering with the phospholipid tissue thromboplastins used for the laboratory determination of the partial thromboplastin time and is not associated with a bleeding tendency in vivo.[38] In fact, patients with a lupus anticoagulant are at risk for thrombotic events. Therefore, long-term anticoagulation should be considered for patients with a lupus anticoagulant who are undergoing valve replacement.[39]

Pulmonary involvement may result in restrictive lung disease, with a diffusion defect and arterial hypoxemia resulting. Chronic renal failure may be a late result of lupus, with well-recognized implications for anesthetic management. Active lupus cerebritis may make conduct of a procedure such as pericardiocentesis difficult or impossible under local anethesia.

Rheumatoid Arthritis. Chronic constrictive pericarditis can occur as a complication of rheumatoid arthritis. Approximately one-third of patients with rheumatoid arthritis will have pericardial thickening or effusion seen by echocardiography.[40] Pericarditis usually is seen only in those patients with otherwise severe manifestations of their disease. When present constrictive pericarditis usually improves after pericardiectomy.[41,42] Conduction system abnormalities may be due to myocardial rheumatoid nodules or from inflammatory changes.

Of importance to the anesthesiologist is frequent involvement of the cervical spine in severe rheumatoid arthritis, including atlantoaxial subluxation and the potential for spinal cord or vertebral artery compression. Of additional interest to the anesthesiologist is the possible involvement of the temporomandibular and cricoarytenoid joints. Most rheumatic pleural effusions will spontaneously resolve, but some will require percutaneous or surgical drainage or decortication for recurrent pleuritis.[43]

Malignancies

Malignant pericardial disease is associated most commonly with cancers of the breast and lung, Hodgkin's disease, and other lymphomas. The spectrum of pericardial disease associated with malignancies ranges from acute hemorrhagic pericardial tamponade, to compression syndromes from tumor masses, to constrictive physiology from a noncompliant pericardium encased with infiltrating tumor. Unlike patients with radiation-induced constrictive pericarditis, patients with pericardial disease secondary to a malignancy may present with signs and symptoms of pericardial tamponade, constrictive disease, or a combination of both.

Hodgkin's Lymphoma. Large anterior mediastinal masses, which can be seen in patients with Hodgkin's lymphoma, pose significant risk of intrathoracic airway compression during the institution of positive pressure ventilation, independent of endotracheal intubation. The physical presence of such masses should be sought by computerized tomography before surgical intervention for pericardial disease.[44] The functional significance of anterior mediastinal masses can be evaluated, in part, by flow–volume spirometry. If functional intrathoracic airway compression is present, there often will be a flattening of the expiratory phase of the flow–volume loop in the supine but not sitting positions.[45] Furthermore, many such patients will report symptoms of air hunger or a sensation of chest compression in the supine but not in the lateral or sitting positions. When such signs or symptoms are present, serious consideration must be given to performing the surgical procedure under local anesthesia or after an effective course of radiation or chemotherapy to reduce the size of the mediastinal mass before the induction of general anesthesia. Fiberoptic intubation with the patient appropriately sedated, but breathing spontaneously, also may reveal the presence of functional airway obstruction that might not be appreciated by routine chest roentgenogram or computerized tomography.[46]

Current chemotherapy for Hodgkin's lymphoma includes such anesthetically relevant agents as bleomycin (pulmonary fibrosis, respiratory failure possibly associated with high inspired concentrations of oxygen[47,48]), doxorubicin (myocardial dysfunction[49-51]), and prednisone (suppression of the pituitary–adrenal axis).

Breast, Lung Cancer. Primary treatment may involve use of chemotherapeutic agents with anesthetic implications. Some of these patients will have received chest irradiation as well.

Radiation Therapy. Pericardial injury, either a chronic effusion or constrictive pericarditis, usually presents months to years after radiation therapy, especially after mantle irradiation for Hodgkin's disease, lymphoma, or other thoracic neoplasms.[52] Typically, patients have received 4500 rads or more. The likelihood of pericardial injury varies with total dose of radiation administered, as well as the amount of heart included in the radiation portal. If echocardiography and cardiac catheterization data reveal a large effusion, it should be drained, initially in the catheterization laboratory. Symptomatic patients with large effusions who are otherwise expected to survive longer than days to weeks should undergo a pericardial window or, less frequently, a formal pericardiectomy. If the primary radiation-induced lesion is symptomatic pericardial constriction, then a full formal pericardiectomy should be considered. At surgery, the pericardium and adjacent tissue will be very friable and densely adherent; bleeding will be a major intraoperative consideration.

Prior Cardiac Surgery

Unlike effusive tamponade from most other causes, in which echocardiography demonstrates the effusion to be homogenous, in the perioperative period, the collection of blood around the heart usually will be loculated (areas of clotted and unclotted blood). Echocardiographic findings typical of effusive tamponade such as right atrial and right ventricular collapse, Doppler flow variation across the mitral and tricuspid valves with respiration, and swinging of the heart within the effusion are not commonly seen in the postoperative period.[53] Localized compression of each of the cardiac chambers, as well as of the pulmonary outflow tract has been reported.[54] Pulsus paradoxus may not be seen due to the presence of hypovolemia. The presence of hemodynamic compromise (hypotension, low urine output, low cardiac output) in combination with the echocardiographic finding of a pericardial separation width of >10 mm has been shown to have 100% sensitivity for detection of postoperative cardiac tamponade.[53]

Postoperative constrictive pericarditis is the most common cause of constrictive pericarditis requiring pericardiectomy in many series, with an overall incidence of 0.2 to 0.3% of all patients undergoing cardiac surgery.[55,56] Constrictive physiology may present in the immediate postoperative period or, more typically, months to years later. Povidone-iodine irrigation around the heart may be one etiologic factor in postoperative constrictive pericarditis.[55]

Pericardial closure at the time of the original procedure decreases the incidence of perioperative cardiac tamponade from blood pooling,[57] as well as subsequent constrictive pericarditis that results from organized hematoma around the posterior aspect of the heart.[58] Furthermore, closure of the pericardium greatly facilitates reexploration during subsequent cardiac surgery by preventing the right ventricle and anteriorly placed grafts from becoming densely adherent to the anterior chest wall. This not only reduces the amount of bleeding during subsequent surgery but makes catastrophic entry into cardiac chambers in reexploration much less likely to occur. However, the pericardium is not closed routinely at the end of cardiac surgery by all surgeons for a number of reasons. For patients with dilated ventricles or those who have developed myocardial edema while supported by cardiopulmonary bypass, closure of the pericardium may restrict ventricular diastolic filling enough to be hemodynamically significant, especially if preexisting left ventricular compliance is low (as with aortic stenosis).[59,60] Furthermore, some surgeons are concerned that pericardial closure may kink or otherwise mechanically distort anteriorly or laterally placed coronary grafts, compromising both short-term flow and perhaps long-term patency.

■ SURGERY FOR PERICARDIAL EFFUSION OR TAMPONADE

The indications and timing of surgery for a pericardial effusion depend on the etiology of the effusion, its rate of accumulation, and the severity of resultant hemodynamic compromise.

There are three surgical options for permanent drainage of recurrent pericardial effusions: a pericardial "window," a partial pericardiectomy, or a full pericardiectomy. A pericardial "window" creates a continuity between the pericardium and pleura or the pericardium and peritoneum. It can be performed under local anesthesia, with the patient in the semisitting position. Its advantages include obtaining a pericardial specimen for formal pathologic examination and minimal physiologic trespass for the often marginally compensated patient. For these reasons, it is the approach taken most often for patients with malignant pericardial effusions, whose life expectancy from their underlying disease is measured in weeks to months, or for patients with hemodynamically significant uremic pericardial effusions who are awaiting initiation or intensification of hemodialysis. The operative mortality is approximately 0 to 5% and is primarily a function of the patient's underlying disease.[61,62] The drawbacks to a pericardial "window" include a significant incidence of reaccumulation of the effusion, as well as the potential development of constrictive pericarditis as a late sequelae.

An operative adjunct to the creation of a pericardial "window" is pericardioscopy, which allows visualization of much of the epicardial surface, as well as examination of the intrapericardial structures.[63] It is useful in directing intraoperative biopsy for diagnostic purposes. Because of the possibility of mechanically induced dysrhythmias during periocardioscopy, preparations for emergent electrical cardioversion or defibrillation must be made before the induction of anesthesia.

In as many as 75% of patients undergoing pericardiectomy, the indication for the procedure is refractory pericardial effusion.[55] Of these, the most common etiologies are neoplastic disease and uremia, although the incidence of pericardial tamponade in the period immediately after cardiac surgery may be as high as 1 to 5%.[64,65]

■ ANESTHETIC TECHNIQUE FOR SURGERY FOR PERICARDIAL EFFUSION

Goals

1. In cases of tamponade, relieve the restriction to diastolic filling before the induction of anesthesia.

2. Avoid positive pressure ventilation until tamponade physiology has been relieved.
3. Maintain filling pressures high enough to overcome diastolic filling restrictions: central venous pressure or pulmonary capillary wedge pressure may need to be 20 to 30 torr.
4. Avoid vasodilation.
5. Avoid bradycardia.
6. If compromised, support myocardial contractility.

Patients undergoing pericardiostomy or pericardiectomy for tamponade or recurrent effusion present a unique constellation of problems for the anesthesiologist. Ventricular filling in diastole is limited to a varying degree by the effusion; this can range from trivial compromise to an intrapericardial pressure high enough to be life-threatening. Any maneuver that reduces venous return has the potential of further diminishing diastolic filling to the point at which stroke volume becomes inadequate to sustain life. Such maneuvers potentially include positive-pressure ventilation, an intravascular volume inadequate to overcome the limitation on diastolic filling imposed by the effusion, and systemic venodilatation.

For these reasons, it is essential that the cardiac anesthesiologist have a preoperative assessment of the absolute magnitude of the effusion and, more importantly, its hemodynamic effect. Except when the patient's condition has not allowed time for preoperative echocardiography and/or catheterization, this information should be available.

Initial Management of Patients With an Effusion

Patients with an effusion require meticulous assessment and management before induction of anesthesia. The degree of right atrial (RA) and right ventricular (RV) collapse is assessed easily with echocardiography, and this information usually is available before induction. Patients with tamponade will require volume infusion to raise CVP and improve RV filling. It may be necessary to increase the CVP to 20 or 30 mm Hg in severe cases. Most patients with tamponade will have complete emptying of the RV and left ventricle (LV) in systole as a compensatory measure. If echocardiographic examination or previous history suggests systolic impairment, inotrope infusion is warranted to optimize stroke volume. An agent that is not associated with vasodilation such as epinephrine is the best choice. Vasodilation must be avoided. It reduces RV filling and reduces systemic blood pressure in patients who have a fixed stroke volume. Alpha-adreneric support may be necessary to maintain perfusion pressure. Heart rate must be maintained to maintain cardiac output in the setting of a reduced, fixed SV. Patients with tamponade generally are tachycardic.

Definitive treatment for tamponade is drainage. Patients in extremis or those who are minimally responsive to the above measures should undergo pericardiocentesis with local anesthesia, preferably with echocardiographic or fluoroscopic guidance, before the induction of general anesthesia and initiation of positive-pressure ventilation.[66] Although blind pericardiocentesis using an electrocardiogram (ECG) lead on the exploring needle to detect injury current has been used in the past, the ready availability of echocardiography at the present time makes its use preferred, especially considering the risks of unguided pericardiocentesis. Reference to the pericardial compliance curve (*see* Fig. 8–2) indicates that the entire effusion need not be drained before induction of general anesthesia. It is necessary to remove only a small volume of fluid to place the patient below the "knee" of the pericardial pressure–volume curve and effect a dramatic improvement in hemodynamics.

Premedication

Because drainage of pericardial fluid usually is an urgent or emergent procedure for patients with some degree of hemodynamic compromise, judicious premedication in the holding area while under the direct care of the anesthesiologist is warranted. Midazolam in increments of 0.015 to 0.02 mg/kg is a reasonable approach.

Preinduction

As for other cardiac surgical procedures, ECG leads for I, II, III, aVR, aVL, aVF, and V_5 should be in place before induction, as well as the confirmed ability to defibrillate and electrically cardiovert the heart. Adequate intravenous (IV) access with at least one large-bore (14- or 16-gauge) IV catheter should be obtained. A radial artery catheter is placed before induction. A pulmonary artery catheter is useful before pericardiocentesis and during induction of general anesthesia, both to document that preinduction pericardiocentesis has relieved tamponade physiology and to allow optimization of diastolic filling pressures during induction and surgery. The case should not be unnecessarily delayed to obtain central venous access, however.

Induction and Maintenance

For the patient with a small, hemodynamically insignificant effusion who is undergoing pericardial biopsy or pericardioscopy for diagnostic purposes or for the creation of a pericardial window to prevent a reaccumulation of fluid, the anesthetic management will be dictated primarily by the patient's underlying medical condition, as discussed above.

For patients with tamponade, induction of general anesthesia may begin after partial drainage of the effusion has been accomplished. The presence of central venous or a pulmonary artery catheter will document the relief of tamponade physiology and indicate the safety of proceeding with induction. If thermodilution cardiac output determinations are possible, then optimization of the patient's intravascular volume to maximize stroke volume can be accomplished before and during the anesthetic. Transthoracic echocardiography also can be used to quickly assess the degree of improvement with drainage of fluid.

The patient should be prepped and drapped before induction in case emergent surgical decompression is needed after induction. Unless all of the fluid has been removed, the patients will continue to exhibit some degree of tamponade physiology. In addition, reaccumulation of fluid may have occurred since drainage. Induction with agents with minimal cardiovascular effects is warranted. Etomidate 0.3 mg/kg in combination with fentanyl 5 to 10 μg/kg or sufentanil 1 to 2 μg/kg is appropriate. Ketamine 1 to 2 mg/kg IV[67] may be used because it maintains heart rate, contractility, and systemic vascular resistance (SVR). Caution must be exercised for patients who have high existing sympathetic tone because the negative inotropic effects will predominate. Muscle relaxants should be chosen to offset any vagotonic effects of the narcotics. Pancuronium is a good choice if large narcotic doses are chosen. Amnesia can be maintained with benzodiapines or low doses of inhalational agents. After the effusion has been removed, the choice of anesthetic agents should be guided by the patient's underlying disease state and consideration of postoperative ventilatory requirements.

A transesophageal echocardiography (TEE) probe is inserted after induction and tracheal intubation. This allows on-line assessment of ventricular filling and compression and assessment of contractility. In addition, the completeness of fluid evacuation can be assessed easily. This may be important when loculated effusions exist.

Drainage of a large effusion and relief of tamponade generally produces a marked improvement in hemodynamics, but it also may produce pulmonary venous congestion or pulmonary edema due to the sudden increase in pulmonary venous return to the left atrium (LA) and LV. This is particularly likely if there is reduced LV systolic function, lesions that predispose an elevation of LAP (MR, MS, poor LV compliance), or LV afterload mismatch due to a high SVR. Treatment will require vasodilation with IV nitroglycerin.

In the unusual situation in which preinduction drainage of the effusion is not possible, either because of loculations or adhesions, induction of anesthesia can be accomplished by spontaneous ventilation and the use of a volatile agent or small doses of ketamine. Sevoflurane or halothane is preferred in this circumstance, because it is better tolerated for mask induction and is less likely to generate coughing, which will impede venous return and worsen the hemodynamic effects of the effusion. Positive-pressure ventilation should be avoided until surgical drainage of the effusion is accomplished, and the patient should be intubated for airway protection, if indicated, while breathing spontaneously. Attention must be paid to ventricular filling pressures, and intravascular volume may need to be supplemented to allow generation of an adequate stroke volume.

■ SURGERY FOR CONSTRICTIVE PERICARDITIS

Patients with constrictive pericarditis do not present emergently for pericardiectomy. A thorough review of the cardiac catheterization data by the anesthesiologist before the induction of anesthesia is mandatory, so that an informed judgment concerning optimal filling pressures, stroke volume, and possible need for inotropic support can be made. Patients undergoing pericardiectomy for constrictive disease present a spectrum of anesthetic challenges different from the patient with pericardial tamponade. Etiologies of constrictive pericarditis requiring formal pericardiectomy include idiopathic (40% of patients in some series); before cardiac surgery (30%); viral, bacterial, or less frequently, fungal pericarditis in a small percentage; pericardial involvement with a malignancy, either contiguous or distant; or pericarditis due to a connective tissue disorder. Unlike anesthetizing a patient with a pericardial effusion, during which the most difficult aspects of the anesthetic occur before induction and during the early part of an otherwise brief procedure, pericardiectomy for constrictive disease requires ongoing vigilance and often endurance during a long and difficult surgery.

Pericardiectomy for constrictive disease usually involves extensive dissection of tissue that is densely adherent, often to thin-walled cardiac chambers, the great vessels, coronary arteries, or aortocoronary saphenous vein grafts. Perioperative mortality can be as high as 10%, with hemorrhage being a significant or primary cause of death.[68] Massive hemorrhage can occur from inadvertent entry into cardiac chambers, or the patient can bleed more slowly, but continuously, from raw dissected surfaces. It is imperative that venous access be adequate to guarantee timely volume, blood, and coagulation factor replacement, as needed. Usually, patients undergoing pericardiectomy for constrictive disease are explored through a median sternotomy. Many will have undergone prior cardiac surgery, and although pump oxygenator standby is typical, cardiopulmonary bypass actually is required in only 10% of such patients.[55] The primary reason for avoiding the use of cardiopulmonary bypass for constrictive pericardiectomy is the need for systemic anticoagulation. In patients with constriction secondary to prior cardiac surgery, dense adhesions around the heart may incorporate epicardial saphenous vein or internal mammary coronary grafts, and damage during pericardiectomy, with either bleeding or myocardial ischemia, can result.[56]

When constrictive pericarditis is the result of prior cardiac surgery, the primary physiologic defect, whether a valvular lesion or myocardial ischemia, has been ameliorated or fully corrected. Although this might argue against placement of a pulmonary artery catheter with cardiac output capability, there are other reasons for the use of invasive monitoring. Some patients will be explored to resolve the differential diagnosis of constrictive pericarditis versus restrictive cardiomyopathy. Here, the diagnosis might require measurement of the end-diastolic pressures in both atrium and ventricle, preferably both right and left, before and after pericardiectomy. Some patients undergoing pericardiectomy for constrictive disease require inotropic support during and after surgery. Furthermore, in some patients with a densely adherent pericardium, or with an underlying coagulopathy, the ability to assess filling pressures during significant blood and intravascular volume replacement is essential.

Although some surgeons will approach the heart through a left lateral thoracotomy and remove pericardium from the left ventricle only, most will use a median sternotomy and resect as much pericardium as is possible. Pericardial resection usually will extend over the entire anterior surface, exclusive of pericardium that overlies coronary artery grafts, laterally to the phrenic nerves, and inferiorly to the diaphragmatic surface.[69] When cardiopulmonary bypass is not used, the anesthesiologist must expect frequent mechanically induced dysrhythmias, and therefore have the capability of electrically cardioverting or defibrillating the patient. In addition, frequent manipulation and displacement of the heart during the dissection will cause wide swings in stroke volume and blood pressure. If the extent of the dissection or the potential complications of reentering the chest of a patient who has undergone prior cardiac surgery requires the institution of cardiopulmonary bypass, then the anesthesiologist must be prepared to deal with ongoing hemorrhage, with surgical hemostasis difficult to achieve. Adequate reserves of red cells, as well as platelets and other blood products, must be immediately available.

■ ANESTHETIC TECHNIQUE

Goals

1. Maintain adequate central venous volume, as guided by the cardiac catheterization data.

2. Avoid bradycardia; diastolic filling is limited by the constricting pericardium, and slow heart rates will result in low cardiac output.

3. Establish generous venous access. Prolonged, continuous bleeding is common and a major cause of mortality.

4. Aggressively treat platelet, red cell, and clotting factor depletion.

5. Positive-pressure ventilation is not detrimental; changes in intrathoracic compliance are poorly transmitted through a stiff, adherent pericardium.

6. Be prepared for a long, tedious surgery.

Premedication

The principal determinant of preoperative sedation will be the patient's underlying medical condition. For example, a young, otherwise healthy patient with constrictive pericarditis secondary to mantle irradiation for Hodgkin's disease years earlier should be premedicated as for any other major operation. The premedication of a patient with severe rheumatoid arthritis undergoing pericardiectomy for constrictive disease who also has an unstable cervical spine will be determined primarily by the need for sedation and topical anesthesia for an awake intubation. If the patient is undergoing pericardiectomy secondary to prior cardiac surgery, premedication will be determined primarily by the adequacy of myocardial revascularization and the presence of residual angina or ischemia. If the patient has residual myocardial ischemia, then premedication considerations are similar to those for primary revascularization (*see* Chapter 4).

Except when myocardial ischemia is likely, relative tachycardia need not be avoided, because an increased heart rate is a primary compensatory mechanism to overcome the restriction of diastolic filling, thereby maintaining cardiac output. There is little filling in the mid-to-late period of diastole, due to the restraining influence of the noncompliant pericardium. For this reason, sinus rhythm is somewhat less critical to ventricular filling than in aortic stenosis, where diminished ventricular compliance can be partially overcome by appropriately timed atrial systole (*see* Chapter 5). Nonetheless, sinus rhythm should be maintained when possible.

Preinduction

Patients are prepared as for coronary artery bypass graft (CABG) or valve surgery (*see* Chapter 4), with even more emphasis on adequate IV access, including central venous catheterization. A pulmonary artery catheter with thermodilution capability usually is indicated, independent of the etiology of the constrictive disease. The ability to measure cardiac output, as well as right- and left-sided filling pressures, is extremely useful, even though myocardial contractility will be normal in many patients with constrictive pericarditis.

Induction and Maintenance

With pericardiocentesis under local anesthesia, the primary hemodynamic defect of a pericardial effusion is at least temporarily corrected before the induction of general anesthesia. In contrast, the patient with constrictive pericarditis has no such physiologic remedy available, with markedly compromised ventricular function during and often for a lengthy time after pericardiectomy. Delayed recovery in ventricular function may be due to an incomplete removal of the pericardium or the result of underlying ventricular dysfunction from chronic pericardial constriction. Furthermore, complete pericardiectomy is not always possible, due to the absence of a cleavage plane between the adherent pericardium and underlying epicardium.[69]

The specific conduct of induction of anesthesia depends on the etiology of the patient's constrictive pericarditis and the anticipated duration of surgery. Induction may be similar to that used for coronary artery bypass surgery (*see* Chapter 4), if the duration of surgery is expected to be lengthy and significant residual ventricular dysfunction is anticipated in the immediate postoperative period. This would include a combination of fentanyl 25 to 50 µg/kg or sufentanil 5 to 10 µg/kg, together with a benzodiazepine or inhalational agent. If the etiology of constrictive pericarditis is secondary to prior coronary revascularization, then a significant potential for perioperative myocardial ischemia exists and ongoing vigilance for myocardial ischemia must be maintained throughout the anesthetic. Reopening of the chest and dissection and removal of the pericardium itself can injure entrapped coronary bypass grafts as well as an engrafted internal mammary artery.

Unlike the patient with a pericardial effusion, changes in intrathoracic pressure are not transmitted to the heart through the thickened pericardium in constrictive disease. This eliminates the need to avoid positive-pressure ventilation and makes induction and maintenance quite similar to that for coronary revascularization. The primary difference between surgery for revascularization and constrictive pericarditis is that the latter is of shorter duration, with a greater risk of severe hemorrhage and a greater likelihood of needing inotropic support (*see* Chapter 4). In fact, many of these patients will require inotropic support both during and for a period of time after surgery. In addition, unlike the patient undergoing revascularization, the patient with constrictive pericarditis may take as long as a month to regain normal hemodynamics and ventricular function.[70]

Anesthetizing patients for pericardiectomy for constrictive disease is particularly challenging, requiring close coordination between surgeon and anesthesiologist, as well as full cognizance of the extracardiac anesthetic implications of the patient's underlying illness.

■ REFERENCES

1. Nathan MRP, Lipat G, Sanders M: Unusual echocardiographic findings in pericardial tamponade. *Am Heart J* 1979; **98**:225-227.
2. Lorell B: Pericardial disease, in Braunwald E (ed): *Heart Disease.* 3rd ed. Philadelphia, WB Saunders, 1988.
3. Rousou JA, Parker T, Engelman RM, et al: Phrenic nerve paresis associated with the use of iced slush and the cooling jacket for topical hypothermia. *J Thorac Cardiovasc Surg* 1985; **89**:921-925.
4. Shabetai R: *The Pericardium.* New York, Grune & Stratton, 1981.
5. Brenner JI, Waugh RA: Effect of phasic respiration on left ventricular dimension and performance in a normal population. *Circulation* 1978; **57**:122-127.
6. Southworth H, Stevenson CS: Congenital defects of pericardium. *Arch Intern Med* 1938; **61**:223.
7. Mangano D: The effect of the pericardium on ventricular systolic function in man. *Circulation* 1980; **61**:352-357.
8. Mangano DT, et al: Significance of the pericardium in human subjects: Effects on left ventricular volume, pressure and ejection. *J Am Coll Cardiol* 1985; **6**:290-295.
9. Beck CS: Two cardiac compression triads. *JAMA* 1935; **104**:714-716.
10. Fowler NO, Gabel M, Buncher CR: Cardiac tamponade: A comparison of right versus left heart compression. *J Am Coll Cardiol* 1988; **12**:187-193.
11. Antman EM, Cargill V, Grossman W: Low-pressure cardiac tamponade. *Ann Intern Med* 1979; **91**:403-406.
12. Come P: Echocardiographic recognition of pericardial disease, in Come P (ed): *Diagnostic Cariology: Noninvasive Imaging Techniques.* Philadelphia, JB Lippincott, 1985.
13. Parameswaran R, Goldberg H: Echocardiographic quantification of pericardial effusion. *Chest* 1983; **83**:767-770.
14. Schiller NB, Botvinick EH: Right ventricular compression as a sign of cardiac tamponade: An analysis of echocardiographic ventricular dimensions and their clinical implications. *Circulation* 1977; **56**:774-779.
15. Cosio FG, et al: Abnormal septal motion in cardiac tamponade with pulsus paradoxus. *Chest* 1977; **71**:787-788.
16. D'Cruz IA, et al: Diagnosis of cardiac tamponade by echocardiography: Changes in mitral valve motion and ventricular dimensions, with special reference to paradoxical pulse. *Circulation* 1975; **52**:460-465.
17. Singh S, Wann LS, Schuchard GH, et al: Right ventricular and right atrial collapse in patients with cardiac tamponade — A combined echocardiographic and hemodynamic study. *Circulation* 1984; **70**:966-971.
18. Settle HP, Adolph RJ, Fowler NO, et al: Echocardiographic study of cardiac tamponade. *Circulation* 1977; **56**:957-959.
19. Appleton CP, Hatle LK, Popp RL: Cardiac tamponade and pericardial effusion: respiratory variation in transvalvular flow velocities studied by Doppler echocardiography. *J Am Coll Cardiol* 1988; **11**:1020-1030.
20. Cunningham MJ, Safian RD, Come PL, et al: Absence of pulsus paradoxus in a patient with cardiac tamponade and coexisting pulmonary artery obstruction. *Am J Med* 1987; **83**:973-976.
21. Wong B, Murphy J, Chang CJ, et al: The risk of pericardiocentesis. *Am J Cardiol* 1979; **44**:1110-1114.
22. Moore JW, Bricker JT, Mullins CE, et al: Infusion of blood from pericardial sac into femoral vein: A technique for survival until operative closure of a cardiac perforation during balloon septostomy. *Am J Cardiol* 1985; **56**:494-495.

23. Gregory MA, Whitton ID, Cameron EW: Myocardial ischemia in constrictive pericarditis: A morphometric and electron microscopic study. *Br J Exp Path* 1984; **65**:365-376.

24. Luft LC, Gilman JK, Weyman AE: Pericarditis in the patient with uremia: Clinical and echocardiographic evaluation. *Nephron* 1980; **25**:160-166.

25. DePace NL, Nestico PF, Schwartz AB, et al: Predicting success of intensive dialysis in the treatment of uremic pericarditis. *Am J Med* 1984; **76**:38-46.

26. Watson AJS, Keogh JAB: Effect of 1-deamino-8-d-arginine vasopressin on the prolonged bleeding time in chronic renal failure. *Nephron* 1982; **32**:49-52.

27. Salzman EW, Weinstein MJ, Weintraub RM, et al: Treatment with desmopressin acetate to reduce blood loss after cardiac surgery. *N Engl J Med* 1986; **314**:1402-1406.

28. Hunter JM, Jones RS, Utting JE: Comparison of vecuronium, atracurium and tubocurarine in normal patients and in patients with no renal function. *Br J Anaesth* 1984; **56**:941-950.

29. Powell DR, Miller RD: The effect of repeated doses of succinylcholine on serum potassium in patients with renal failure. *Anesth Analg* 1975; **54**:746-748.

30. Sagrista-Sauleda J, Permanyer-Miralda G, Soler-Soler J: Tuberculous pericarditis: Ten year experience with a prospective protocol for diagnosis and treatment. *J Am Coll Cardiol* 1988; **11**:724-728.

31. Quale JM, Lipschik GY, Heurich AE: Management of tuberculous pericarditis. *Ann Thorac Surg* 1987; **43**:653-655.

32. Larrieu AJ, Tyers FO, Williams EH, et al: Recent experience with tuberculous pericarditis. *Ann Thorac Surg* 1980; **29**:464-468.

33. Carson TJ, Murray GF, Wilcox BR, et al: The role of surgery in tuberculous pericarditis. *Ann Thorac Surg* 1974; **17**:163-167.

34. Strang JIG, Gibson DG, Mitchison DA, et al: Controlled clinical trial of complete surgical drainage and prednisolone in treatment of tuberculous pericardial effusion in Transkei. *Lancet* 1988; **2**:759-763.

35. DelRio A, Vazquez JJ, Sobrino JA, et al: Myocardial involvement in systemic lupus erythematosis. *Chest* 1978; **74**:414-417.

36. Stevens MB: Lupus carditis (editorial). *N Engl J Med* 1988; **319**:861-862.

37. Galve E, Candell-Riera J, Pigran C, et al: Prevalence, morphologic types and evolution of cardiac valvular disease in systemic lupus erythematosus. *N Engl J Med* 1988; **319**:817-823.

38. Asherson RA, Lubbe WF: Cerebral and valve lesions in SLE: Association with antiphospholipid antibodies (editorial). *J Rheumatol* 1988; **15**:539-541.

39. Dajee H, Hurley EJ, Szarnicki RJ: Cardiac valve replacement in systemic lupus erythematosus: A review. *J Thorac Cardiovasc Surg* 1983; **85**:718-726.

40. MacDonald WJ, Crawford MH, Klippel JH, et al: Echocardiographic assessment of cardiac structure and function in patients with rheumatoid arthritis. *Am J Med* 1977; **63**:890-896.

41. Burney DP, Martin CE, Thomas CS, et al: Rheumatoid pericarditis: Clinical significance and operative management. *J Thorac Cardiovasc Surg* 1979; **77**:511-515.

42. John JT, Hough A, Sergent JS: Pericardial disease in rheumatoid arthritis. *Am J Med* 1979; **66**:385-390.

43. Yarbrough JW, Sealy WC, Miller JA: Thoracic surgical problems associated with rheumatoid arthritis. *J Thorac Cardiovasc Surg* 1975; **69**:347-354.

44. Northrip DR, Bohman BK, Tsueda K: Total airway occlusion and superior vena cava syndrome in a child with an anterior mediastinal tumor. *Anesth Analg* 1986; **65**:1079-1082.

45. Neuman GG, Weingarten AE, Abramowitz RM, et al: The anesthetic management of the patient with an anterior mediastinal mass. *Anesthesiology* 1984; **60**:144-147.

46. Sperry RJ, Lake CL, Mentzer RM, et al: Case conference. *J Cardiothorac Anesth* 1987; **1**:71-79.

47. Gilson AJ, Sahn SA: Reactivation of bleomycin lung toxicity following oxygen administration. *Chest* 1985; **88**:304-306.

48. LaMantia KR, Glick JH, Marshall BE: Supplemental oxygen does not cause repiratory failure in bleomycin-treated surgical patients. *Anesthesiology* 1984; **60**:65-67.

49. Bristow MR, Mason JW, Billingham ME, et al: Doxorubicin cardiomyopathy: Evaluation by phonocardiography, endomyocardial biopsy and cardiac catheterization. *Ann Intern Med* 1978; **88**:168-175.

50. Isner JM, Ferrans UJ, Cohen SR, et al: Clinical and morphologic cardiac findings after anthracycline chemotherapy. *Am J Cardiol* 1983; **51**:1167-1174.

51. Freter CE, Lee TC, Billingham ME, et al: Doxorubicin cardiac toxicity manifesting seven years after treatment. *Am J Med* 1986; **80**:483-485.

52. Applefield MM, Wiernik PH: Cardiac disease after radiation therapy for Hodgkin's disease: Analysis of 48 patients. *Am J Cardiol* 1983; **51**:1679-1681.

53. Bommer WJ, Follette D, Pollock M, et al: Tamponade in patients undergoing cardiac surgery: A clinical-echocardiographic diagnosis. *Am Heart J* 1995; **130**:1216-1223.

54. D'Cruz IA, Kensey K, Campbell C, et al: Two-dimensional echocardiography in cardiac tamponade occurring after cardiac surgery. *J Am Coll Cardiol* 1985; **5**:1250-1252.

55. Miller JI, Mansour KA, Hatcher CR: Pericardiectomy: Current indications, concepts and results in a university center. *Ann Thorac Surg* 1982; **34**:40-45.

56. Kutcher MA, King SB III, Alimurung BN, et al: Constrictive pericarditis as a complication of cardiac surgery: Recognition of an entity. *Am J Cardiol* 1982; **50**:742-748.

57. Cunningham JN, Spencer FC, Zeff R, et al: Influence of primary closure of the pericardium after open-heart surgery on the frequency of tamponade, postcardiotomy syndrome, and pulmonary complications. *J Thorac Cardiovasc Surg* 1975; **70**:119-125.

58. Cohen MV, Greenberg MA: Constrictive pericarditis: Early and late complication of cardiac surgery. *Am J Cardiol* 1979; **43**:657-661.

59. Jarvinen A, Peltola K, Rasanen J, et al: Immediate hemodynamic effects of pericardial closure after open-heart surgery. *Scand J Thorac Cardiovasc Surg* 1987; **21**:131-134.

60. Fanning J, Vasko JS, Kilman JW: Delayed sternal closure after cardiac surgery. *Ann Thorac Surg* 1987; **44**:169-172.

61. Little AG, Kresmer PC, Wade JL, et al: Operation for diagnosis and treatment of pericardial effusions. *Surgery* 1984; **96**:738-744.

62. Piehler JM, Pluth JR, Schaff HV, et al: Surgical management of effusive pericardial disease. *J Thorac Cardiovasc Surg* 1985; **90**:506-516.

63. Little A, Ferguson MK: Pericardioscopy as adjunct to pericardial window. *Chest* 1986; **89**:53-55.

64. Bahn CH, Annest LS, Miyamoto M: Pericardial closure. *Am J Surg* 1986; **151**:612-615.

65. Nandi P, Leung SM, Cheung KL: Closure of pericardium after open heart surgery: A way to prevent postoperative cardiac tamponade. *Br Heart J* 1976; **38**:1319-1323.

66. Stanley TH, Weidauer HE: Anesthesia for the patient with cardiac tamponade. *Anesth Analg* 1973; **52**:110-114.

67. Kaplan JA, Bland JW Jr, Dunbar RW: The perioperative management of pericardial tamponade. *South Med J* 1976; **69**:417-419.

68. Cameron J, Oesterle SN, Baldwin JC, et al: The etiologic spectrum of constrictive pericarditis. *Am Heart J* 1987; **113**:354-360.

69. Culliford AT, Lipton M, Spencer FC: Operation for chronic constrictive pericarditis: Do the surgical approach and degree of pericardial resection influence the outcome significantly? *Ann Thorac Surg* 1980; **29**:146-152.

70. Viola AR: The influence of pericardiectomy on the hemodynamics of chronic constrictive pericarditis. *Circulation* 1973; **48**:1038-1042.

Anesthesia for Surgery of the Thoracic Aorta

Brian J. Cammarata

■ INTRODUCTION

Thoracic aorta lesions are among the most clinically challenging and acutely life-threatening lesions encountered by the cardiac anesthesiologist. These lesions, which have a high incidence in patients older than 60 years of age, carry an intraoperative mortality of 9.4%[1] and an overall mortality rate of 10 to 35%.[2] Preoperative risk factors for death include preexisting lung and renal disease, type II repairs, and emergency procedures. Postoperative risk factors include reoperation, dialysis, and prolonged ventilation.[2] Approximately 30% of these patients have coexisting pulmonary, vascular, renal, and coronary artery disease, whereas up to 70% have coexisting hypertension.[3] Therefore, a significant percentage of this population is at high risk for intraoperative and postoperative complications. Although aortic lesions often affect older patients, younger patients sustaining blunt chest trauma also may present with lesions of the aorta.

Because these patients are critically ill, surgical urgency often affords the anesthesiologist little time for pertinent history and preoperative studies before the patient's arrival into the operating suite. Nevertheless, a brief review of all available laboratories, cardiac studies, and radiographic studies is crucial. Preparation should be made for massive blood transfusion, blood salvage techniques, and replacement of coagulation components, because more than one-third of intraoperative deaths may be attributed to coagulopathy and bleeding.[2] Appropriate hemodynamic and neurological monitoring for the operation is essential.

The anesthesiology team should have an established plan for induction and maintenance of anesthesia. Induction of general anesthesia should cause minimal hemodynamic perturbations. Airway management must balance concerns for airway protection and surgical exposure. Hemodynamic stability and adequate end-organ perfusion are optimal goals. Familiarity with the use of vasoactive agents is vital because a pharmacologic intervention that supports one organ system may be detrimental to another. The intraoperative care team also must consider the role of extracorporeal circulatory techniques during the procedure. The success of this operation depends on communication between the anesthetic and surgical teams. This chapter will focus on the pathophysiologic mechanisms and perioperative management of thoracic aortic lesions.

■ CLASSIFICATION OF AORTIC LESIONS

Aortic lesions may be classified into three pathophysiologic subtypes: aortic dissection, aortic aneurysm, and aortic rupture.[4] Aortic rupture and acute aortic dissections are surgical emergencies requiring immediate intervention. Aortic aneurysms and chronic aortic dissections often are repaired in a nonemergent fashion.

Aortic Dissection

Aortic dissection may occur by stressing or manipulating a vessel that is predisposed to injury.[5-7] Risk factors for aortic dissection include hypertension, aortic medial disease, Marfan syndrome, congenital bicusid aortic valve, aortic atherosclerosis, and blunt chest trauma.[8] Approximately 70% of patients with aortic dissections have a history of hypertension.[9] Frequently, the acute event precipitating the dissection is never determined. However, iatrogenic injuries resulting from surgical manipulation of the aorta[6] and placement of diagnostic or therapeutic devices into the aorta[9-11] have been documented. The ratio of males to females with aortic dissection is between 2 and 4 to 1; peak incidence is in the fifth to seventh decades of life.[1,12] A dissection less than 14 days old is defined as acute, and a dissection older than 2 weeks is defined as chronic.[13,14] Approximately 33% of all thoracic aneurysms will present as an acute dissection.[15] Anatomically, 60% of dissections involve the ascending aorta, 20% involve the transverse arch, and 20% involve the descending aorta.[16,17]

Although the pathophysiologic mechanism of aortic dissection remains uncertain, two major theories have been proposed.[8,18,19] The first theory involves an intimal tear with ensuing intramedial dissection.[7,18] This separation usually occurs between the middle and outer thirds of the media with subsequent progression throughout the aorta.[12] The second theory cites rupture of the vasa vasorum as the mechanism of injury with subsequent intramedial hemorrhage and dissection of the vessel.[15]

Aortic dissections are described according to either the De Bakey or Stanford classification. De Bakey organized these lesions based on the initial site of injury and the location of aortic extension (see Fig. 9–1).[20] In Type I

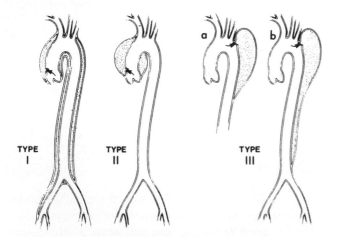

FIGURE 9–1. De Bakey classification for aortic dissections (Types I, II, and III and subtypes A and B). De Bakey Types I, II, and III A correspond to Stanford Type A while DeBakey Type III B corresponds to Stanford Type B. *(From: DeBakey ME. The development of vascular surgery. Am J Surg 1979; **137**:697–738.)*

and II dissections, the inciting lesion occurs in the ascending aorta. Type I lesions extend into the descending aorta with potential infradiaphragmatic aortic involvement, whereas Type II lesions are limited to the ascending aorta, stopping before the takeoff of the innominate artery. Both types of lesions may render the aortic valve incompetent due to retrograde dissection and mechanical deformation of the aortic valve annulus. Type III lesions commence with an intimal tear in the descending aorta, commonly in the distal aortic arch or proximal descending aorta distal to the takeoff of the left subclavian artery.[8] Type III lesions are further subdivided into subtype A, which has a retrograde extension into the proximal aortic arch, and subtype B, which has antegrade extension into the descending aorta. Another, perhaps simpler, classification is that described by the Stanford Group.[21] Type A dissections are those with any involvement of the ascending aorta, and Type B dissections involve only the descending aorta distal to the left subclavian artery. Younger patients with underlying connective tissue abnormalities are prone to Type A dissections, whereas older patients with muscular degeneration will commonly present with a Type B dissection.[14]

Management of these patients depends on the location of the lesion and extent of the dissection. Medical management involves controlling blood pressure and myocardial contractility, but this often is a temporizing measure until the patient can undergo surgical repair.[1] Patients with a Type I or II lesion who undergo surgical repair have a significantly lower hospital mortality rate than patients who are managed medically.[6] In comparison, patients with a Type III lesion do not have a significant difference in mortality with either medical or surgical management.[4-6] The hospital mortality rate remains a remarkable 23.5% for surgically managed Type I or II lesions and approximately 35% for medically or surgically managed Type III lesions.

Aortic Rupture

Rupture of the aorta often results from nonpenetrating chest injuries sustained in trauma.[22] Although prompt diagnosis and treatment are crucial for survival, this lesion may remain clinically silent and thus untreated.[23] Anatomically, the heart and distal aorta are mobile components, whereas the aortic arch is fixed by the great vessels.[24] During the deceleration phase of an acceleration–deceleration injury, the arch motion slows with the body while the remaining aortic components continue in motion. This energy creates a shearing force on the aorta, leading to injury. Up to 95% of aortic injuries will occur at the isthmus,[22] where the aorta is tethered by the ligamentum arteriosum.[9] Additional sites that commonly sustain injury include the aortic hiatus in the diaphragm, midthoracic descending aorta, and origin of the left subclavian artery. Multiple sites of aortic injury occur in up to 20% of patients.[25]

The mortality rate for repair of this lesion is approximately 20%.[24] As of the mid-1970s, an estimated 10 to 16% of fatal accident victims experienced aortic rupture. Eighty to 90% of these patients died instantaneously. Survivors often have acute self-containment of the rupture until repair is performed. Among the 10 to 20% who survive 1 hour after the injury, 30% die within 6 hours, 49% die within 24 hours, and 72% die within 8 days.

Aortic Aneurysm

Aneurysms are classified by their etiology, location, and shape.[5] The most common etiology for aortic aneurysms is dissection.[26] Aortic pathology predisposing aneurysm includes atherosclerosis, aortitis, cystic medial necrosis, syphilitic aortitis, trauma, postoperative false aneurysms, connective tissue disorders, and congenital aortic anomalies.[1,26] Dissecting aneurysms are more common to the ascending aorta, whereas atherosclerotic aneurysms are primarily localized to the descending aorta.[27] The De Bakey and Stanford classifications, which were discussed under aortic dissections, are commonly used to describe the location and extent of this lesion. Aneurysms are described morphologically as fusiform or saccular (*see* Fig. 9–2).[1] Fusiform aneurysms have a higher operative mortality than saccular aneurysms. The male:female ratio with this lesion is approximately 2:1, although women have a higher incidence of rupture.[27] This disorder tends to affect older patients; the mean age for diagnosis is in the sixth decade of life. Additionally, the incidence of aortic rupture is higher with dissecting aneurysms than with atherosclerotic aneurysms and with ascending aortic aneurysms than with descending aortic aneurysms.

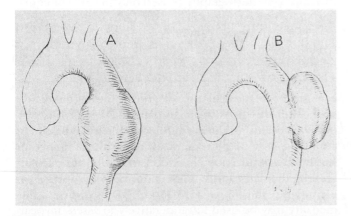

FIGURE 9–2. Types of thoracic aortic aneurysms. **A.** Fusiform. **B.** Saccular. *(Reprinted with permission from: Magilligan DJ Jr, Ullyot DJ: The heart. I. Acquired diseases, in Way LW (ed):* Current Surgical Diagnosis and Treatment. *Norwalk, CT: Appleton and Lange, 1991, p 359.)*

Aortic aneurysm is a disease necessitating surgical intervention.[2,21] Patients without surgical intervention have a 2-year survival rate of less than 25%.[2] The operative mortality for repair is 20 to 34% for acute dissections and 8 to 22% for chronic dissections.[21] These patients have a high incidence of coexisting pulmonary, cardiac, and vascular disease complicating their intraoperative and postoperative care.[28,29]

■ DIAGNOSIS OF AORTIC LESIONS

Aortic lesions often present with a constellation of symptoms suggesting the ongoing events. These symptoms are a result of expansion, dissection, or rupture of the aorta.[1] Table 9–1 provides a comprehensive list of symptoms in patients with aortic lesions. Severe anterior chest or back pain is the most common presenting symptom.[1,27] This symptom may occur directly from aortic expansion or from involvement of juxta-aortic structures and extend into the neck, shoulders, or abdomen. The intensity of pain may not correlate with the size of the lesion. Up to one-half of patients with aortic injury will be asymptomatic. Possible explanations for the lack of symptoms might include distracting injuries in the patient with trauma, chronic nature of the dissection, or acute coexisting cardiac ischemia with associated dysfunction. Therefore, suspected aortic lesions often will require further diagnostic evaluation for diagnosis.

Chest radiography is a rapid and easily accessible method for diagnosing aortic lesions. Table 9–2 lists eight classic radiographic signs consistent with aortic injury. Loss of the aortic knob contour is the most consistent finding on chest radiograph for patients with aortic injury.[30,31] However, radiograph underpenetration or venous mediastinal bleeding may cause false-positive studies. The next most common finding is superior mediastinal widening. Specifically, radiographs are assessed for the ratio of mediastinal to chest width (M/C). An M/C ratio of greater than 0.25 is consistent with an aortic injury. The remainder of the findings are considered nonspecific. While left hemothorax is described as a classic radiographic sign of aortic injury, isolated right hemothoraces secondary to posterior mediastinal erosion also have been described.[32,33] Figure 9–3 shows some of these classic radiographic findings in a patient with an aneurysm of the transverse aortic arch.

Using more sophisticated imaging techniques such as angiography, computerized tomography (CT), magnetic resonance imaging (MRI), aortography, transthoracic echocardiography (TTE), and transesophageal echocardiography (TEE) provides superior specificity and sensitivity of diagnosis over chest radiographs. Table 9–3 lists the sensitivity, specificity, and accuracy of each

TABLE 9–1. Presenting signs and potential etiologies for patients with thoracic aortic lesions. The frequency of these findings, as calculated from previous studies is indicated when obtainable)

Symptom/Clinical Finding	Possible Etiology	Frequency
Chest or back pain	active aortic dissection	>50%
No clinical findings	distracting injuries, chronic dissection	5–50%
Angina	aortic dissection into coronary arteries	5.8%
Acute myocardial infarction	aortic dissection into coronary arteries/thrombus	
Aortic regurgitation	aortic valve injury/ascending arch injury	10–50%
Assymetric upper extremity pulse amplitude	arch interruption	9–45%
Hypertension of the upper extremities	distal aortic occlusion/rupture	37%
Distant heart sounds	pericardial tamponade/pericardial effusion	
Hypotension	hypovolemia/aortic dissection	
Pulmonary edema	lung contusion/myocardial contusion/acute aortic insufficiency	
Hemothorax	traumatic injury/descending thoracic injury	3%
Respiratory difficulty	bronchial or tracheal compression/atelectasis/pneumonitis/acute aortic insufficiency with pulmonary edema rib fractures	8%
Pneumothorax		
Confusion	hypotension/acute head injury	
Horner's syndrome		
Paraplegia	spinal cord ischemia/trauma	2.3–2.6%
Hemoptysis	erosion of bronchus/pulmonary contusion trauma	
External chest wall abnormalities		35%
Jaw pain	referred secondary to dissection	8.8%
Hoarseness	stretching/compression of laryngeal nerve	8.6%
Dysphasia	esophageal compression or erosion	5%
Hematemasis	esophageal compression or erosion	5%
Melena	direct intestinal injury/intestinal infarction	
Anuria or hematuria	renal injury/renal infarction/hypovolemia	2–3%

(Compiled from references 1, 5, 15, 16, 18, 24, 27, and 41.

modality. Historically, aortography has been considered the "gold standard" in assessing lesions of the aorta.[34] However, this modality is costly, relatively invasive, and time consuming.[35,36] Additionally, aortography subjects patients to potentially nephrotoxic contrast agents. Although aortography remains the superior diagnostic modality for coronary artery anatomy evaluation and branch vessel involvement, numerous studies have evaluated diagnostic alternatives with promising results.[35,37-41] Several series have shown MRI to be 100% sensitive and specific in diagnosing aortic lesions.[42,43] Furthermore, MRI or CT in combination with TTE has equivalent sensi-

TABLE 9–2. Chest radiograph findings in thoracic aortic lesions

Loss of aortic contour
Mediastinal widening
Displacement of the right paraspinous interface
Deviation of the trachea to the right
Displacement of the nasogastric tube to the right
Left hemothorax
Depression of the left main-stem bronchus below 40° from horizontal
Left apical cap

Compiled from: Sefczek DM, Sefczek RJ, Deeb ZL: Radiographic signs of acute tranumatic rupture of the thoracic aorta. Am J Roentgenol 1983; 141:1259–1262.

tivity and specificity to aortography for evaluating such lesions.[35] The limited ability of CT and MRI to evaluate the aortic valve is well supplemented by adding echocardiography. Figure 9–4 represents a proposed algorithm for evaluating a suspected aortic injury. The suspected location of the lesion will determine whether echocardiography or MRI/CT are used for the initial evaluation. With this approach, aortography is used only in cases of equivocal findings from other diagnostic techniques.

TEE provides excellent resolution of intrathoracic structures in a rapid, relatively noninvasive fashion[41,42,44-49] and is discussed in detail in Chapter 3. For patients with a thoracic aortic injury, intraoperative TEE can make or confirm the diagnosis, locate dissection sites, evaluate the surgical repair, and assess the adequacy of perfusion during cardiopulmonary bypass.[50] In comparison with aortography, TEE provides a higher sensitivity, significantly shorter examination time for assessing thoracic aortic dissection and is superior in identifying thrombus formation.[51] Furthermore, this modality may be used intraoperatively to assess myocardial performance, signs of ischemia, heart valve status, and postrepair aortic integrity. For patients with trauma, TEE is highly sensitive and specific for evaluation of aortic injuries. Therefore, some authors believe that trans-

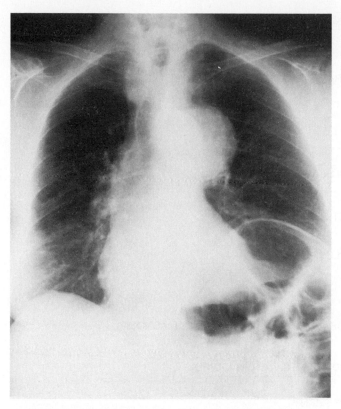

FIGURE 9–3. Posteroanterior roentgenogram of a patient presenting with a chronic transverse arch aortic aneurysm. The aneurysm itself, as well as the consequences of its presence, are illustrated. Note the deviation of the trachea, as well as the elevation of the left hemidiaphragm. At surgery, the left phrenic nerve was stretched and splayed by the aneurysm.

bronchus.[38,52] Furthermore, examination of the subdiaphragmatic descending aorta is limited. Ultrasonic artifacts sometimes are confused with sites of intimal tears and lead to an incorrect diagnosis[50] (*see* Chapter 3). Finally, examination of the thoracic aorta requires views from the upper esophagus. In awake, sedated patients, extensive examination at this level may not be well tolerated.[45] Chapter 3 provides a list of relative and absolute contraindications to placement of the TEE probe.[53] Despite these limitations, TEE is a widely used perioperative and intraoperative diagnostic modality for evaluating patients with aortic injuries.

■ TRACHEAL AND BRONCHIAL COMPRESSION FROM AORTIC LESIONS

As diagrammed in Figure 9–6, the aortic arch "saddles" the left main-stem bronchus as the vessel makes the transition from ascending to transverse to descending aorta.[54] Ultimately, the descending aorta assumes its location along the posterior wall of the bronchus. A thoracic aortic lesion can impinge upon and damage the trachea or main-stem bronchus, leading to tracheomalacia and respiratory distress.[55-59] Whereas thoracic aortic lesions usually cause compression or deviation of the left main-stem bronchus, the right main-stem bronchus and trachea also may be compromised.[55-62]

Symptoms of airway compression may be exacerbated by or induced by changes in body position. A recent case report describes a patient in whom a thoracic aneurysm compressed the left main-stem bronchus and right pulmonary artery.[60] This combination of lesions caused the patient to function well while in the supine position but to decompensate rapidly with ventilation-to-perfusion mismatch in the left lateral position.

A preoperative history and examination revealing stridor, wheezing, cough, or tracheal deviation should raise suspicion of aortic impingement and possible tracheomalacia.[61] Unilateral vocal cord paralysis, which results from compression of the recurrent laryngeal nerve between the aorta and trachea, may present clinically as

esophageal echocardiography should be a first-line modality for patients with suspected thoracic aortic injury.[37] Furthermore, a negative TEE study would exclude the diagnosis of aortic injury. Figure 9–5 shows the transesophageal echocardiography findings in a patient with an aortic aneurysm at the junction of the transverse and descending aorta.

TEE has several limitations. Lesions of the distal ascending aorta may be difficult to visualize with TEE secondary to interference of the trachea and left main stem

TABLE 9–3. Sensitivities, specificities, predictive values, and accuracies of imaging techniques for the diagnosis of thoracic aortic dissection

Technique	Sensitivity (%)	Specificity (%)	PPV (%)	NPV (%)	Accuracy (%)
Angiography	77–88	94–100	95–100	71–84	86
CT	80–83	88–100	83–100	71–88	86
MRI	100	100	100	100	100
TEE	97–99	98–100	98–100	96–99	—

CT = computed tomography; MRI = magnetic resonance imaging; NPV = negative predictive value; PPV = positive predictive value; TEE = transesophageal echocardiography.
*From: Barbant SD, Eisenberg MJ, Schiller NB: The diagnostic value of imaging techniques for aortic dissection. Am Heart J 1992; **124:**541–543.*

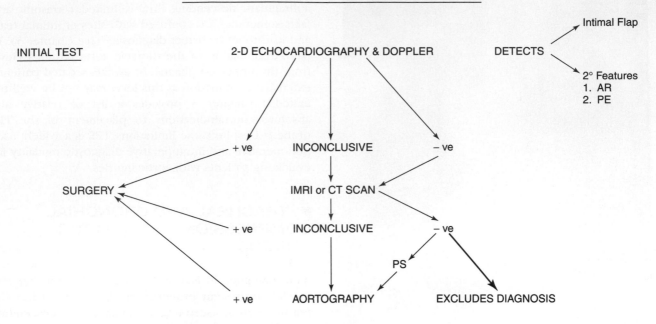

TYPE I OR II SUSPECTED (ASCENDING AORTA INVOLVED)

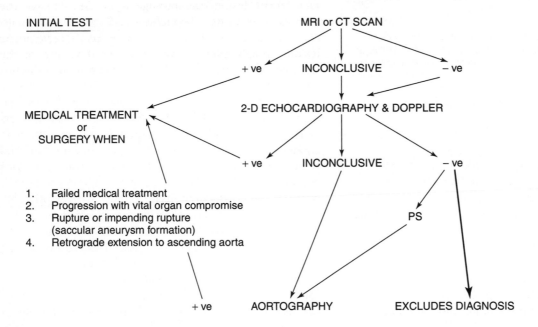

FIGURE 9–4. Diagnostic approach to suspected thoracic aortic lesions. *(Reprinted with permission from: Goldman AP, et al: The complementary role of magnetic resonance imaging, Doppler echocardiography, and computed tomography in the diagnosis of dissecting thoracic aneurysms. Am Heart J 1986; 111:970–981.)*

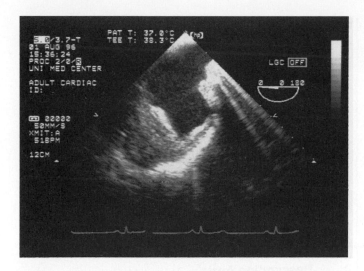

FIGURE 9–5. Transesophageal echocardiographic image of a large Type B aortic aneurysm. The lesion is located inferior to the junction of the transverse and descending aorta.

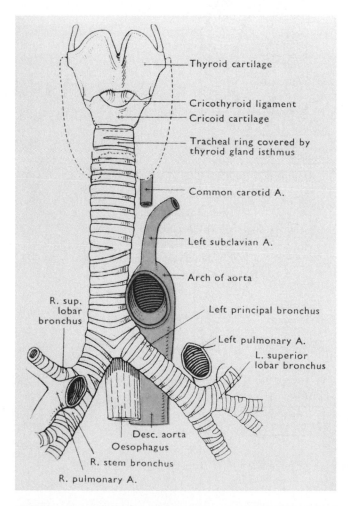

FIGURE 9–6. Schematic diagram representing anatomical relationship of great vessels to the tracheobronchial tree. *(Reprinted with permission from: Cunningham DJ: Manual of Practical Anatomy. 13th ed. London, Oxford, 1966.)*

voice hoarseness.[58] Preoperative pulmonary function testing with flow–volume loop analysis will reveal an intrathoracic obstructive process in severe cases. Finally, radiographic studies may be useful in delineating the extent of airway compromise caused by aortic lesions.

■ SURGICAL APPROACH AND MANAGEMENT

Management of Ventilation

The location of the aortic lesion will dictate the surgical approach necessary for repair. Ascending and transverse aortic arch lesions are repaired through a median sternotomy without the requirement for one-lung ventilation (OLV). These patients can be managed with a single-lumen endotracheal tube. Lesions of the distal transverse arch and descending aorta are repaired through a left thoracotomy. Surgical exposure is enhanced and trauma to the left lung is minimized by providing OLV with the left lung collapsed. However, caution is indicated as endotracheal intubation in patients with tracheal or bronchial obstruction from an aortic lesion can result in trachea/bronchial damage or frank aortic rupture.[55,56,63,64]

Consequences of Aortic Cross-Clamping

Aortic cross-clamping at some level is required for repair of all thoracic aortic lesions. The placement of the aortic cross-clamps for repair of various aortic lesions is summarized in Figure 9–7. Aortic cross-clamping creates potential for end-organ ischemia. The organs at risk vary with the position of the cross-clamps. The consequences of ischemia to the heart and brain and management of this ischemia are covered in detail elsewhere (*see* Chapters 12 and 13).

Spinal Cord Ischemia. Spinal cord ischemia is a potential consequence of aortic cross-clamping.

VASCULAR ANATOMY OF THE SPINAL CORD. Anatomically, the blood supply to the spinal cord is derived from several sources. A single anterior spinal artery arises from the vertebral arteries at the level of the foramen magnum and supplies the anterior two-thirds of the spinal cord.[65] A pair of posterior spinal arteries arise from the posterior inferior cerebellar arteries and supply the remainder of the cord. The vertebral, deep cervical, intercostal, and lumbar arteries also contribute to spinal cord perfusion as the anterior and posterior radicular arteries (*see* Fig. 9–8).[66] The largest radicular artery is the *arteria radicularis magna* or artery of Adamkiewicz, which supplies the majority of blood to the lower two-thirds of the spinal cord. The origin of

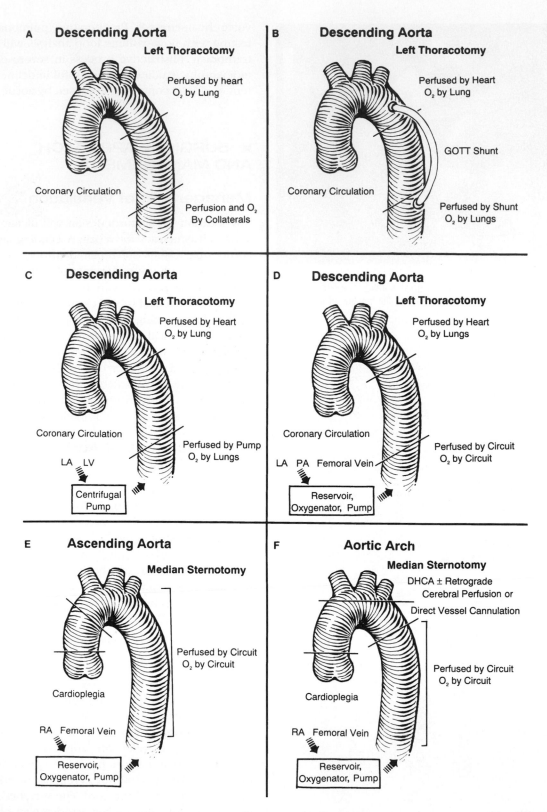

FIGURE 9–7. Circulatory adjuvants for the repair of thoracic aortic lesions. See text for relative merits and disadvantages of each technique.

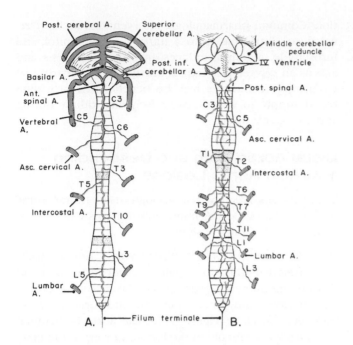

FIGURE 9–8. Schematic diagram representing arterial blood supply to the spinal cord. **A.** Anterior surface and arteries. **B.** Posterior surface and arteries. Shaded areas represent common areas of ischemia. *(Reprinted with permission from: Carpenter MB: Human Neuroanatomy. 7th ed. Baltimore, Williams & Wilkins, 1976, p 602.)*

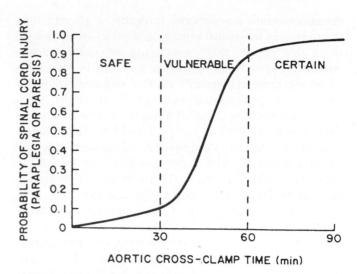

FIGURE 9–9. Relative risk of ischemic spinal cord injury as correlated with aortic cross-clamp duration. *(Reprinted with permission from: Svensson LG, Loop FD: Prevention of spinal cord ischemia in aortic surgery, in Bergan JJ, Yao JST (eds): Arterial Surgery: New Diagnostic and Operative Techniques. New York, Grune and Stratton, 1988, pp 273–285)*

this vessel is localized to T-9 to T-12 in over 60% of patients.[67,68] Therefore, in contrast to the upper spinal cord, the lower cord has a relatively limited blood supply with few collaterals and is at risk for ischemia during aortic cross-clamping or hypotensive periods.[69,70]

DETERMINANTS OF SPINAL CORD PERFUSION. Spinal cord perfusion pressure (SCPP) is the difference between mean arterial pressure, at any segment of the spinal cord, and cerebrospinal fluid (CSF) pressure. Efforts to improve perfusion necessitate either an increase in mean arterial pressure or a reduction in CSF pressure. Lumbar drains have been advocated to reduce CSF volume and thus pressure in an effort to augment SCPP. However, studies of this therapeutic intervention suggest no significant reduction in the incidence of postoperative neurological deficits.[68,71,72] More recent work has focused on selective cooling of the spinal cord via lavage of the subarachnoid space.[73] Corticosteroids, thiopental, N-methyl-D-aspartate receptor antagonists, papaverine, and magnesium also have undergone limited studies regarding their protective effects on the spinal cord.[74]

CONSEQUENCES OF SPINAL CORD ISCHEMIA. Among the most common perioperative injuries associated with repair of thoracic aorta lesions is postoperative paraplegia. The incidence of paraplegia after thoracic aortic repair ranges from 2 to 40%, depending on the site of the lesion and the degree of aortic involvement and aortic dissec-

tion.[74] Patients with dissection have at least a 2-fold greater incidence of postoperative paraplegia when compared with those without dissection. Despite numerous animal and human studies, the precise mechanism of spinal cord injury during aortic cross-clamping remains uncertain. Contributing factors include duration of spinal ischemia, inadvertent ligation of the artery of Adamkiewicz, elevations in CSF pressure, preexisting collateral blood vessels, and perioperative hyperglycemia.[67,69,74,75] The spinal cord will tolerate a limited period of ischemia before irreversible cellular injury occurs. Figure 9–9 depicts the relative risk of aortic cross-clamp periods.[76] A cross-clamp time of less than 30 minutes is considered safe and carries a minimal risk for postoperative paraplegia. Thirty to 60 minutes of cross-clamp time leaves patients more vulnerable to injury, whereas times greater than 60 minutes approach a 90% incidence of paraplegia.[69] Therefore, for repairs exceeding 30 minutes, patients may benefit from extracorporeal circulatory techniques to augment end-organ perfusion.

MONITORING FOR SPINAL CORD ISCHEMIA. Somatosensory-evoked potentials (SSEPs) and motor-evoked potentials (MEPs) are used to detect intraoperative spinal cord ischemia.[77,78] SSEP monitoring involves stimulation of upper or lower extremity peripheral nerves with signal observation at the cervical spine and scalp.[79] The electrical signal, which is carried by the dorsal columns, assesses the integrity of afferent long tracts within the spinal cord.[80] In a series of studies using a dog model, SSEP monitoring detected clinically significant spinal cord ischemia within 3 to 5 minutes of aortic cross-clamping.[81] At 8.5 minutes, complete loss of the SSEP signal occurred. Furthermore, limiting the cross-clamp time to 5 minutes after the loss of SSEP signal resulted in no postoperative neurological deficits. In contrast, noncollateralized canines subjected to 10 minutes of cross-clamp time after the loss of the SSEP signal experienced a 67% incidence of neurological complications. SSEP monitoring also may be helpful in assessing the adequacy of distal perfusion via extracorporeal circula-tion.[82] In a series of 33 human subjects, the benefit of SSEP monitoring was evaluated.[83] SSEP monitoring was beneficial for assessing the adequacy of spinal cord perfusion and alerting the intraoperative team of impending neurological injury. SSEP was also useful in evaluating the effectiveness of distal perfusion via shunts or bypass during the procedure.[77] Furthermore, cellular death occurs 15 to 45 minutes after sustained hypotension and disappearance of the SSEP signal.

Some investigators have questioned the efficacy of SSEP as a monitoring device. Some have found no reduction in postoperative neurological deficits associated with the use of SSEP monitoring.[84] Also, the predominantly efferent anterior horn area seems to be most sensitive to ischemia.[85] SSEP directly assesses the dorsal column but can only indirectly monitor these motor areas within the cord.[86] Additionally, SSEP monitoring cannot differentiate between peripheral and central ischemia causing observed changes.[78] Investigators have advocated epidurally placed stimulating electrodes to avoid false results from peripheral nerves.[87]

Renal Ischemia.   The most dreaded consequence of renal ischemia is acute renal failure. Acute renal failure after thoracic aneurysm surgery occurs in 3.6 to 27% of cases.[88] Up to 33% of survivors become dialysis-dependent.[2] Reported risk factors for postoperative renal failure include heart disease, need for reoperation, renal ischemic time exceeding 30 minutes, postoperative respiratory insufficiency, preexisting renal dysfunction, urgent or emergency procedures, and large volumes of blood loss during the procedure.[2,28] A recent series using a statistical model to evaluate a patient's risk revealed advanced patient age and preoperative serum creatinine level as key predictors of postoperative renal failure.[88]

Several therapeutic interventions to avoid this complication have been used. Although intraoperative urine output of 0.5 to 1 mL/kg/hr has been considered a measure of adequate renal perfusion and function, this assumption may be invalid.[89] Adequate hydration and renal perfusion pressure are important for renal protec-tion. Common pharmacologic interventions include "renal dose" dopamine (2 to 4 μg/kg/min), mannitol, and furosemide. Mannitol induces an osmotic diuresis and acts as an oxygen-free radical scavenger. Extracorporeal circulatory techniques may be beneficial in providing blood supply to an otherwise ischemic kidney during aortic cross-clamping.

Distal Aortic Arch and Descending Thoracic Aortic Lesions

These lesions are repaired through a left thoracotomy with the aid of OLV. A number of options exist in the management of these lesions.

Simple Aortic Cross-clamping.   Conceptually, the simplest method for repairing distal aortic arch and descending thoracic aortic lesions involves cross-clamping the aorta and proceeding with the surgical procedure. As shown in Figure 9–7A, the aorta is clamped proximally and distally to the lesion. Coronary and cerebral perfusion are uninterrupted by this arrangement, whereas distal aortic perfusion is either temporarily interrupted or occurs via collateral vessels. Pulmonary blood flow continues normally. This method produces proximal aortic hypertension, which may produce left ventricular (LV) afterload mismatch, LV distension and mitral regurgitation (MR), and myocardial ischemia. Pharmacologic management of LV function during this period is challenging and will be discussed in detail later. Aortic cross-clamp time ideally is limited to less than 30 minutes.[69,90] As shown in Figure 9–9, this minimizes the risks of spinal cord injury.

To provide flow to the areas distal to the distal clamp, several techniques have been developed. The concept behind all of them is diversion of blood from the heart for distribution to the distal aorta. This serves two purposes: it provides blood flow to the areas distal to the aortic cross-clamp and it offers a nonpharmacologic method to control proximal aortic hypertension and LV distension during the cross-clamp period. The available methods are described below.

Gott Shunt.   The work of Gott and colleagues developed the tridodecymethyl ammonium chloride–heparin shunt consisting of sized, non-thrombogenic plastic tubing.[91] The segment of tubing is placed into the aorta between the proximal clamp and the aortic valve, and the other end of the tubing is placed into the aorta beyond the distal clamp (*see* Fig. 9–7B). This method has several advantages and disadvantages:

ADVANTAGES

- The shunt provides a method for distal perfusion without the need for systemic heparinization.[92]
- The shunt is easily placed.

DISADVANTAGES

- Precise control of the amount of blood that is shunted is impossible because proximal decompression and distal perfusion are shunt-diameter-dependent.[69] The 7- and 9-mm shunts that are available commercially may not provide adequate distal aortic flow.[93,94]
- Other problems include bleeding from the insertion sites, accidental dislodgement during the procedure, migration of the proximal end of the shunt across the innominate or left carotid artery, blockage of the surgeon's field of view, kinking of the shunt, embolic stroke, and death.[15,69,70,95]

Several series have demonstrated postoperative neurological injuries despite the use of a shunt.[93,94,96,97] Advocates of the Gott shunt report low morbidity and mortality with this technique.[98,99]

Left Heart Bypass. Left heart bypass removes a fraction of oxygenated blood from either the left atrium or, occasionally, the left ventricle, for delivery to a distal aortic site or to the femoral artery (*see* Fig. 9-7C). A centrifugal pump (*see* Chapters 3 and 11) is used in this arrangement. No oxygenator is needed because oxygenated blood from the left heart is used. A perfusionist must be present to run the system. This technique offers several advantages and disadvantages:

ADVANTAGES

- The amount of blood diverted form the LA to distal aorta can be precisely controlled. Communication with the perfusionist is essential.
- The system is relatively easy to insert.
- Minimal heparization is needed (ACT = 150 sec)
- Patients undergoing left heart bypass have smaller differences between the upper and lower extremity mean arterial pressure, higher intraoperative urine output, lower incidence of postoperative azotemia, and less blood loss in comparison with patients undergoing Gott shunt bypass.[100]

DISADVANTAGES

- No blood or fluid can be added to the bypass system because there is no reservoir. Large-bore peripheral or central venous access is a necessity.
- The absence of a heat exchanger does not allow the patient to be actively warmed or cooled.

A 4% incidence of postoperative renal failure is associated with left heart bypass, as compared with 9% and 11% for simple cross-clamping and CPB, respectively.[29] However, left heart bypass has not eliminated complications from aortic surgery. A 3% early mortality

rate, 1.5% reversible renal failure rate, and 2.3% incidence of permanent spinal cord injury have been reported despite using left heart bypass for patients undergoing repair of descending thoracic aortic lesions.[101]

Partial CPB. Partial CPB (*see* Chapter 10) can be used in the repair of distal arch or descending aortic lesions (*see* Fig. 9-7D). Partial CPB exists when only a portion of the systemic venous drainage to the heart is captured and returned to the CPB circuit. During partial CPB, the remaining portion of systemic venous return is to the RA. This blood makes its way to the pulmonary bed, where gas exchange occurs. The blood then returns to the left atrium (LA) and LV, where it is ejected into the systemic circulation. For partial CPB to be effective, two things must be true:

1. The heart must be beating and ejecting — if ejection is ineffective or nonexistent, distention of the heart will occur and systemic blood flow will be inadequate.
2. The lungs must be ventilated — in the absence of ventilation, systemic venous blood that enters the RA ultimately will reach the systemic circulation without gas exchange having occurred. This will result in hypercarbia and hypoxemia.

The source of venous blood for this technique can be the femoral vein, LA, or pulmonary artery. The RA is poorly accessible from a left thoracotomy. Arterial outflow from the CPB circuit is delivered to a distal aortic site or to the femoral artery. The CPB circuit contains a venous reservoir, a heat exchanger, and an oxygenator. The oxygenator portion of the circuit is redundant when the LA is used as the source of venous blood. This approach has several advantages and disadvantages.

ADVANTAGES

- The patient can be actively warmed. This is a major advantage if hypothermia becomes a problem.
- Blood and fluid can be added easily to the system via the venous reservoir. In addition, the patient can be transfused with warm fluid from the venous reservoir very quickly by having the perfusionist make CPB arterial outflow exceed venous inflow.
- All shed blood can be scavenged by the cardiotomy suction and returned to the venous reservoir without the need for a cell-saver system.
- Precise control of the amount of blood diverted from the heart to the distal aorta is possible. The perfusionist partially occludes the venous drainage line with a clamp that controls arterial outflow with the pump head to determine the

balance between proximal and distal blood flow. Close communication is essential.

DISADVANTAGES

• Full systemic anticoagulation with heparin is necessary.

Although hypoperfusion may be the primary mechanism of end-organ injury during aortic cross-clamping,[102] providing distal circulatory support has not reduced the incidence of paraplegia in all series.[96] Therefore, the etiology of spinal cord injuries in these patients probably is multifactorial.

Ascending Aorta and Aortic Arch Lesions

To be repaired these lesions require initiation of full cardiopulmonary bypass (CPB) (see Chapter 10). They are repaired through a median sternotomy. The clamps are placed such that coronary circulation is terminated and the heart must be arrested and protected with cardioplegia (see Chapter 12). As a result, systemic circulation must be provided by full CPB. All of the systemic venous drainage to the heart is captured and returned to the CPB circuit and subsequently to the patient. In lesions of the ascending aorta (see Fig. 9–7E), arterial cannulation for return of oxygenated blood to the patient can be obtained in the distal ascending aorta, aortic arch, or femoral artery. This arrangement allows cerebral perfusion to be maintained. Venous cannulation usually is obtained via the right atrium (RA).

Lesions of the ascending aorta and aortic arch (see Fig. 9–7F) or of just the aortic arch require full CPB as well. The site of arterial cannulation is the femoral artery as the ascending aorta and arch are involved in the repair. Venous cannulation usually is obtained via the RA. In this arrangement, there is no source of cerebral blood flow. As a result, some modifications must exist to provide either cerebral blood flow or to minimize the effects of cerebral ischemia during the cross-clamp period.

Cerebral blood flow can be provided antegrade by cannulation of one or more of the arch vessels and diversion of a portion of the arterial output from the CPB circuit to these cannulation sites. Sites for selective cannulation with anterograde perfusion have included the carotid, innominate, and subclavian arteries.[103] However, experts continue to disagree regarding the optimal site of cannulation, perfusion rate, perfusion temperature, and perfusion pressure and methods to evaluate adequacy of perfusion.[104] Furthermore, selective cannulation carries the risk of embolic event or arterial damage at the site of cannulation. Nevertheless, selective cerebral perfusion may prevent cerebral ischemia in patients undergoing long surgical repairs.[103]

In the absence of cerebral perfusion, mitigation of the effects of cerebral ischemia can be accomplished through the use of deep hypothermia circulatory arrest (DHCA).[105] This modality and it practical application are discussed in detail in Chapters 10 and 13. Combining DHCA with continuous retrograde cerebral perfusion (CRCP) may extend the safe arrest limit to between 65 and 90 minutes[106,107] and reduce the risk of neurologic injury during the surgical procedure. CRCP is accomplished by low pressure delivery (<20 to 30 mm Hg) of hypothermic (<20°C), oxygenated blood from the CPB circuit to the superior vena cava with venting of the effluent via the aortic arch.[106,108] This approach has many advantages, including its technical ease, ability to easily visualize blood returning from the great vessels, and removal of particulate material from arterial sites.[109]

■ ANESTHETIC TECHNIQUE

Goals

1. Obtain a thorough understanding of the type and location of the lesion. Review the operative plan and prepare for use of OLV and adjuvant methods to provide distal perfusion where indicated.
2. Prepare for potential blood loss, including pharmacologic measures to reduce bleeding.
3. Determine necessary invasive and noninvasive monitoring.
4. Minimize hemodynamic perturbations during induction and maintenance of general anesthesia.

Evaluation

As discussed previously, review of the patient's medical history and prior radiographic, echocardiographic, and angiographic studies is critical for the anesthesiologist's understanding of preexisting conditions and current injuries. Information regarding the patient's prior lung status may provide insight into his ability to tolerate OLV for long periods. Evaluation of existing radiological studies will help determine the surgical approach, which, in turn, dictates monitoring and the need for OLV.

Control of both blood pressure and ejection velocity are the mainstays of hemodynamic optimization of the patient with an aortic lesion. Increased blood pressure and ejection velocity are capable of extending an existing dissection or causing a contained aortic rupture to progress to frank rupture. It should be kept in mind that aggressive control of blood pressure with vasodilators is likely to cause a reflex tachycardia and an increase in LV dp/dt, thereby increasing ejection velocity and the sheer forces on the aortic lesion. This scenario is particularly likely in otherwise healthy patients with trauma who may already have a hyperdynamic LV secondary to blood loss and high catecholamine levels. Simultaneous control of both blood pressure and ejection velocity is best obtained with a combination of beta blockers and vasodilators.

Premedication

Patients who present for elective repair of lesions often are hemodynamically optimized before surgery. Oral antihypertensive agents may include beta blockers, calcium channel blockers, diuretics, and angiotensin-converting enzyme (ACE) inhibitors. Calcium channel- and beta-blocking agents may be advantageous in providing simultaneous blood pressure and heart rate control. Treatment with anxiolytic agents will further assist in controlling hypertension and tachycardia and, therefore, will minimize aortic wall tension. Commonly used sedatives include lorazepam 1 to 2 mg PO, midazolam 1 to 4 mg IV, and morphine 0.05 to 0.1 mg/kg IM.

Patients who present emergently for repair of an aortic lesion may be somewhat more difficult to manage. Beta-blocking agents along with vasodilators are the mainstay of therapy.[14] Esmolol, metoprolol, or propranolol commonly are used intravenous beta-receptor-blocking agents in this setting. The advantages of esmolol include its high specificity for the $beta_1$ receptor and its short duration of action. Options for vasodilator therapy include nitroprusside, nitroglycerin, trimethaphan, and halogenated inhalational anesthetic agents. Nitroprusside causes relaxation of resistance vessel vascular smooth muscle and, as such, is a potent vasodilator.[110,111] Nitroprusside may induce coronary steal and subsequent myocardial ischemia. Additionally, distal organ and spinal cord perfusion may be further compromised in patients receiving nitroprusside during aortic cross-clamping.[83,112] Nitroglycerin is primarily a venodilator.[111] This medication generally is easier to titrate and provides dilation of the large coronary arteries. However, nitroglycerin may not provide adequate arterial relaxation and blood pressure reduction. Both drugs may compromise oxygenation during OLV by blunting hypoxic pulmonary vasoconstriction.[113] The clinical use of trimethaphan is limited by its side effect profile[114] and tachyphylaxis.

Preinduction

Preparation for massive blood loss is crucial. Bilateral upper-extremity 14- or 16-gauge intravenous catheters should be placed. If the patient has poor peripheral venous access, large-bore central venous access is an alternative approach. The location for arterial line placement will depend on the location of the lesion. Distal aortic lesions (Stanford Type B) will necessitate placement of a right upper extremity (radial) arterial line. In repairing this lesion, the proximal aortic cross-clamp will probably be placed distal to the innominate artery. Therefore, the patency of the right subclavian artery will be preserved throughout the procedure. Proximal aortic lesions (Stanford Type A) will necessitate placement of a left upper extremity arterial line. The left subclavian artery probably will be distal to the distal aortic clamp site. If all of the arch vessels are excluded from circulation by placement of the clamps, femoral artery cannulation should be used. Femoral artery cannulation is used in conjunction with right radial artery cannulation in patients undergoing repair of distal arch or descending thoracic aortic lesions with distal perfusion. The femoral artery cannula is necessary to monitor the adequacy of distal perfusion. Communication with the surgeon is necessary to determine which femoral artery can be used for monitoring pressure when a femoral artery also is going to be used for perfusion.

All necessary pressor and vasodilatory agents and six units of typed and cross-matched blood should be available in the operating room before induction. Additionally, an antithrombolytic agent, such as aminocaproic acid or aprotinin is often used prophylactically to reduce bleeding. There is question regarding whether use of aprotinin is safe in the setting of DHCA (*see* Chapter 10).

Epidural catheters often are used in nonanticoagulated patients undergoing nonemergent procedures. Caution must be exercised as inadvertent vascular placement of the catheter is consideration for delaying the procedure. A test dose with 3 to 5 mL of 1.5% lidocaine with 1:200,000 epinephrine is prudent to confirm correct placement of the catheter. Additionally, confirming normal coagulation status before epidural catheter removal is recommended.

Induction

For nonemergent procedures, a high-dose narcotic induction with fentanyl (50 to 100 µg/kg) or sufentanyl (10 to 12 µg/kg) will minimize hemodynamic disturbances. An intermediate-acting, nondepolarizing neuromuscular blocker such as vecuronium (0.1 mg/kg), rocuronium (0.6 mg/kg), or cis-atracurium (0.2 mg/kg) will provide adequate muscle relaxation. Providing small doses of muscle relaxant during the narcotic infusion will minimize opioid-induced chest wall rigidity. Pancuronium generally is avoided during induction secondary to its vagolytic and norepinephrine-releasing effects, which can produce hypertension and tachycardia. However, smaller (1 to 2 mg) doses of pancuronium for maintenance relaxation usually is well tolerated.

Patients undergoing emergent procedures may be considered to have "full stomachs" and require a rapid sequence induction. A sedative hypnotic such as sodium thiopental (3 to 5 mg/kg), propofol (2 to 2.5 mg/kg), or etomidate (0.2 to 0.3 mg/kg) in combination with a smaller narcotic dose (fentanyl 10 μg/kg or sufentanyl 1.0 μg/kg) will blunt the hemodynamic effects of laryngoscopy and will provide rapid induction of general anesthesia. Succinylcholine 1 to 2 mg/kg is used for rapid muscle relaxation, although large doses of nondepolarizing agents are an alternative. Protection of the airway and the potential for aspiration must be weighed against the undesirable hemodynamic response to direct laryngoscopy. The addition of beta blockade and vasodilator therapy before laryngoscopy will help attenuate this undesirable response. After the airway is secured, deepening the anesthetic with a supplemental narcotic dose will improve hemodynamic stability.

Lesions of the ascending and transverse aortic arch are managed with a single-lumen endotracheal tube of appropriate size. As discussed previously, aortic lesions may cause both tracheal and bronchial compression and caution should be exercised in tube placement.

Repair of lesions of the distal aortic arch and descending thoracic aorta are facilitated by provision of OLV. The options available for providing OLV are discussed in detail in Chapter 7. The preferred technique uses a left-sided double-lumen endotracheal tube (DLT) unless collapse of the left main-stem bronchus has occurred. In these instances, a right-sided DLT is used. Achieving and maintaining proper positioning of the right upper lobe bronchus lumen can be problematic.[58] This is particularly true when surgical manipulation of the tracheal bronchial tree is necessary to mobilize the aorta. As discussed in detail in Chapter 7, the left-sided DLT is placed using fiberoptic bronchoscopy. This approach virtually guarantees proper tube position.[58,63] This approach, although very useful for all patients requiring DLT placement, is particularly important for patients with thoracic aortic lesions in whom unsuspected compression of the left main stem bronchus may exist. Blind advancement of the left-sided DLT under these circumstances may result in bronchial or aortic disruption. In addition, if unsuspected left main-stem bronchus compression is diagnosed fiberoptically, a right-sided DLT may be chosen.

A rapid-sequence induction with cricoid pressure may be necessary for some patients presenting with aortic lesions. Placement of a DLT under these circumstances may be difficult because of their large size and the propensity of the tracheal cuff to catch and tear on the patient's teeth as the tip of the tube is manuevered to align with the larynx. Under these circumstances, placement of a Univent tube may be easier (*see* Chapter 7). This system consists of a single-lumen tube with a built-in bronchial blocker. The bronchial blocker can be directed into either main-stem bronchus. In addition to being easier to place in the trachea than a DLT, this tube eliminates the need for exchanging a DLT to a single-lumen endotracheal tube at the end of the surgical procedure for patients who require postoperative ventilation. As discussed in Chapter 7, disadvantages of this device include high bronchial cuff occlusion pressures[64] and compromised ability to actively deflate, apply continuous positive airway pressure (CPAP) to, or suction the nondependent lung.

Intraoperative Management

After induction of general anesthesia, additional venous access or monitoring lines are placed. Monitoring includes a 5-lead electrocardiogram (a V_5 lead is not possible in left thoracotomy patients), as well as arterial and pulmonary artery catheters. Additionally, many centers use intraoperative TEE to monitor for myocardial ischemia and to provide on-line assessment of ventricular and valvular function. The patient is then positioned. If a DLT is used, the tube position should be checked with the fiberoptic bronchoscope after the patient has been positioned laterally to ensure that the tube remains optimally positioned.

As coagulopathy and bleeding are a common cause of death,[2] preparation for massive transfusion and red cell salvage before incision is recommended. Six units of compatible blood should be present throughout the procedure. Immediate availability of platelets and fresh frozen plasma also is crucial. A rapid transfusion device, although often unnecessary, can be indispensable, particularly when full or partial CPB is not used.

Ascending Aortic and Aortic Arch Repairs. These lesions require full CPB and may require DHCA. Management of those entities is discussed in detail in Chapters 10 and 13. Management of patients with acute aortic insufficiency in association with aortic dissection and a dilated aortic root is discussed in Chapter 5. These patients also may have myocardial ischemia if the dissection involves the coronary ostia.

Distal Aortic Arch and Descending Thoracic Aortic Lesions. If the approach is cross-clamp without distal circulatory support, vigorous afterload control with an intravenous or inhalational agent will be necessary. Reduction of mean arterial blood pressure to approximately 20% below baseline with nitroglycerin or nitroprusside before aortic cross-clamping will minimize wall tension in the proximal aortic segment after the clamp is placed. Isoflurane also has been advocated as a vasodilatory agent in this setting. Patients have received up to 2.5 +/- 0.3% isoflurane for hemodynamic control during aortic cross-clamping without negative consequence.[115] Blood pressure manipulation must always consider the potential detrimental effects on end-organ perfusion.

After cross-clamp application, blood pressure is maintained at the individual's normotensive state. Placement of the cross-clamp causes an acute increase in LV afterload and reduction in cardiac output.[116] However, the pulmonary artery occlusion pressure and central venous pressure usually will remain unchanged. Although LV afterload mismatch should be anticipated, several series have shown that diastolic dysfunction is a more common sequela to cross-clamp placement.[117,118] If pulmonary capillary wedge pressure (PCWP) increases with cross-clamp application, three etiologies must be entertained:

1. LV afterload mismatch with LV dilation — LV dilation may be accompanied by development of a new V wave on the PCWP trace, suggesting functional MR. TEE is valuable in assessing LV size and function during this period. LV dilatation with or without functional MR is an indication for immediate intervention with vasodilators. If LV dilation persists despite afterload reduction, initiation of inotropic support is warranted. A dobutamine infusion (5 to 10 μg/kg/min) will reduce LV size with no increase in myocardial oxygen consumption.

2. Myocardial ischemia — myocardial ischemia may be accompanied by ST segment changes, but monitoring of ischemia is hampered by the lack of a V_5 lead. TEE will likely reveal new regional wall motion abnormalities at this point (*see* Chapters 3 and 4). Treatment of myocardial ischemia is outlined in detail in Chapter 4.

3. Impaired LV diastolic function due to impaired relaxation — determination of impaired relaxation requires TEE to obtain Doppler spectra of the mitral valve inflow (*see* Chapter 3). This should resolve with afterload reduction and is the diagnosis of exclusion after LV dilatation and ischemia.

Acidosis may be treated with bolus administration of sodium bicarbonate, although a continuous infusion (0.05 mEq/kg/min) during cross-clamping may be more efficacious.[119] Large doses of sodium bicarbonate administered immediately before cross-clamp release will cause a transient iatrogenic hypercarbia, which when combined with a metabolic acidosis, can result in profound acidemia.[120]

The physiologic changes associated with cross-clamp removal include hypotension, pulmonary hypertension, and metabolic acidosis.[74] Preparation for cross-clamp removal will help minimize or attenuate these undesirable consequences. Several minutes before cross-clamp removal, the patient should be volume loaded to a PCWP of 10 to 20 torr.[121] With TEE, adequate LV volume can be assessed visually. Additionally, all vasodilating agents are discontinued and the cross-clamp is removed over a several-minute period. Hyperventilation before cross-clamp removal will help minimize the acidosis and, therefore, pulmonary hypertension, associated with clamp removal. Despite these measures, patients may require variable periods of vasopressor support after removal of the aortic cross-clamp. Intractable hypotension after cross-clamp removal is an indication for reapplication of the cross-clamp.

If a shunt or assisted circulatory method is used, attention to the proximal and distal perfusion pressures is critical. In the case of Gott shunts, attention is focused on adequacy of flow and patency of the shunt. Little titratable control of proximal and distal pressure is possible. Proximal hypertension with the shunt patent requires pharmacologic interventions as described for simple cross-clamping. Distal hypotension with a patent shunt is problematic. Interventions to elevate proximal blood pressure, such as vasopressors and volume infusion, may work, but they also may produce unacceptably high proximal pressures.

Left heart bypass and partial CPB provide more proximal hemodynamic control and predictable distal perfusion than a Gott shunt. With left heart bypass and partial CPB, the easiest initial approach is to decide, in conjunction with the perfusionist, the amount of flow that will be diverted to the distal aorta after cross-clamp

TABLE 9–4 Clinical scenarios and therapeutic interventions during left heart bypass

PP	DP	PCWP	TEE	INTERVENTION
↑	↓	↑	↑ LVEDA	increase pump flow
↑	↓	↓	↓ LVEDA	increase pump flow, volume infusion
↑	↑	⇄	⇄ LVEDA	vasodilation in conjunction with volume infusion
↑	↑	↑	↑ LVEDA	vasodilator, maintain pump flow, allow venous drainage to temporarily exceed arterial outflow when using partial CPB circuit
↓	↓	↓	↓ LVEDA	volume infusion, temporary vasopressor support
↓	↓	↑	↑ LVEDA	increase pump flow, inotropic support if resolution of LV distention does not improve LV performance and proximal pressure
↓	↑	↑	↑ LVEDA	institution of inotropic support followed by incremental decrease of pump flow to avoid further LV distention
↓	↑	↓	↓ LVEDA	decrease pump flow, if proximal pressure is low after desired distal pressure is reached then volume infusion

PP = proximal pressure; CPB = cardiopulmonary bypass; DP = distal pressure; LVEDA = left ventricular end-diastolic area; PCWP = pulmonary capillary wedge pressure; TEE = transesophageal echocardiography.

application. This will depend on the size of the patient and the desired distal perfusion pressure. Usually, distal perfusion pressure is maintained at 40 to 60 mm Hg.

After this has been established, the balance of proximal and distal pressure is fine tuned and managed as shown in Table 9–4 using proximal pressure, distal pressure, PCWP, and TEE.

Remember that, when using left heart bypass, volume must be infused directly into the patient. During partial CPB, volume can be infused directly into the patient or added directly into the venous reservoir. The severity of hypotension after cross-clamp removal when distal perfusion is supplied tends to be less than that seen with simple cross-clamping. Nonetheless, close attention to acid–base status, renal function, and a short cross-clamp time are still important.

■ REFERENCES

1. De Bakey ME, McCollum CH, Graham JM: Surgical treatment of aneurysms of the descending thoracic aorta. Long-term results in 500 patients. *J Cardiovasc Surg* 1978; **19:**571-576.

2. Gilling-Smith GL, Worswick L, Knight PF, et al: Surgical repair of thoracoabdominal aortic aneurysm: 10 years' experience. *Br J Surg* 1995; **82:**624-629.

3. Shenaq SA, Chelly JE, Karlberg H, et al: Use of nitroprusside during surgery for thoracoabdominal aortic aneurysm. *Circulation* 1984; **70:**1-7.

4. Kwitka G, Rosenberg JN, Nugent M: Thoracic aortic disease, in Kaplan JA (ed): *Cardiac Anesthesia*. 3rd ed. Philadelphia, WB Saunders Company, 1993, pp 758, 760.

5. Ergin MA, Galla JD, Lansman S, Griepp RB: Acute dissections of the aorta. Current surgical treatment. *Surg Clin North Am* 1985; **65:**721-741.

6. Appelbaum A, Karp RB, Kirklin JW: Ascending vs descending aortic dissections. *Ann Surg* 1976; **183:**296-300.

7. Murray CA, Edwards JE: Spontaneous laceration of ascending aorta. *Circulation* 1973; **47:**848-858.

8. Larson EW, Edwards WD: Risk factors for aortic dissection: A necropsy study of 161 cases. *Am J Cardiol* 1984; **53:**849-855.

9. Roberts WC: Aortic dissection: Anatomy, consequences and causes. *Am Heart J* 1981; **101:**195-214.

10. Benedict JS, Buhl TL, Henney RP: Acute aortic dissection during cardiopulmonary bypass. *Arch Surg* 1974; **108:**810-813.

11. Sakamoto I, Hayashi K, Matsunaga N, et al: Aortic dissection caused by angiographic procedures. *Radiology* 1994; **191:**467-471.

12. De Bakey ME, Cooley DA, Creech O Jr: Surgical considerations of dissecting aneurysm of the aorta. *Ann Surg* 1955; **112:**586-610.

13. DeSanctis RW, Doroghazi RM, Austen WG, Buckley MJ: Aortic dissection. *N Engl J Med* 1987; **317:**1060-1067.

14. Miller DC: Aortic dissection of the aorta — continuing need for earlier diagnosis and treatment. *Mod Concepts Cardiovasc Dis* 1985; **54:**51-55.

15. Schwartz MJ: Anesthesia for emergency cardiac surgery, in DiNardo JA, Schwartz MJ (eds): *Anesthesia for Cardiac Surgery*. Norwalk, CT, Appleton and Lange, 1990, pp 205-212.

16. Lindsay J Jr, Hurst JW: Clinical features and prognosis in dissecting aneurysm of the aorta. A re-appraisal. *Circulation* 1967; **35:**880-888.

17. Magilligan DJ Jr, Ullyot DJ: The heart: I. Acquired diseases, in Way LW (ed): *Current Surgical Diagnosis and Treatment*. Norwalk, CT, Appleton and Lange, 1991, p 359.

18. Hirst AE Jr, Johns VJ, Kime SW: Dissecting aneurysm of the aorta: A review of 505 cases. *Medicine* 1958; **37:**217-279.

19. Wilson SK, Hutchins GM: Aortic dissecting aneurysms: Causative factors in 204 subjects. *Arch Pathol Lab Med* 1982; **106:**175-180.

20. De Bakey ME: The development of vascular surgery. *Am J Surg* 1979; **137:**697-738.

21. Miller DC, Stinson EB, Oyer PE, et al: Operative treatment of aortic dissections. *J Thorac Cardiovasc Surg* 1979; **78:**365-382.

22. Parmley LF, Mattingly TW, Manion WC, Jahnke EJ: Nonpenetrating traumatic injury to the aorta. *Circulation* 1958; **17:**1086-1101.

23. Wilson RF: Accidental and surgical trauma, in Shoemaker WC, Ayres S, Grenvik A, et al (eds): *Textbook of Critical Care*. 2nd ed. Philadelphia, WB Saunders Company, 1989, pp 1230-1271.

24. Kirsh MM, Behrendt DM, Orringer MB, et al: The treatment of acute traumatic rupture of the aorta. A 10-year experience. *Ann Surg* 1976; **184:**308-315.

25. Greendyke RM: Traumatic rupture of aorta. Special reference to automobile accidents. *JAMA* 1966; **195:**527-530.

26. Bickerstaff LK, Pairolero PC, Hollier LH, et al: Thoracic aortic aneurysms: A population-based study. *Surgery* 1982; **92:** 1103-1108.

27. Pressler V, McNamara JJ: Thoracic aortic aneurysm. Natural history and treatment. *J Thorac Cardiovasc Surg* 1980; **79:**489-498.

28. Hollier LH, Symmonds JB, Pairolero PC, et al: Thoracoabdominal aortic aneurysm repair. Analysis of postoperative mortality. *Arch Surg* 1988; **123:**871-875.

29. Svensson LG, Crawford ES, Hess KR, et al: Variables predictive of outcome in 832 patients undergoing repairs of the descending thoracic aorta. *Chest* 1993; **104:**1248-1253.

30. Sefczek DM, Sefczek RJ, Deeb ZL: Radiographic signs of acute traumatic rupture of the thoracic aorta. *Am J Roentgenol* 1983; **141:**1259-1262.

31. Strum JT, Marsh DG, Bodily KC: Ruptured thoracic aorta: Evolving radiological concepts. *Surgery* 1979; **85:**363-367.

32. Gandelman G, Barzilay N, Krupsky M, Resnitzky P: Left pleural hemorrhagic effusion. A presenting sign of thoracic aortic dissecting aneurysm. *Chest* 1994; **106:**636-638.

33. van der Vliet JA, Heijstraten FMJ, van Roye SFS, Buskens FGM: Spontaneous right haemothorax secondary to aortic rupture. *Eur J Vasc Surg* 1994; **8:**634-638.

34. Stein HL, Steinberg I: Selective aortography, the definitive technique for diagnosis of dissecting aneurysm of the thoracic aorta. *Am J Roentgenol* 1968; **102:**333.

35. Goldman AP, Kotler MN, Scanlon MH, et al: The complementary role of magnetic resonance imaging, Doppler echocardoigraphy and computed tomography in the diagnosis of dissecting thoracic aneurysms. *Am Heart J* 1986; **111:**970-981.

36. Cigarroa JE, Isselbacher EM, DeSanctis RW, Eagle KA. Diagnostic imaging in the evaluation of suspected aortic dissection. *N Engl J Med* 1993; **328:**35-43.

37. Buckmaster MJ, Kearney PA, Johnson SB, et al: Further experience with tranesophageal echocardiography in the evaluation of thoracic aortic injury. *J Trauma* 1994; **37:**989-995.

38. Simon P, Owen AN, Havel M, et al: Transespohageal echocardiography in the emergency surgical management of patients with aortic dissection. *J Thorac Cardiovasc Surg* 1992; **103:** 1113-1117.

39. Nienaber CA, von Kodolitsch Y, Nicolas V, et al: The diagnosis of thoracic aortic dissection by noninvasive imaging procedures. *N Engl J Med* 1993; **328:**1-9.

40. Barbant SD, Eisenberg MJ, Schiller NB: The diagnostic value of imaging techniques for aortic dissection. *Am Heart J* 1992; **124:**541-543.

41. Ballal RS, Nanda NC, Gatewood R, et al: Usefulness of transesophageal echocardiography in assessment of aortic dissection. *Circulation* 1991; **84:**1903-1914.

42. Nienaber CA, Spielmann RP, von Kodolitsch Y, et al: Diagnosis of thoracic aortic dissection. Magnetic resonance imaging versus transesophageal echocardiography. *Circulation* 1992; **85:**434-447.

43. Fruewald FXJ, Neuhold A, Fezoulidis J, et al: Cine MR in dissection of the thoracic aorta. *Eur J Radiol* 1989; **9:**37-41.

44. Iliceto S, Antonelli G, Sorino M, et al: Two-dimensional echocardiographic recognition of complications of cardiac invasive procedures. *Am J Cardiol* 1984; **53:**846-848.

45. Bjerke RJ: Intraoperative diagnosis of aortic dissection using transesophageal echocardiography. *J Cardiothorac Vasc Anesth* 1992; **6:**720-723.

46. Neustein SM, Lansman SL, Quintana CS, et al: Transesophageal Doppler echocardiographic monitoring or malperfusion during aortic dissection repair. *Ann Thorac Surg* 1993; **56:**358-361.

47. Ileceto S, Nanda NC, Rizzon P, et al: Color Doppler evaluation of aortic dissection. *Circulation* 1987; **75:**752-755.

48. Laissy J-P, Blanc F, Soyer P, et al: Thoracic aortic dissection: Diagnosis with transesophageal echocardiography versus MR imaging. *Radiology* 1995; **194:**331-336.

49. Nishino M, Tanouchi J, Tanaka K, et al: Transesophageal echocardiography diagnosis of thoracic aortic dissection with the completely thrombosed false lumen: Differentiation from true aortic aneurysm with mural thrombus. *J Am Soc Echocardiog* 1996; **9:**79-85.

50. O'Connor CJ, Rothenberg DM: Anesthetic consideration for descending thoracic aortic surgery: Part I. *J Cardiothorac Vasc Anesth* 1995; **9:**581-588.

51. Chirillo F, Cavallini C, Longhini C, et al: Comparative diagnostic value of transesophageal echocardiography and retrograde aortography in the evaluation of thoracic aortic dissection. *Am J Cardiol* 1994; **74:**590-595.

52. Konstadt SN, Reich DL, Quintana C, Levy M: The ascending aorta: How much does transesophageal echocardiography see? *Anesth Analg* 1994; **78:**240-244.

53. Khandheria BK, Tajik AJ, Freeman WK: Transesophageal echocardiographic examination. Technique, training and safety, in Freeman WK, Sweard JB, Khandheria BK, Tajik AJ (eds): *Transesophageal Echocardiography.* New York, Little, Brown and Company, 1994, p 49.

54. Cunningham DJ: *Manual of Practical Anatomy.* 13th ed. London, Oxford, 1966.

55. Charrette EJP, Winton TL, Salerno TA: Acute respiratory insufficiency from an aneurysm of the descending thoracic aorta. *J Thorac Cardiovasc Surg* 1983; **85:**467-470.

56. Nishiwaki K, Komatsu T, Shimada Y, et al: Severe tracheal compression caused by false aneurysm arising from the ascending aorta: Successful airway management using induced hypotension and bronchoscopy. *Anesthesiology* 1993; **73:**1047-1049.

57. Gorman RB, Merritt WT, Greenspun H, et al: Aneurysmal compression of the trachea and right mainstem bronchus complicating thoracoabdominal aneurysm repair. Anesthesiology 1993; **79;**1424-1427.

58. Cohen JA, Denisco RA, Richards TS, et al: Hazardous placement of a Robertshaw-Type endobronchial tube. *Anesth Analg* 1986; **65:**10-101.

59. Lukanich JM, Conlan AA: Left hilar mass with obstruction of the main bronchus due to localized pseudoaneurysm of the thoracic aorta. *Can J Surg* 1996; **39:**63-66.

60. Mori M, Chuma R, Kiichi Y, et al: The anesthetic management of a patient with a thoracic aortic aneurysm that caused compression of the left mainstem bronchus and the right pulmonary artery. *J Cardiothorac Vasc Anesth* 1993; **7:**579-584.

61. Schwartz AJ, Hensley FA Jr: Case conference. *J Thorac Cardiovasc Anesth* 1990; **4:**631-645.

62. Penner C, Myacher B, Light RB: Compression of the left main bronchus between a descending thoracic aortic aneurysm and an enlarged right pulmonary artery. *Chest* 1994; **106:**959-961.

63. Smith GB, Hirsch NP, Ehrenwerth J: Placement of double-lumen endobronchial tubes: Correlation between clinical impressions and bronchoscopic findings. *Br J Anaesth* 1986; **58:** 1317-1320.

64. Kelley JG, Gaba DM, Brodsky JB: Bronchial cuff pressures of two tubes used in thoracic surgery. *J Cardiothorac Vasc Anesth* 1992; **6:**190-192.

65. Lake CL: Cardiovascular anatomy and physiology, in Barash PG, Cullen BF, Stoelting RK (eds): *Clinical Anesthesia.* Philadelphia, JB Lippincott Company, 1992, p 993.

66. Carpenter MB: *Human Neuroanatomy.* 7th ed. Baltimore, Williams & Wilkins, 1976, p 602.

67. Djindjian R, Faure C: Accidents medullaries de aortogram. *J Belge Radiol* 1967; **50:**207-213.

68. Wadouh F, Lindemann E-M, Arndt CF, et al: The arterial radicularis magna anterior as a decisive factor influencing spinal cord damage during aortic occlusion. *J Thorac Cardiovasc Surg* 1984; **88:**1-10.

69. Shenaq SA, Svensson LG: Paraplegia following aortic surgery. *J Cardiothorac Vasc Anesth* 1993; **7:**81-94.

70. Livesay JJ, Cooley DA, Ventemiglia RA, et al: Surgical experience in descending thoracic aneurysmectomy with and without adjuncts to avoid ischemia. *Ann Thorac Surg* 1985; **39:**37-45.

71. Crawford ES, Svensson LG, Hess KR, et al: A prospective randomized study of cerebrospinal fluid drainage to prevent paraplegial after high-risk surgery on the thoracoabdominal aorta. *J Vasc Surg* 1990; **13:**36-46.

72. Murray MJ, Bower TC, Olover WC, et al: Effects of cerebrospinal fluid drainage in patients undergoing thoracic and thoracoabdominal aortic surgery. *J Cardiothorac Vasc Anesth* 1993; **7:**266-272.

73. Wojewska PA: Spinal cord protection during thoracoabdominal aneurysm resection. *J Thorac Cardiovasc Surg* 1995; **109:**1244-1246.

74. O'Connor CJ, Rothenberg DM: Anesthetic consideration for descending thoracic aortic surgery: Part II. *J Cardiothorac Vasc Anesth* 1995; **9:**734-747.

75. Kazui T, Komatsu S, Yokoyama H: Surgical treatment of aneurysms of the thoracic aorta with the aid of partial cardiopulmonary bypass: An analysis of 95 patients. *Ann Thorac Surg* 1987; **43:**622-627.

76. Svensson LG, Loop FD: Prevention of spinal cord ischemia in aortic surgery, in Bergan JJ, Yao JST (eds): *Arterial Surgery: New Diagnostic and Operative Techniques.* New York, Grune and Stratton, 1988, pp 273-285.

77. Kaplan BJ, Friedman WA, Alexander JA, Hampson SR: Somatosensory evoked potential monitoring of spinal cord ischemia during aortic operations. *Neurosurgery* 1986; **19:**82-90.

78. Gugino LD, Kraus KH, Heino R, et al: Peripheral ischemia as a complicating factor during somatosensory and motor evoked potential monitoring of aortic surgery. *J Cardiothorac Vasc Anesth* 1992; **6:**715-719.

79. Gilbert HC, Vender JS: Monitoring the anesthetized patient, in Barash PG, Cullen BF, Stoelting RK (eds): *Clinical Anesthesia.* Philadelphia, JB Lippincott Company, 1992, pp 760-761.

80. Stoelting RK, Dierdorf SF: Diseases of the nervous system, in: *Anesthesia and Co-Existing Disease.* New York, Churchill Livingstone, 1993, p 200.

81. Laschinger JC, Cunningham JN Jr, Cooper MM, et al: Monitoring of somatosensory evoked potentials during surgical procedures on the thoracoabdominal aorta. I. Relationship of aortic cross-

clamp duration, changes in somatosensory evoked potentials, and incidence of neurologic dysfunction. *J Thorac Cardiovasc Surg* 1987; **94**:260-265.

82. Laschinger JC, Cunningham JN Jr, Baumann FG, et al: Monitoring of somatosensory evoked potentials during surgical procedures on the thoracoabdominal aorta. II. Use of somatosensory evoked potentials to assess adequacy of distal aortic bypass and perfusion after thoracic aortic cross clamping. *J Thorac Cardiovasc Surg* 1987; **94**:266-270.

83. Cunningham JN Jr, Laschinger JC, Spencer FC: Monitoring of somatosensory evoked potentials during surgical procedures on the thoracoabdominal aorta. IV. Clinical observations and results. *J Thorac Cardiovasc Surg* 1987; **94**:275-285.

84. Crawford ES, Mizrahi EM, Hess KR, et al: The impact of distal aortic perfusion and somatosensory evoked potential monitoring on prevention of paraplegia after aortic aneurysm operation. *J Thorac Cardiovasc Surg* 1988; **95**:357-367.

85. Hollier LH: Protecting the brain and spinal cord. *J Vasc Surg* 1987; **5**:524-528.

86. McNulty S, Arboosh V, Goldberg M: The relevance of somatosensory evoked potentials during thoracic aortic aneurysm repair. *J Cardiothorac Vasc Anesth* 1991; **5**:262-265.

87. Matsui Y, Goh K, Shiiya N, et al: Clinical application of evoked spinal cord potentials elicited by direct stimulation of the cord during temporary occlusion of the thoracic aorta. *J Thorac Cardiovasc Surg* 1994; **107**:1519-1527.

88. Schepens MA, Defauw JJ, Hamerlijnck RP, Verneulen FE: Risk assessment of acute renal failure after thoracoabdominal aortic aneurysm surgery. *Ann Surg* 1994; **219**:400-407.

89. Alpert RA, Roizen MF, Hamilton WK, et al: Intraoperative urinary output does not predict postoperative renal function in patients undergoing abdominal aortic revascularization. *Surgery* 1984; **95**:707-711.

90. Katz NM, Blackstone EH, Kirklin JW, Karp RB: Incremental risk factors for spinal cord injury following operation for acute traumatic aortic transection. *J Thorac Cardiovasc Surg* 1981; **81**:669-674.

91. Gott VL, Wippen JD, Dutton RC: Heparin bonding on colloidal graphite surfaces. *Science* 1963; **142**:1297.

92. Gott VL: Heparinized shunts for thoracic vascular operations. *Ann Thorac Surg* 1972; **14**:219-220.

93. Lawrence GH, Hessel EA, Savvage LR, et al: Results of the use of the TDMAC-heparin shunt in the surgery of aneurysms of the descending thoracic aorta. *J Thorac Cardiovasc Surg* 1977; **73**:393-398.

94. Molina JE, Cogordan J, Einzig S, et al: Adequacy of ascending aorta-descending aorta shunt during cross-clamping of the thoracic aorta for preventing of spinal cord ischemia. *J Thorac Cardiovasc Surg* 1985; **90**:126-136.

95. Schepens MAAM, Defauw JJAM, Hamerlijnck RPHM, et al: Use of left heart bypass in the surgical repair of thoracoabdominal aortic aneurysms. *Ann Vasc Surg* 1995; **9**:327-338.

96. Crawford ES, Rubio PA: Reappraisal of adjuncts to avoid ischemia in the treatment of aneurysms of descending thoracic aorta. *J Thorac Cardiovasc Surg* 1973; **66**:693-703.

97. Brewer LA, Fosburg RG, Mulder GA, et al: Spinal cord complications following surgery for coarctation of the aorta. *J Thorac Cardiovasc Surg* 1972; **64**:368-379.

98. Verdant A, Page A, Cossette R, et al: Surgery of the descending thoracic aorta: Spinal cord protection with the Gott shunt. *Ann Thorac Surg* 1988; **45**:147-154.

99. Verdant A, Page A, Cossette R, et al: Surgery of the descending thoracic aorta: spinal cord protection with the Gott shunt. *Ann Thorac Surg* 1995; **60**:1151-1152.

100. Ataka K, Okada M, Yamashita C, et al: Beneficial circulatory support by left heart bypass with a centrifugal (BioMedicus) pump for aneurysms of the descending aorta. *Artificial Organs* 1993; **17**:300-306.

101. Borst HG, Jurmann M, Buhner B, Laas J: Risk of replacement of descending aorta with a standardized left heart bypass technique. *J Thorac Cardiovasc Surg* 1994; **107**:126-132.

102. Hassan N, Javid H, Hurter J, et al: Descending aortic aneurysmectomy without adjuncts to avoid ischemia. *Ann Thorac Surg* 1980; **30**:326-332.

103. Tabayashi K, Ohmi M, Togo T, et al: Aortic arch aneurysm repair using selective cerebral perfusion. *Ann Thorac Surg* 1994; **57**:1305-1310.

104. Alamanni F, Agrifoglio M, Pompilio G, et al: Aortic arch surgery: Pros and cons of selective cerebral perfusion. *J Cardiovasc Surg* 1995; **36**:31-37.

105. Subramanian S: Management of cardiopulmonary bypass in infants and children, in Glenn WWL (ed): *Thoracic and Cardiovascular Surgery.* 4th ed. Norwalk, CT, Appleton-Century-Crofts, 1983.

106. Murase M, Maeda M, Koyama T, et al: Continuous retrograde cerebral perfusion for protection of the brain during aortic arch surgery. *Eur J Cardiothorac Surg* 1993; **7**:597-600.

107. Deeb GM, Jenkins E, Bolling SF, et al: Retrograde cerebral perfusion during hypothermic circulatory arrest reduces neurologic morbidity. *J Thorac Cardiovasc Surg* 1995; **109**:259-268.

108. Safi HJ, Brien HW, Winter JN, et al: Brain protection via cerebral retrograde perfusion during aortic arch aneurysm repair. *Ann Thorac Surg* 1993; **56**:270-276.

109. Coselli JS: Retrograde cerebral perfusion vial a superior vena caval cannula for aortic arch aneurysm operations. *Ann Thorac Surg* 1994; **57**:1668-1669.

110. Mann T, Cohn PF, Holman L, et al: Effect of nitroprusside on regional myocardial blood flow in coronary artery disease. Results in 25 patients and comparison with nitroglycerin. *Circulation* 1978; **57**:732-738.

111. Stoelting RK: Peripheral vasodilators, in: *Pharmacology and Physiology in Anesthetic Practice.* 2nd ed. Philadelphia, J.B. Lippincott Company, 1991, pp 324-334.

112. Gelman S, Reves JG, Fowler K, et al: Regional blood flow during cross-clamping of the thoracic aorta and infusion of sodium nitroprusside. *J Thorac Cardiovasc Surg* 1983; **85**:287-291.

113. Benumof JL: Hypoxic pulmonary vasoconstriction and infusion of sodium nitroprusside. *Anesthesiology* 1979; **50**:481-483.

114. Benowitz NL: Antihypertensive agents, in Katzung BG (ed): *Basic and Clinical Pharmacology.* Englewood Cliffs, NJ, Prentice Hall, 1992, p 146.

115. Godet G, Bertrand M, Coriat P, et al: Comparison of isoflurane with sodium nitroprusside for controlling hypertension during thoracic aortic cross-clamping. *J Cardiothorac Anesth* 1990; **4**:177-184.

116. Gelman S, McDowell H, Varner PD, et al: The reason for cardiac output reduction after aortic cross-clamping. *Am J Surg* 1988; **155**:578-586.

117. Connelly GP, Arkoff H, Dempsey A, et al: Left ventricular diastolic dysfunction associated with infrarenal arotic crossclamp. *Anesthesiology* 1993; **79**:A86.

118. Tokioka H, Saeki S, Koyama Y, et al: The effect of aortic cross-clamping on left ventricular filling dynamics during anesthesial of abdominal aortic surgery. *Anesthesiology* 1992; **77**:A571.

119. Saleh SA, Crawford ES, Bomberger RS, et al: Intraoperative acid-base management for the resection of thoraco-abdominal aortic aneurysms: A comparison of the bolus vs continuous infusion of sodium bicarbonate. *Anesth Analg* 1982; **61**:213.

120. O'Rourke JK, Beattie C, Walman AT, et al: Acidosis during high aortic cross clamp surgery. *Anesthesiology* 1985; **63**:A266.

121. Silverstein PR, Caldera DL, Cullen DJ, et al: Avoiding the hemodynamic consequences of aortic cross-clamping and unclamping. *Anesthesiology* 1979; **50**:462-466.

10

Management of Cardiopulmonary Bypass

James A. DiNardo

The cardiac anesthesiologist must be closely involved with commencing, maintaining, and terminating cardiopulmonary bypass (CPB). It is essential for the anesthesiologist to have a working knowledge of the CPB circuit to aid the surgeon and perfusionist in diagnosing and treating the problems that may be associated with extracorporeal circulation.

■ THE CPB CIRCUIT

The CPB circuit is intended to isolate the cardiopulmonary system so that optimal surgical exposure can be obtained for operations on the heart and great vessels. For this isolation to be effective, the CPB circuit must be able to perform the functions of the intact cardiopulmonary system for a finite period. At a minimum, the circuit must be capable of adding oxygen and removing carbon dioxide from blood and of providing adequate perfusion of all organs with this blood. In addition, the circuit must be able to fulfill these requirements without doing permanent damage to the cardiopulmonary system, the blood, or any of the patient's end organs.

The components of a typical CPB circuit are illustrated in Figure 10–1. The components of the circuit are described in the following sections.

Venous Drainage

For the cardiopulmonary system to be isolated, all venous return to the heart must be made available to the CPB circuit. Blood is collected from the venous circulation and then drains by a siphon into a reservoir that lies on the floor, well below the patient. For a given mean systemic venous pressure and venous resistance, maximum venous return is reached when the right atrial (RA) pressure falls to zero. When the RA pressure is less than zero, the superior vena cava (SVC) and inferior vena cava (IVC) collapse and the heart acts as a Starling resistor.[1]

Total (also complete or full) CPB is said to occur when all of the systemic venous drainage to the heart is captured and returned to the CPB circuit and subsequently to the patient. *Partial CPB* is said to occur when only a portion of the systemic venous drainage to the heart is captured and returned to the CPB circuit. During partial CPB, the remaining portion of systemic venous return is to the RA. Ideally, this blood makes its way to the right ventricle (RV) and pulmonary bed, where gas exchange occurs. The blood then returns to the left atrium (LA) and left ventricle (LV), where it is ejected into the systemic circulation. For partial CPB to be effective, two things must be true:

1. The heart must be beating and ejecting — if ejection is ineffective or nonexistent, distention of the heart will occur and systemic blood flow will be inadequate.
2. The lungs must be ventilated — in the absence of ventilation, systemic venous blood that enters the RA will ultimately reach the systemic circu-

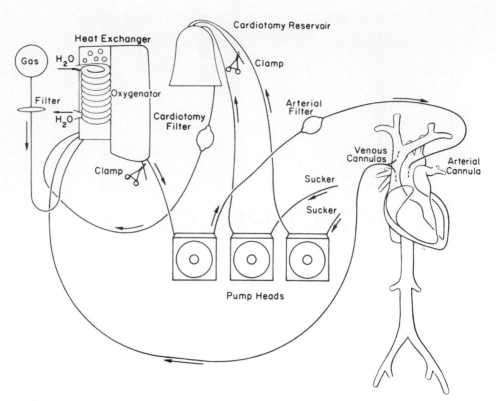

FIGURE 10-1. Typical cardiopulmonary by-pass circuit. *(From: Lake CL: Pediatric Cardiac Anesthesia. Norwalk, CT, Appleton and Lange, 1988, p 157.)*

lation without gas exchange having occurred. This will result in hypercarbia and hypoxemia.

During partial CPB, the patient's systemic blood flow is provided in part by the CPB circuit and in part by the patient's heart. The patient's arterial pH, Po_2, and Pco_2 are a reflection of the quantity and effectiveness of these two sources of blood. Therefore, during partial CPB, blood for blood gas analysis must be drawn from the patient and not from the CPB circuit.

When blood from both the SVC and IVC is collected by cannulae of the proper size, RA pressure will approach zero.[2] Various cannula are shown in Figure 10-2. Total CPB is best accomplished with either direct cannulation of both the SVC and IVC or with use of two-stage single venous cannula in the RA.

- Direct cannulation of the SVC and IVC — this is accomplished through two separate incisions at the caval RA junctions. In patients with a persistent left SVC draining to the coronary sinus, direct cannulation of this vessel will be necessary as well. The advantage of the two-cannula system is that when tapes are tightened around the cannulae in the SVC and IVC, the right heart can be isolated completely. It is essential that the tapes are tightened during procedures in which the right heart is opened so that air is not entrained continuously in the venous drainage system.

Tightening the tapes also is necessary when the left atrium must be exposed because it allows retraction of an empty right atrium. If the right heart is not opened, the tapes must be left loose so that blood return to the right atrium from the coronary sinus can be collected. Normally, for adults, cannulae of 11 to 12 mm in outer diameter are used. Pediatric cannulae range from 4.0 to 7.0 mm in outer diameter. A larger cannula is used in the IVC as compared with the SVC, because a larger portion of systemic venous return (two-thirds) is from the IVC.

- Two-stage single venous cannula in the RA — for adults and larger children, venous drainage also can be accomplished with one larger-bore cannula with two orifices. One orifice (32- to 36-French outer diameter) lies directly in the IVC and the other (40- to 51-French outer diameter) lies in proximal to the SVC–RA junction. This cannula is inserted via one incision in the right atrial appendage. The single-cannula system requires only one atriotomy and is satisfactory for procedures that do not require opening the atriae or ventricles, such as coronary artery bypass grafting or aortic valve replacement. In addition, coronary sinus and persistent left SVC return is collected continuously via the orifice that lies at the SVC–RA junction.

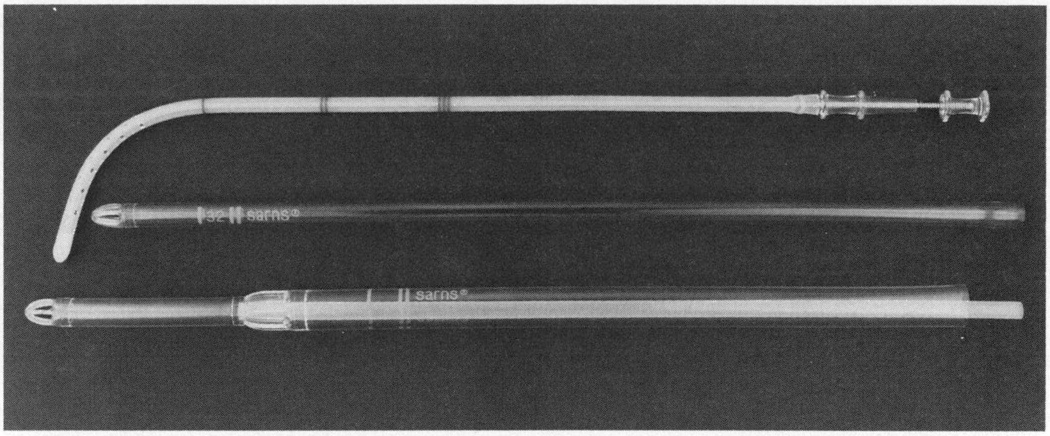

FIGURE 10–2. Top. Vent line with stylet inserted. This type of line commonly is used to vent left ventricle via left atrium. **Middle.** 11-mm outer diameter venous cannula used in adults for cannulation and drainage of superior vena cava (SVC) and inferior vena cava (IVC). **Bottom.** Two-stage venous cannula (12-mm and 17-mm outer diameter) used for drainage of both SVC and IVC via single incision in right atrial appendage.

Partial CPB can be accomplished with the previously described cannulation techniques simply by partially impeding venous return to the CPB circuit with a clamp on the venous drainage line. More commonly, partial CPB is the result of venous cannulation via the femoral venous system. In this situation, a cannula is inserted retrograde up a femoral vein toward the heart, preferably into the IVC or RA. This system is much less effective than caval cannulation via the right atrium. The femoral vein limits the size of the cannula, which can be inserted (20-French outer diameter for adults). This inhibits optimal systemic venous drainage because of the large pressure drop across the long, narrow cannula. This, in turn, elevates RA pressure, which for a given mean arterial pressure and systemic venous resistance, further compromises venous return. For these reasons, with femoral venous cannulation, it usually is impossible to divert all venous return to the CPB circuit.

The major advantage of femoral venous cannulation is that it can be provided emergently and quickly without a sternotomy. Partial CPB commonly is used under the following circumstances:

- During repair of thoracic aortic lesions (*see* Chapter 9).
- As temporary support for cardiogenic shock after invasive cardiac catheterization or electrophysiologic laboratory procedures.
- To provide partial decompression of the heart during difficult surgical dissection in patients who had previous heart surgery.

Even with appropriate cannulation techniques, there may be compromise of venous return to the CPB circuit. Air lock may occur when large bubbles of air become lodged in the venous drainage lines. This air usually is entrained into the venous drainage lines from around loose cannulation sites. This can occur even when the right heart is not directly open to air. Air lock acutely disrupts the siphon effect. This causes right atrial pressure to rise above zero and venous return to the venous reservoir to fall. Malposition of the venous cannula, such as in the portal vein rather than in the IVC, will compromise venous return. Surgical manipulation of the heart may cause kinking of the venous cannulae or sequestration of blood in the right atrium and compromise venous return.

Arterial Inflow

Normally, arterial inflow is obtained via a cannula placed in the lesser curve of the ascending aorta proximal to the innominate artery. This arrangement allows perfusion of all vessels of the arch and distal aorta, as well as perfusion of the coronary ostia. In adults, aortic cannulas in the range of 6.5 to 8 mm in outer diameter are used. Pediatric cannulas range from 2.0 to 5.0 mm in outer diameter. An aortic cannula is shown in Figure 10–3. Because the distal end of the arterial cannula is significantly smaller than the arterial inflow line, a large pressure drop exists across the arterial cannula. Figure 10–4 illustrates the pressure drop across various-sized cannulas. At normal bypass flows of 2.0 L/min/m², a gradient in excess of 120 mm Hg may exist across a 6.5-mm-outer diameter cannula in an adult. In addition, the small distal end of the cannula causes a jet of blood to be propelled. It is essential that this jet is directed down the lumen of the

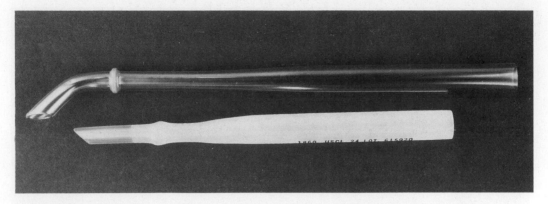

FIGURE 10–3. **Top.** Aortic cannula for use in adults. **Bottom.** Femoral artery cannula for use in adults.

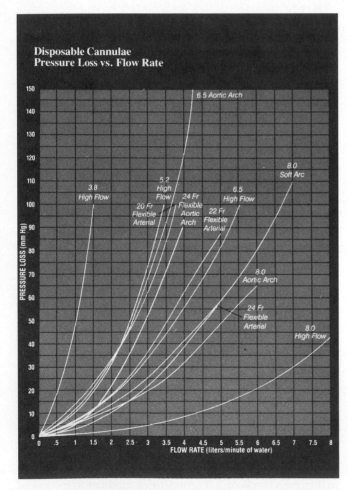

FIGURE 10–4. Pressure drop across arterial cannula is plotted against flow rate through cannula for several different sizes. It is clear that as flow rate increases, pressure drop across any size cannula will increase. Furthermore, the smaller the cannula, the greater the pressure drop at any flow rate. *(Used courtesy of Sarns, Inc./3M.)*

aorta and not up into the innominate artery so that a cerebral overperfusion injury does not occur.

In some circumstances, it may be necessary to obtain arterial inflow via a femoral artery. Placement of the cannula in the femoral artery provides perfusion to the proximal aorta and coronary ostia in a retrograde fashion. A femoral artery cannula is shown in Figure 10–3. This route has several limitations. The smaller caliber of the femoral vessel limits the size of the arterial cannula that can be used without risk of damage to the artery. The smaller the cannula, the larger will be the pressure drop across it. If the pressure drop is severe, flow will be limited after the safe maximum arterial perfusion line pressure (about 300 mm Hg) has been reached. Perfusion to the leg in which the cannula is placed is limited by the fact that the cannula occupies the entire lumen of the femoral artery and is directed proximally. This may result in an ischemic leg and a persistent metabolic acidosis. When these cannulas are removed, there often is a washout of lactic acid, which results in a profound systemic metabolic acidosis that may require treatment with sodium bicarbonate and hyperventilation.

Pumps

There currently are two types of pumps used on modern CPB machines to provide nonpulsatile flow: the double-headed nonocclusive roller pump (*see* Fig. 10–5) and the centrifugal blood pump (*see* Figs. 10–6 and 10–7).

The double-headed roller pump is the most commonly used. The double-headed roller pump is a positive volume displacement pump. At least one head is in contact with the pump boot at all times to push blood forward and ensure continuous forward flow. The pump boot is the piece of tubing in contact with the pump

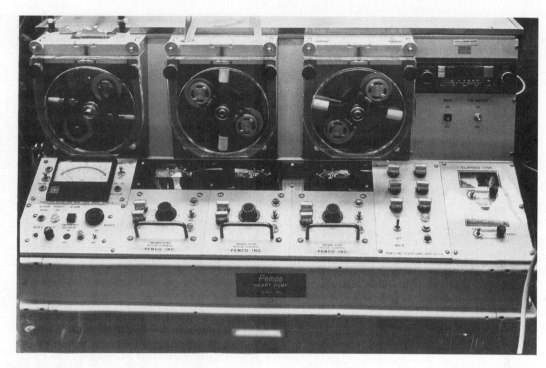

FIGURE 10–5. Three nonocclusive roller pumps. In the two pumps to the left, it can be seen that at least one pump head is in contact with the pump boot at all times. The pump boot is a piece of tubing designed to be in contract with roller heads. In the pump to the far left, connections between the pump boot and inflow and outflow lines can be seen.

heads. It generally is thicker and more durable than the other sections of tubing in the CPB circuit.

Roller pumps are driven by a load-independent electric motor. After the pump speed has been set, the pump will continue the forward displacement of the same volume of blood, even if the resistance to flow is increased by kinking or clamping the arterial line. This will result in a large pressure increase in the arterial inflow line, which can result in the rupture of connections between sections of tubing. To avoid this type of disaster, some centers use pressure gauges on the arterial inflow line. If arterial line pressure rises to dangerous levels (300 mm Hg) pump flow can be reduced to allow line pressure to fall until the problem is sorted out.

The centrifugal pump (*see* Chapter 11) is a kinetic pump. It operates on the constrained vortex principle. Blood is driven through the pump by centrifugal forces generated by a vortex in the pump.[3,4] It has been suggested that this causes less trauma to blood components than the roller pump.[3] Although the pump is driven by a load-independent electric motor, this pump does not behave like the roller pump. When line resistance is increased, blood flow falls as the shear forces between the layers of blood are increased and less forward displacement of blood occurs. This resistance dependence prevents increases in arterial line pressure when clamping or kinking occurs.

The pump is said to be inflow-responsive as well. If a large quantity of air is introduced into this pump, cohesive forces will no longer exist between layers of blood and pumping will cease. In addition, the risk of micro air embolization is reduced because small, low-

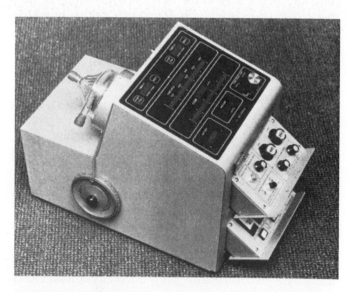

FIGURE 10–6. Bio-Medicus centrifugal pump inserted in driving mechanism. (*Used courtesy of Bio-Medicus.*)

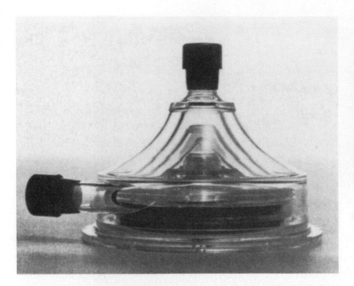

FIGURE 10–7. Closeup of Bio-Medicus centrifugal pump. Inflow is at apex of pyramidal-shaped pump while outflow is at left side of base. *(Used courtesy of Bio-Medicus.)*

density air bubbles become trapped in the center of the vortex. This allows the pump to be used safely without a reservoir for left atrial to femoral artery bypass,[4] aortoaortic bypass,[5] or aortic to femoral artery bypass[5] in the repair of thoracic aneurysms. With heparin-bonded tubing and without an oxygenator, the centrifugal pump has been used safely with minimal systemic heparinization (activated clotting time 150 to 200 seconds) for these repairs.[4,5]

Oxygenators

Oxygenators are intended to perform the gas exchange functions of the lung in the CPB circuit. Despite the fact that oxygenators are incorporated in a system in which blood is pumped under pressure, all gas exchange occurs at atmospheric pressure because the oxygenators are vented to the atmosphere. There currently are two types of oxygenators used: bubble oxygenators and membrane oxygenators.

Bubble Oxygenators. Bubble oxygenators allow oxygen delivery to and carbon dioxide removal from blood via a gas bubble–blood interface. A typical bubble oxygenator is illustrated in Figure 10–8. Venous blood from the venous drainage line and blood from the cardiotomy lines drain to the proximal portion of a bubble column. The proximal portion of the bubble column is separated from the gas entry chamber by a dispersion plate. The dispersion plate breaks up the bulk gas (100% O_2 or an O_2/CO_2 mixture) into bubbles of appropriate size for gas exchange. This gas is bubbled through blood in the bubble chamber so that gas exchange may occur. The blood gas mixture then passes through a debub-

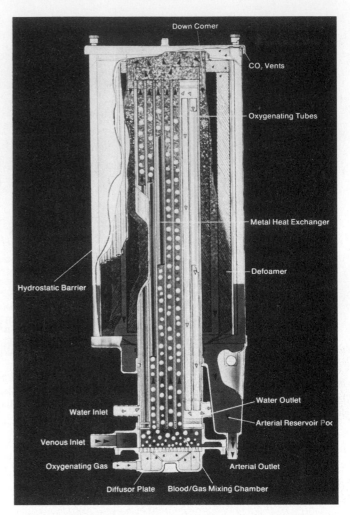

FIGURE 10–8. Cutaway view of typical bubble oxygenator. Water inlet and outlet for heat exchange coils are located at the bottom of the oxygenator. Oxygen inflow also is located at the bottom. Venous blood passively enters oxygenator via venous cannulas and venous drainage line. O_2, CO_2, and heat exchange all occur as blood–gas mixture is carried to the top of the oxygenator. Blood–gas mixture then spills over into defoaming chamber before entering arterial reservoir. From the arterial reservoir, blood is pumped into the patient via arterial inflow line and arterial cannula.

bler/defoamer. The chamber has a large surface area of polyurethane mesh sponge coated with an antifoaming agent and covered with polyester fabric. This arrangement serves to eliminate a major source of gaseous microemboli. The antifoaming agent causes bubbles to collapse by reducing surface tension and the other components mechanically disrupt the bubbles. From here, the blood falls into an arterial reservoir. The reservoir provides an area for further elimination of bubbles by allowing them to rise to the top of the blood. Blood in the arterial reservoir is then pumped to the patient. The volume in the reservoir provides a volume buffer, which allows the perfusionist to react to changes in venous return without pumping the reservoir dry and then pumping air into the patient.

Oxygen is relatively less soluble and diffusible in blood than carbon dioxide (ratio of 1:25). Therefore, oxygen delivery is enhanced by small bubbles where the surface area available for gas exchange is large. Carbon dioxide removal, on the other hand, is enhanced by large bubbles where the volume of the gas bubbles is large. In reality, the bubble size is somewhere between these two extremes (3 to 7 microns). For a given bubble size, increasing the flow of bubbles through blood results in enhanced CO_2 removal. Therefore, arterial P_{CO_2} is controlled by the gas to blood flow ratio (GBFR). Some additional control of CO_2 can be obtained by using an O_2/CO_2 mixture instead of 100% O_2 as the bulk gas. Independent control of arterial P_{O_2} is difficult as the FI_{O_2} is fixed (100% O_2) or very nearly fixed (O_2/CO_2). Removal of nitrogen (N) bubbles is difficult and, therefore, O_2/N mixtures are not used.

The blood–gas interface is not physiologic due to the constantly changing blood–gas interface. This results in traumatization of the blood. Increasing gas flow to enhance gas exchange results in further traumatization of the blood. In addition, increasing gas flow increases the number and decreases the size of the bubbles generated. This increases the risk that gaseous microemboli will reach the arterial circulation.

Membrane Oxygenators. Membrane oxygenators allow oxygen delivery to and carbon dioxide removal from blood across a thin membrane, eliminating any direct blood gas contact. Membrane oxygenators generally are of two types: microporous membranes and solid membranes. Microporous membranes are made of polypropylene or Teflon with small, nonwettable pores (0.3 to 0.7 microns in diameter) that blood cannot pass through. Upon exposure to blood, these pores become covered with a thin proteinaceous layer through which gas exchange occurs without blood and gas coming in direct contact. These microporous membranes offer no limitation to the diffusion of CO_2 or O_2. Solid membranes generally are constructed of methyl silicon rubber that must be thin enough (less than 25 microns) to permit diffusion. These membranes do offer some limitation to the diffusion of CO_2 and O_2 with CO_2 diffusing five times as easily as O_2.

A typical microporous membrane is illustrated in Figure 10–9. In this particular device, the microporous membrane is arranged in parallel sheets with blood flowing on one side of the membrane and gas on the other. In some devices, the microporous or solid material is arranged in capillary tubes (200 to 300 microns in diameter) with blood inside or outside the capillaries flowing in one direction and the gas outside or inside of the capillaries following in the opposite direction. In others, the membrane is arranged as a scrolled envelope. All of these arrangements of microporous material

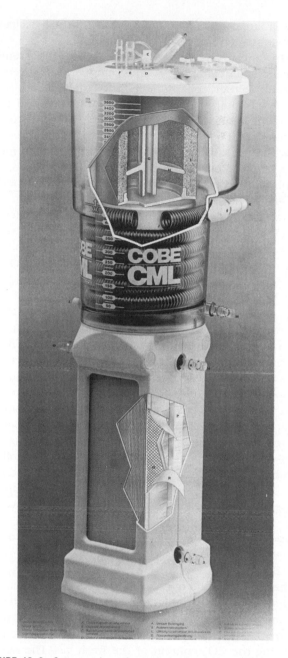

FIGURE 10–9. Cutaway view of a typical microporous membrane oxygenator. Venous reservoir and heat exchange coils are located at the top of the device, whereas the membrane portion is located at the bottom. Cutaway of membrane portion shows membrane to be arranged in sheets. Venous blood passively enters venous reservoir at top of oxygenator via venous drainage line **(A)**. Venous blood then flows down over heat exchange coils before leaving reservoir **(M)** and entering pump. Heat exchanger coil inflow and outflow ports can be seen **(K and L)**. Pump then pumps blood through membrane and out arterial inflow line into patient. Venous blood is pumped into top of membrane **(N)**. Oxygenating gas also enters membrane at top **(O)**. Gas exchange occurs as blood is pumped from top to bottom of membrane. Arterial blood leaves membrane via arterial inflow line at bottom **(S)**.

allow a large surface area (2 to 4 m²) for gas exchange to be contained in a relatively small space.

In most membrane oxygenators the venous drainage and cardiotomy lines empty into a venous reservoir (either collapsible or hard shell, noncollapsible) and is pumped through the membrane and then out to the patient via the arterial line. This is because the high resistance inherent in the membrane does not allow gravity flow of venous blood through the membrane into an arterial reservoir. Currently, there is one membrane oxygenator (Terumo Capiox E) that does allow gravity flow-through.

Although modern membranes themselves offer little impedance to the diffusion of gas, there are other characteristics of membrane oxygenators that limit gas exchange. The primary determinants of O_2 and CO_2 exchange across a membrane are the solubility and diffusibility of O_2 and CO_2 in blood and their partial-pressure gradient across the membrane. Because O_2 is relatively less soluble and diffusible in blood than CO_2 (ratio of 1:25), oxygen exchange is dependent on the thickness of the blood film and the pressure gradient for O_2 across the membrane. The pressure gradient for O_2 can be increased by increasing the O_2 content of the fresh gas flow. However, because of the low diffusibility of O_2 in blood, a thick blood film will result in poor O_2 delivery to the cells most distant from the membrane, even when the pressure gradient for O_2 is high. Modern membranes have design features to keep the blood film thin. In addition, the intentional hemodilution that is a consequence of asanguineous CPB primes also serves to keep the blood film thin. Modern membranes have such a large surface area that maximal oxygenation can occur at low gas flows as long as the blood film is thin.

Because CO_2 is relatively more soluble than O_2, CO_2 exchange is dependent only on the pressure gradient for CO_2 across the membrane. Normally, fresh gas flow to the membrane oxygenator contains no CO_2, and thus, the gradient for CO_2 removal cannot be increased by lowering the CO_2 content of the fresh gas. The rate of CO_2 removal can be increased by increasing the rate of fresh gas flow or sweep rate; this is analogous to increasing alveolar ventilation.

Membrane oxygenators offer several advantages over bubble oxygenators:

1. Traumatization of blood is greatly reduced because there is not a constantly changing direct blood–gas interface. Numerous studies have shown bubble oxygenators to be more traumatic to blood (particularly platelets) than membrane oxygenators; however, the relevance of this finding to clinical outcome and post-CPB transfusion requirements in both long (>2 hours) and short (<2 hours) CPB runs remains controversial.[6-10]

2. No defoaming stage is needed because bubbles are not directly added to blood.
3. Oxygen and carbon dioxide exchange can be varied independently. This allows gas flow to be increased to improve carbon dioxide elimination without substantially affecting oxygenation.
4. Oxygen–air mixtures can be used instead of 100% oxygen. In a bubble oxygenator, bubbles containing nitrogen may be absorbed slowly into the systemic circulation, increasing the risk of gaseous microemboli. In a membrane oxygenator, this risk does not exist. Air–oxygen mixtures allow greater control of the oxygen partial pressure (Po_2) on CPB.

Heat Exchangers

Most procedures are performed on CPB in conjunction with systemic hypothermia to reduce systemic, particularly cerebral, oxygen consumption and to aid in maintaining myocardial hypothermia during aortic cross-clamping. Heat exchangers are necessary to produce the active cooling and rewarming of the patient's blood required for systemic hypothermia on CPB.

Heat exchange is accomplished by a countercurrent flow of water and the patient's blood. Water of a predetermined temperature is pumped into a spiral metal coil as blood flows in the opposite direction over the coil (see Figs. 10-8 and 10-9). The countercurrent flow arrangement provides the most efficient method of heat exchange. Water input temperature is determined by mixing various proportions of hot and cold water before its introduction into the tube. A device capable of accurately producing water of the appropriate temperature and pumping it to the heat exchange coils is a necessary component of the CPB circuit. Such a device is shown in Figure 10-10.

Heat exchanger coils generally are located in the CPB circuit before the oxygenator because the solubility of gases in blood is reduced as blood temperature rises. This arrangement reduces the risk of systemic gaseous microemboli that may be produced during rewarming. As the temperature gradient between the venous blood input and water input decreases, heat exchange slows exponentially. Nonetheless, the temperature gradient between venous blood input and water input is kept lower than 10°C to avoid large changes in gas solubility. During warming, the heated water input temperature never exceeds 40°C to avoid heat damage to blood and myocardial tissue.

Cardiotomy Suction

Cardiotomy or pump suction is incorporated into most CPB circuits, where it serves as an important source of blood conservation. Most systems use a roller pump to

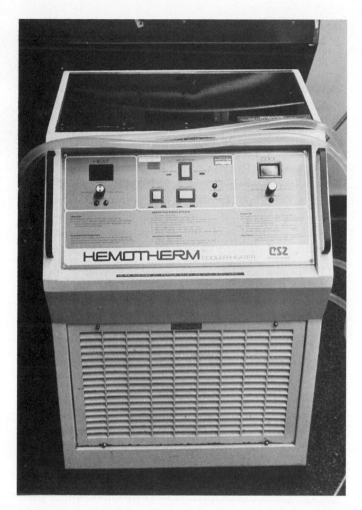

FIGURE 10-10. Heat exchange device, capable of accurately generating water of the desired temperature and pumping it to heat exchange coils of an oxygenator.

provide the necessary suction. The collected blood goes either to a filtered cardiotomy reservoir and then to the venous reservoir or directly to a venous reservoir that contains a filter. Cardiotomy suction has been implicated as the major source of blood traumatization in CPB. Although the interaction of blood with the pericardial surface has been implicated in causing platelet and leukocyte aggregation, the major source of blood trauma is the simultaneous aspiration of air and blood.[11,12] For this reason, it is important that the pump head on the cardiotomy suction turns only fast enough to allow aspiration of blood. If a sucking sound is heard from the cardiotomy, sucker aspiration of air is occurring and the pump head rotation should be slowed.

Often, the cardiotomy suction is used before initiation of CPB during cannula placement. It is essential that adequate heparinization is obtained before use of cardiotomy suction so that clot is not introduced into the cardiotomy or venous reservoir (see "Assess Anticoagulation" later in this chapter).

Vent Line

Venting is intended to prevent blood from collecting in the ventricles during CPB. When blood collects in the ventricles, distension of the ventricles and warming of the heart may occur. Distension causes mechanical damage to the heart from subendocardial compression and also compromises surgical exposure. The risk of distension is greatest when the blood return to the right or left heart is high and when the ventricles are no longer effectively ejecting blood. As CPB commences, bradycardia, ventricular fibrillation, or asystole may occur and prevent effective ventricular ejection. Myocardial hypothermia during cardioplegic arrest will be compromised by warm blood collecting in the ventricles during aortic cross-clamping in the unvented heart.

Figure 10–11 illustrates the most common causes of continued blood return to the right and left ventricles after institution of CPB with all IVC and SVC return diverted to the circuit. Blood flow to the right heart during CPB usually is the result of coronary blood flow. Most

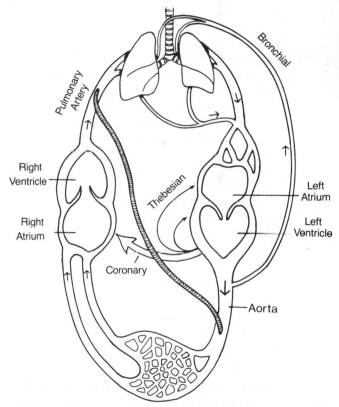

FIGURE 10–11. Potential sources of continued blood flow to right and left heart during CPB. Bronchial flow is derived from aorta and returns to left atrium. Coronary blood flow returns to the right atrium via coronary sinus but variable proportions may return to the left atrium and ventricle via thebesian veins. Shunt is seen between the aorta and pulmonary artery. This shunt may be anatomical (patent ductus arterious) or surgical (Blalock–Taussig, Potts, Waterston). Finally, aortic regurgitation may be responsible for blood flow into left ventricle on CPB before aortic cross-clamping.

coronary blood flow comes from coronary arteries and their collaterals. A small portion comes from noncoronary collaterals, usually of pericardial and mediastinal origin. Coronary venous blood returns to the coronary sinus, which is located near the junction of the IVC and the RA. Coronary sinus return can be captured by a properly positioned two-stage cannula or with separate IVC and SVC cannulas with the tapes loosened. For procedures in which the right heart is opened, coronary sinus blood can be captured with the cardiotomy suction. Coronary sinus blood flow (except that contributed by noncoronary collaterals) will cease when the aortic cross-clamp is applied and coronary arterial blood flow ceases.

Blood flow to the left heart during CPB stems from several sources:

1. Thebesian veins. These veins drain a very small portion of the coronary circulation into the left atrium and ventricle. This flow will cease when the aortic cross-clamp terminates coronary blood flow.

2. Bronchial veins. The bronchial veins drain into the pulmonary veins and subsequently into the left atrium and ventricle. The bronchial circulation may be very large in patients with cyanotic heart disease.

3. Extracardiac left-to-right shunts. For patients with congenital heart disease, a large portion of pulmonary blood flow may be supplied by large systemic-to-pulmonary artery shunts such as a Blalock–Taussig (subclavian artery to pulmonary artery), Waterston (ascending aorta to right pulmonary artery), Potts (descending aorta to left pulmonary artery), or patent ductus arterious (PDA). If these shunts are not ligated before institution of CPB, the blood return to the pulmonary artery, and subsequently to the left atrium and left ventricle, may be very large.

4. Aortic valve incompetence. Flow return to the left ventricle also may result from an incompetent aortic valve. In this instance, retrograde filling of the left ventricle with blood from the aortic cannula will occur until the aortic cross-clamp is applied.

Normally, right ventricular venting is unnecessary because coronary sinus flow can be captured. Several sites are available for left ventricular venting. The right superior pulmonary vein provides relatively easy retrograde access to the left atrium and the ventricle via the mitral valve. The insertion site subsequently can be used for placement of a transthoracic LA pressure line. Direct venting of the left ventricular apex is possible, but this route requires careful repair and may result in damage to the left ventricle. Direct venting via the left atrium is also possible. The pulmonary artery can be used to vent

both the right heart and the left heart (*see* Fig. 10–11). However, a competent mitral valve will limit effective venting of the left ventricle via this route.

The vent line collects blood from the ventricular vent and returns it either to the filtered cardiotomy reservoir and then to the venous reservoir or directly to a venous reservoir that contains a filter. The vent line may allow passive drainage of the ventricular vent or the vent line may pass through a roller pump to allow active venting. The risk of active venting is that after the ventricle has been emptied of blood, continued active venting may result in entrainment of air into the ventricular cavity. In procedures in which the heart is not opened (such as coronary artery bypass grafting), this entrainment of air will require the additional step of evacuating air from the heart before termination of bypass. Close communication between surgeon and perfusionist are necessary to avoid this complication.

Micropore Filters.   Most CPB circuits are equipped with both cardiotomy and arterial microporous filters. These filters serve two purposes: (1) to remove particulate contaminants such as bone, tissue, and fat fragments from blood; and (2) to prevent micro and macro air emboli. Screen filters are made of a woven polyester mesh. These filters have a 30- to 40-micron pore size and a large working surface area. This pore size makes these filters useful for trapping both air and particulate microemboli without high resistance to flow or damage to cellular blood elements. Depth filters are composed of packed fibers of Dacron and filter by impaction of particles on their wetted surface. These filters tend to lose their air-filtering capabilities over time, cause more hemolysis, and are more damaging to platelets.

Screen filters commonly are used on the arterial side of the circuit to prevent delivery of emboli to the arterial circulation. Figure 10–12 illustrates a typical arterial line filter. The vent at the top of the filter allows air to be vented directly back to the venous reservoir so that it is not trapped in the filter. This is important in cases of massive air emboli, in which the presence of trapped air will greatly reduce the filter surface area and allow the pressure in the filter to become high enough to translocate air across the filter and into the arterial circulation of the patient. The arterial filter also has a bypass line so that it can be excluded from the circuit if it becomes clogged with debris. A combination of depth and screen filters are used in most cardiotomy reservoirs.

Ultrafiltrators.   Ultrafiltrators are devices commonly added to the CPB circuit to remove excess fluid and produce hemoconcentration. When used in conjunction with CPB, these devices produce an ultrafiltrate that occurs as the result of a hydrostatic pressure gradient across a semipermeable membrane. These are the same devices that can be used for hemodialysis when they are

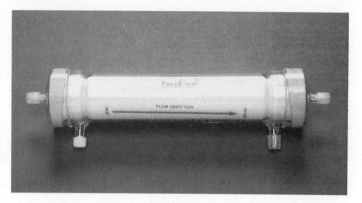

FIGURE 10–13. A typical hollow-fiber microporous ultrafiltration device used for hemoconcentration during and after cardiopulmonary bypass.

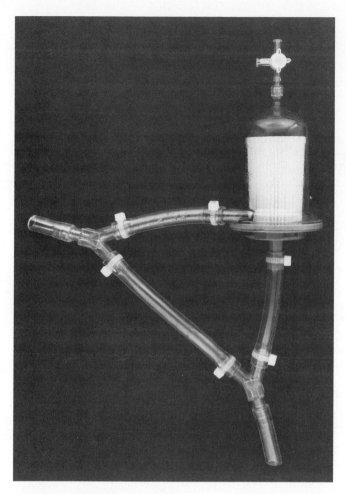

FIGURE 10–12. 40-μm screen filter for use on arterial inflow line. Arterial blood enters the filter at the very bottom and exits at the lower left. Line to bypass filter is included in the setup. Normally, this line is clamped. The stopcock at the top of the filter usually is connected to line that drains into venous reservoir. This allows any air that becomes trapped in filter to be vented before entry into the patient's circulation.

used in conjunction with a dialysate. When used in conjunction with CPB, they are commonly called hemoconcentrators.

These devices consist of a core of microporous hollow fibers made of polysulfone, polyamide, or polyacrylnitrile material arranged in a bundle. The pore size generally is 0.30 to 0.40 microns. A typical ultrafiltration device used for hemoconcentration is shown in Figure 10–13. Blood inflow to the device is obtained from the arterial side of the CPB circuit whole blood outflow from the device is diverted to the cardiotomy reservoir or venous reservoir. The ultrafiltrate is collected in a container connected to a vacuum source. Two possible arrangements of an ultrafiltration device in the CPB circuit are shown in Figure 10–14.

The ultrafiltrate is discarded and has the composi-

tion of glomerular filtrate. The rate at which ultrafiltrate is produced is dependent on the transmembrane pressure gradient (TMP). TMP is determined by the arterial inlet pressure (Pa), the venous outlet pressure (Pv), the absolute value of applied suction at the outlet (Pn), the oncotic pressure at the inlet (Pi), and the oncotic pressure at the outlet (Po):

$$TMP = \frac{Pa + Pv}{2} + Pn - \frac{Pi + Po}{2}$$

Pn is increased by using the regulated vacuum source connected to the outlet of the device. TMP should not exceed 500 mm Hg.

From a practical point of view, the amount of fluid that can be removed by this method is limited by the level of blood in the venous reservoir. In children, this may not allow the hematocrit to be raised to the desired level using ultrafiltration. Modified ultrafiltration (MUF) allows hemoconcentration to continue after weaning from CPB and is particularly useful for children. Inflow to the ultrafiltrator during MUF is from the aortic cannula. Outflow from the ultrafiltrator is to the right atrium. The child's blood volume is kept constant as ultrafiltrate is lost by replacing it with blood from the CPB circuit, which passes through the ultrafiltrator before being delivered to the right atrium. In this way, the CPB circuit can remain primed and the patient's blood, as well as the CPB blood, can be hemoconcentrated. This method allows a hematocrit approaching 40% to be reached and may improve clinical outcome by removing inflammatory mediators and reducing postoperative blood loss.[13]

Circuit Prime

Generally, priming solutions are asanguineous, except when severe anemia exists. Early hematic primes were associated with the "homologous blood syndrome" char-

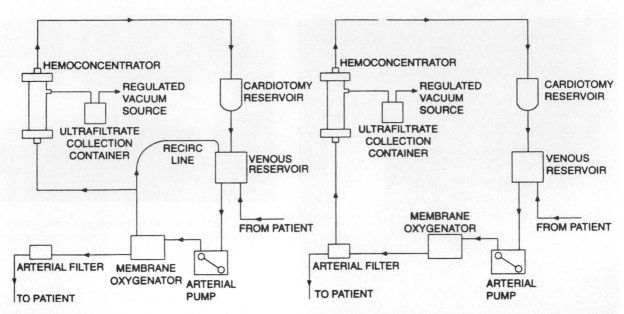

FIGURE 10–14. Two possible arrangements for use of an ultrafiltration device for hemoconcentration during cardiopulmonary bypass with a membrane oxygenator.

acterized by a shock-like syndrome with pooling of blood in the splanchnic bed.[14] This probably was due to incompatibility reactions between both donor and recipient blood and between the multiple donor units.[15] Basic prime solutions are either crystalloid or crystalloid–colloid combinations. Crystalloid primes usually are lactated Ringer's. Crystalloid–colloid primes usually are either 5 or 25% albumin added to lactated Ringer's or 6% hydroxyethyl starch (hetastarch) added to lactated Ringer's. Blood may be added to the prime if the hematocrit on CPB is lower than desired.

Comparisons of crystalloid and crystalloid–colloid primes have not shown to be either clearly superior. Weight gain and pulmonary shunt fraction is greater during the immediate postoperative period in patients receiving crystalloid primes compared with those receiving crystalloid–colloid primes.[16] Hydroxyethyl starch as a component of prime has been shown to cause clinically insignificant elevations in the prothrombin time and reductions in platelet count.[15] Albumin as a component of prime has been implicated in causing a decrease in urine volume and free water clearance on CPB.[17] Both albumin/lactated Ringer's and hydroxyethyl starch/lactated Ringer's primes are more expensive than lactated Ringer's prime; the albumin prime is four times more expensive than the hydroxyethyl starch prime.

Heparin generally is a component of the pump prime. Most centers add between 3000 and 10,000 units of heparin to the prime, depending on the size of the prime volume. This allows heparin to be distributed over the thrombogenic surfaces of the CPB circuit.

Priming with asanguineous solutions results in normovolemic hemodilution as the patient's red cell mass is diluted with prime solution when CPB commences. Hemodilution on CPB in conjunction with systemic hypothermia offers several advantages:

1. Large increases in viscosity (a major determinant of peripheral vascular resistance) accompany hypothermia. In contrast, hemodilution results in a viscosity reduction due to a decrease in red cell mass. With a hematocrit of 40%, a decrease in temperature from 37 to 27°C increases viscosity by approximately 25%. Decreasing the hematocrit from 40 to 20% at 27°C decreases viscosity by approximately 40%. Hemodilution in the presence of systemic hypothermia allows microvascular flow to be maintained without the need for the high-line pressures that accompany high peripheral vascular resistance.

2. Systemic hypothermia reduces whole-body oxygen consumption. Each 1°C decrease in body temperature results in a 5 to 6% reduction in both whole-body and cerebral oxygen consumption.[18] In contrast, hemodilution reduces oxygen delivery by reduction of red cell mass and oxygen-carrying capacity. Normovolumic hemodilution level lower than a hematocrit level of 20% has been shown to result in a decrease in total body oxygen consumption despite high flow rates on CPB.[19] Therefore, in combination with systemic hypothermia, hematocrit levels in the 20 to 25%

range allow maximal advantage of hemodilution to be made without compromising whole-body oxygen delivery in children and adults.

3. Hemodilution with hematocrit levels in the 20% range are more effective than hematocrits in the 30% range in reducing post-CPB transfusion requirements in children with cyanotic heart disease.[20]

■ PREPARATION FOR CPB

The anesthesiologist has several important responsibilities in ensuring safe preparation for CPB. These are described in the following sections.

Assess Anticoagulation

Before use of cardiotomy suction, cannulation, and commencing bypass, it is essential that adequate anticoagulation be obtained. Inadequate anticoagulation in the most dramatic form will result in overt thombus formation on the cannulas during cannulation and on the oxygenator once CPB commences. Less dramatic but equally life-threatening is a state of disseminated intravascular coagulation, which results from inadequate anticoagulation on CPB and which becomes apparent when CPB is terminated. Heparin currently is the primary anticoagulant used for CPB. It generally is acknowledged that an activated clotting time (ACT) in excess of 400 seconds is necessary to ensure adequate anticoagulation for the safe conduct of CPB.[21,22] It should be remembered that a heparin dose does not reliably result in a predictable plasma heparin concentration and that the plasma heparin concentration does not necessarily correlate with the anticoagulant effect of heparin. For this reason, a test such as the ACT, which quantitates the anticoagulant effect of heparin, must be used to safely initiate systemic anticoagulation.

Heparin should always be given into a central line through which venous return can be demonstrated easily or directly into the heart (usually the right atrium) by the surgeon. This is necessary to ensure that the heparin dose has reached the central circulation. The CVP port of a pulmonary artery catheter or of a central venous catheter works well in this regard. The ACT should be measured after heparin administration. Due to the redistribution of heparin into capillary endothelium, the ACT, 2 minutes after heparinization, is significantly higher than the 5-, 10-, and 15-minute ACTs, whereas the ACT at 20 minutes is significantly lower than the 5-, 10-, and 15-minute ACTs.[23]

Generally, a 300-units/kg dose of heparin is effective in prolonging the ACT to more than 400 seconds. Approximately 50% of patients who have been receiving preoperative IV heparin therapy will have an ACT of less than 400 seconds after a 300-units/kg dose of heparin.[24,25] The etiology of this resistance is unknown, and doses of heparin as high as 1,000 units/kg may be needed for these patients.[24] Heparin resistance has been observed in elderly patients due to decreased antithrombin-III levels and in patients with thrombocytosis.[26] Platelet factor 4 (which neutralizes heparin) may be released in excess in patients with thrombocytosis after heparin administration.[25] Other sources of heparin resistance include antithrombin-III deficiency, infective endocarditis, intracardiac thrombus, shock, and low-grade disseminated intravascular coagulation.[27] Fresh frozen plasma (a source of antithrombin-III) administration has been used as a method of improving heparin response in patients with documented antithrombin-III deficiency.[28] It also has been used to reduce the heparin requirement in cases in which the source of heparin resistance is unknown.[27,29,30] When the initial dose of heparin fails to produce an ACT of more than 400 seconds, the use of fresh frozen plasma does not guarantee such an ACT and additional heparin may still be necessary.[30] Therefore, it may be more prudent to reserve fresh frozen plasma use for documented cases of antithrombin-III deficiency and cases in which large doses of heparin (>600 units/kg) fail to produce an ACT of more than 400 seconds.

Infants and children will have higher heparin requirements than adults when dose is calculated based on weight.[31] This may be due to lower antithrombin-III levels and/or the larger surface-area-to-weight ratio present in infants and children.[31]

Administration of heparin for CPB may result in hypotension due to calcium binding and can be treated with calcium administration (1 to 2 mg/kg). If heparin is administered over 1 to 2 minutes and adequate intravascular volume is maintained, calcium administration usually is unnecessary.

Recommendations

1. A baseline ACT is not necessary because adequate hemostasis post-CPB will require neuralization of heparin and correction of platelet and coagulation factor deficiencies. The goal is a normal ACT in the post-CPB period, regardless of the baseline ACT. If a baseline ACT is drawn, the following factors must be taken into consideration:

   • An ACT drawn after incision will be shorter than one drawn before incision.[33]
   • Patients on preoperative heparin infusions and those with factor deficiencies that impair the intrinsic and common coagulation pathways will have prolonged ACTs.

2. Administer 300 units/kg of heparin via a free-flowing central venous catheter and obtain an

ACT 2 to 3 minutes later. Alternatively, the heparin dose can be injected directly into the right atrium by the surgeon.

3. If the ACT is more than 400 seconds, no additional heparin is necessary. The ACT should be checked every 20 minutes until CPB commences. Additional heparin may be necessary if an extended period of time elapses.

4. If the ACT is less than 400 seconds after the initial heparin dose, additional heparin will be necessary. By constructing a heparin dose–response curve, the required heparin dose can be determined.[33] Most centers no longer use this cumbersome method; instead, an additional 100 units/kg of heparin is administered and the ACT is checked 5 minutes later.

5. Step 4 should be repeated until an ACT level greater than 400 seconds is reached or until the total heparin dose equals 600 units/kg. Before reaching the 600-units/kg dose it may be prudent to make certain that the heparin is reaching the central circulation, that the heparin is really heparin and is not outdated, and to try a different lot of heparin.

6. When the heparin dose reaches 600 units/kg without an ACT of more than 400 seconds, 0.015 to 0.03 units/kg of fresh frozen plasma should be administered and the ACT should be rechecked.

7. If the ACT is still less than 400 seconds, additional heparin in 100-units/kg increments should be administered.

8. In patients deemed to be at high risk for heparin resistance, it is best to begin the heparinization process as early as possible so that the commencement of CPB will not be unduly delayed.

Arterial Cannulation

Arterial cannulation generally is accomplished before venous cannulation. Prior placement of the arterial cannula allows prompt commencement of CPB if severe hemodynamic compromise occurs with venous cannulation. The arterial cannula usually is placed in the ascending aorta via an aortotomy encircled by two purse-string sutures after adequate heparinization has been obtained. Transesophageal echocardiography (TEE) is useful in guiding cannula placement; this is discussed in detail in Chapter 3. So the aortotomy does not extend and so a hematoma or intimal dissection does not develop at the cannulation site, arterial blood pressure and aortic wall tension must be carefully controlled. Generally, a systolic blood pressure less than 120 mm Hg or a mean blood pressure less than 70 mm Hg is sought. It may be necessary to use vasodilator therapy

to accomplish this. Nitroprusside or nitroglycerin started at 0.15 to 0.30 µg/kg/min and titrated upward is a useful strategy. The anesthesiologist should aid the surgeon in visually examining the arterial cannula and arterial inflow line for air bubbles after they are connected and before bypass commences. These bubbles must be eliminated before bypass starts by disconnecting the cannula and the inflow line, holding them upright, and tapping them with clamps. This allows the bubbles to float upward, where they can be flushed out before the inflow line and cannula are reconnected.

Obstruction of the lumen of the aorta may occur if the cannula is introduced too far into the aorta. This is particularly likely in infants and children, in whom the arterial cannula is large relative to the lumen of the aorta. If dampening of the arterial trace and/or distension of the systemic ventricle occurs with placement of the arterial cannula, the surgeon should immediately be made aware of the situation so the cannula can be repositioned.

Venous Cannulation

Placement of the venous cannula requires that the surgeon manipulate the right atrium. This manipulation may result in a variety of atrial dysrhythmias occurring, such as atrial premature beats, atrial fibrillation, or atrial flutter. These dysrhythmias may result in hemodynamic compromise. For this reason, it is essential that the internal cardioversion paddles be on the surgical field, ready to be synchronized before atrial cannulation commences. Placement of the venous cannula also may result in rapid blood loss. This blood can be collected with the cardiotomy suction and rapid transfusion of prime solution can occur via the arterial cannula.

Assess the Priming Volume

Most CPB circuits have a prime volume of 500 to 2000 mL. The volume will vary with the size of the oxygenator, venous reservoir, and tubing. The smaller volumes generally are used for infants and children. The hematocrit (Hct) on CPB can be predicted accurately in the following manner when the pump is primed with an asanguineous solution:

$$\text{Estimated blood volume (EBV)} = \text{patient's weight in kg} \times F$$

where F = 80 mL/kg for weight < 10 kg, 75 mL/kg for weight 10 to 20 kg, and 70 mL/kg for weight > 20 kg.

$$\text{Red cell mass (RCM)} = \text{Hematocrit (Hct)} \times \text{EBV}$$
$$\text{Hct on CPB} = \text{RCM}/(\text{EBV} + \text{prime volume}).$$

If the predicted hematocrit falls below 20 to 25%, blood will have to be substituted for the asanguineous solution in the prime. This will be particularly likely in infants, children, and small adults, in whom the prime volume will be large relative to the patient's RCM. The RCM necessary to obtain the desired hematocrit on CPB is determined as follows:

$$RCM\ needed = [(desired\ Hct\ on\ CPB) \times (EBV + prime)] - RCM\ existing.$$

The volume of blood prime necessary to obtain the desired RCM will depend on whether whole blood or packed cells is used in the prime. The RCM of a blood product is determined by multiplying the Hct of the blood product by its volume. Therefore, the RCM of a unit of packed cells might be 0.7 × 350 mL or 245 mL, whereas that of whole blood will be 0.4 × 350 mL or 140 mL.

If the predicted Hct is higher than 20 to 25%, blood may be withdrawn from the patient before commencement of CPB. This will be likely to occur in large patients with high Hct values in whom the prime volume is small relative to the patient's RCM. To maintain normovolemia volume replacement with a crystalloid or colloid solution will be necessary as blood is withdrawn. Normally, 3 mL of a crystalloid solution, or 1 mL of a colloid solution, is used to replace each 1 mL of withdrawn whole blood. The amount of whole blood that can be withdrawn from the patient before CPB can be determined as follows:

$$Desired\ RCM = (desired\ Hct\ on\ CPB) \times (EBV + prime\ volume)$$

$$Desired\ pre\text{-}CPB\ Hct = desired\ RCM/EBV$$

$$Volume\ of\ whole\ blood\ to\ be\ withdrawn = EBV \times \{(Pre\text{-}CPB\ Hct - desired\ pre\text{-}CPB\ Hct)/(Pre\text{-}CPB\ Hct + desired\ pre\text{-}CPB\ Hct)/2\}$$

Various site are available for monitoring body temperature. The core is considered to be the well perfused organs; the shell is an intermediate area that consists mainly of less well perfused muscle and fat. Shell temperature will lag behind core temperature during cooling and rewarming. Homogenous cooling and rewarming should result in a minimal temperature gradient between core and shell temperature.

Tympanic Membrane. This is a core temperature site. These probes provide close correlation to the temperature at the base of the brain during cooling and rewarming and to actual brain temperature during stable hypothermia. These probes are associated with some risk of tympanic membrane damage.

Esophagus. This is a core temperature site. During rapid cooling and rewarming and during CPB, temperature measurements in the esophagus must be interpreted with caution. Because of their proximity to the mediastinum, probes in the esophagus will reflect changes in the CPB perfusate temperature and the tem-

perature of blood or fluid in the pericardial space not detected in other core sites. Esophageal temperatures will fall quickly during cooling and rise rapidly during rewarming and may not accurately reflect the patient's temperature in other core sites. The blood temperature, as measured by the pulmonary artery catheter, closely approximates esophageal temperature. The reliability of pulmonary artery (PA) catheter temperature monitoring on CPB is limited because there is little or no pulmonary blood flow at this time.

Nasopharynx. These probes, like tympanic membrane probes, provide close correlation to the temperature at the base of the brain during cooling and rewarming and to actual brain temperature during stable hypothermia. There is little risk associated with placement of these probes and, as a result, this site is preferable to the tympanic membrane. This site is not influenced by acute changes in mediastinal temperature changes and will more closely reflect actual core temperature changes.

Rectum and Urinary Bladder. Rectal temperature is not a core temperature but a measure of shell temperature. Bladder temperature and rectal temperature correlate closely. High urine output creates closer correlation between bladder temperature and core temperature. Temperature changes in the rectum and bladder will lag behind temperature changes in the core sites. These probes are therefore very useful in determining whether the core and shell temperatures have equilibrated after cooling and rewarming.

Baseline Assessment of the Pupils

The pupils should be checked for symmetry, and any asymmetry due to iridectomies or the like should be noted.

■ COMMENCING CPB

The anesthesiologist must work in concert with the perfusionist and surgeon to ensure that CPB commences smoothly. The anesthesiologist must remain alert to help solve problems.

Assess Venous Drainage

When the clamps are taken off the venous line, there should be continuous flow of venous blood from the venous cannula(s) into the pump reservoir. If this does not occur, the venous line must be examined for air lock, residual clamps, or mechanical obstruction of the cannula due to malposition. The surgeon and perfusionist must be alerted if they are not aware of the situation. The head and neck should be assessed for adequate venous drainage, and the pupils should be rechecked for symmetry. Poor SVC drainage will result in engorgement and cyanosis of the head and neck. If poor SVC drainage is suspected, the surgeon should be alerted so that the cannula can be repositioned. Transducing the sideport of the pulmonary artery catheter introducer will allow measurement of the pressure in the SVC and is useful in detecting poor SVC drainage.

Pulmonary artery catheters migrate further out into the pulmonary arterial system during CPB and ventricular apical retraction. The pulmonary artery catheter should be pulled back 5 cm as CPB commences to prevent it from lodging in the wedge position when CPB is terminated.[35]

Assess Arterial Inflow

When the pump head begins to turn, there should be continuous flow of the crystalloid prime followed by oxygenated blood into the aorta. The arterial waveform will take on a nonpulsatile flat line form punctuated by intermittent small pulsations as the LV ejects its small residual volume. When an extremely low (less than 30 mm Hg) or nonexistent pressure is observed as CPB commences, dissection at the site of aortic cannulation must be excluded immediately. If is heralded by dilation of the cannulated vessel, a reduction in arterial pressure, and an increase in the pump line pressure. An aortic dissection requires immediate attention. The dissection site must be repaired and an alternate cannulation site must be found.

Misdirection of the aortic cannula into one of the arch vessels should be assessed as CPB commences. A high arterial perfusion line pressure (when measured) is likely to result but is not uniformly observed.[36] If the subclavian or innominate artery is cannulated, the blood pressure measured in the ipsilateral radial artery will be abnormally high with wider-than-normal pulsations, whereas that measured in the contralateral radial artery will be abnormally low (below 30 mm Hg). Cannulation of either carotid artery will result in an abnormally low pressure, regardless of which radial artery pressure is being monitored. Unilateral otorrhea, rhinorrhea, conjunctival edema, facial edema, and facial coldness are later signs of arch vessel cannulation and are the result of cerebral overperfusion.[36,37] Misdirection has been reported into the innominate artery,[36] left subclavian artery,[35] and left carotid artery.[37,38] In one of the cases of left carotid cannulation, a fatal cerebral overperfusion injury occurred.[37] If misdirection is suspected, immediate action to correct the placement is necessary.

The risk of misdirection of the arterial cannula into one of the arch vessels is higher in reoperative procedures because the surgeon may need to cannulate the aorta higher to avoid the previous cannulation site. TEE is not reliable in visualizing the ascending aortic cannulation site due to the blind spot created by the trachea and bronchus (*see* Chapter 3). However, longitudinal plane imaging reliably allows visualization of the left subclavian and left carotid arteries. In conjunction with color flow Doppler imaging, it is possible to detect preferential direction of the jet of blood out of the cannula into one of these arteries.

Assess Oxygenator Function

After CPB has commenced the oxygenator function must be assessed rapidly. There should be immediate visual assessment of whether arterialized blood leaves the oxygenator and is pumped to the patient. Infrared oxygen saturation monitors on the venous and arterial lines will verify that the blood leaving the oxygenator is saturated with oxygen. Optical fluorescence technology allows on-line monitoring of both venous and arterial Po_2, Pco_2, and pH but is expensive. Blood gas analysis is routine at most hospitals and will provide information on oxygenation, CO_2 elimination, and acid–base status. If arterialized blood does not leave the oxygenator, it must be assessed immediately for malfunction. The most likely cause of failure is an inadequate supply of fresh gas to the oxygenator from a flow meter malfunction, gas line switch, or gas line leak.[38]

Inadequate oxygenation also may occur if the maximum flow capacity of the oxygenator is exceeded. Maximum flow capacity is defined as the maximum volume of blood with an hemoglobin (Hb) of 12% at a temperature of 37°C that can enter an oxygenator with an oxygen saturation of 65% and leave the oxygenator with an oxygen saturation of at least 95%. For most oxygenators, this maximal flow capacity is 6 L/min. If blood flow through the oxygenator exceeds this maximal flow capacity, arterial desaturation may result. Arterial desaturation may occur at flow rates less than the maximal flow capacity if a very low mixed venous saturation exists as bypass commences. The most common causes of a low mixed venous oxygen saturation as CPB commences are as follows:

1. Low prebypass cardiac output.
2. Oxygen consumption that is abnormally high due to shivering, light anesthesia, or hyperthermia.
3. The surface area of the oxygenator being too small to meet the metabolic demands of a large patient.

Discontinue Ventilation

Ventilation should be discontinued after bypass has commenced unless partial CPB is initiated and a significant volume of blood continues to flow through the pulmonary arteries. Complete collapse of the lungs provides optimal surgical exposure, whereas continuous positive airway pressure potentially inhibits exposure and has no proven benefit in the post-CPB period.[40,41]

Assess Need for Venting

The anesthesiologist can aid the surgeon in the decision to vent by observing the right and left heart for dilation with TEE and by examining the right atrial and pulmonary artery pressure traces on CPB. An elevation of the right atrial pressure suggests continued blood return to and dilation of the right heart. An elevation of the pulmonary artery pressure suggests significant left ventricular distension with mitral valve incompetence and retrograde flow of blood into the pulmonary artery.

Supplement Neuromuscular Blockade

It is important to administer a muscle relaxant as CPB commences to prevent the large increases in systemic oxygen consumption that accompany shivering and to prevent the diaphragmatic movement that compromises surgical exposure during the operative procedure.

The effect of hypothermic CPB on nondepolarizing neuromuscular blockade is complex. Hypothermic CPB in the absence of neuromuscular blockade enhances electrochemical neuromuscular transmission, assessed by electromyogram (EMG), but attenuates mechanical function, assessed by twitch tension development.[42] Clinically, the goal is attentuation of the mechanical response with neuromuscular blocking agents. Vecuronium neuromuscular blockade as assessed by twitch tension is enhanced and prolonged by hypothermic CPB, whereas pancuronium and d-tubocurarine neuromuscular blockade as assessed by twitch tension is unaltered.[43] Atracurium neuromuscular blockade as assessed by twitch tension development also is enhanced by hypothermic CPB.[44]

From a practical point of view, any of the nondepolarizing muscle relaxants can be utilized to ensure muscle relaxation during CPB. It has been demonstrated that pancuronium requirements are increased at the initiation of CPB and during rewarming.[45] Presumably, hemodilution at the onset of CPB reduces the plasma concentration of neuromuscular blocking agents, whereas rewarming reverses hypothermia-induced depression of twitch tension development. Pancuronium 0.05 mg/kg at the start of cardiopulmonary bypass, followed by pancuronium 0.01 mg/kg/hr while on CPB, is sufficient. When circulatory arrest is used, a large enough dose of relaxant to last the entire arrest period must be administered at the outset. It obviously is better to err on the side of overdosing the patient in this regard.

■ CONDUCT OF CPB

After CPB has commenced, the perfusionist assumes primary responsibility for its safe conduct with the cooperation of the surgeon and anesthesiologist. It is necessary to be familiar with the effects of CPB on various organ systems to make rational management decisions.

Temperature

CPB can be conducted in conjunction with systemic normothermia but is most commonly conducted in conjunction with systemic hypothermia. Systemic hypothermia reduces systemic O_2 consumption. Likewise, cerebral hypothermia reduces cerebral O_2 consumption. Q_{10} defines the ratio of O_2 consumption at a defined temperature to the O_2 consumption at temperature 10°C lower. Systemic Q_{10} is approximately 2.5, whereas cerebral Q_{10} is approximately 2.1 to 3.5. Reductions in O_2 consumption permit reductions in O_2 supply to be tolerated. Levels of hypothermia have been defined as follows: mild (32 to 35°C), moderate (26 to 31°C), deep (20 to 25°C), and profound (< 20°C). Unfortunately, not all authors adhere to this classification and care must be taken when comparing data from studies. For instance, it is not uncommon for temperatures < 20°C used in conjunction with pediatric cardiac surgery to be called "deep hypothermia."

Systemic Blood Flow

Systemic blood flow on CPB is determined by the rate at which the perfusionist rotates the arterial pump head and can be varied instantaneously. In the steady state, systemic blood flow and venous return must be equal, just as they are in the intact circulatory system. If venous return is compromised for any reason, then systemic blood flow may transiently exceed venous return and the volume of blood in the venous reservoir will diminish. As the volume of blood in the venous reservoir falls, the perfusionist must decrease systemic blood flow by decreasing the speed of pump rotation. Simultaneously, volume is added to the venous reservoir while the source of compromised venous return is aggressively pursued and corrected. If the venous reservoir is inadvertently emptied, massive arterial air embolization may occur. This disastrous complication is preventable in several ways:

1. Vigilance on the part of the perfusionist and anesthesiologist.
2. Alarm systems on the venous reservoir that sound when a predetermined reservoir volume is reached.
3. Bubble sensors on the arterial perfusion line that shut down the arterial pump head before massive transfusion of air occurs.

Optimal flow rates for CPB have yet to be defined clearly, although the obvious goal is to maintain systemic and particularly cerebral oxygen delivery. Flows of 2 to 2.4 L/min/m² commonly are used for infants, children, and adults during mild to moderate systemic hypothermia. Due to age-related differences in the relationship of surface area to weight, this corresponds to flow rates of 50 to 70 mL/kg/min in adults, 80 to 100 mL/kg/min in children, and 150 mL/kg/min in infants. Nonetheless, it has been demonstrated that flows as low as 1.2 L/min/m² will not compromise whole-body oxygen delivery when moderate systemic hypothermia is employed.[46,47] At such low flow rates, systemic oxygen delivery is maintained by increased peripheral extraction of oxygen. Because low mixed venous oxygen saturations result, oxygen delivery reserve is compromised.

Systemic Blood Pressure

Mean arterial pressure (MAP) on CPB is determined by the relationship between pump flow and systemic vascular resistance (SVR):

$$SVR = [(MAP - CVP) \times 80]/\text{pump flow rate}.$$

Recall that the central venous pressure (CVP) on CPB with adequate venous drainage will be zero and that 80 is a conversion factor. It is obvious that for a given SVR, the MAP can be instantaneously increased or decreased by increasing or decreasing pump flow. Likewise, the perfusionist is able to maintain MAP when acute increases or decreases in SVR occur by decreasing or increasing pump flow. It is not uncommon for MAP to decrease to 30 to 50 mm Hg as CPB commences despite pump flow rates of 2.0 to 2.4 L/min/m² or approximately 4 L/min in a 70-kg patient.

This is due, in part, to the enormous decrease in viscosity that occurs when the patient's blood volume and the asanguineous prime first mix.[48] Viscosity, as discussed previously, is a major determinant of SVR. Several other factors have been identified which influence SVR on CPB.[49]

- Temperature — the incidence of low SVR is significantly higher during normothermic compared with hypothermic CPB. This may be caused by vasoconstriction induced by hypothermia or release of vasodilator substances during normothermia. Long periods of rewarming during reperfusion also seem to contribute to low SVR.
- Age and peripheral vascular disease — older patients and patients with peripheral vascular disease are less likely to exhibit low SVR during CPB secondary to a less compliant arterial system.
- Diabetes — diabetics are less likely to exhibit low SVR during CPB secondary to coexisting vascular disease, sympathetic neuropathy with near maximum vasodilation at rest, and reduced baroreceptor sensitivity.

- Left ventricular function — patients with LV ejection fraction (EF) < 40% are less likely to exhibit low SVR during CPB. These patients tend to be receiving vasodilator therapy to improve systolic fucntion and may have near-maximal vasodilation at rest.

Cerebral Blood Flow

The control of cerebral blood flow on CPB is dependent on several factors, as described in the following sections.

Cerebral Autoregulation. It has been demonstrated that cerebral blood flow autoregulation is altered by hypothermic nonpulsatile CPB. Cerebral blood flow is autoregulated between MAP values of 30 and 110 mm Hg during CPB in patients without cerebrovascular disease or preexisting hypertension.[49] In contrast, in the intact circulation of normal, nonhypertensive patients, cerebral blood flow is autoregulated between MAP values of 50 and 150 mm Hg. Unfortunately, there are no data on the lower limit of cerebral autoregulation on CPB in patients with coexisting cerebrovascular disease. It may be prudent to maintain a slightly higher MAP (higher than 50 mm Hg) on CPB in patients with known cerebrovascular disease although there is no evidence to support or refute this recommendation (*see* Chapter 13).

Aging has not been shown to have an effect on cerebral autoregulation during CPB[51] but diabetics appear to have impaired cerebral autoregulation during CPB.[52] Cerebral autoregulation is lost and cerebral vascular responses to PCO₂ are attenuated under conditions of deep (18–20°C) hypothermia CPB in infants and children.[53,54] This is felt to be due to cold induced vasoparesis.

Acid–Base Management. Electrochemical neutrality seems to be important in preservation of cellular protein and enzyme structure and maintenance of the constant transcellular hydrogen (H⁺) ion gradient necessary for many cellular processes. In addition, optimal functioning of the imidazole buffering system is dependent on maintenance of cellular electrochemical neutrality. The imidazole group of the amino acid histidine is present on many blood and cellular proteins and is an important buffer. Electrochemical neutrality occurs when there are equal concentrations of hydroxyl (OH⁻) and hydrogen (H⁺) ions.[54] As temperature decreases, the dissociation constant (pK) of aqueous systems such as those found in cells increases. This results in a reduction in the concentrations of OH⁻ and H⁺ ions as temperature decreases. If there are equal concentrations of OH⁻ and H⁺, then electrochemical neutrality will be maintained. Recall that pH is the inverse log of the H⁺ ion concentration; as the H⁺ ion concentration falls, pH rises. Thus, for electrochemical neutrality to be maintained, pH must increase as temperature decreases. In an electrochemically neutral cell at 37°C, the measured pH will be 7.40, whereas in an electrochemically neutral cell at 20°C, the measured pH will be 7.80.

Changes in cellular pH during hypothermia are mediated through P_{CO_2} homeostasis. As temperature decreases, the solubility of CO_2 in blood increases. If the total CO_2 content of blood is held constant, this increase in CO_2 solubility will result in a reduction in P_{CO_2}. For example, if the total CO_2 content is held constant and the measured P_{CO_2} at 37°C is 40 mm Hg, then the measured P_{CO_2} at 20°C will be 16 mm Hg. This will cause pH to increase as temperature decreases and electrochemical neutrality will be maintained.

pH-stat and alpha-stat acid–base management are commonly discussed in association with management of CPB. pH-stat and alpha-stat regulation are acid–base management methods that directly influence blood flow to the brain and other organs. Although pH-stat and alpha-stat acid–base management commonly are mentioned in association with temperature-corrected and temperature-uncorrected blood gases, it must be emphasized that these are entirely different concepts. The method of blood gas interpretation (corrected or uncorrected) does not dictate the method of acid–base management (pH-stat or alpha-stat).

When a blood gas sample is drawn from a patient at 25°C and sent to the blood gas laboratory, the sample is warmed to 37°C before measurement. The values obtained at 37°C are called the temperature-uncorrected values. These values are converted to temperature-corrected values using a computer nomogram. The nomogram accounts for temperature-induced changes in pH, O_2 solubility, and CO_2 solubility in a closed-blood system. When pH and P_{CO_2} are measured at 37°C and then corrected to a lower temperature, the electrochemically neutral pH will be higher and the correct P_{CO_2} will be lower than the normal values at 37°C. Therefore, electrochemical neutrality is maintained by keeping pH alkalotic in temperature-corrected blood gases and normal in temperature-uncorrected gases. This is known as alpha-stat regulation. For practical purposes, it is easier to use uncorrected gases and keep pH and P_{CO_2} in the range considered normal at 37°C. It has been demonstrated that cerebral blood flow and oxygen consumption are appropriately coupled when alpha-stat regulation is used.[50,56-58]

pH stat regulation refers to maintaining pH and P_{CO_2} at normal values for 37°C when temperature-corrected gases are used and at acidotic values when temperature-uncorrected gases are used. For practical purposes, pH stat is maintained by adding CO_2 to the ventilating gas during hypothermic CPB to elevate the P_{CO_2} and decrease the pH. In contrast to alpha-stat regulation, in which total CO_2 content is kept constant, pH

stat regulation results in an increase in total CO_2 content. It has been demonstrated that hyperperfusion relative to cerebral oxygen demand (uncoupling of cerebral blood flow and metabolism) occurs when pH-stat regulation is used with hypothermic CPB.[56,59,60] This hyperperfusion state is the result of an inappropriately high P_{CO_2} for the degree of hypothermia present. It results from the ability of the cerebral vasculature to maintain vasomotor responses to varying P_{CO_2} during hypothermic cardiopulmonary bypass. As with normothermia hypercarbia causes cerebral vasodilation.

The potential danger of this hyperperfused state is that it may result in increased delivery of microemboli into the cerebral circulation.

An initial study demonstrated no difference in neurologic outcome in patients undergoing open heart procedures or coronary artery bypass grafting using hypothermic CPB with alpha-stat regulation as compared with pH-stat regulation.[61] A number of subsequent studies have clearly demonstrated a higher incidence of neurologic dysfunction in patients managed with pH-stat regulation as compared with alpha-stat management for coronary bypass surgery using hypothermic CPB.[62-64] The apparent discrepancy can be explained, in part, by the fact that patients in the initial study underwent both open and closed procedures, unfiltered bubble oxygenators were used, and pH-stat regulation may not have been achieved in the treatment group.[61] Presently, it seems that alpha-stat regulation is the most prudent course during moderately hypothermic CPB. This topic is discussed in detail in Chapter 13.

Temperature. Normothermic CPB for coronary artery bypass grafting has been associated with an increased incidence of postoperative neurologic dysfunction as compared with hypothermic CPB in two trials.[65,66] A third trial was unable to demonstrate a difference in neurologic outcome in normothermic versus hypothermic CPB.[67] This discrepancy may be because in the two studies demonstrating a difference between normothermia and hypothermia, patient temperature was rigorously maintained at 37°C in the normothermic group, whereas in the study demonstrating no difference, the normothermic group was allowed to drift between 34° and 36°C. These studies suggest that active, aggressive warming with perfusate temperatures of 40° to 42°C may produce cerebral hyperthermia and adverse neurologic outcome. This topic is discussed in detail in Chapter 13.

Pump Flow Rates. Cerebral blood flow and oxygen delivery are maintained with flow rates as low as 1.0 L/min/m² and perhaps as low as 0.5 L/min/m² when moderately hypothermic CPB (26° to 29°C) and alpha-stat regulation are used.[68,69] There seems to be a preferential distribution of blood flow to the brain when low pump flows are used. Despite this, cerebral oxygen delivery at these flows is maintained at the expense of increased cerebral extraction of oxygen and a decreased jugular venous oxygen saturation. In addition, despite the fact that somatosensory neural transmission remains intact when moderate systemic hypothermia is used and pump flow is reduced to 0.5 L/min/m², significant cerebral lactate accumulation is seen to develop after 15 minutes.[70]

Low flow rates are used most commonly in conjunction with pediatric open-heart procedures to improve exposure. In neonates, infants, and children, cerebral blood flow and cerebral metabolism are unaffected by reductions in conventional pump flow rates less than 45%.[71] When conventional flow rates (150 mL/kg/min for neonates and 100 mL/kg/min for infants and children) are reduced 45% to 70% at moderate hypothermia (26° to 29°C) with alpha-stat acid–base management, cerebral blood flow and metabolic rate decrease with a compensatory increase in oxygen extraction.[71] Similar reductions during deep hypothermia (18° to 22°C) do not produce increased oxygen extraction.[71] Minimal acceptable low flows on CPB for pediatric patients are not yet clearly defined, but cellular oxygen debt seems to occur at 5 to 30 mL/kg/min at 18°C and at 30 to 35 mL/kg/min at 28°C.[71] A recent randomized trial of low-flow (50 mL/kg/min or 0.7 L/min/m²) CPB and hypothermic circulatory arrest for repair of D-transposition of the great vessels in infants demonstrated better perioperative[72] and 1-year[73] neurologic outcome in the low-flow group.

Deep Hypothermic Circulatory Arrest (DHCA). To improve exposure during complex repairs in neonates and children and during aortic arch repairs in adults, DHCA may be used. DHCA allows cessation of blood flow, cannula removal, and exsanguination of the patient into the venous reservoir. DHCA has been studied most extensively in pediatric patients, and the subject has been extensively reviewed elsewhere.[74,75] The following guidelines have been recommended for use of DHCA in children:

1. Surface cooling as well as core cooling with CPB
2. Hemodilution to a hematocrit of 20%
3. Reduction of whole-body oxygen consumption with muscle relaxants administered before arrest
4. Possible use of electroencephalogram (EEG) to monitor suppression of brain activity with hypothermia and anesthetic agents (*see* Chapter 13)
5. Attentuation of stress responses
6. Avoidance of severe hyperglycemia before and after arrest
7. Limitation of DHCA to 30-minute intervals. If a longer period of arrest is required, a reperfusion

period of 5 minutes every 20 to 30 minutes is recommended.

Surface cooling usually is accomplished during the pre-CPB period by placing the patient on a cooling blanket at 3 to 4°C using unwarmed intravenous fluids and unhumidified gases, reducing the room temperature, and packing the patient's head in ice. These techniques allow the patient to be cooled to 30° to 32°C before beginning CPB and core cooling. Some centers administer steroids (methylprednisolone 30 mg/kg or decadron 8 mg/kg) before CPB and arrest.

Core cooling is accomplished on CPB. Some centers administer phentolamine 0.2 mg/kg as core cooling commences to promote vasodilation and more homogenous cooling. Phentolamine also may be used before core rewarming. Nasopharyngeal and rectal temperature should be allowed to equilibrate at <18°C. This normally requires 15 to 20 minutes of core cooling but may require up to 30 minutes of core cooling. Longer intervals of core cooling should be used for patients with extensive systemic to pulmonary collaterals because these shunts delay the rate of cerebral cooling on CPB.[76,77] Finally, recent evidence suggests that aggressive surface cooling and rapid core cooling with the heat exchanger water bath set at 4° to 5°C at the onset of CPB provide better suppression of cerebral metabolism than less aggressive surface and core cooling.[78]

Previously, alpha-stat acid–base management had been recommended for core cooling and rewarming during DHCA. However, a retrospective analysis of children undergoing DHCA revealed a poorer developmental outcome in patients managed with alpha stat as compared with pH stat.[79] This has prompted debate as to the best approach.[80,81] Those who favor pH stat point to the developmental study and to the fact that the luxury cerebral perfusion afforded by pH stat may promote better brain cooling and subsequent metabolic recovery.[82] Those who are opposed suggest that inadequate brain cooling secondary to a short interval of core cooling is responsible for the poorer developmental outcomes and that pH stat would be unnecessary if better core cooling were performed. Furthermore, pH-stat management may promote development of intracellular acidosis, which impairs subsequent cerebral metabolic recovery.[83] It has been suggested that an initial period of core cooling using pH stat followed by a short period of alpha-stat cooling before arrest is optimal.[83] The controversy is far from resolved and the results of a randomized trial comparing pH-stat and alpha-stat management for DHCA are pending. This topic is discussed in detail in Chapter 13.

Ideally, profound systemic hypothermia dramatically reduces cerebral metabolic rate and results in production of an isoelectric EEG. However, residual cerebral electrical activity may persist despite the use of profound systemic hypothermia. In these instances, further suppression of brain activity and cerebral metabolic rate can be accomplished with anesthetic agents such as thiopental (5 to 10 mg/kg during core cooling and before arrest). The efficacy of such interventions remains to be demonstrated in clinical trials.

Myocardial Blood Flow

On CPB, the coronary ostia are provided with hemodiluted, nonpulsatile blood flow until the aortic cross-clamp is applied. Aortic cross-clamping for cardiac surgery involves placing a completely occlusive clamp across the ascending aorta between the aortic perfuser and the aortic valve/coronary ostia such that the coronary circulation is excluded from the CPB circulation. Aortic cross-clamping has evolved as the method of choice for providing an immobile, bloodless field for the cardiac surgeon. The advantages and disadvantages of this technique will be discussed in detail in Chapter 11. Depending on the operative procedure and technique, variable periods of time may pass from the onset of CPB until placement of the aortic cross-clamp. It is therefore necessary to be familiar with the effects of CPB, hemodilution, and hypothermia on myocardial oxygen delivery and demand.

Myocardial Oxygen Delivery. Myocardial oxygen delivery is the product of coronary blood flow and the oxygen-carrying capacity of the blood. Coronary blood flow in turn is dependent on the pressure gradient between the aorta and the myocardial tissue. For the subendocardium, the tissue most likely to be hypoperfused, this gradient is equal to the MAP minus the right or left ventricular intracavitary pressure. The factors described in the following sections play a major role in determining oxygen and substrate delivery to the myocardium, particularly the subendocardium, during CPB.

CORONARY STENOSIS. Due to the pressure drop across stenoses, perfusion to the area supplied by the stenosed artery will be compromised if MAP is reduced. Therefore, whereas cerebral blood flow can be maintained with perfusion pressures as low as 30 mm Hg, myocardium supplied by stenosed arteries is poorly perfused at this pressure. Such low perfusion pressures should not be tolerated for more than a few minutes in patients with critical stenoses. Subendocardial ischemia in the distribution of a critical coronary stenosis is avoided if MAP is maintained at 80 mm Hg in the beating, empty heart.[84] However, subendocardial ischemia is inevitable in the distribution of a critical coronary stenosis when ventricular fibrillation exists despite maintenance of MAP.[84,85] This ischemia is seen to develop after as little as 15 minutes of ventricular fibrillation with MAP values as high as 80 mm Hg.[85]

VENTRICULAR DISTENSION. Ventricular distension markedly elevates intracavitary pressure and compromises subendocardial perfusion for a given MAP. The causes of ventricular distension have been discussed previously. If ventricular distension is likely to persist, then ventricular venting is necessary. Ventricular distension can be terminated promptly when aortic insufficiency exists by placing the aortic cross-clamp.

VENTRICULAR FIBRILLATION. As systemic cooling on CPB progresses, the heart becomes progressively more bradycardic. When the temperature of the heart reaches approximately 28°C, coarse ventricular fibrillation ensues and myocardial wall tension increases. As the temperature of the heart continues to drop, the ventricular fibrillation becomes finer, myocardial oxygen consumption decreases, and ventricular wall tension diminishes.[85] Ventricular fibrillation, particularly in hypertrophied myocardium, results in poor perfusion of the subendocardium due to increased myocardial wall tension and a reduced perfusion gradient.[86] When the MAP is less than 50 to 60 mm Hg, subendocardial perfusion will be compromised when ventricular fibrillation exists.[87-89]

HEMODILUTION. In the presence of adequate perfusion pressures, myocardial oxygen delivery is potentially compromised by the reduced oxygen-carrying capacity of the hemodiluted systemic perfusate despite the fact that the decreased temperature allows more oxygen to be carried in solution. Oxygen delivery to the nonhypertrophied ejecting myocardium is unlikely to be compromised unless the Hct is less than 15%.[90] In the presence of coronary stenoses or concentric hypertrophy, Hct values in the 20 to 30% range may be needed to prevent ischemia in the normothermically bypassed heart.

HYPOTHERMIA. Hypothermia reduces coronary vasodilator reserve capacity and potentially limits myocardial oxygen delivery. Therefore, despite the fact that hypothermia reduces myocardial oxygen consumption (described later), subendocardial ischemia develops in the beating, empty heart when MAP is lower than 50 mm Hg at 28°C due to attenuated coronary vasodilator reserve.[91]

ACID–BASE MANAGEMENT. Alpha-stat acid–base management has been shown to result in better myocardial oxygen delivery, lactate extraction, and post-CPB function than pH-stat management.[92,93]

Myocardial Oxygen Demand. CPB provides a state of hypothermic, hemodiluted, nonpulsatile flow during which the heart is called upon to do little or no mechanical work in the form of generating pulsatile flow. The two major determinants of myocardial oxygen consumption on CPB are temperature and the functional status of the myocardium.

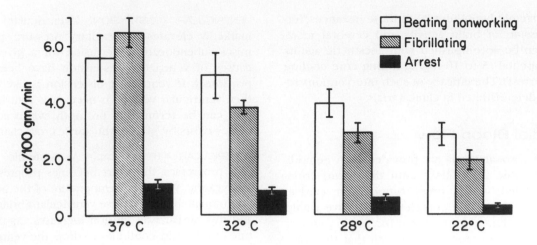

FIGURE 10–15. Left ventricular oxygen consumption during three functional states (beating empty, fibrillating, and arrested) and at four temperatures. Hypothermia clearly reduces myocardial oxygen consumption for any functional state. Below 37°C, the beating, empty heart consumes the most oxygen, followed in decreasing order by the fibrillating and arrested heart. *(From: Buckberg GD, Brazier JR, Nelson RL, et al: Studies on the effects of hypothermia on regional myocardial blood flow and metabolism during cardiopulmonary bypass I. The adequately perfused beating, fibrillating, and arrested heart. J Thorac Cardiovasc Surg 1977; **73:89**.)*

TEMPERATURE. As Figure 10–15 illustrates, the lower the temperature of the heart, the less oxygen it consumes per minute for a given functional state. For the beating empty heart, oxygen consumption per beat increases as temperature decreases due to the positive inotropic effect of cold on the myocardium. However, this increase in oxygen consumption per beat is overshadowed by the larger relative decrease in heart rate induced by cold, such that oxygen consumption per minute falls.[86]

FUNCTIONAL STATUS. The functional status of the myocardium — whether beating and empty, fibrillating, or arrested — plays an important role in determining myocardial oxygen consumption (*see* Fig. 10–13). Below 37°C, the heart consumes less oxygen fibrillating than it does beating and empty. Recall, however, that subendocardial perfusion is compromised by fibrillation due to increased wall tension.

Renal Function

Normally, renal blood flow is autoregulated between renal artery pressures of 80 and 180 mm Hg. Despite this, it has been demonstrated that systemic flows as low as 1.6 to 1.8 L/m²/min and sustained MAP as low as 50 mm Hg during hypothermic, hemodiluted, nonpulsatile CPB do not result in a deterioration of post-CPB renal function.[94,95]

In addition, pH management, pulsatile versus nonpulsatile flow, and CPB temperature do not influence renal function during or after CPB.[96–98] The quantity of urine output on CPB has not consistently been found to be a predictor of post-CPB renal dysfunction.[94,95,99] The

presence of preexisting renal dysfunction, post-CPB ventricular dysfunction and low cardiac output, use of intra-aortic balloon pump (IABP), emergency operative procedures, DHCA, and advanced age have all been identified as independent predictors of post-CPB renal dysfunction and acute renal failure.[99,100] In fact, the presence of post-CPB ventricular dysfunction and low cardiac output is a major risk factor in the development of post-CPB renal dysfunction and failure.[94,95]

Generally, a urine output of 1 mL/kg/hour is considered adequate while on CPB. Although urine output on CPB has not consistently been correlated with post-CPB renal function, oliguria (urine output less than 0.5 mL/kg/hr) must be considered a harbinger of renal hypoperfusion and ischemia.

Recommendations

Lower Limits of Mean Arterial Pressure. The safe lower limits of MAP on CPB must be determined with all organ systems in mind. If the aortic cross-clamp is applied within 1 to 2 minutes after the start of CPB, a MAP greater than 30 mm Hg with a pump flow of 2.0 to 2.4 L/min/m² is acceptable for patients without cerebrovascular disease. For patients with known cerebrovascular disease, a MAP in excess of 50 mm Hg may be more prudent (*see* Chapter 13). If there is a delay in placing the aortic cross-clamp, then attention should be directed toward optimal perfusion of the myocardium. A MAP of at least 50 mm Hg should be maintained for perfusion of the beating, empty heart. If ventricular fibrillation develops and is likely to persist for more than a few minutes, then MAP must be elevated to at least 60 to 80 mm Hg to ensure subendocardial perfusion. Likewise, if ventricular fibrillation is likely to persist, myocardial temperature should be decreased to reduce oxygen consumption and improve perfusion by lowering wall tension. A vent must be placed if left ventricular distension occurs. If coronary stenosis or ventricular hypertrophy also exists, MAP must be elevated to 80 to 100 mm Hg and the cross-clamp should be applied as soon as possible.

If high pump flows are needed to maintain the desired MAP, the maximal flow capacity of the oxygenator may be exceeded. If this is likely, then SVR can be increased and pump flow can be decreased to maintain MAP. SVR can be increased by transfusion of blood into the venous reservoir to increase viscosity. Generally, this strategy is reserved for those instances in which the Hct is less than 20%. SVR can also be increased by increasing arteriolar tone. The simplest way to accomplish this is by infusing an alpha agonist such as phenylephrine into the pump. As a rule, as CPB progresses, arteriolar tone will increase and the phenylephrine can be stopped.

Maintenance of Mean Arterial Pressure. Generally, a mean arterial blood pressure less than 70 mm Hg is sought to remain within the limits of cerebral autoregulation and to reduce noncoronary collateral blood flow after the aortic cross-clamp has been applied. Because the noncoronary collaterals originate from the mediastinum and pericardium, the blood they deliver to the heart will be at the same temperature as the patient (25° to 30°C). While the aortic cross-clamp is in place and the heart is arrested with cardioplegia, optimal myocardial temperature is usually between 8° and 15°C. Excessive noncoronary collateral flow will cause the heart to rewarm and compromise myocardial preservation. Excessive noncoronary collateral flow also will compromise surgical exposure by causing bleeding from the incised coronary artery. There are several strategies available to reduce MAP and each has its own advantages and disadvantages:

1. Reduction of pump flow is useful as a temporizing maneuver, but a prolonged reduction may result in systemic and cerebral hypoperfusion.
2. Sodium nitroprusside is a very effective arteriolar dilator and thus very useful in reducing SVR. It is easily titratable, has no negative inotropic properties, and has a short half-life. It has, however, been implicated in causing reversible platelet dysfunction.[101]
3. Nitroglycerin does not cause platelet dysfunction, is easily titratable, and has a short half-life and no negative inotropic properties but is much less effective than nitroprusside. This decreased effectiveness is because nitroglycerin is primarily a venodilator and actively adheres to the plastic components of the CPB circuit.[102]

4. Volatile anesthetic agents such as halothane, enflurane, and isoflurane are very effective, easily titratable arteriolar dilators. To be used, the vaporizer must be spliced into the fresh gas flow line of the oxygenator. This gives the anesthesiologist one more vaporizer to worry about maintaining and filling on a piece of equipment that is not his or her primary responsibility (the pump). Damage has occurred when isoflurane has been spilled accidentally on both bubble[103] and membrane[104] oxygenators. In addition, the volatile agents have negative inotropic effects that can compromise separation from CPB. During CPB with a bubble oxygenator, isoflurane is completely eliminated from the circulation 10 minutes after it is discontinued.[105] Nonetheless, it is prudent to discontinue these agents before removal of the aortic cross-clamp to allow adequate time for their elimination before coronary blood flow resumes.

Acid–Base Management. Alpha-stat management of acid–base status should be used for patients undergoing normothermic and hypothermic CPB. This is accomplished most easily by using temperature-uncorrected blood gases with pH maintained at 7.42 to 7.45. The best acid–base management strategy for patients undergoing DHCA remains to be elucidated. Some centers use alpha stat, others use pH stat, and others use pH stat during the initial core cooling period followed by a short period of continued core cooling with alpha stat before arrest.

Urine Output. A urine output of at least 1.0 mL/kg/min is desirable on CPB. Urine output should be assessed every 15 minutes while on CPB. If urine output falls below 0.1 mL/kg/15 min (0.5 mL/kg/hr), action is necessary. Aortic perfusion pressure should be increased to at least 50 mm Hg. If this fails to increase urine output or if aortic perfusion pressure is already optimized, a diuresis with furosemide 0.5 to 1.0 mg/kg or mannitol 0.5 to 1.0 g/kg should be instituted. The volume expansion that occurs after mannitol infusion does not present a problem while on CPB. Induction of a brisk diuresis will result in obligate potassium losses in urine. This can result in hypokalemia before termination of CPB, which may require potassium supplementation.

Monitoring of Anticoagulation. Maintenance of anticoagulation must continue on CPB. The anticoagulant effect of heparin is prolonged by the presence of hemodilution, the anticoagulant effect of hypothermia, and the prolonged half-life of heparin associated with hypothermia.[106] Nonetheless, the anticoagulation status of the patient should be monitored every 30 minutes with an ACT. Care must be taken to ensure adequate anticoagulation during rewarming.

■ PREPARATION FOR TERMINATION OF CPB

It is essential that an organized approach be taken to preparing for the termination of CPB so that a smooth transition is ensured. The anesthesiologist has the following responsibilities:

Ensure Rewarming

After induced systemic hypothermia, it is necessary to ensure that adequate core rewarming has occurred before termination of CPB. The perfusionist will assume responsibility for using the heat exchanger to rewarm the patient when instructed to do so by the surgeon. Generally, rewarming will take place for 30 to 60 minutes before termination of CPB, depending on the degree of the hypothermic state and its length. As with cooling, the site of temperature measurement is important in assessing homogeneous core rewarming. Equilibration of the bladder or rectal temperature and the nasopharyngeal temperature at 36° to 37°C is desired.

The rate of rewarming is important as jugular venous desaturation, indicative of increased cerebral oxygen extraction, has been noted in adults during rewarming.[107] Furthermore, increased cerebral O_2 extraction during rewarming may be associated with subsequent cognitive defects, particularly in elderly patients.[108,109]

Despite homogeneous core rewarming, it is not uncommon for the patient's core temperature to drop 2° to 3°C in the hour after termination of CPB. This is due to reperfusion of the cold extremities, which results in a reequilibration of the patient's temperature at a lower-than-ideal core temperature. The greater the difference between the nasopharyngeal and the rectal or urinary bladder temperature when CPB is terminated, the greater will be the expected temperature "afterdrop." This temperature afterdrop may result in arterial vasoconstriction and shivering, which will increase myocardial oxygen consumption. Infusing sodium nitroprusside and maintaining MAP greater than or equal to 70 mm Hg by increasing pump flow has been advocated as a method of decreasing afterdrop.[110] This method allows the poorly perfused cold extremities to be perfused with warmed blood before termination of CPB. Therefore, the caloric load of peripheral rewarming is in large part assumed by the heat exchanger and not the patient. Warmed, humidified airway gases have not been found to be beneficial in decreasing afterdrop in adults because humidifiers contribute relatively little heat to the large heat deficit that exists at the termination of CPB.[111] Likewise, the use of warming blankets has not been found to be beneficial in preventing afterdrop in adults[110] but probably is of benefit for children due to their larger surface-area-to-volume ratio.

Ensure Adequate Anesthesia and Muscle Relaxation

Awareness is unlikely to exist during systemic hypothermia but may occur during rewarming. Unfortunately, this has not been well studied. In one study, 2% of patients had awareness for events late in the operative procedure (after CPB) when the primary amnesic agent was lorazepam 0.05 mg/kg given at induction.[112] Common sense dictates that some provision for amnesia be made as rewarming occurs. Volatile anesthetic agents, if used during CPB, should not be relied on because they will be terminated before termination of CPB. A benzodiazepine such as midazolam 0.05 to 0.15 mg/kg, diazepam 0.075 to 0.15 mg/kg, or lorazepam 0.025 to 0.05 mg/kg, administered as rewarming commences, is advocated. A muscle relaxant should be titrated to ensure adequate relaxation as the hypothermic attenuation of mechanical muscle function is reversed.

Perform an Air Drill

After procedures in which the heart chambers are opened, or in closed procedures in which air may have entered a heart chamber, it is necessary to evacuate all intracardiac air before termination of CPB to avoid systemic air embolism. The following steps are important in an air drill.[113]

1. The patient is placed in the head-down position.
2. The lungs are ventilated and the table is rolled from side to side to help remove sequestered air from the pulmonary veins.
3. With the open atrium under a pool of blood, the venous line is partially clamped and the lungs are ventilated so that the ventricle becomes filled with blood. The ventricle is then freed of air either by aspiration on a vent line or by apical needle aspiration while the heart is elevated and massaged.
4. The atriotomy or vent insertion site is closed under a pool of blood.
5. The proximal aorta is evacuated of air either through the cardioplegia cannula or through a needle placed in the aorta.
6. The aortic cross-clamp is not removed until the heart and aorta are free of air so that no air is ejected systemically.

TEE is valuable during deairing as it allows the effectiveness of the previously described procedures to be monitored on line. Air is particularly likely to be retained in the LV apex, LA, right coronary sinus, and the pulmonary veins; the right upper pulmonary vein in particular.[114,115] Removal of retained air requires flow through the pulmonary circulation and the heart. TEE surveillance, combined with the joint efforts of the surgeon, anesthesiologist, and perfusionist, are necessary to prevent systemic air emboli during evacuation procedures.

Determine Factors That May Make Termination of CPB Difficult

Communication with the surgeon is essential here. It is best to know about the possibility of residual defects or incomplete revascularization before termination of CPB. Such information will affect the management of the patient if termination of CPB is difficult or impossible. Factors that increase the likelihood of a need for inotropic support to terminate CPB are discussed in detail in Chapters 4 to 7. In general, poor preoperative systolic function, particularly where pre- or intraoperative inotropic support is needed; poor myocardial preservation and/or a long cross-clamp time; and incomplete revascularization; all increase the likelihood that post-CPB inotropic support will be needed.

Defibrillation

After rewarming and removal of the aortic cross-clamp, it may be necessary to defibrillate the heart. Several factors have been shown to be important in determining the ease of defibrillation after aortic cross-clamp removal:

1. A serum potassium level of approximately 5 mEq/L decreases the defibrillation threshold compared with levels approximately 0.5 mEq/L lower.[116] In many institutions where potassium cardioplegia solution is used, serum potassium levels are in the 5-mEq/L range at the time of aortic cross-clamp removal. If defibrillation is unsuccessful in the presence of a low serum potassium, infusion of potassium should be considered.
2. Aortic perfusion pressure and the duration of reperfusion after aortic cross-clamp removal are important. Recall that subendocardial perfusion is compromised during ventricular fibrillation on CPB. A longer reperfusion period after aortic cross-clamp removal allows for washout of the products of anaerobic metabolism and for replenishment of energy stores. For these reasons, a mean aortic blood pressure of at least 50 mm Hg for greater than 5 minutes is likely to increase the success of defibrillation.[116]
3. Myocardial temperature at the time of defibrillation should be greater than 30°C.[116] Recall that spontaneous fibrillation occurs at a myocardial temperature of 28°C.
4. Patients with valvular heart disease are more likely to need multiple defibrillation attempts compared with patients without valvular disease.[116] This is not due to the increased heart

weight and size often associated with valvular heart disease.[116,117]

5. Lidocaine has been shown to reduce the number and the energy dose of DC shocks required for ventricular defibrillation.[118] Lidocaine 1 mg/kg is given 5 minutes before aortic cross-clamp removal. Prophylaxic lidocaine infusions do not seem to be necessary. Lidocaine infusions initiated after CPB in coronary artery bypass patients have been shown to slightly decrease the incidence of nonsustained ventricular tachycardia with no apparent clinical benefit.[119] Infusions of lidocaine are warranted for treatment of high-grade ventricular ectopy. Hypomagnesemia has been demonstrated in up to 70% of patients after CPB and may predispose ventricular and supraventricular tachyarrhythmias.[120] As a result, some centers supplement magnesium (2.4 to 4.8 g or 100 mg/kg in children) before or immediately after termination of CPB.

After optimization of conditions as described above, ventricular defibrillation is accomplished by the use of internal paddles. Much lower energy levels are required than for transthoracic defibrillation; 2.5 to 20 joules or watt-seconds using internal paddles is sufficient to defibrillate most hearts. Defibrillation energy is started at 2.5 joules and increased in 2.5- to 5-joule increments.

Inability to defibrillate a heart of a patient in whom conditions have been optimized suggests ongoing myocardial ischemia from poor revascularization or from coronary air or particulate emboli. Coronary air embolus is particularly common in procedures in which the left heart has been opened. When coronary air embolus is suspected, efforts should be made to increase perfusion pressure to break up bubbles and move them through to the venous side of the circulation. This can be performed in several ways. Obviously, the less aggressive methods should be tried first:

1. Increasing MAP on CPB will increase coronary perfusion pressure.
2. Placing a partially occluding clamp distal to the aortic perfuser will increase coronary perfusion pressure further.
3. Re-cross-clamping the aorta and reinfusing a small dose of cardioplegia will deliver a low-viscosity solution at high pressure into the coronary arteries.

Potassium and Acid–Base Balance

Hypokalemia will compromise defibrillation and has been discussed. Hyperkalemia presents other problems. As the serum potassium level climbs greater than 5 mEq/L, the PR and QT intervals shorten and the T waves become peaked. A serum potassium level greater than 6 mEq/L will increase the incidence of dysrhythmias and conduction abnormalities due to a reduction in the threshold for membrane depolarization. This may predispose the patient to pacemaker-induced dysrhythmias. Pacing may not be possible as the serum potassium approaches 7 mEq/L. As levels reach 9 to 10 mEq/L, idioventricular rhythms progress to ventricular asystole and fibrillation.

Immediate treatment of an elevated serum potassium with electrocardiogram (ECG) changes is indicated. Calcium chloride 10 mg/kg, sodium bicarbonate 0.5 to 1.0 mEq/kg, or 1 mL/kg of 50% dextrose and 0.1 units/kg of regular insulin IV all work immediately to reduce serum potassium by shifting it intracellularly. Where severe hyperkalemia exists, diuretic therapy will be necessary to increase the excretion of potassium as well. In patients with compromised renal function, efforts must be made to avoid hyperkalemia resulting from use of potassium cardioplegia. It is possible to scavenge the cardioplegic solution from the coronary sinus so that it does not end up in the pump and elevate the serum potassium.[121] In addition, it also is possible to use cold crystalloid cardioplegia without potassium in these patients.

Alpha-stat pH management should continue as the patient is warmed. Total CO_2, PCO_2, and pH should be corrected if necessary before termination of CPB. It may be necessary to give sodium bicarbonate to treat a metabolic acidosis or to adjust oxygenator gas flow to correct PCO_2.

Obtain Pacing

After the aortic cross-clamp has been removed, the heart has been defibrillated, and potassium and acid–base status has been corrected, it may be necessary to obtain pacing. This is normally accomplished with the aid of epicardial pacing wires.

Epicardial pacing can be bipolar (two wires on the heart) or unipolar (one wire on the heart, one through the skin of the epigastric area). Atrial, ventricular, or atrial and ventricular wires may be placed. Atrial wires usually are placed at or near the right atrial appendage. Ventricular wires are placed on the free wall of the right ventricle. The wires are brought out through the skin in the epigastric area and can be removed easily postoperatively. By convention, the atrial wires are brought out on the right side of the epigastric area and the ventricular wires are brought out on the left side. The combination of atrial and ventricular wires allows atrial, ventricular, or atrial ventricular sequential pacing when used in combination with a dual output (atrial and ventricular) sequential external pacemaker (*see* Fig. 10–16).

The current output (milliamperes) of the pacemaker is increased slowly until the desired cardiac

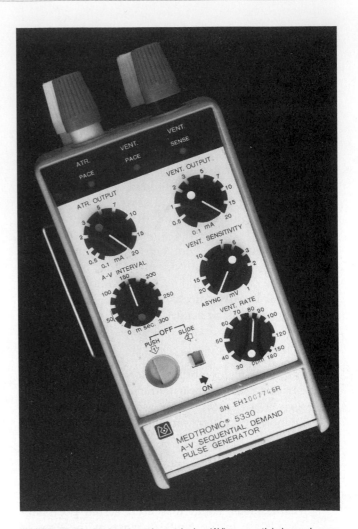

FIGURE 10–16. Medtronic atrioventricular (AV) sequential demand pacemaker. This pacemaker can be used for atrial, ventricular, or AV sequential demand pacing. Two atrial and two ventricular output ports are seen at top. In this photograph, atrial and ventricular current output are maximal at 20 mA. The AV interval (time lag between atrial and ventricular pulses) is 150 msec. The pacemaker rate is set at 80 pulses per minute (ppm); thus, atrial and ventricular pulses will be delivered 150 msec each at a rate of 80 per minute. Ventricular sensitivity is set to asynchronous mode. In this mode, the pacemaker will not sense electrical activity and will continue to pace at the set rate regardless of the patient's underlying rhythm. Pacemaker threshold for detection of electrical activity can be increased by reducing ventricular sensitivity toward a minimum value of 1 mV.

chamber is captured. Each pacemaker spike must result in appropriate atrial and/or ventricular capture and contraction. There also must be appropriate sequential contraction of the atria and ventricles when atrial ventricular sequential pacing is desired. It is necessary to look at both the ECG trace and the heart to ensure capture. After the minimum current output necessary for capture has been determined (usually 5 to 10 milliamperes), the current output is increased by 5 more milliamperes to ensure continued capture. In patients having undergone previous cardiac surgery (redos), atrial and ventricular scarring may necessitate higher current outputs than normal to obtain capture. In some instances, capture may not be possible until the epicardial pacer wire is moved to a site with less scarring. When atrial ventricular sequential pacing is required, the optimal PR interval will need to be determined. Generally, an interval of 150 msec is chosen to start and then varied within the 120- to 200-msec range as needed to optimize ventricular filling and cardiac output. Because electrocautery is used extensively in the post-CPB period, the sensing threshold (millivolts) of the pacemaker may have to be increased toward the nonsensing or asynchronous mode to prevent inhibition of the pacemaker by electrocautery radiofrequency current.

Arterial Pressure and Pump Flow

After the aortic cross-clamp has been removed the MAP should be maintained in the 60 to 80 mm Hg range to allow adequate reperfusion of the heart to replenish adenosine 5′-triphosphate (ATP) stores and remove anaerobic metabolites. In preparation for termination of CPB, it is best to accomplish this by maintaining a calculated SVR in the range of 1000 to 1500 dynes/sec/cm^{-5} and adjusting pump flows accordingly. SVR can be varied with the use of either phenylephrine or nitroprusside as needed.

Hematocrit

Generally, an Hct greater than 20% is sought as CPB terminates. Advance planning is needed to achieve this goal. Reduction of the prime volume may be needed for some patients, as described previously. Vigorous diuresis during CPB may result in hemoconcentration; likewise, the use of a hemoconcentrating device during CPB will achieve the same end. Transfusion of red blood cells may be necessary if these methods fail or are not appropriate due to low venous reservoir levels on CPB. Hct levels in the low 20s as CPB terminates at 37°C should be expected to result in low SVR due to decreased viscosity.

Resume Ventilation

Before terminating CPB, it is necessary to be certain that the lungs are easily reinflated, that if the pleural cavity is not opened no pneumothorax exists, and that all fluid is sucked out of open chest cavities. Caution should be exercised when reinflating the lungs of patients with internal mammary artery (IMA) grafts to avoid stretching or avulsing the grafts. It also is necessary to resume ventilation at a minute ventilation that will prevent hypercarbia after CPB terminates. Large increases in pulmonary vascular resistance are seen with small elevations in arterial CO_2 after cardiac surgery.[122] Such elevations in pulmonary vascular resistance may cause RV failure in patients with compromised RV systolic function. It should be remembered that CO_2 production is likely to be higher at the termination of CPB than it was before initiation of CPB due to the differences in body temperature.

For children, it may be desirable to maintain mild hypercarbia in certain instances. In patients undergoing systemic to pulmonary artery shunt procedures, pulmonary overperfusion may occur if the shunt is large and pulmonary vascular resistance is low. Hypercarbia may provide protection from overperfusion by increasing pulmonary vascular resistance. Conversely, high pulmonary vascular resistance and high airway pressures will compromise pulmonary blood flow in children having undergone the Fontan procedure (right atrial to pulmonary artery anastomosis) due to the low driving pressure for pulmonary blood flow (see Chapter 6).

■ TERMINATION OF CPB

Termination of CPB requires very close cooperation between the anesthesiologist, surgeon, and perfusionist. CPB should not be terminated until each of these three individuals involved is satisfied with the status of the patient. Specific recommendations for termination of CPB are given in Chapters 4 through 7. The following basic principles should be remembered.

The range of filling pressures expected to provide optimal preload for a particular patient should be discussed before termination of CPB. It is best to err on the side of underfilling the heart to avoid ventricular distension. Distension will compromise subendocardial perfusion and elevate wall tension. Visual inspection of the heart will provide information on distension and wall motion but it must be remembered that it is primarily the free wall of the right ventricle that is visible through a median sternotomy. The functional status of the right ventricle is not necessarily the same as that of the left ventricle.

If inotropic support is anticipated to be necessary for termination of CPB, it is best not to start infusing the agent into the heart any earlier than 5 minutes before termination of CPB. Early infusion of inotropic agents increases myocardial oxygen consumption while the heart is being reperfused on CPB. This compromises replenishment of energy stores and serves no useful purpose.

CPB should be terminated at a pump flow and SVR that are reasonable for the patient. If the perfusionist is pumping 5 L/min with a MAP of 50 mm Hg, then the patient will have to have a cardiac output greater than 5 L/min to maintain a MAP of 70 mm Hg after CPB has been terminated. If such an output is an unreasonable expectation, then efforts must be made to increase SVR to a normal range before termination of CPB. This will allow termination of CPB at the desired MAP with a cardiac output that the patient can realistically produce. Recall that on CPB, SVR = (MAP × 80)/pump flow, with the normal range 1000 to 1500 dynes × sec × cm^{-5}.

CPB is terminated by gradually clamping the venous line so that venous return to the reservoir is impeded. Simultaneously, the perfusionist slows the rate of the arterial pump head. This results in gradual transfusion of the patient via the arterial cannula. The volume of blood in the venous reservoir will slowly drop as the process continues. When adequate preload is obtained as assessed by pulmonary capillary wedge pressure, central venous pressure, visual inspection of the heart, and TEE the transfusion is terminated.

As the heart fills with blood, ejection should begin. The simplest way to assess this is by observing the arterial waveform. Elevation of filling pressures with evidence of poor ejection is indicative of afterload mismatch. There is either poor systolic function or a level of afterload that is excessive for the inotropic state of the heart. If SVR has been normalized before termination of CPB, efforts can be directed toward increasing the contractile state of the heart with inotropes.

In some institutions, calcium chloride 5 to 10 mg/kg is used as the first intervention in this setting. Calcium chloride increases the inotropic state of the myocardium and induces an increase in SVR that outlasts the inotropic effects. Often, this intervention is all that is required to complete termination of CPB. Others believe that calcium chloride administration is contraindicated at this time because of the compromised calcium homeostasis that accompanies the insult of aortic cross-clamping (*see* Chapter 11). Administration of calcium may exacerbate ischemic damage by causing accumulation of intracellular calcium. Beta-adrenergic agents, on the other hand, increase intracellular calcium but also promote its reuptake into the sarcoplasmic reticulum and may be more appropriate in this setting.

Before therapy for low arterial pressure is initiated, the possibility that a discrepancy exists between the intra-arterial radial arterial pressure and the central aortic or femoral artery pressure should be investigated. This can be determined by simultaneous observation of the central aortic and radial artery pressures and will prevent unnecessary therapeutic interventions from being made. Central aortic pressure can be monitored easily by having the surgeon place a small needle in the ascending aorta or aortic cannula attached to a length of pressure tubing that can be passed over the drapes to a transducer. It has been demonstrated that after CPB, intra-arterial radial arterial systolic pressure may underestimate central aortic, brachial, or femoral artery systolic pressure by 10 to 34 mm Hg in a significant number of both children[123] and adults.[124-128] The etiology of this discrepancy is unclear with both arterial-to-venous shunting in forearm blood vessels and peripheral vas-

ospasm implicated.[128,129] It has been demonstrated that the gradient develops upon initiation of CPB and is not affected by vasodilators or vasopressors.[127] Because this discrepancy may persist for up to 90 minutes after the termination of CPB,[124,129] it may be necessary to place a femoral arterial line for continued monitoring.

If the patient separates from CPB with high filling pressures, ventricular distension, low cardiac index (below 2 L/min/m²), and low MAP (under 40 mm Hg), prolonged efforts to correct the hemodynamics of CPB should not be made. Reinstitution of CPB will prevent the downward spiral induced by subendocardial ischemia and elevated wall tension. In addition, it will allow reperfusion of the heart during a low energy consumption state. After CPB has been reinstituted several questions must be addressed:

- Was the ventricular failure biventricular or was only one ventricle involved?
- Was there pulmonary artery hypertension and RV failure?
- Was there RV or LV ischemia?
- Is the prosthetic valve working properly?
- Is all of the monitoring equipment functioning properly and giving accurate information?
- Are there unsuspected lesions in evidence, such as previously unsuspected MR?
- Is the repair of the congenital lesion complete and successful? Is there a residual defect that requires repair? (*See* Chapter 6.)
- Is the heart rate optimized?
- Is the appropriate type of pacing being performed and is the pacemaker capturing the desired chambers?

Having addressed these questions, therapy directed toward specific problems (Chapters 4 through 7) can be instituted, and another attempt can be made to terminate CPB.

■ POST-CPB MANAGEMENT

After termination of CPB, it is necessary to stabilize the patient and to reverse heparinization to allow decannulation and chest closure.

Protamine Administration

Protamine is a polyvalent cation derived from salmon sperm that is currently used to neutralize systemic heparinization. Protamine normally is given after stable hemodynamics are maintained after termination of CPB. It should not be administered until the likelihood that having to reinstitute CPB is small. After protamine neutralization of heparin begins, the cardiotomy suction should not be used and removal of the arterial and venous cannulas should proceed. This prevents contamination of the heparinized CPB circuit with protamine should prompt reinstitution of CPB be necessary and prevents thrombus formation on the cannulas.

There are several approaches to the neutralization of heparin with protamine, all with reportedly good clinical results. Some centers use 1.0 to 1.3 mg of protamine for each 100 units of heparin determined to exist at the termination of CPB. This ratio is based on the in-vitro protamine to heparin neutralization ratio of 1.3:1.0.[34] The amount of heparin present is determined by obtaining an ACT when CPB terminates and using reverse extrapolation of the patient's heparin dose-response curve to correlate ACT and heparin dose. This method has been criticized because the ACT obtained at the termination of CPB is prolonged by factors other than heparin, such as CPB-induced platelet dysfunction and hemodilution.[130,131] This may result in an overestimation of the heparin present at the termination of CPB and a larger than necessary protamine dose.

Some centers simply administer a fixed dose of protamine based on the patient's weight (3 to 4 mg/kg) regardless of the heparin dose administered, whereas others administer 1.0 to 1.3 mg of protamine for each 100 units of heparin administered. Obviously, these methods do not rely on any post-CPB assessment of residual heparin effect (ACT) to determine the protamine dose. Nonetheless, these methods have been shown to result in adequate heparin reversal.[131] In the case of the fixed-dose regimen, heparin reversal is obtained at much lower protamine doses than predicted by the reverse extrapolation method.[131]

In a different approach, some centers use heparin assays and then calculate the protamine dose based on the patient's blood volume and a neutralization ratio of 1.0 to 1.3.[132] Despite the fact that not all heparin present in blood exerts an anticoagulant effect and need be neutralized, this method has been shown to provide adequate heparin reversal with low doses of protamine.

Other centers use in-vitro protamine titration. This method requires ACT tubes containing protamine, creation of a dose response–neutralization curve, and an estimate of the patient's blood volume.[133] This method results in adequate heparin reversal at lower doses of protamine than predicted by the reverse extrapolation method.

The ACT should be checked after administration of the selected protamine dose. The goal is to return the ACT to a normal value. There are several adverse reactions associated with protamine administration. These protamine reactions are well documented in adults but it must be emphasized that they occur in pediatric patients as well.[133] The reactions associated with protamine administration are described in the sections that follow.

Pulmonary Hypertension. Pulmonary hypertension after protamine reversal of heparin may be so profound as to result in RV failure and circulatory collapse.[135,136] This reaction seems to be idiosyncratic and is associated with high levels of thromboxanes and C5a anaphylatoxins, which result in bronchoconstriction and pulmonary vasoconstriction in susceptible patients after protamine administration.[137] Recent evidence suggests that heparin–protamine complexes are the initiating mechanism.[138] This reaction seems to occur in susceptible patients regardless of whether the protamine is infused into the right or left atrium,[136] administered as a bolus,[135] or given as a slow infusion.[136] To date, there is no good evidence to suggest that patients with preexisting pulmonary hypertension are at greater risk for this reaction.[139] Fortunately, this reaction is rare, occurring in less than 3% of cases.[137,138]

Systemic Hypotension. This is a much more common reaction to protamine administration.[140,141] The decrease in systemic blood pressure is due to a decrease in SVR. Pulmonary histamine release has been implicated in causing this SVR reduction.[141,142] Systemic hypotension is more common in patients with poor ventricular function secondary to their inability to compensate for the decrease in SVR.[141] The incidence of this reaction is related to the speed of infusion. Regardless of the infusion site (right atrium, left atrium, aorta, peripheral vein) this reaction can be avoided or at least decreased in severity when a slow infusion (over more than 3 minutes) of protamine is used.[140,143]

Protamine-induced platelet aggregation and release of vasoactive substances also may produce systemic hypotension, particularly when platelet concentrates are infused in association with protamine.[144]

True Allergic (Anaphylactic and Anaphylactoid) Reactions. True allergic reactions require the presence of IgE or IgG antibodies to the substance in question. Typical manifestations of this type of reaction include: hypotension, flushing, urticaria, bronchospasm, and pulmonary edema secondary to capillary leak. IgE-mediated reactions are the result of IgE–antigen complex causing mast cells to degranulate. IgG-mediated reactions are the result of activation of the complement cascade by the IgG–antigen complex.

Formation of these antibodies is enhanced in patients who have been exposed previously to the allergen or to a substance that is similar to the allergen. An increased incidence of protamine reactions has been reported to occur in patients taking NPH insulin. These patients are presumed to be presensitized to protamine from the insulin preparation. An incidence of reactions as high as 27% has been reported,[145] but prospective studies suggest an incidence of approximately 0.6%.[146,147] An increased incidence of reactions also has been suggested in patients with fish allergies[148]; however, prospective analysis does not support this contention.[147] Theoretically, vasectomized men might be at an increased risk secondary to the existence of antisperm (protamine) antibodies. IgG antibodies to protamine were found in 29% of vasectomized men.[149] One case of an allergic protamine reaction has been reported in a vasectomized man in whom high titers of protamine specific IgG antibody were subsequently found.[149]

Therefore, the risk of true allergic reactions in patients who were previously sensitized to protamine seems to be low. Of note is the fact that a case–control study demonstrated that the risk of an adverse response to protamine was 25 times higher in patients with protamine-specific IgG antibody and 95 times higher in patients with protamine-specific IgE antibody.[150] One must conclude from these data and the prospective data that the percentage of patients exposed to protamine or protamine-like substances who go on to develop IgG or IgE antibodies is low. Furthermore, not all patients with IgG antibodies to protamine develop reactions to protamine.

Efforts have been made to identify patients at risk for protamine reactions by testing for IgE and IgG antibodies in those patients likely to be presensitized to protamine. Skin testing commonly is used to test for IgE-mediated hypersensitivity. Enzyme-linked immunosorbent assays (ELISAs) and radioallergosorbent tests (RASTs) are used to detect minute quantities of circulating IgG and IgE to an allergen. Recently, both skin testing and ELISA in patients at risk for protamine reactions have been shown to have a high false-positive rate or poor specificity. In other words, many patients with a positive test for protamine antibodies do not go on to develop a reaction.[151] This severely limits the value of this type of testing.

Noncardiogenic Pulmonary Edema. This reaction has been reported to occur as a delayed reaction (more than 20 minutes after administration) to protamine in a small number of patients (approximately 30%).[143] It is not entirely clear that protamine alone is responsible for this reaction as concomitant blood product administration also has been implicated.[143]

Heparin Rebound. Rarely, heparin rebound may occur after protamine administration. This phenomenon has received much attention and is defined as a reprolongation of the ACT occurring 1 to 8 hours after adequate heparin neutralization, which renormalizes with protamine. Several etiologies have been suggested. A large quantity of heparin remains bound to plasma proteins for up to 6 hours after clinically adequate neutralization of heparin with protamine. As protamine is cleared, the protein-bound heparin dissociates slowly and binds to antithombin III to produce an anticoagulant effect.[152] It is not surprising, then, that the inci-

dence of heparin rebound has been shown to be reduced when a heparinization protocol that uses lower heparin doses is compared with one that uses higher doses.[153] Concurrent protamine metabolism also may be a factor.[154] Heparin rebound also may be due to enhancement of residual heparin by infusion of blood components such as fresh frozen plasma that elevate antithrombin-III levels.[155]

Recommendations

1. Slow administration (25 mg/min) of the chosen protamine dose into the right atrium via a central venous catheter. The central venous route is chosen over peripheral venous administration to ensure that the drug reaches the central circulation just as with heparin administration. The slow infusion rate will obviate the need for left atrial or aortic infusion, which may cause systemic air and particulate emboli.

2. If systemic hypotension due to a decrease in SVR occurs, the protamine infusion should be stopped. The SVR should be elevated with an alpha agonist (phenylephrine, norepinephrine) and preload should be optimized with volume infusion. The protamine infusion can then be restarted slowly while SVR and preload are maintained.

3. If pulmonary hypertension occurs, immediate action is necessary. The protamine should be stopped in an effort to reduce pulmonary vascular resistance while the circulation is supported. Infusion of epinephrine may be necessary to provide inotropic support of the RV. If pulmonary hypertension persists, infusion of nitroglycerin, or prostaglandin E_1 (started at 0.01 to 0.02 µg/kg/min) into the right atrium will help reduce pulmonary vascular resistance and improve RV function. If large doses of vasodilating agents are needed, vasopressor agents may be necessary to treat systemic vasodilation. The vasopressor agents should then be infused through a left atrial catheter to limit their effects on the pulmonary vasculature. Protamine infusion may have to continue with continued vasopressor/vasodilator therapy. In severe cases, reinstitution of CPB may be necessary.

4. If an anaphylactic or anaphylactoid reaction occurs in association with protamine administration, therapy with epinephrine, steroids, and bronchodilators is warranted.

5. An ACT should be repeated after protamine infusion. If the ACT remains elevated above normal, an additional 0.25 to 0.5 mg/kg of protamine should be administered and the ACT rechecked.

6. If heparin rebound is suspected, the ACT should be rechecked. If the ACT is elevated, additional protamine 0.25 to 0.5 mg/kg should be administered. This usually is adequate to treat heparin rebound.

Assessment of Coagulation Status

Bleeding or oozing that continues after appropriate protamine reversal of heparin must be investigated. The most likely causes are listed below.

Surgical Bleeding. The surgical field must be assessed carefully for bleeding sites. This inspection must include the cut sternal edges, the harvest site of the mammary artery, and the back of the heart.

Platelet Function Defects. This is the most common cause of a bleeding problem after CPB after heparin has been reversed and surgical bleeding has been controlled.[156-158] Transient defects in platelet plug formation and aggregation are seen in all patients put on CPB.[156-158] Generally, platelet function returns to near-normal status 2 to 4 hours after CPB.[158]

This transient dysfunction is caused by platelet surface glycoprotein (GP) receptors that are redistributed internally into platelets during CPB.[159,160] The presence of plasmin is responsible for this inactivation or redistribution of GP receptors. These GP receptors are essential for platelet adhesion and aggregation. Platelet adhesion is mediated through von Willebrand's factor, which binds to the platelet GP Ib-IX complex and to exposed endothelial elements. Platelet-to-platelet aggregation is mediated through fibrinogen binding to the GP IIb-IIIa complex.

These defects are exacerbated and prolonged by drugs that inhibit platelet function. Aspirin inhibits thromboxane A2 production for 5 days after ingestion, whereas nonsteroidal anti-inflammatory drugs (NSAIDs) have similar effects only as long as significant blood levels are maintained. This impairs platelet activation and aggregation. Preoperative aspirin ingestion has been shown to increase blood loss after CPB by exacerbating CPB-induced platelet dysfunction (*see* Chapter 1). Additionally, 15 to 20% of patients who ingest aspirin are hyperresponders, which further contributes to platelet dysfunction.[161]

Platelet functional defects tend to compound hemostasis problems from all other causes as well. Whether CPB-induced platelet dysfunction results in clinical problems with hemostasis depends on the extent of the defects, the patient's preexisting platelet function, and the presence or absence of additional coagulation defects.

Desmopressin acetate (DDAVP) in a dose of 0.3 µg/kg increases levels of factor VIII and von Willebrand's factor and shortens bleeding time induced by disease states (uremia, chronic liver disease) and a variety of congenital and acquired platelet function defects (aspirin,[162] NSAIDs). von Willebrand's factor is known to mediate platelet aggregation and adherence on thrombogenic surfaces. The increased levels of von Willebrand's factor that result from DDAVP infusion may be responsible for improving platelet function post-CPB. Despite this, DDAVP has not been shown to be consistently effective in reducing blood loss or homologous transfusion requirements in pediatric[163] and adult cardiac surgical patients when given after CPB and protamine administration.[164] Meta-analysis of a number of studies suggests that DDAVP is most effective in reducing blood loss as compared with placebo in a subset of cardiac surgical patients who experience excessive blood loss.[164] Which patients constitute this subset and whether this reduction in blood loss is associated with a reduced homologous transfusion requirement are as yet undetermined.

Some patients who can benefit from DDAVP have been identified. Thromboclastography can be used to identify patients who will benefit from DDAVP after CPB.[165] Patients with an MA < 50 mm (*see* Chapter 3) indicative of reduced platelet function demonstrate less blood loss and a reduction in homologous transfusion requirements after coronary artery bypass graft (CABG) surgery with DDAVP compared with placebo. Patients taking preoperative aspirin have been shown to have reduced blood loss after CABG with DDAVP compared with placebo[166-168] with two of the studies demonstrating a reduced requirement for homologous transfusions.[167,168]

DDAVP relaxes vascular smooth muscle[169] and should be administered slowly (over 20 to 30 minutes) to avoid reductions in SVR with subsequent hypotension.[170]

Thrombocytopenia. Platelet counts do decrease on and after CPB, but generally they do not fall below 100,000.[156-158] In general, the fall in platelet counts on CPB is slightly greater than what would be expected with hemodilution, with the difference being due to platelet adherence to synthetic surfaces, platelet destruction, platelet sequestration in the lungs, and platelet consumption in wounds.[159] Because platelet function defects are so prevalent, thrombocytopenia, when it does exist, is an important cause of altered hemostasis.

Dilution of Clotting Factors. There is a dilutional reduction in the levels of factor II, factor V, factor VII, factor X, and factor XI for up to 48 hours after CPB.[156,158] Levels of factor VIII:C have been shown to decrease[156] and increase[158] during and after CPB. In general, factor levels rarely fall below the 30% level, which compromises hemostasis.[156,158] Likewise, the fibrinogen level is reduced by dilution during and after CPB but rarely falls below the critical 100-mL/dL level.[156,158] It is not surprising, then, that the prophylactic administration of fresh frozen plasma has not been shown to reduce bleeding after routine CPB procedures in adult patients without preexisting coagulopathies.[171] Obviously, if preexisting deficiencies in factor levels or activities are present, CPB-induced reductions in factors levels may become clinically significant and factor replacement may be required.

Infants and small children are at risk for significant dilution of coagulation factors when the prime volume is large relative to their blood volume. Dilution of coagulation factors is particularly likely to occur when the patient is polycythemic (reduced plasma volume) and when large volumes of asanginous or packed red cell primes are used in place of whole blood primes. Children whose transfusion requirements in the immediate post-CPB period are met with whole blood that is less than 48 hours old have total transfusion requirements 85% less than those treated with component therapy.[172]

Fibrinolysis. It generally is agreed that enhanced fibrinolytic activity occurs during CPB.[156-158] This is a direct consequence of compliment activation and contact activation of the instrinic clotting cascade that occurs with commencement of CPB despite adequate heparinization.[173] Fibrinolysis occurs as the result of plasmin breaking down insoluble fibrin. Plasmin is generated when factor-XII-dependent plasminogen activator stimulates conversion of plasminogen to plasmin. Release of tissue plasminogen activator from endothelial sources also stimulates this conversion. Three antifibrinolytic agents currently are in use and have been shown, to varying degrees, to improve hemostasis after CPB. Ideally, these agents are administered before CPB and before stimulation of the coagulation and fibrinolytic processes. The three agents epsilon-aminocaproic acid (EACA), tranexamic acid (TA), and aprotinin are summarized below.

Mechanism of Action

EACA. This drug is a synthetic analog of lysine. There are five lysine binding domains or kringles within the structure of plasminogen. EACA inhibits fibrinolysis by occupying these sites and preventing the interaction of plasminogen with fibrin.

TA. This drug also is a synthetic analog of lysine. It is 6 to 10 times more potent than EACA with a similar mechanism of action.

Aprotinin. Aprotinin is naturally occurring (bovine lung) 59-amino-acid polypeptide that is a serine protease inhibitor. Plasma concentrations of aprotinin inhibit the action of plasmin and kallikrein by reversible binding to the active serine sites of these enzymes. Because aprotinin binds 30 times more avidly to plasmin than kallikrein, a higher plasma concentration of aprotinin is needed to inhibit kallikrein as compared with plasmin. Concentrations of aprotinin high enough to inhibit kallikrein are not maintained throughout CPB, even when high doses are used. Therefore, inhibition of the contact activation system probably is not as important to the action of aprotinin as inhibition of plasmin-induced fibrinolysis. Administration of aprotinin to patients undergoing CPB results in reduced formation of fibrin degradation products, increased alpha$_2$ antiplasmin (an inhibitor of plasmin) and plasminogen activator inhibitor activities, and decreased tissue plasminogen activator release.[1] Neutralization of plasmin by aprotinin prevents translocation of GP Ib from the platelet surface and may allow normal platelet adhesive function to be maintained.[174]

Aprotinin also seems to be capable of blunting the inflammatory response induced by CPB and heart and lung reperfusion in a manner similar to that of methylprednisolone by inhibiting release of interleukins and tumor necrosis factor.[175]

Dosage and Administration

EACA. This drug should be given as 100 to 150 mg/kg IV after induction and 10 to 15 mg/kg/hr, usually for 5 to 6 hours.[176] Higher doses (as much as 40 g) have been used, but no dose–response data exist to support them. The drug is renally concentrated and the infusion rate should be decreased in accordance with creatinine clearance.

TA. This drug is given as 10 mg/kg IV after induction and 1 mg/kg/hr, usually for 5 to 6 hours.[176] Dose-response data support use of this dose, although doses higher than 40 mg/kg were not investigated.[177] Recently, much higher doses of TA (10 g) have been used. The drug is renally concentrated and the infusion rate should be decreased in accordance with creatinine clearance.

Aprotinin. Aprotinin is dosed in kallikrein inactivation units (KIU). One KIU is the quantity of aprotinin that produces 50% inhibition of 2 kallikrein units; 100,000 KIU of aprotinin is equivalent to 14 mg of aprotinin. Current packaging of aprotinin contains 10,000 KIU/mL or 1.4 mg/mL.

High-dose aprotinin (Hammersmith protocol) is defined as:

- 2 million KIU (280 mg) as an IV loading dose over 30 minutes after induction
- 500,000 KIU/hr (70 mg/hr) as an intraoperative infusion
- 2 million KIU (280 mg) in the pump prime

Some centers modify the high-dose protocol based on patient weight as follows:

- 20,000 KIU/kg (2.8 mg/kg) to a maximum of 2 million KIU as an IV loading dose over 30 minutes after induction

- 20,000 KIU/kg (2.8 mg/kg) to a maximum of 2 million KIU infused over 5 hours intraoperatively (4,000 KIU/kg/hr for 5 hours)
- 20,000 KIU/kg (2.8 mg/kg) to a maximum of 2 million KIU in the pump prime

Low-dose aprotinin is defined as:

- 1 million KIU (140 mg) as an IV loading dose over 30 minutes after induction
- 250,000 KIU/hr (35 mg/hr) as an intraoperative infusion
- 1 or 2 million KIU (140 or 280 mg) in the pump prime

An alternate lower-dose protocol is the addition of 2 million KIU (280 mg) to the pump prime alone.

The incidence of severe allergic reactions to aprotinin seems to be approximately 0.5% on initial exposure.[153] It is recommended that a test dose of aprotinin 0.5 or 1.0 mL be administered before commencement of therapy. If there is no reaction after 10 minutes, the bolus dose can be given.

The incidence of severe allergic reactions in patients with previous exposure is approximately 2.8 to 10%.[178,179,180] Both fatal and nonfatal anaphylactic shock have occurred during secondary exposure with the documented presence of IgE and IgM antibodies. Patients who are likely to have previous exposure are those who have undergone prior cardiac surgical procedures. In particular, bridge to cardiac transplant patients are likely to have prior exposure because aprotinin has been demonstrated to reduce blood loss and transfusion requirements after placement of mechanical assist devices (*see* below and Chapter 11). A second exposure is likely at the time of device explantation and cardiac transplantation (*see* Chapter 7). Aprotinin use also has been extended to noncardiac surgical procedures (orthopedics, ENT) and previously was used for treatment of pancreatitis. Patients who have had a previous exposure within 6 months have a 3-fold increase in the incidence (4.5% versus 1.5%) of adverse reactions upon reexposure.[180]

For patients with previous exposure, it is recommended that a skin prick test or intradermal test be performed before administration of a very dilute (<1 μg/mL) intravenous test dose.[182] Patients with previous exposure may benefit from pretreatment with steroids and a histamine H_1/H_2 receptor antagonist. In addition, some recommend delaying injection of the bolus dose until the surgeon is ready to commence CPB so that circulatory support can be initiated immediately in case of a reaction. Aprotinin should not be added to the CPB pump prime until it is certain that the patient has not reacted to the test dose or bolus dose.

Efficacy

Many studies examining the efficacy of EACA, TA, and aprotinin in reducing blood loss and homologous transfusion requirements have been performed. Most studies compare these agents to placebo, but some head-to-head comparison studies exist. Comparisons are complicated by the fact that not all groups use comparable dosages of these agent. Doses of EACA as high as 40 g and doses of TA as high as 10 g have been used. Comparisons are further complicated by the fact that the "trigger" criteria for transfusion of homogolous blood products varies from study to study. Some of these studies have been compiled previously.[159,160,183-185] The existing literature is summarized here.

EACA.   EACA has been shown to reduce blood loss after both primary pediatric[186] and adult[187-189] cardiac surgical procedures. EACA has not been studied in association with repeat cardiac surgical procedures to date. EACA has not been demonstrated consistently to reduce the requirement for homologous transfusions despite reductions in postoperative bleeding.[160,183,185] Direct comparisons of EACA (5 to 10 g loading dose followed by 2 g/hr for 5 hours) and high-dose aprotinin showed aprotinin to be more effective than EACA in reducing postoperative blood loss and the need for homologous transfusions.[190,191]

TA.   TA has been shown to reduce bleeding and homologous transfusions requirements after primary and repeat adult cardiac surgical procedures.[192-194] TA, like EACA, has not been shown consistently to reduce homologous blood requirements despite reductions in postoperative bleeding.[160,195] High-dose aprotinin is more effective than TA (10 mg/kg followed by an infusion) in reducing blood loss and the need for homologous transfusions.[183,185,196] High-dose TA (10g) is effective in reducing blood loss and autologous transfusion requirements compared with placebo[197] and may be as effective as high-dose aprotinin in reducing blood loss and transfusion requirements in repeat valve replacement patients.[198] TA (5 g) and low-dose aprotinin reduced homologous transfusion requirements and blood loss comparably in another study.[199]

Aprotinin.   High-dose and low-dose aprotinin have been shown consistently to reduce bleeding and homologous transfusion requirements in patients undergoing primary and repeat cardiac surgery.[159,160] Postoperative chest-tube output is reduced 35 to 80% as compared with controls and the percentage of patients requiring donor–blood transfusions is reduced from 40 to 100% in controls to 20 to 60% in aprotinin treated patients.[159,160] Aprotinin added to the pump prime (2 million KIU or 280 mg) also has been shown to reduce bleeding and homologous transfusion requirements in patients undergoing primary and repeat cardiac surgery; however, the reductions are not as dramatic as for high- and low-dose regimens.[159,160,200] High-dose and low-dose aprotinin also have been demonstrated to reduce blood loss and homologous transfusion requirements in patients taking preoperative aspirin.[159,201] High-dose aprotinin has been demonstrated to reduce blood loss and transfusion requirements in patients undergoing heart, heart–lung, and lung transplantation (*see* Chapter 7).[202-204] In addition, aprotinin reduces blood loss and transfusion requirements in patients receiving mechanical circulatory assist devices (*see* Chapter 11).[205,206]

The efficacy of aprotinin in children is less clear, partly because of large variations in the dose of aprotinin studied.[207-211] Three studies have demonstrated no benefit to the use of aprotinin.[208-210] Two studies, one using 2.8 mg/kg as a bolus, 2.8 mg/kg in the pump prime, and an infusion of 1.4 mg/kg/hr during CPB[201] and the other using 3.9 mg/kg as a bolus, 4.0 mg/kg in the pump prime, and an infusion of 1.0 mg/kg/hr during CPB[211] have demonstrated reduced postoperative blood loss and reduction in the number of patients requiring homologous transfusions as compared with placebo and control, respectively. Both low-dose aprotinin (120-mg/m^2 bolus, 120 mg/m^2 in the pump prime, and an infusion of 28 mg/m^2/h) and high-dose aprotinin (240-mg/m^2 bolus, 240 mg/m^2 in the pump prime, and an infusion of 56 mg/m^2/h) have been demonstrated to be superior to placebo in reducing homologous blood product requirements in children undergoing repeat heart surgery.[212]

Special Considerations Regarding Aprotinin

The use of aprotinin involves some special considerations:

- Effects on whole blood clotting times — aprotinin is known to prolong the whole-blood activated partial thromboplastin time (APTT) but not whole blood prothrombin time.[213] Nonactivated whole blood clotting time (WBCT) is prolonged by aprotinin as well and this prolongation is aprotinin-dose-dependent and enhanced by heparin.[214] In addition, aprotinin prolongs the celite-activated ACT and, to a much lesser extent, the kaolin activated ACT.[214] As with the WBCT, heparin enhances this effect. It was believed previously that this prolongation of APTT and celite ACT was the result of aprotinin inhibition of the bean phosphatide activator in the APTT assay and of the celite activator in the ACT assay. Kaolin ACT was believed to be unaffected because aprotinin is bound by kaolin or because kaolin has greater potency to activate coagula-

tion than celite. Therefore, it was conceivable that a prolonged celite ACT in the presence of aprotinin might occur in the presence of inadequate heparinization. Based on these conclusions, it was recommended that to avoid under-anticoagulation on CPB, celite ACT should not be used. Instead, a kaolin ACT, a thrombin-based test such as the high-dose thrombin time (HiTT), a heparin assay such as automated protamine titration assay, or a high-dose thromboplastin time (HiPT) is recommended.[215-217]

- Recent evidence suggests that aprotinin has an anticoagulant effect due to inhibition of contact phase activation and that the prolongation of the celite ACT corresponds to enhanced anticoagulation obtained with aprotinin.[214,218] Reliable anticoagulant in the presence of aprotinin using the celite ACT has been documented.[218] Until this issue is resolved, adherence to the previously described recommendations is the most prudent course.

Perhaps most important is the fact that the APTT should not be used in algorithms to detect post-CPB coagulopathies or heparin effect in patients receiving aprotinin.

- Renal function — aprotinin is filtered and rapidly bound to the brush border of the proximal convoluted tubules, where it remains until metabolized. 90% of the administered dose appears in the kidney in a few hours and remains there for 12 to 14 hours.[219] In addition, the deleterious effects of aprotinin seem to be exacerbated by hypothermia. All of these issues have raised concerns about renal function in patients undergoing cardiac surgery with hypothermic CPB. A large body of data to date indicates that although high-dose aprotinin administration is associated with tubular proteinuria and transient mild plasma creatinine elevations (0.5 mg/dL), it has minimal adverse clinical effects on renal function.[159,160,220] Similar creatinine elevations have been seen with low-dose aprotinin (30,000 KIU/kg in the pump prime) in pediatric cardiac surgical patients.[221] Considering its effects on renal function, aprotinin should be used at a reduced dosage in patients with preexisting renal dysfunction.

- Coronary artery bypass graft patency — concerns that aprotinin use may contribute to early graft occlusion have not been substantiated. A few studies have detected a small, statistically insignificant decrease in IMA and saphenous vein patency in aprotinin-treated patients, whereas other studies have detected no difference between aprotinin-treated patients and controls.[159]

Deep Hypothermic Circulatory Arrest (DHCA)

— Concern has been raised regarding the use of aprotinin in association with DHCA due to reports of increased mortality, renal failure, myocardial infarction, disseminated intravascular coagulation, and death.[222,223] Others report significant reductions in homologous blood requirements and a trend toward improved outcome with aprotinin despite significant, transient renal dysfunction.[224,225] The discrepancy between these reports may be due, in part, to inadequate heparinization in the groups reporting complications. Use of aprotinin the setting of DHCA requires further elucidation.

Post-CPB Bleeding

The following scheme is suggested for patients who exhibit persistent bleeding after what should be adequate heparin reversal with protamine.

1. Check for surgical bleeding. This is more difficult than it sounds, because it may involve significant manipulation of the heart to visualize distal coronary anastomoses, the posterior portions of aortic and pulmonic suture lines, or atrial suture lines.

2. Administer additional protamine 0.5 to 1.0 mg/kg. If available, an ACT with heparinase is valuable at this point. Medtronic supplies a two-chamber cartridge. Both chambers contain kaolin and calcium chloride. One chamber contains highly purified heparinase capable of rapidly neutralizing 6 units/mL of heparin.

   - If the heparinase ACT is normal (120 + 20) and the nonheparinase ACT is within 10% of this value, then the heparin has been neutralized and no additional protamine is necessary.
   - If the heparinase ACT is normal and the nonheparinase ACT is elevated, then the patient is heparinized and more protamine is warranted.
   - If both the heparinase ACT and the nonheparinase ACT are elevated above normal and are within 10% of each other, the patient should be evaluated for other causes of an elevated ACT besides heparin such as factor deficiencies (intrinic and common pathway). No further protamine is necessary.
   - If both the heparinase ACT and the nonheparinase ACT are elevated above normal and the nonheparinase ACT is elevated more than 10% above the value of the heparinase ACT, the patient has both heparin and other factors as a cause. Additional protamine and evaluation for factor deficiencies both are warranted.

3. Consider platelet dysfunction. Prophylactic platelet transfusion after CPB does not seem to be warranted;[226] however, when there is post-CPB bleeding that warrants treatment and residual heparin and surgical bleeding have been eliminated as causes, platelets should always be administered as a first-line treatment. A unit of platelets contains 5.5×10^{10} platelets; 0.1 units/kg generally will raise the platelet count by 50,000 to 80,000. In most cases, this will control the bleeding.[158] For cases in which other deficiencies exist, platelet therapy will prevent platelet defects from compounding the problem. Platelet dysfunction is particularly likely if the CPB time > 2 hours or if the patient has had recent aspirin or NSAID ingestion. Significant dysfunction can exist in the presence of a normal platelet count, but thrombocytopenia will exacerbate the problem. Dilutional thrombocytopenia should be considered in neonates, infants, and children in whom the CPB prime volume, although reduced, is large relative to the patient's blood volume. A platelet count < 80,000 to 100,000 with continued bleeding is an indication for platelet transfusion.

   As discussed previously, DDAVP may be considered as an alternative to platelet transfusion in certain subsets of patients. Because this therapy has not proved to be consistently reliable, there should be a low threshold to initiate platelet transfusion if continued platelet dysfunction is suspected.

4. When platelet therapy fails to correct the problem, a coagulation profile should be obtained. An ACT, prothrombin time (PT), activated partial thromboplastin time (aPTT), thrombin time (TT), platelet count, fibrinogen level, and fibrin degradation products (FDP) should be measured. It should be kept in mind that these values may take up to 1 hour to obtain. Data from a thromboelastograph (TEG) (*see* Chapter 3), when available, are extremely valuable.

   - aPTT > 1.5 control
   - PT > 1.5 control
   - TEG R and K prolonged with R >>> K

All of these findings point to factor deficiencies. Initial therapy is fresh frozen plasma (FFP) 10 to 15 mL/kg.

   - fibrinogen < 100 mg/dL
   - TT > 1.5 control
   - TEG R and K slightly prolonged with MA < 40

These findings are compatible with hypofibrinogenemia. Initial therapy can be with cryoprecipitate 0.25 units/kg. Cryoprecipitate is the best source of fibrinogen, factor VIII, and factor XIII. One unit of cryoprecipitate contains approximately 150 mg of fibrinogen and 80 units of factor VIII in 15 mL.

It should be remembered that hypofibrinogenemia rarely exists in the post-CPB setting in the absence of factor deficiencies. Factor deficiencies will be treated with FFP, which contains 2 to 4 mg of fibrinogen/mL or 500 to 1000 mg of fibrinogen/250 mL. This is equivalent to 3.5 to 7 units of cryoprecipitate. When large quantities of FFP are used, cryoprecipitate may not be needed to treat hypofibrinogenemia.

Finally, platelet dysfunction and thrombocytopenia also will reduce the TEG MA and, in severe cases, also prolong the R and K. The TEG, in combination with a fibrinogen level and platelet count, will allow differentiation of the two etiologies.

- D-dimers > 1.0 μg/mL
- fibrin split products > 40 μg/mL
- TEG A_{60} < CMA, LYS60 > 15%

These findings implicate fibrinolysis and use of one of the three antifibrinolytic agents discussed earlier should be considered.

This scheme is complicated by the use of aprotinin, which prolongs the aPTT, the celite ACT (and to lesser extent the kaolin ACT), and the R of the TEG.[227]

Decannulation

Generally, the venous cannula is removed first. With the arterial cannula in place, urgent reinstitution of CPB can be accomplished quickly. Hemodynamic compromise due to atrial dysrhythmias and volume loss may accompany removal of the atrial cannula. As long as only a small portion of the protamine has been infused, volume infusion via the arterial cannula can be undertaken safely.

To avoid undue stress on the aortotomy and to allow its easy closure, the aortic systolic blood pressure should be 120 mm Hg or less for arterial decannulation. Nitroprusside infusion may be necessary to achieve this goal.

Pericardial and Chest Closure

The pericardium is not routinely closed after all cardiac surgical procedures. When a normal pericardium, small ventricular volumes, and low filling pressures exist, pericardial closure does not affect left ventricular diastolic or systolic function.[228] For patients with distended ventricles, myocardial edema, and poor systolic function after CPB, pericardial closure may further compromise hemodynamics secondary to extrinsic reduction in diastolic filling. Chest closure may produce the same effects.[229] In patients with severe post-CPB ventricular dysfunction, this compromise may prohibit pericardial and/or chest closure despite initiation or acceleration of inotropic and vasodilator therapy. In these patients, the chest is left open and covered with a piece of latex rubber or an adhesive plastic drape,[229] with closure accomplished 2 to 3 days after the procedure.

On occasion, one or both of the epicardial pacer wires may "short out" and become nonfunctional when the chest is closed. Therefore, atrial and ventricular epicardial pacing should be checked after the sternal edges are allowed to fall together but before chest closure. If the wires become nonfunctional, it may be necessary for the surgeon to move them to alternate sites on the atrium and ventricle before chest closure.

■ MANAGEMENT OF UNUSUAL PROBLEMS ON CPB

For patients requiring CPB, there are several conditions that present difficult management problems.

Dialysis

Hemodialysis-dependent patients have successfully undergone cardiac surgery employing CPB.[230] In addition, dialysis has been performed successfully on CPB.[231] Dialysis performed on CPB offers several advantages by obviating the need for dialysis in the immediate pre- and postoperative period. Hemodynamic instability often accompanies dialysis. This instability can be detrimental to cardiac surgical patients in the immediate pre- and postoperative period. Dialysis on CPB allows this instability to be avoided. Hemolysis, blood transfusions, and the use of cardioplegia solution create a large potassium load, which in hemodialysis-dependent patients may result in severe hyperkalemia after CPB. Dialysis on CPB allows control of serum potassium as well as of intravascular volume. Finally, anticoagulation for dialysis in the immediate postoperative period can be avoided.

Generally, dialysis on CPB can be accomplished easily.[230] We have, however, encountered two major problems with intraoperative dialysis:

1. Bicarbonate and not acetate should be used as the buffer source for CPB dialysis. We have encountered persistent metabolic acidosis during dialysis using acetate. Acetate must be metabolized to bicarbonate to provide buffering. Acetate metabolism and bicarbonate production is compromised when hepatic perfusion is poor,[232] as might be expected with hypothermic CPB.

2. Patients who are dialyzed with reusable dialyzers may develop anaphylactoid reactions to ethylene oxide used to sterilize the dialyzers. This is believed to be secondary to development of IgE antibodies.[233] To avoid this reaction, reusable dialyzers are normally carefully flushed clean of ethylene oxide with priming fluid before use.[234] In one such patient, we took precautions to flush the dialyzer; however, nearly fatal hypotension and bronchospasm developed when the patient

was exposed to the membrane oxygenator, which had been sterilized with ethylene oxide and had not been flushed clean. Therefore, in these patients, it is important to flush both the dialyzer and the oxygenator clean of ethylene oxide.

Cold-Reactive Proteins

Cold-reactive proteins are proteins that, when cooled below a specific temperature (their thermal amplitude or critical temperature), precipitate or cause red cell agglutination. The subsequent microvascular occlusion can lead to cerebral and myocardial ischemia and infarction as well as hepatic and renal dysfunction. Subsequent hemolysis also can complicate the picture. Patients with these proteins present difficult management problems for procedures in which systemic hypothermia and cold cardioplegic solutions are normally used. Cold reactive proteins can be classified as follows[235-238]:

1. Cold aggutinins (CA) — these are monoclonal or polyclonal IgM antibodies directed against the I or i antigen of the red cell membrane. These antibodies react most efficiently with red cells at low temperatures. The result is agglutination of red cells, complement fixation with subsequent microvascular occlusion, and ischemia. Antibody binding occurs best at low temperatures, whereas complement fixation occurs best at high temperatures. Hemolysis occurs in the thermal range of 10° to 30°C because this is the optimal range of overlap between antibody binding and complement fixation.

    CA are more common in patients with infectious or lymphoproliferative diseases as well as in HIV-positive patients but an idiopathic form of CA disease exists. The idiopathic form is more common in older patients and is more common in women and usually involves monoclonal IgM antibodies to the I antigen of the red cell membrane. The infectious forms such as *Myoplasma pneumonia* tend to involve polyclonal IgM antibodies while the lymphoproliferative disorders involve monoclonal IgM antibodies. Normal persons have low titers of anti-I antibodies that react at low temperatures (< 20°C) and are not clinically significant.[239]

    Most cases involving cold-reactive proteins and CPB are in patients with CA.
2. Cryoglobulins — these are serum proteins or protein complexes that undergo reversible precipitation at low temperatures. The result is multiorgan ischemia and dysfunction from microvascular occlusion. Type I cryoglobulins consist of monoclonal IgG (multiple myeloma) or IgM (Waldenstrom's macroglobulinemia). Type II cryo-

globulins consists of monoclonal IgM directed against polyclonal IgG and usually are associated with autoimmune, infectious, and lymphoproliferative disorders. Type III cryoglobulins consist of polyclonal IgM directed against polyclonal IgG and are associated with infections and autoimmune diseases.

    There is limited experience (three reported cases) in patients with cryoglobulins undergoing procedures requiring CPB.
3. Paroxysmal cold hemoglobinuria — these IgG antibodies are associated with syphilis, have a critical temperature below 20°C, and are potent hemolysins. There are no case reports of CPB in patients with this disorder.

Recommendations for Patients With CA

1. Detection of CA over clinically relevant temperatures can be accomplished at the time of crossmatching by direct Coombs' tests done at 4°C, 25°C, and 37°C. If this is positive, titers at the various temperatures can be performed. This will give an accurate but not precise determination of thermal amplitude and titers preoperatively. Alternatively, intraoperative detection can be accomplished when a sample of patient blood is added to the cardioplegia solution (4°C) before systemic cooling. If agglutination occurs, it is easily visualized. This will document the presence of a CA at a low thermal amplitude but provides no titers. Furthermore, the information is not available preoperatively.
2. Systemic temperatures are kept above the thermal amplitude of the CA. If DHCA is planned, the thermal amplitude of the CA must be known to determine whether temperatures <20°C are feasible.
3. Myocardial preservation can be accomplished as follows:

   - Cardioplegia can be avoided entirely and warm ischemic arrest can be used. This method is unacceptable when long cross-clamp times are expected or when preoperative myocardial dysfunction exists.
   - Warm crystalloid or blood cardioplegia can be used, but the advantages of hypothermia in reducing myocardial oxygen consumption are lost. In addition, frequent instillations of cardioplegia will be needed to keep the heart arrested.
   - Cold crystalloid cardioplegia can be used as in normal circumstances. However, the temperature of the cardioplegia (4° to 8°C) generally is below the critical temperature and will initiate

autoagglutination. This may result in micovascular thombus formation and infarction, nonhomogenous delivery of cardioplegia, and hemolysis.

- Delivery of warm cardioplegia followed by delivery of cold cardioplegia.[240] The right heart is completely isolated with the use of bicaval cannulation and tapes. The right atrium is then opened to allow visualization of the coronary sinus. Warm crystalloid cardioplegia is infused until all of the blood is washed out of the coronaries. Cold crystalloid cardioplegia is then delivered. The presence of noncoronary collaterals may add blood to the coronary circulation despite aortic cross-clamping. Therefore, efforts must be made to reduce noncoronary collateral flow by keeping perfusion pressures on CPB low as discussed previously.

3. For patients who have CA detected preoperatively and in whom the thermal amplitude and titers are high, plasmapheresis may be used to decrease the cold agglutinin titer and increase the margin of safety for use of hypothermia. Plasmapheresis carries the risk of large volume shifts in patients with limited cardiac reserve, is expensive, carries an infectious risk, and is of uncertain efficacy.

4. Efforts should be made to warm all intravenous fluids.

5. Efforts to avoid nonautologous transfusions should be made because donor red cells will not be coated with C3d. C3d is a component of the complement system, which coats some of the patient's red cells after an episode of agglutination and affords some protection from subsequent agglutination and lysis.[240]

6. Steroids may help prevent or mitigate the agglutination and lysis process.[240]

Sickle Cell Disease

Concern centers around the use of hypothermic CPB in patients with sickle cell disease. Hypothermia without the benefit of hemodilution increases blood viscosity, reduces capillary perfusion, promotes stasis, and thus increases the risk of sickling. Furthermore, hypoxia and acidosis promote sickling because sickling occurs when the red cell is in the deoxygenated state. Exchange transfusions to replace Hb S with normal Hb B before CPB have been suggested as a method of addressing these issues. Patients who are heterozygous for the Hb S gene (sickle cell trait) have been treated with exchange transfusions,[241,242] but recent experience with these patients indicates that hypothermic CPB can be used without prior exchange transfusions if hemodilution is used and hypoxia and acidosis are avoided.[243,244] There is a case report of a child with sickle cell trait undergoing profound hypothermia and circulatory arrest without benefit of exchange transfusion.[245] In patients who are homozygous for the Hb S gene, exchange transfusions either preoperatively or intraoperatively to reduce the quantity of Hb S before hypothermic CPB has been the reported technique of choice.[246,247] Exchange transfusions to reduce Hb S to at least 50% (the level present in trait patients) and perhaps as low as 20%[248] seem warranted.

■ REFERENCES

1. Guyton AC, Jones CE, Coleman TG: Regulation of venous return, in: Guyton AC (ed): *Circulatory Physiology: Cardiac Output and Its Regulation.* Philadelphia, WB Saunders, 1973.

2. Bennet EW, Fewel JG, Ybarra J, et al: Comparison of flow differences among venous cannulas. *Ann Thorac Surg* 1983; **36:** 59-65.

3. Lynch MF, Peterson D, Baker V: Centrifugal blood pumping for open heart surgery. *Minn Med* 1978; **61:**536-537.

4. Diehl JT, Payne DD, Rastegar H, Cleveland RJ: Arterial bypass of the descending thoracic aorta with the Bio-Medicus centrifugal pump. *Ann Thorac Surg* 1987; **44:**422-423.

5. Oliver HF, Maher TD, Liebler GA, et al: Use of the Bio-Medicus centrifugal pump in traumatic tears of the thoracic aorta. *Ann Thorac Surg* 1984; **38:**586-591.

6. Van Oeveren W, Kazatchins MD, Descamps-Latscha B, et al: Deleterious effects of cardiopulmonary bypass. A prospective study of bubble versus membrane oxygenation. *J Thorac Cardiovasc Surg* 1985; **89:**888-899.

7. Van den Dungen JJ, Karliczek GF, Brenken U, et al: Clinical study of blood trauma during perfusion with membrane and bubble oxygenators. *J Thorac Cardiovasc Surg* 1982; **83:**108-116.

8. Sade RM, Bartles DM, Dearing JP, et al: A prospective randomized study of membrane versus bubble oxygenators in children. *Ann Thorac Surg* 1980; **29:**502-511.

9. Clark RE, Beauchamps RA, Magrath RA, et al: Comparison of bubble and membrane oxygenators in short and long perfusions. *J Thorac Cardiovasc Surg* 1978; **78:**655-666.

10. Hessel EA, Johnson DD, Ivey TD, Miller DW: Membrane versus bubble oxygenator for cardiac operations. A prospective randomized trial. *J Thorac Cardiovasc Surg* 1980; **80:**11.

11. De Jong JCF, ten Duis HJ, Smit Sibinga CT, Wildevuur CRH: Hematologic aspects of cardiotomy suction in cardiac operations. *J Thorac Cardiovasc Surg* 1980; **79:**227-236.

12. Wright G, Sanderson JM: Cellular aggregation and trauma in cardiotomy suction systems. *Thorax* 1979; **34:**621-628.

13. Journois D, Pouard P, Greeley WL, et al: Hemofiltration during cardiopulmonary bypass in pediatric cardiac surgery. *Anesthesiology* 1994; **81:**1181-1189.

14. Dow JW, Dickson JF, Hamer NA, Gadboys HL: Anaphylactoid shock due to homologous blood exchange in the dog. *J Thorac Cardiovasc Surg* 1960; **39:**449-456.

15. Gadboys HL, Slomin R, Litwak RS: Homologous blood syndrome: 1. Preliminary observations on its relationship to clinical cardiopulmonary bypass. *Ann Surg* 1962; **156:**793-804.

16. Sade RM, Stroud MR, Crawford FA, et al: A prospective randomized study of hydroxyethel starch, albumin, and lactated Ringer's solution as priming fluid for cardiopulmonary bypass. *J Thorac Cardiovasc Surg* 1985; **89:**713-722.

17. Utley JR, Stephens DB, Wachtel C, et al: Effect of albumin and mannitol on organ blood flow, oxygen delivery, water content, and renal function during hypothermic hemodilution cardiopulmonary bypass. *Ann Thorac Surg* 1982; **33**:250-257.

18. Michenfelder JD, Theye RA: Hypothermia: Effect on canine brain and whole body metabolism. *Anesthesiology* 1968; **29**:1107-1112.

19. Kawashima Y, Yamamoto Z, Manabe H: Safe limits of hemodilution in cardiopulmonary bypass. *Surgery* 1972; **76**:391-397.

20. Milam JD, Austin SF, Nihill MR, et al: Use of sufficient hemodilution to prevent coagulopathies following surgical correction of cyanotic heart disease. *J Thorac Cardiovasc Surg* 1985; **89**:623-629.

21. Bull BS, Korpman RA, Huse WM, Briggs BD: Heparin therapy during extracorporeal circulation: I. Problems inherent in existing heparin protocols. *J Thorac Cardiovasc Surg* 1975; **69**:674-684.

22. Young JA, Kisker CT, Doty DB: Adequate anticoagulation during cardiopulmonary bypass determined by activated clotting time and the appearance of fibrin monomer. *Ann Thorac Surg* 1978; **26**:231-240.

23. Gravlee GP, Angert KC, Tucker WY, et al: Early anticoagulation peak and rapid redistribution after intravenous heparin. *Anesthesiology* 1987; **68**:126-129.

24. Cloyd GM, D'Ambra MN, Akins CW: Diminished anticoagulant response to heparin in patients undergoing coronary artery bypass grafting. *J Thorac Cardiovasc Surg* 1987; **94**:535-538.

25. Leckie RS, DiNardo JA: Comparative effects of preoperative intravenous heparin and nitroglycerin therapy on heparin response in patients undergoing CABG surgery (abstract 79), in: Proceedings of the Tenth Annual Meeting of the Society of Cardiovascular Anesthesia, Society of Cardiovascular Anesthesia, 1988, p 79.

26. Gravlee GP, Braurer SD, Roy RC, et al: Predicting the pharmacodynamics of heparin: A clinical evaluation of the Hepcon System 4. *J Cardiothorac Anesth* 1987; **1**:379.

27. Anderson EF: Heparin resistance prior to cardiopulmonary bypass. *Anesthesiology* 1986; **64**:504-507.

28. Soloway H, Christiansen TW: Heparin anticoagulation during cardiopulmonary bypass in an antithrombin-III deficient patient. *Am J Clin Pathol* 1980; **73**:23.

29. Sabbagh AH, Chung GKT, Shuttleworth, P, et al: Fresh frozen plasma: A solution to heparin resistance during cardiopulmonary bypass. *Ann Thorac Surg* 1984; **37**:466-468.

30. Barnette RE, Shupak RC, Pontius J, Rao AK: In vitro effect of fresh frozen plasma on the activated coagulation time in patients undergoing cardiopulmonary bypass. *Anesth Analg* 1988; **67**:57-60.

31. Dauchot PJ, Berzina-Moettus L, Rabinovitch A, Ankeney JL: Activated coagulation and activated partial thromboplastin times in assessment and reversal of heparin-induced anticoagulation for cardiopulmonary bypass. *Anesth Analg* 1983; **62**:710-719.

32. Urban P, Scheidegger D, Buchmann B, Skarvan K: The hemodynamic effects of heparin and their relation to ionized calcium levels. *J Thorac Cardiovasc Surg* 1986; **91**:303-306.

33. Mark L, Whitaker C, Gravlee G, et al: When should a control ACT be taken? (abstract) *Soc Cardiovasc Anesth* 1989.

34. Bull BS, Huse WM, Brauer FS, Korpman RA: Heparin therapy during extracorporeal circulation. II. The use of a dose-response curve to individualize heparin and protamine dosage. *J Thorac Cardiovasc Surg* 1975; **69**:685-689.

35. Johnson WE, Royster RL, Choplin RH, et al: Pulmonary artery catheter migration during cardiac surgery. *Anesthesiology* 1986; **64**:258-262.

36. McLeskey CH, Cheney FW: A correctable complication of cardiopulmonary bypass. *Anesthesiology* 1982; **56**:214-216.

37. Watson BG: Unilateral cold neck: A new sign of misplacement of the aortic cannula during cardiopulmonary bypass. *Anaesthesia* 1983; **38**:659-681.

38. Ross WT, Lake CL, Wellons HA: Cardiopulmonary bypass complicated by inadvertent carotid cannulation. *Anesthesiology* 1981; **54**:85-86.

39. Massagee JT: Cardiopulmonary bypass oxygenator failure, in Reves JG, Hall KD (eds): *Common Problems in Cardiac Anesthesia*. Chicago, Year Book, 1987.

40. Stanley TH, Wen-Shin L, Gentry S: Effects of ventilatory techniques during cardiopulmonary bypass on post-bypass and post-operative pulmonary compliance and shunt. *Anesthesiology* 1977; **46**:391-395.

41. Svennevig JL, Lindberg H, Geiran O, et al: Should the lungs be ventilated during cardiopulmonary bypass? Clinical, hemodynamic, and metabolic changes in patients undergoing elective coronary artery surgery. *Ann Thorac Surg* 1984; **37**:295-300.

42. Buzello W, Pollmaecher T, Schuluermann D, Urbanyi B: The influence of hypothermic cardiopulmonary bypass on neuromuscular transmission in the absence of muscle relaxants. *Anesthesiology* 1986; **64**:279-281.

43. Buzello W, Schluermann D, Pollmaecher T, Spillner G: Unequal effects of cardiopulmonary bypass-induced hypothermia on neuromuscular blockade from constant infusion of alcuronium, d-tubocurarine, pancuronium, and vecuronium. *Anesthesiology* 1987; **66**:842-846.

44. Flynn PJ, Hughes R, Walton B: Use of atracurium in cardiac surgery involving cardiopulmonary bypass with induced hypothermia. *Br J Anaesth* 1984; **56**:967-972.

45. D'Hollaner AA, Duvaldestin P, Henzel D, et al: Variations in pancuronium requirement, plasma concentration, and urinary excretion induced by cardiopulmonary bypass with hypothermia. *Anesthesiology* 1983; **58**:505-509.

46. Hickey RF, Hoar PF: Whole-body oxygen consumption during low flow hypothermic cardiopulmonary bypass. *J Thorac Cardiovasc Surg* 1983; **86**:903-906.

47. Fox LS, Blackstone EH, Kirklin JW, et al: Relationship of whole body oxygen consumption to perfusion flow rate during hypothermic cardiopulmonary bypass. *J Thorac Cardiovasc Surg* 1982; **83**:239-248.

48. Gordon RJ, Ravin M, Rawitscher RE, Daicoff GR: Changes in arterial pressure, viscosity, and resistance during cardiopulmonary bypass. *J Thorac Cardiovasc Surg* 1975; **69**:552-561.

49. Christakis GT, Fremes SE, Koch JP, et al: Determinants of low systemic vascular resistance during cardiopulmonary bypass. *Ann Thorac Surg* 1994; **58**:1040-1049.

50. Govier AV, Reves JG, McKay RD, et al: Factors and their influence on regional cerebral blood flow during nonpulsatile cardiopulmonary bypass. *Ann Thorac Surg* 1984; **38**:592-600.

51. Newman MF, Croughwell MD, Blumenthal JA, et al: Effect of aging on cerebral autoregulation during cardiopulmonary bypass. Association with postoperative cognitive dysfunction. *Circulation* 1994; **90**(II):243-249.

52. Croughwell N, Lyth M, Quill TJ, et al: Diabetic patients have abnormal cerebral autoregulation during cardiopulmonary bypass. *Circulation* 1990; **82**:(suppl IV):IV-407-IV-412.

53. Greeley WJ, Ungerleider RM, Smith R, et al: The effects of deep hypothermic cardiopulmonary bypass and total circulatory arrest on cerebral blood flow in infants and children. *J Thorac Cardiovasc Surg* 1989; **97**:737-745.

54. Kern FH, Ungerleider RM, Quill TJ, et al: Cerebral blood flow response to changes in arterial carbon dioxide tension during hypothermic cardiopulmonary bypass in children. *J Thorac Cardiovasc Surg* 1991; **101**:618-622.

55. Rahn H, Reeves RB, Howell BJ: Hydrogen ion regulation, temperature and evolution. *Am Rev Respir Dis* 1975; **112**:165-172.

56. Murkin JM, Farrar JK, Tweed WA, et al: Cerebral autoregulation and flow/metabolism coupling during cardiopulmonary bypass: The influence of Pa_{CO_2}. *Anesth Analg* 1987; **66**:825-832.

57. Prough DS, Stump DA, Roy RC, et al: Response of cerebral blood flow to changes in carbon dioxide tension during hypothermic cardiopulmonary bypass. *Anesthesiology* 1986; **64:**576–581.

58. Johnsson P, Messeter K, Ryding E, et al: Cerebral blood flow and autoregulation during hypothermic cardiopulmonary bypass. *Ann Thorac Surg* 1987; **43:**386–390.

59. Murkin JM, Farrar JK, Tweed WA, et al: Relationship between cerebral blood flow and O_2 consumption during high-dose narcotic anesthesia for cardiac surgery. *Anesthesiology* 1985; **63:**A44.

60. Lundar T, Lindegaard KF, Froysaker T, et al: Dissociation between cerebral autoregulation and carbon dioxide reactivity during nonpulsatile cardiopulmonary bypass. *Ann Thorac Surg* 1985; **40:**582–587.

61. Bashein G, Townes BD, Nessly ML, et al: A randomized study of carbon dioxide management during hypothermic cardiopulmonary bypass. *Anesthesiology* 1990; **72:**7–15.

62. Stephan H, Weyland A, Kazmaier S, et al: Acid-base management during hypothermic cardiopulmonary bypass does not affect cerebral metabolism but does affect blood flow and neurologic outcome. *Br J Anaesth* 1992; **69:**51–57.

63. Venn GE, Patel RL, Chambers DJ, et al: Cardiopulmonary bypass: Perioperative cerebral blood flow and postoperative cognitive deficit. *Ann Thorac Surg* 1995; **59:**1331–1335.

64. Murkin JM, Martzke JS, Buchan AM, et al: A randomized study of the influence of perfusion technique and pH management strategy in 316 patients undergoing coronary artery bypass surgery. II. Neurologic and cognitive outcomes. *J Thorac Cardiovasc Surg* 1995; **110:**349–362.

65. Martin TD, Craver JM, Gott JP, et al: Prospective, randomized trial of retrograde warm blood cardioplegia: myocardial benefit and neurologic threat. *Ann Thorac Surg* 1994; **57:**298–304.

66. Mora CT, Henson MB, Weintraub WS, et al: The effect of temperature management during cardiopulmonary bypass on neurologic and neuropsychologic outcomes in patients undergoing coronary revascularization. *J Cardiovasc Thorac Surg* 1996; **112:**514–522.

67. The Warm Heart Investigators: Randomized trial of normothermic versus hypothermic coronary bypass surgery. *Lancet* 1994; **343:**559–563.

68. Murkin JM, Farrar JK, Cleland A, et al: The influence of perfusion flow rates on cerebral blood flow and oxygen consumption during hypothermic cardiopulmonary bypass. *Anesthesiology* 1987; **67:**A9.

69. Fox LS, Blackstone EH, Kirklin JW, et al: Relationship of brain blood flow and oxygen consumption to perfusion flow rate during profoundly hypothermic cardiopulmonary bypass. *J Thorac Cardiovasc Surg* 1984; **87:**658–664.

70. Rebeyka IM, Coles JG, Wilson GJ, et al: The effect of low-flow cardiopulmonary bypass on cerebral function: An experimental and clinical study. *Ann Thorac Surg* 1987; **43:**391–396.

71. Kern FH, Ungerleider RM, Reeves JG, et al: Effect of altering pump flow rate on cerebral blood flow and metabolism in infants and children. *Ann Thorac Surg* 1994; **56:**1366–1372.

72. Newberger JW, Jonas RA, Wernovsky G, et al: A comparison of the perioperative neurologic effects of hypothermic circulatory arrest versus low-flow cardiopulmonary bypass in infant heart surgery. *N Engl J Med* 1993; **329:**1057–1064.

73. Bellinger DC, Jonas RA, Rappaport LA, et al: Developmental and neurologic status of children after heart surgery with hypothermic circulatory arrest or low-flow cardiopulmonary bypass. *N Engl J Med* 1995; **332:**549–555.

74. Hickey PR, Andersen NP: Deep hypothermic circulatory arrest: A review of pathophysiology and clinical experience as a basis for anesthetic management. *J Cardiothorac Anesth* 1987; **1:**137–155.

75. Jonas RA: Hypothermia, circulatory arrest, and the pediatric brain. *J Cardiothorac Vasc Anesth* 1996; **10:**66–74.

76. Wong PC, Barlow CF, Hickey PR, et al: Factors associated with choreoathetosis after cardiopulmonary bypass in children with congenital heart disease. *Circulation* 1992; **86**(suppl II):II-118–II-126.

77. Kirshbom PM, Sharyak LA, DiBernardo LR, et al: Effects of aortopulmonary collaterals on cerebral cooling and cerebral metabolic recovery after circulatory arrest. *Circulation* 1995; **92**(suppl II):II-490–II-494.

78. Kern FH, Ungerleider RM, Schulamn SR, et al: Comparing two strategies of cardiopulmonary bypass cooling on jugular venous oxygen saturation in neonates and infants. *Ann Thorac Surg* 1995; **60:**1198–1202.

79. Jonas RA, Bellinger DC, Rappaport LA, et al: Relation of pH strategy and developmental outcome after hypothermic circulatory arrest. *J Thorac Cardiovasc Surg* 1993; **106:**362–368.

80. Kern FH, Greeley WJ; Pro: pH-stat management of blood gases is not preferable to alpha-stat in patients undergoing brain cooling for cardiac surgery. *J Cardiothorac Vasc Anesth* 1995; **9:**215–218.

81. Burrows FA: Con: pH-stat management of blood gases is preferable to alpha-stat in patients undergoing brain cooling for cardiac surgery. *J Cardiothorac Vasc Anesth* 1995; **9:**219–221.

82. Hiramatsu T, Miura T, Forbess JM, et al: pH strategies and cerebral energetics before and after circulatory arrest. *J Thorac Cardiovasc Surg* 1995; **109:**948–958.

83. Skaryak LA, Chai PJ, Kern FH, et al: Blood gas management and degree of cooling: effects of cerebral metabolism before and after circulatory arrest. *J Thorac Cardiovasc Surg* 1995; **110:**1649–1657.

84. Schaff HV, Ciardullo RC, Flaherty JT, Gott VL: Development of regional myocardial ischemia distal to a critical coronary stenosis during cardiopulmonary bypass: Comparison of the fibrillating vs the beating nonworking states. *Surgery* 1978; **83:**57–66.

85. Ciadullo RC, Schaff HV, Flaherty JT, Gott VL: Myocardial ischemia during cardiopulmonary bypass. The hazards of ventricular fibrillation in the presence of a critical coronary stenosis. *J Thorac Cardiovasc Surg* 1977; **73:**746–757.

86. Buckberg GD, Brazier JR, Nelson RL, et al: Studies on the effects of hypothermia on regional myocardial blood flow and metabolism during cardiopulmonary bypass I. The adequately perfused beating, fibrillating, and arrested heart. *J Thorac Cardiovasc Surg* 1977; **73:**87–94.

87. Brazier JR, Cooper N, McConnell DH, Buckberg GD: Studies on the effects of hypothermia on regional myocardial blood flow and metabolism during cardiopulmonary bypass III. Effects of temperature, time, and perfusion pressure in fibrillating hearts. *J Thorac Cardiovasc Surg* 1977; **73:**102–109.

88. Cox JL, Anderson RW, Pass HI, et al: The safety of induced ventricular fibrillation during cardiopulmonary bypass in nonhypertrophied hearts. *J Thorac Cardiovasc Surg* 1977; **74:**423–432.

89. Spadaro J, Bing OHL, Gaasch WH, et al: Effects of perfusion pressure on myocardial performance, metabolism, wall thickness, and compliance. *J Thorac Cardiovasc Surg* 1982; **84:**398–405.

90. Brazier J, Cooper N, Buckberg G: The adequacy of subendocardial oxygen delivery. The interaction of determinants of flow, arterial oxygen content and myocardial oxygen need. *Circulation* 1974; **49:**968–977.

91. McConnell DH, Brazier JR, Cooper N, Buckberg GD: Studies of the effects of hypothermia on regional myocardial blood flow and metabolism during cardiopulmonary bypass II. Ischemia during moderate hypothermia in continually perfused beating hearts. *J Thorac Cardiovasc Surg* 1977; **73:**95–101.

92. McConnell DH, White F, Nelsom RL, et al: Importance of alkalosis in maintenance of "ideal" blood pH during hypothermia. *Surg Forum* 1975; **26:**263.

93. Becker H, Vinten-Johansen J, Buckberg GD, et al: Myocardial damage caused by keeping pH 7.40 during systemic deep hypothermia. *J Thorac Cardiovasc Surg* 1981; **82:**810–820.

94. Hiberman M, Derby GC, Spencer RJ: Sequential pathophysiologic changes characterizing the progression from renal dysfunction to acute renal failure following cardiac operations. *J Thorac Cardiovasc Surg* 1980; **79:**838-844.

95. Hiberman M, Myers BD, Carrie BJ: Acute renal failure following cardiac surgery. *J Thorac Cardiovasc Surg* 1979; **77:**880-888.

96. Badner NH, Murkin JM, Lok P: Differences in pH management and pulsatile/nonpulsatile perfusion during cardiopulmonary bypass do not influence renal function. *Anesth Analg* 1992; **75:**696-701.

97. Regragui IA, Izzat MB, Birdi I, et al: Cardiopulmonary bypass perfusion temperature does not influence perioperative renal function. *Ann Thorac Surg* 1995; **60:**160-164.

98. Lema G, Meneses G, Urzua J, et al: Effects of extracorporeal circulation on renal function in coronary surgical patients. *Anesth Analg* 1995; **81:**446-451.

99. Zanardo G, Michielson P, Paccagnella A: Acute renal failure in the patient undergoing cardiac operation, prevalence, mortality rate, and main risk factors. *J Thorac Cardiovasc Surg* 1994; **107:**1489-1495.

100. Corwin HL, Spraque SM, DeLaria GA, et al: Acute renal failure associated with cardiac operations: A case-control study. *J Thorac Cardiovasc Surg* 1989; **98:**1107-1112.

101. Harris SN, Rinder CS, Rinder HM, et al: Nitroprusside inhibition of platelet function is transient and reversible by catecholamine priming. *Anesthesiology* 1995; **83:**1145-1152.

102. Dasta JF, Jacobi J, Wu LS: Loss of nitroglycerin to cardiopulmonary bypass circuit. *Crit Care Med* 1983; **11:**50-52.

103. Maltry DE, Eggers GWN: Isoflurane-induced failure of the Bentley-10 oxygenator. *Anesthesiology* 1987; **66:**100-101.

104. Cooper S, Levin R: Near catastrophic oxygenator failure. *Anesthesiology* 1987; **66:**101-102.

105. Price SL, Brown DL, Carpenter RL, et al: Isoflurane elimination via a bubble oxygenator during extracorporeal circulation. *J Cardiothorac Anesth* 1988; **2:**41-44.

106. Hughes DR, Faust RJ, Didisheim P: Heparin monitoring during human cardiopulmonary bypass: Efficacy of activated clotting time vs the fluorimetric heparin assay. *Anesth Analg* 1982; **61:**189-191.

107. Croughwell ND, Frasco P, Blumenthal J, et al: Warming during cardiopulmonary bypass is associated with jugular bulb desaturation. *Ann Thorac Surg* 1992; **53:**827-832.

108. Croughwell ND, Newman MF, Blumenthal J, et al: Jugular bulb desaturation and cognitive dysfunction following cardiopulmonary bypass. *Ann Thorac Surg* 1994; **58:**1702-1708.

109. Newman MF, Kramer D, Croughwell ND, et al: Differential age effects of mean arterial pressure and rewarming on cognitive dysfunction after cardiac surgery. *Anesth Analg* 1995; **81:**236-242.

110. Noback C, Tinker JH: Hypothermia after cardiopulmonary bypass in man. *Anesthesiology* 1980; **53:**277-280.

111. Ralley FE, Ramsay JG, Wylands JE, et al: Effect of heated humidified gases on temperature drop after cardiopulmonary bypass. *Anesth Analg* 1984; **63:**1106-1110.

112. Robinson RJS, Boright WA, Ligier B, et al: The incidence of awareness, and amnesia for perioperative events, after cardiac surgery with lorazepam and fentanyl anesthesia. *J Cardiothorac Anesth* 1987; **1:**524-530.

113. Effective measures in the prevention of intraoperative aeroembolus. *J Thorac Cardiovasc Surg* 1971; **62:**731-735.

114. Tingleff J, Joyce FS, Pettersson G: Intraoperative echocardiographic study of air embolism during cardiac operations. *Ann Thorac Surg* 1995; **60:**673-677.

115. Orihashi K, Matsuura Y, Hamanaka Y, et al: Retained intracardiac air in open heart operations examined by transesophageal echocardiography. *Ann Thorac Surg* 1993; **55:**467-471.

116. Lake CL, Sellers TD, Nolan SP, et al: Energy dose and other variables possibly affecting ventricular defibrillation during cardiac surgery. *Anesth Analg* 1984; **63:**743-751.

117. Kerber RE, Sarnat W: Factors influencing the success of ventricular defibrillation. *Circulation* 1979; **60:**226-230.

118. Lake CL, Kron IL, Mentzer RM, Crampton RS: Lidocaine enhances intraoperative ventricular defibrillation. *Anesth Analg* 1986; **65:**337-340.

119. Johnson RG, Goldberger AL, Thurer RL, et al: Lidocaine prophylaxis in coronary revascularization patients: A randomized, prospective trial. *Ann Thorac Surg* 1993; **55:**1180-1184.

120. Karmy-Jones R, Hamilton A, Dzavik V, et al: Magnesium sulfate prophylaxis after cardiac operations. *Ann Thorac Surg* 1995; **59:**502-507.

121. Kopman EA: Scavenging of potassium cardioplegic solution to prevent hyperkalemia in hemodialysis-dependent patients. *Anesth Analg* 1983; **62:**780-782.

122. Salmenpera M, Heinonen J: Pulmonary vascular responses to moderate changes in $Paco_2$ after cardiopulmonary bypass. *Anesthesiology* 1986; **64:**311-315.

123. Gallagher JD, Moore RA, McNicholas KW, Jose AB: Comparison of radial and femoral arterial blood pressures in children after cardiopulmonary bypass. *J Clin Monit* 1985; **1:**168-171.

124. Stern DH, Gerson JI, Allen FB, Parker FB: Can we trust the direct radial artery pressure immediately following cardiopulmonary bypass? *Anesthesiology* 1985; **62:**557-561.

125. Mohr R, Lavee J, Goor DA: Inaccuracy of radial arterial pressure measurement after cardiac operations. *J Thorac Cardiovasc Surg* 1987; **94:**286-290.

126. Bazaral MB, Welch M, Golding LAR, et al: Comparison of brachial and radial arterial pressure monitoring in patients undergoing coronary artery bypass surgery. *Anesthesiology* 1990; **73:**38-45.

127. Rich GF, Lubanski RE, McLoughlin TM: Differences between aortic and radial artery pressure associated with cardiopulmonary bypass. *Anesthesiology* 1992; **77:**63-66.

128. Gravlee GP, Wong AB, Adkins TG, et al: A comparison of radial, brachial, and aortic pressures after cardiopulmonary bypass. *J Cardiothorac Anesth* 1989; **3:**20-26.

129. Pauca AL, Meredith JW: Possibility of A-V shunting upon cardiopulmonary bypass discontinuation. *Anesthesiology* 1987; **67:**91-94.

130. Culliford AT, Gitel SN, Starr N, et al: Lack of correlation between activated clotting time and plasma heparin during cardiopulmonary bypass. *Ann Surg* 1981; **193:**105-111.

131. Esposito RA, Culliford AT, Colvin SB, et al: The role of the activated clotting time in heparin administration and neutralization for cardiopulmonary bypass. *J Thorac Cardiovasc Surg* 1983; **85:**174-185.

132. Umlas J, Taft RH, Gauvin G, Swierk P: Anticoagulation monitoring and neutralization during open heart surgery — A rapid method for measuring heparin and calculating safe reduced protamine doses. *Anesth Analg* 1983; **62:**1095-1099.

133. LaDuca F, Mills D, Thompson S, Larson K: Neutralization of heparin using a protamine titration assay and the activated clotting time. *J Extra-Corpor Technol* 1987; **19:**358-364.

134. Ullman DA, Bloom BS, Danker PR, et al: Protamine-induced hypotension in a two-year-old child. *J Cardiothorac Anesth* 1988; **2:**497-499.

135. Lowenstein E, Johnson WE, Lappas DG, et al: Catastrophic pulmonary vasoconstriction associated with protamine reversal of heparin. *Anesthesiology* 1983; **59:**470-473.

136. Kronenfeld MA, Garguilo R, Weinberg P, et al: Left atrial injection of protamine does not reliably prevent pulmonary hypertension. *Anesthesiology* 1987; **67:**578-580.

137. Morel DR, Zapol WM, Thomas SJ, et al: C5a and thromboxane generation associated with pulmonary vaso- and broncho-constriction during protamine reversal of heparin. *Anesthesiology* 1987; **66:**597-604.

138. Horiguchi T, Enzan K, Mitsuhata H, et al: Heparin-protamine complexes cause pulmonary hypertension in goats. *Anesthesiology* 1995; **83:**786-791.

139. Konstadt SN, Thys DM, Kong D, et al: Absence of prostaglandin changes associated with protamine administration in patients with pulmonary hypertension. *J Cardiothorac Anesth* 1987; **1:**388-391.

140. Horrow JC: Protamine: A review of its toxicity. *Anesth Analg* 1985; **64:**348-361.

141. Michaels IALM, Barash PG: Hemodynamic changes associated with protamine administration. *Anesth Analg* 1983; **62:**831-835.

142. Casthely PA, Goodman K, Fyman PN, et al: Hemodynamic changes after the administration of protamine. *Anesth Analg* 1986; **65:**78-80.

143. Horrow JC: Protamine allergy. *J Cardiothorac Anesth* 1988; **2:**225-242.

144. Bjoraker DG, Ketcham TR: In vivo platelet response to clinical protamine sulfate infusion. *Anesthesiology* 1982; **57:**A7.

145. Stewart WJ, McSweeney SM, Kellett MA: Increased risk of severe protamine reactions in NPH insulin-dependant diabetics undergoing cardiac catheterization. *Circulation* 1984; **70:**788-792.

146. Levy JH, Zaidan JR, Faraj B: Prospective evaluation of risk of protamine reactions in patients with NPH insulin-dependant diabetes. *Anesth Analg* 1986; **65:**739-749.

147. Levy JH, Schwieger IM, Zaidan JR, et al: Evaluation of patients at risk for protamine reactions. *J Cardiovasc Thorac Surg* 1989; **98:**200-204.

148. Knape JTA, Schuller JT, DeHaan P: An anaphylactic reaction to protamine in a patient allergic to fish. *Anesthesiology* 1981; **55:**324-325.

149. Adourian U, Shampaine EL, Hirshman CA, et al: High-titer protamine-specific IgG antibody associated with anaphylaxis: Report of a case and quantitative analysis of antibody in vasectomized men. *Anesthesiology* 1993; **78:**368-372.

150. Weiss ME, Nyhan D, Peng Z, et al: Association of protamine IgE and IgG antibodies with life threatening reactions to intravenous protamine. *N Engl J Med* 1989; **320:**886-892.

151. Horrow JC, Pharo GH, Levit LS, et al: Neither skin tests nor serum enzyme-linked immunosorbent assay tests provide specificity for protamine allergy. *Anesth Analg* 1996; **82:**386-389.

152. Teoh KHT, Young E, Bradley CA, et al: Heparin binding proteins. Contribution to heparin rebound after cardiopulmonary bypass. *Circulation* 1993; **88:**420-425.

153. Gravlee GP, Rogers AT, Dudas LM, et al: Heparin management protocol for cardiopulmonary bypass influences postoperative heparin rebound but not bleeding. *Anesthesiology* 1992; **76:**393-401.

154. Fabian I, Aronson M: Mechanism of heparin rebound. In vitro study. *Thromb Res* 1980; **18:**535-542.

155. Soloway HB, Christansen TW: Heparin anticoagulation during cardiopulmonary bypass in an antithrombin 3 deficient patient: Implications relevant to the etiology of heparin rebound. *Am J Clin Pathol* 1980; **73:**723-725.

156. Mammen EF, Koets MH, Washington BC, et al: Hemostasis changes during cardiopulmonary bypass surgery. *Semin Thromb Hemost* 1985; **11:**281-292.

157. Bick RL: Hemostasis defects associated with cardiac surgery, prosthetic devices, and other extracorporeal devices. *Semin Thromb Hemost* 1985; **11:**249-280.

158. Harker LA, Malpass TW, Branson HE, et al: Mechanism of abnormal bleeding in patients undergoing cardiopulmonary bypass: Acquired transient platelet dysfunction associated with selective alpha-granule release. *Blood* 1980; **56:**824-834.

159. Davis R, Whittington R: Aprotinin. A review of its pharmacology and therapeutic efficacy in reducing blood loss associated with cardiac surgery. *Drugs* 1995; **49:**954-983.

160. Yost CS: Clinical utility and cost effectiveness of aprotinin to reduce operative bleeding. Comparison with other antifibrinolytics. *Am J Anesthesiol* 1996; **23:**233-241.

161. Fiore LD, Brophy MT, Lopez A, et al: The bleeding time response to aspirin. Identifying the hyper-responder. *Am J Clin Pathol* 1990; **94:**292-296.

162. Lethagen S, Rugarn P: The effect of DDAVP and placebo on platelet function and prolonged bleeding time induced by oral acetylsalicylic acid intake on volunteers. *Thromb Haemostasis* 1992; **67:**185-186.

163. Reynolds LM, Nicolson SC, Jobes DR, et al: Desmopressin does not decrease bleeding after cardiac operation in young children. *J Thorac Cardiovasc Surg* 1993; **106:**954-958.

164. Cattaneo M, Harris AS, Stromberg U, et al: The effect of desmopressin on reducing blood loss in cardiac surgery — A meta-analysis of double-blind, placebo-controlled trials. *Thromb Haemost* 1995; **74:**1064-1070.

165. Mongan PD, Hosking MP: The role of desmopressin acetate in patients undergoing coronary artery bypass surgery. A controlled clinical trial with thromboelastographic risk stratification. *Anesthesiology* 1992; **77:**38-46.

166. Gratz I, Koehler J, Olsen D, et al: The effect of desmopressin acetate on postoperative hemorrhage in patients receiving aspirin therapy before coronary artery bypass operations. *J Thorac Cardiovasc Surg* 1992; **104:**1417-1422.

167. Dilthey G, Dietrich W, Spannagl M, et al: Influence of desmopressin acetate (DDAVP) on homologous blood requirement in cardiac surgical patients pretreated with platelet-inhibiting drugs. *J Cardiothorac Vasc Anesth* 1993; **7:**425-430.

168. Sheridan DP, Card RT, Pinilla JC, et al: Use of desmopressin acetate to reduce blood transfusion requirements during cardiac surgery in patients with acetylsalicyclic acid induced platelet dysfunction. *Can J Surg* 1994; **37:**33-36.

169. Johns RA: Desmopressin is a potent vasorelaxant of aorta and pulmonary artery isolated from rabbit and rat. *Anesthesiology* 1990; **72:**858-864.

170. Frankville DD, Harper GB, Lake CL, et al: Hemodynamic consequences of desmopressin administration after cardiopulmonary bypass. *Anesthesiology* 1991; **74:**988-996.

171. Roy RC, Stafford MA, Hudspeth AS, et al: Failure of prophylaxis with fresh frozen plasma after cardiopulmonary bypass. *Anesthesiology* 1988; **69:**254-257.

172. Manno CS, Hedberg KW, Kim HC, et al: Comparison of the hemostatic effects of fresh whole blood, stored whole blood and components after open heart surgery in children. *Blood* 1991; **77:**930-936.

173. Chen RH, Frazier OH, Cooley DA: Antifibrinolytic therapy in cardiac surgery. *Tex Heart Inst J* 1995; **22:**211-215.

174. Lu H, Soria C, Soria J, et al: Reversible translocation of glycoprotein Ib in plasmin-treated platelets: Consequences for platelet function. *Eur J Clin Invest* 1993; **23:**785-793.

175. Hill GE, Alonso A, Stammers AH, et al: Aprotinin and methylprednisolone equally blunt cardiopulmonary bypass-induced inflammation in humans. *J Thorac Cardiovasc Surg* 1995; **110:**1658-1662.

176. Verstraete M: Clinical application of inhibitors of fibrinolysis. *Drugs* 1985; **29:**236-261.

177. Horrow JC, Van Riper DF, Strong MD, et al: The dose-response relationship of tranexamic acid. *Anesthesiology* 1995; **82:**383-392.

178. Goldstein DJ, Oz MC, Smith CR, et al: Safety of repeat aprotinin administration for LVAD recipients undergoing cardiac transplantation. *Ann Thorac Surg* 1996; **61:**692-695.

179. Diefenbach C, Abel M, Limpers B, et al: Fatal anaphylatic shock after aprotinin reexposure in cardiac surgery. *Anesth Analg* 1995; **80:**830-831.

180. Dietrich W, Spath P, Ebell A, et al: Prevalence of anaphylactic reactions to aprotinin: Analysis of two hundred forty-eight reexposures to aprotinin in heart operations. *J Cardiovasc Thorac Surg* 1997; **113**:194-201.

181. Wuthrich B, Schmid P, Schmid ER et al: IgE-mediated anaphylactic reaction to aprotinin during anaesthesia. *Lancet* 1993; **340**:173-174.

182. Levy JH: Antibody formation after drug administration during cardiac surgery: Parameters for aprotinin use. *J Heart Lung Transplant* 1993; **12**:S26-32.

183. Hardy JF, Belisle S: Natural and synthetic antifibrinolytics in adult cardiac surgery: Efficacy, effectiveness and efficiency. *Can J Anesth* 1994; **41**:1104-1112.

184. Westaby S: Aprotinin in perspective. *Ann Thorac Surg* 1993; **55**: 1033-1041.

185. Fremes SE, Wong BI, Lee E, et al: Metanalysis of prophylatic drug treatment in the prevention of postoperative bleeding. *Ann Thorac Surg* 1994; **58**:1580-1588.

186. McClure PD, Izsak J: The use of epsilon-aminocaproic acid to reduce bleeding during cardiac bypass in children with congenital heart disease. *Anesthesiology* 1974; **40**:604-608.

187. Vander Salm TJ, Ansell JE, et al: The role of epsilon-aminocaproic acid in reducing bleeding after cardiac operations: A double-blind study. *J Thorac Cardiovasc Surg* 1988; **95**:538-540.

188. Daily PO, Lampherc JA, Dembitsky WP, et al: Effect of prophylactic epsilon aminocaproic acid on blood loss and transfusion requirements in patients undergoing first-time coronary artery bypass grafting. A randomized, prospective, double-blind study. *J Thorac Cardiovasc Surg* 1994; **108**:99-108.

189. Jordan D, Delphin E, Rose E: Prophylactic epsilon-aminocaproic acid (EACA) administration minimizes blood replacement therapy during cardiac surgery. *Anesth Analg* 1995; **80**:827-829.

190. Menichetti A, Tritapepe L, Ruvolo G, et al: Changes in coagulation patterns, blood loss and blood use after cardiopulmonary bypass: aprotinin vs tranexamic acid vs epsilon aminocaproic acid. *J Cardiovasc Surg* 1996; **37**:401-407.

191. dc Peppo AP, Pierri MD, De Paulis R, et al: Intraoperative antifibrinolysis and blood saving techniques in cardiac surgery. Prospective trial of 3 antifibrinolytic drugs. *Tex Heart Inst* 1995; **22**:231-236.

192. Shore-Lesserson L, Reich DL, Vela-Cantos F, et al: Tranexamic acid reduces transfusions and mediastinal drainage in repeat cardiac surgery. *Anesth Analg* 1995; **83**:18-26.

193. Horrow JC, Van Riper DF, Strong MD, et al: The dose-response relationship of tranexamic acid. *Anesthesiology* 1995; **82**:383-392.

194. Horrow JC, Van Riper DF, Strong MD, et al: Hemostatic effects of tranexamic acid and desmopressin during cardiac surgery. *Circulation* 1991; **84**:2063-2070.

195. Coffey A, Pittman J, Halbrook H, et al: The use of tranexamic acid to reduce postoperative bleeding following cardiac surgery: a double-blind randomized trial. *Am Surg* 1995; **61**:566-568.

196. Blauhut B, Harringer W, Bettelheim P, et al: Comparison of the effects of aprotinin and tranexamic acid on blood loss and related variables after cardiopulmonary bypass. *J Thorac Cardiovasc Surg* 1994; **108**:1083-1091.

197. Karski JM, Teasdale SJ, Norman P, et al: Prevention of bleeding after cardiopulmonary bypass with high-dose tranexamic acid. Double-blind, randomized clinical trial. *J Thorac Cardiovasc Surg* 1995; **110**:835-842.

198. Jamieson WRE, Dryden PJ, O'Connor JP, et al: The beneficial effect of both tranexamic acid and aprotinin on blood loss reduction in reoperative valve replacement surgery. *Circulation* 1996; **94** (suppl I):I-720.

199. Pugh SC, Wielogorski AK: A comparison of the effects of tranexamic acid and low-dose aprotinin on blood loss and homologous blood usage in patients undergoing cardiac surgery. *J Cardiothorac Vasc Anesth* 1995; **9**:240-244.

200. Levy JH, Pifarre R, Schaff HV, et al: A multicenter, double-blind, placebo-controlled trial of aprotinin for reducing blood loss and the requirement for donor-blood transfusion in patients undergoing repeat coronary artery bypass grafting. *Circulation* 1995; **92**:2236-2244.

201. Tabuchi N, Huet RCG, Sturk A, et al: Aprotinin preserves hemostasis in aspirin-treated patients undergoing cardiopulmonary bypass. *Ann Thorac Surg* 1994; **58**:1036-1039.

202. Rosston D: Aprotinin therapy in heart and heart-lung transplantation. *J Heart Lung Transplant* 1993; **12**:S19-25.

203. Jaquiss RDB, Huddleston CB, Spray TL: Use of aprotinin in pediatric lung transplantation. *J Heart Lung Transplant* 1995; **14**: 302-307.

204. Kesten S, de Hoyas A, Chaparro C, et al: Aprotinin reduces blood loss in lung transplant recipients. *Ann Thorac Surg* 1995; **59**: 877-879.

205. Goldstein DJ, Seldomridge A, Chen JM: Use of aprotinin in LVAD recipients reduces blood loss, blood use, and perioperative mortality. *Ann Thorac Surg* 1995; **59**:1063-1068.

206. Pae WE, Aufiero TX, Miller CA, et al: Aprotinin therapy for insertion of ventricular assist devices for staged heart transplantation. *J Heart Lung Transplant* 1994; **13**:811-816.

207. Herynkopf F, Lucchese F, Pereira E, et al: Aprotinin in children undergoing correction of congenital heart defects. *J Thorac Cardiovasc Surg* 1994; **108**:517-521.

208. Boldt J, Knothe C, Zickman B, et al: Aprotinin in pediatric cardiac operations: Platelet function, blood loss, and use of homologous blood. *Ann Thorac Surg* 1993; **55**:1460-1466.

209. Dietrich W, Mossinger H, Spannagi M, et al: Hemostatic activation during cardiopulmonary bypass with different aprotinin dosages in pediatric patients having cardiac operations. *J Thorac Cardiovasc Surg* 1993; **105**:712-720.

210. Boldt J, Knothe C, Zickman B, et al: Comparison of two aprotinin dosage regimes in pediatric patients having cardiac operations. Influence on platelet function and blood loss. *J Thorac Cardiovasc Surg* 1993; **105**:705-711.

211. Penkoske PA, Entwistle LM, Marchak E et al: Aprotinin in children undergoing repair of congenital heart defects. *Ann Thorac Surg* 1995; **60**:S529-S532.

212. D'Errico CC, Shayevitz JR, Martindale SJ, et al: The efficacy and cost of aprotinin in children undergoing reoperative open heart surgery. *Anesth Analg* 1996; **83**:1193-1199.

213. Despotis GJ, Alsoufiev A, Goodnough LT, et al: Aprotinin prolongs whole blood activated partial thromboplastin time but not whole blood prothrombin time in patients undergoing cardiac surgery. *Anesth Analg* 1995; **81**:919-924.

214. Despotis GJ, Filos KS, Levine V, et al: Aprotinin prolongs activated and nonactivated whole blood clotting time and potentiates the effect of heparin in vitro. *Anesth Analg* 1996; **82**:1126-1131.

215. Despotis GJ, Joist JH, Joiner-Maier D, et al: Effect of aprotinin on activated clotting time, whole blood and plasma heparin measurements. *Ann Thorac Surg* 1995; **59**:106-111.

216. Wang JS, Lin CY, Hung WT, et al: Monitoring of heparin-induced anticoagulation with kaolin activated clotting time in cardiac surgical patients treated with aprotinin. *Anesthesiology* 1992; **77**:1080-1084.

217. Tabuchi N, Njo TL, Tigchelaar I, et al: Monitoring of anticoagulation in aprotinin-treated patients during heart operation. *Ann Thorac Surg* 1994; **58**:774-777.

218. Dietrich W, Dilthey G, Spannagl M, et al: Influence of high-dose aprotinin on anticoagulation, heparin requirement, and celite- and kaolin-activated clotting time in heparin-pretreated patients undergoing open-heart surgery. A double-blind, placebo-controlled study. *Anesthesiology* 1995; **83**:679-689.

219. Westaby S: Aprotinin in perspective. *Ann Thorac Surg* 1993; **55**: 1033-1041.

220. Feindt PR, Walcher S, Volkmer I, et al: Effects of high-dose aprotinin on renal function in aortocoronary bypass grafting. *Ann Thorac Surg* 1995; **60:**1076-1080.

221. Ranucci M, Corno A, Pavesi M, et al: Renal effects of low dose aprotinin in pediatric cardiac surgery. *Minerva Anesthesiol* 1994; **60:**361-366.

222. Sundt TM, Kouchoukos NT, Saffitz JE, et al: Renal dysfunction and intravascular coagulation with aprotinin and hypothermic circulatory arrest. *Ann Thorac Surg* 1993; **55:**1418-1424.

223. Westaby S, Forni A, Dunning J, et al: Aprotinin and bleeding in profoundly hypothermic perfusion. *Eur J Cardio Thorac Surg* 1994; **8:**82-86.

224. Goldstein DJ, DeRosa CM, Mongero LB, et al: Safety and efficacy of aprotinin under conditions of deep hypothermia and circulatory arrest. *J Thorac Cardiovasc Surg* 1995; **110:**1615-1622.

225. Regragui IA, Bryan AJ, Izzat MB, et al: Aprotinin use with hypothermic circulatory arrest for aortic valve and thoracic aortic surgery: renal function and early survival. *J Heart Valve Dis* 1995; **4:**674-677.

226. Consensus Conference: Platelet transfusion therapy. *JAMA* 1987; **257:**1777-1780.

227. Koza MJ, Walenga JM, Khenkina YN, et al: Thromboelastographic analysis of patients receiving aprotinin with comparisons to platelet aggregation and other assays. *Semin Thromb Hemost* 1995; **21:**80-85.

228. Konstadt S, Thys D, Reich D, et al: The normal pericardium does not affect left ventricular function. *J Cardiothorac Anesth* 1987; **1:**284-288.

229. Fanning WJ, Vasko JS, Kilman JW: Delayed sternal closure after cardiac surgery. *Ann Thorac Surg* 1987; **44:**169-172.

230. Love JW, Jahnke EJ, McFadden RB, et al: Myocardial revascularization in patients with chronic renal failure. *J Thorac Cardiovasc Surg* 1980; **79:**625-627.

231. Soffer O, MacDonell RC, Finlayson DC, et al: Intraoperative hemodialysis during cardiopulmonary bypass in chronic renal failure. *J Thorac Cardiovasc Surg* 1979; **77:**789-791.

232. Vreman HJ, Assomull VM, Kaiser BA, et al: Acetate metabolism and acid-base homeostasis during hemodialysis: Influence of dialyzer efficiency and rate of acetate metabolism. *Kidney Int* 1980; **10:**S62-S74.

233. Ethylene oxide (ETO) as a major cause of anaphylactoid reactions in dialysis (A review). *Artif Organs* 1987; **11:**111-117.

234. Ansorge W, Pelger M, Dietrich W, Baurmeister U: Ethylene oxide in dialyzer rinsing fluid: Effect of rinsing technique, dialyzer storage time, and potting compound. *Artif Organs* 1987; **11:**118-122.

235. Diaz JH, Cooper ES, Ochsner JL: Cardiac surgery in patients with cold autoimmune diseases. *Anesth Analg* 1984; **63:**349-352.

236. Park JV, Weiss CI: Cardiopulmonary bypass and myocardial protection: Management problems in cardiac surgical patients with cold autoimmune disease. *Anesth Analg* 1988; **67:**75-78.

237. Bracken CA, Gurkowski MA, Naples JJ, et al: Cardiopulmonary bypass in two patients with previously undetected cold agglutinins. *J Cardiothorac Vasc Anesth* 1993; **7:**743-749.

238. Agarwal SK, Ghosh PK, Gupta D: Cardiac surgery and cold-reactive proteins. *Ann Thorac Surg* 1995; **60:**1143-1150.

239. Moore RA, Geller EA, Mathews ES, Botros SB, Jose AB, Clark DL: The effect of hypothermic cardiopulmonary bypass on patients with low-titer, nonspecific cold agglutinins. *Ann Thorac Surg* 1984; **37:**233-238.

240. Berreklouw E, Moulijn AC, Pegels JG, Meijne NG: Myocardial protection with cold cardioplegia in a patient with cold autoagglutins and hemolysins. *Ann Thorac Surg* 1982; **33:**521-522.

241. Heiner M, Teasdale SJ, David T, et al: Aorto-coronary bypass in a patient with sickle cell trait. *Can Anaesth Soc J* 1979; **26:**428-438.

242. Yacoub MH, Baron J, El-Etr J, Kittle CF: Aortic homograft replacement of the mitral valve in sickle cell trait. *J Thorac Cardiovasc Surg* 1970; **59:**568-573.

243. Metras D, Coulibaly AO, Longechaud A, Millet P: Open-heart surgery in sickle-cell haemoglobinopathies: Report of 15 cases. *Thorax* 1982; **37:**486-491.

244. Fox MA, Abbott TR: Hypothermic cardiopulmonary bypass in a patient with sickle-cell trait. *Anaesthesia* 1984; **39:**1121-1123.

245. Somanathan S: Anaesthesia and hypothermia in sickle cell disease. *Anaesthesia* 1976; **31:**113.

246. Chun PKC, Flannery EP, Bowen TE: Open-heart surgery in patients with hematologic disorders. *Am Heart J* 1983; **105:**835-842.

247. Riethmuller R, Grundy EM, Radley-Smith R: Open heart surgery in a patient with homozygous sickle cell disease. *Anaesthesia* 1982; **37:**324-327.

248. Kingsley CP, Chronister T, Cohen DJ, et al: Anesthetic management of a patient with hemoglobin SS disease and mitral insufficiency for mitral valve repair. *J Cardiothorac Vasc Anesth* 1996; **10:**419-424.

11

Mechanical Circulatory Assist Devices

James A. DiNardo

This chapter focuses on mechanical circulatory support devices currently available for clinical use. The intra-aortic balloon pump (IABP), centrifugal pumps, ventricular assist devices (VADs), and the total artificial heart (TAH) will be covered. The devices to be reviewed are those in current clinical use (*see* Table 11-1).

■ INDICATIONS FOR MECHANICAL CIRCULATORY ASSIST

The indications for mechanical circulatory support are the presence of left ventricular (LV) failure, right ventricular (RV) failure, or both in the setting of maximal intravenous inotropic support. Maximal inotropic support is defined as use of two or more of the following:

- Dobutamine > 10 µg/kg/min
- Dopamine > 10 µg/kg/min
- Epinephrine > 0.2 µg/kg/min
- Amrinone > 10 µg/kg/min, after a loading dose of 0.75–1.5 mg/kg
- Milrinone > 0.75 µg/kg/min, after a loading dose of 50 µg/kg

Ventricular failure is defined as one or both of the following:

LV dysfunction
- cardiac index < 1.8–2.0 L/min/m²

- systolic blood pressure < 90 mm Hg or mean arterial pressure (MAP) < 70 mm Hg
- left atrial (LA) pressure > 18–25 mm Hg

RV dysfunction
- cardiac index < 1.8–2.0 L/min/m²
- systolic blood pressure < 90 mm Hg or MAP < 70 mm Hg
- RA pressure > 18–20 mm Hg

■ DEVICE SELECTION

The type of mechanical circulatory device selected depends, in large part, on the setting in which the device is to be used. Mechanical circulatory assist devices currently are used in four major capacities:

1. As temporary circulatory support in the subset of patients with postcardiotomy cardiac dysfunction in whom recovery of significant myocardial function is expected. Patients in this category receive short-term to intermediate (days to weeks) mechanical circulatory support during a critical interval while ventricular function recovers. The assist device is then weaned and explanted. This is the most common indication for circulatory support. Postcardiotomy cardiogenic shock is estimated to occur in 2 to 6% of all patients undergoing surgery for coronary revascularization or

TABLE 11–1. CURRENTLY AVAILABLE MECHANICAL CIRCULATORY ASSIST DEVICES

Intra-aortic balloon pump
Centrifugal pumps
    Centramed (LVS, RVS, BVS)
    Bio-Medicus (LVS, RVS, BVS)
    Medtronic (LVS, RVS, BVS)
    Terumo (LVS, RVS, BVS)
Ventricular assist devices
    Thoratec (Pierce-Donachy) (LVAD, RVAD, BiVAD)
    TCI (Heartmate) Left Ventricular Assist Device (LVAD)
    Novacor Left Ventricular Assist System (LVAD)
    Abiomed BVS 5000 (LVAD, RVAD, BiVAD)
Total artificial heart
    CardioWest Total Artificial Heart

LVS, left ventricular support; RVS, right ventricular support; BVS, biventricular support; LVAD, left ventricular assist device; RVAD, right ventricular assist device; BiVAD, biventricular assist device.

valve repair/replacement;[1] 1% of all postcardiotomy patients require mechanical circulatory support.[2] The use of centrifugal pumps and VADs as temporary circulatory support in patients with cardiogenic shock after cardiac surgical procedures has been less successful than the bridge to transplantation experience. Although small individual series[3,4] have survival rates as high as 40%, the Combined Registry for the Clinical Use of Mechanical Ventricular Assist Pumps and Artificial Hearts reports that the overall hospital discharge rate for 965 patients is 25%.[5] This low survival rate is similar for patients supported with both VADs and centrifugal pumps. Factors that have been associated with poor outcome are renal failure, perioperative myocardial infarction, and infection.[5,6] Most patients who do survive are New York Heart Association (NYHA) functional class I or II.[5,7,8]

The IABP, centrifugal pumps, the Abiomed BVS system, and the Thoratec VAD with atrial cannulation all can be used for postcardiotomy support. Biventricular support can be provided by centrifugal pumps, the Thoratec VAD, and the Abiomed BVS system.

2. As temporary circulatory support that provides a bridge to cardiac transplantation. In the case of a bridge to transplantation, a mechanical assist device is implanted with the intention of providing intermediate to long-term (weeks to months) support until a suitable donor heart is found or until the patient dies from irreversible damage to other organ systems. Devices used for a bridge to transplantation must allow patient mobilization and discharge from an inten-

sive care unit (ICU) setting because the wait for a donor heart may be long.

At present, the limiting factor in the number of patients who can be offered a heart transplant is the availability of donor hearts. It is estimated that although 15,000 patients per year could benefit from a heart transplant, only 1,100 donor hearts are available per year.[9] Furthermore, 25 to 30% of suitable transplant candidates die before a donor heart can be found.[9,10] As a result, mechanical assist devices and the TAH are being used with greater frequency as a bridge to cardiac transplantation. For transplant candidates at immediate risk of circulatory arrest, these devices provide mechanical circulatory support until a suitable donor heart is found. The first two successful uses of a VAD as a bridge to transplantation were initiated within days of each other in September 1984, using a Novacor LVAD[11] and a Thoretec LVAD.[12] The first long-term clinical success with a TAH serving as a bridge to transplantation took place in 1985 using the predecessor of the CardioWest TAH, the Symbion Jarvik 7-100 TAH.[13]

The outcome after bridge to transplantation is very good. A recent Combined Registry report revealed that of 584 bridged patients, 70% were transplanted and 69% of those patients went on to be discharged from the hospital.[14] A previous Registry report revealed similar findings.[5] Discharge rates were best for patients supported with a left ventricular assist device (LVAD) as compared with patients supported with right ventricular assist devices (RVADs), biventricular assist devices (BiVADs), or the TAH. However, recent experience with the CardioWest TAH demonstrates transplant and survival rates comparable to other assist devices.[15] After hospital discharge, LVAD patients without preexisting organ dysfunction have 1- and 2-year actuarial survival rates, similar to patients receiving orthotopic heart transplantation without mechanical circulatory support.[5,14]

The TCI and Novacor devices are used exclusively for a bridge to transplantation in patients requiring LV support. The Thoratec VAD also can be used in this capacity. Patients with a bridge to transplantation who require biventricular support are candidates for the TAH, the Thoratec VAD, or the Novacor or TCI devices in conjunction with a centrifugal pump or Thoratec VAD for RV support.

3. As permanently implanted mechanical assist devices. Currently, the Novacor and TCI devices are the two devices available for permanent LV mechanical assist.

4. As temporary short-term circulatory support in the setting of acute myocardial infarction. To date, only the IABP has been evaluated in this capacity.

■ COMPLICATIONS

Accumulated experience has consistently identified thromboembolism, perioperative hemorrhage, and infection as the three major complications associated with use of circulatory assist devices and the TAH, particularly when used long term for a bridge to transplantation.[5,16]

■ CLASSIFICATION OF DEVICES

Several classifications of mechanical circulatory support devices exist, and there is considerable overlap between classifications.

Orthotopic and Heterotopic Prosthetic Ventricles

Heterotopic prosthetic ventricles provide mechanical support in parallel or in series with the intact native ventricles. These devices are commonly called ventricular assist devices (VADs). Some VADs are designed only for left ventricular support, whereas others may be used for left ventricular (LVAD), right ventricular (RVAD), or biventricular support (BiVAD). Table 11–1 summarizes the uses of the clinically available devices.

Orthotopic devices provide mechanical support in place of the excised native ventricles. The native atria are surgically placed in continuity with the prosthetic ventricles. Orthotopic prosthetic ventricles are described more commonly as total artificial hearts (TAHs). Worldwide, as of April 1996, 10 different types of TAHs have been implanted. Most (260 of 306) of these implantations have been CardioWest TAHs or its predecessor, the Symbion (Jarvic) J7 TAH. Of the 188 Symbion TAH implants, 41 were the 100-mL stroke volume type (J7-100) and 147 were of the smaller 70-mL stroke volume type (J7-70). There have been 72 CardioWest TAH implants.

Series versus Parallel Circulatory Support

A circulatory support device may be used in parallel or in series with the native ventricular system, depending on how cannulation for the device is achieved. When inflow to the device is achieved via cannulation of the native atrium and outflow is via cannulation of the corresponding great vessel, the device is said to be "in parallel" with the native ventricular system. When inflow to the device is achieved via cannulation of the apex of the native ventricle and outflow is via cannula-

tion of the corresponding great vessel, the device is said to be "in series" with the native ventricle. Some devices always are used in series with the native ventricle (Novacor LVAD and Thermo Cardiosystems LVAD), some are always used in parallel (Abiomed BVS and centrifugal pumps), and one can be used in either a series or parallel arrangement (Thoratec VAD). Figure 11–1 illustrates parallel and series arrangement.

In general, the series arrangement provides better filling and a higher device output for two reasons. First, the device does not compete with the native ventricle for atrial blood the way it must in a parallel arrangement. Second, native ventricular systole serves to fill the prosthetic ventricle. The series arrangement also provides the native ventricle with a low-impedance outflow tract into the prosthetic ventricle, which greatly reduces native ventricular diameter and systolic wall stress. The major disadvantage of a series arrangement is that the ventricular apex will become akinetic or dyskinetic after removal of the ventricular cannula. For patients who are to be transplanted, this is not an important issue. However, it is a very important issue for patients who are ultimately to be weaned off mechanical support.[17]

Pulsatile versus Nonpulsatile Flow

The IABP and both orthotopic and heterotopic prosthetic ventricles provide pulsatile flow, whereas centrifugal pumps provide nonpulsatile flow. Two types of pulsatile prosthetic ventricles are currently in use: pneumatic and electromechanical. Pulsatile pneumatic pumps use

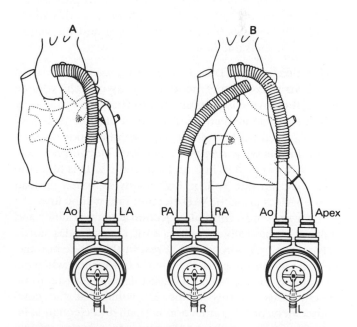

FIGURE 11–1. A. Schematic of a Thoratec VAD in parallel with the left heart. **B.** Schematic of a Thoratec VAD in parallel with the right heart and in series with the left heart.

pressurized air to eject blood from the prosthetic ventricular chamber. Pulsatile electromechanical pumps convert electrical energy to the mechanical energy necessary to eject blood from the prosthetic ventricular chamber.

Extracorporeal versus Implantable Devices

Some devices are extracorporeal, whereas others are implantable. With extracorporeal devices, the pumping device is located outside the body, with both the inflow and outflow conduits entering the patient's thoracic cavity. Implantable devices are implanted in the patient's pericardial cavity or pre-intraperitoneally.

Triggering Modes and Percentage of Systole

Pulsatile pumps have a number of different ways in which ejection can be triggered. In the case of TAH, the ejection rate is set by the operator and is analogous to the heart rate. Because VADs are used in conjunction with the native ventricular system, more options are available to trigger a VADs ejection cycle:

Manual. This mode, also known as the single stroke mode, is used for deairing of the device after implantation. It allows a single ejection with the touch of a button.

Asynchronous. In the asynchronous mode, the VAD ejects at a rate decided upon by the operator. This produces a fixed rate, variable stroke volume mode of operation. At higher device rates, the time available for diastolic filling will be reduced. This can in part be offset by increasing preload to the device. In this mode there will be beats in which the device and the ventricle eject at the same time.

Fill-to-Empty. This is the most commonly used mode for VADs. In this mode, also known as the volume mode, the device is programmed to trigger ejection only when the VAD is filled with blood in diastole. This produces a fixed stroke volume, variable rate mode of operation. In this triggering mode, the VAD ejection rate will vary with preload. When preload to the VAD is high, the VAD ejection rate will be high; likewise, when preload to the VAD is poor, the VAD ejection rate will be low.

Device and ventricular ejection rates will differ and will vary phasically. In the case of series LVADs, aortic valve opening is rarely seen at rest in this mode but may be present during exercise.[18] In a series device, when device filling coincides with LV diastole, filling is said to be synchronous. In this setting, LV volume at the commencement of LV contraction is small and ejection is insufficient to open the aortic valve. In a series device, when device filling coincides with LV systole, filling is said to be countersynchronous. In this setting, there is no ejection out the aortic valve as the low-impedance pathway during native ventricular systole is into the device.

The manner in which filling of the VAD in diastole is detected will be discussed in detail in the section on individual devices. The Novacor device does not have a fill-to-empty mode per se but has a mode that offers similar performance characteristics.

Synchronous. In the synchronous mode, an external electrical signal, usually the R wave of the electrocardiogram (ECG) is used to trigger VAD ejection. Using a programmable delay, the operator can use this mode to reduce ventricular afterload by preventing the device from ejecting into the aorta or pulmonary artery at the same time as the native ventricle.

In addition to having various triggering modes, some devices allow the operator to program the percentage of systole. This allows the operator to decide what percentage of each prosthetic ventricular cycle is devoted to ejection. Obviously, as the prosthetic ventricular ejection rate increases, the time between cycles diminishes. The advantage of reducing the percentage of systole is that it allows a greater proportion of each cycle to be devoted to prosthetic ventricular filling. However, for a given ejection rate, reducing the percentage of systole increases the rapidity of the ejection phase. The more rapid the ejection phase, the more likely are turbulent flow and damage to formed blood elements with resultant hemolysis.[19]

■ DEVICE DESCRIPTION

Intra-aortic Balloon Pump

The intra-aortic balloon pump (IABP), first introduced into clinical use in 1968, has become an important method of providing circulatory support in a wide variety of patients.

The IABP consists of a catheter-mounted balloon, a pump, a gas source, and a microprocessor console. The balloon is thin-walled, measures 2×20 cm, and contains 30 to 40 mL of volume when inflated. The catheter has a hollow central lumen, which allows percutaneous placement over a guidewire, as well as the recording of central aortic pressure. The pump inflates and deflates the balloon at precisely timed intervals, with either CO_2 or helium as the inflating gas. CO_2 carries less of an embolic risk if the balloon ruptures because it is absorbed quickly. Helium has a lower density, allowing faster inflation and deflation, and currently is the preferred gas. The console displays the ECG, the arterial waveform, and the balloon pressure trace. The console controls exactly when the pump inflates and deflates the balloon.

Proper functioning of the IABP depends on the precise timing of balloon inflation and deflation relative to the cardiac cycle. Balloon inflation (*see* Fig. 11–2) optimally occurs immediately after the closure of the aortic valve as represented by the dicrotic notch on the central arterial pressure tracing. The resultant increase in aortic volume increases diastolic arterial pressure (diastolic augmentation) and improves systemic and coronary artery perfusion pressure. The increase in aortic diastolic pressure depends on a number of variables: the nonaugmented aortic diastolic pressure, the compliance of the aorta, the size of the balloon, and the volume of gas in the balloon (from minimal to full volume). Balloon inflation in the noncompliant aorta of an elderly patient will produce a higher augmented diastolic pressure than the same balloon in a compliant aorta.

In the absence of coronary stenoses, augmentation of aortic diastolic blood pressure increases coronary blood flow in both the proximal and distal coronary arteries.[20-22] In the presence of critical coronary stenoses, the IABP does not improve coronary blood flow distal to the stenoses.[20,21] It is conceivable that coronary beds distal to a stenosis could have improved coronary perfusion with IABP counterpulsation if the beds are supplied by collaterals from a nonstenosed coronary artery.

Deflation of the balloon (*see* Fig. 11–3) is adjusted to occur immediately before left ventricular ejection, at the onset of the upstroke of the central arterial waveform. Optimal balloon deflation is established when the arterial diastolic pressure is maximally reduced (unloading). The duration of isovolumic contraction of the left ventricle is determined by the pressure gradient between the left ventricle and the proximal aorta. Balloon deflation quickly lowers proximal aortic pressure, thereby reducing afterload by decreasing the impedance to ejection out the left ventricle. This shortens the duration of isovolumic contraction, which in turn reduces myocardial oxygen consumption. Reduction of myocardial oxygen consumption, rather than augmentation of coronary blood flow, is the primary method by which the IABP ameliorates myocardial ischemia.

In addition to reducing myocardial oxygen consumption, properly timed IABP deflation improves LV systolic function on a beat-to-beat basis by decreasing systolic wall stress.[23] Increases in ejection phase indicates of systolic function, such as ejection fraction, are directly proportional to IABP-induced decreases in systolic wall stress.[23]

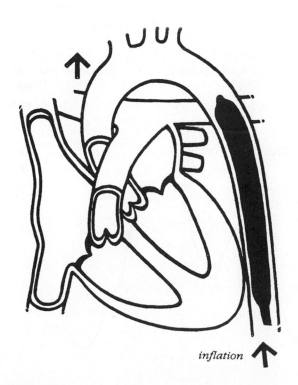

FIGURE 11–2. A properly positioned balloon pump inflating in the descending aorta.

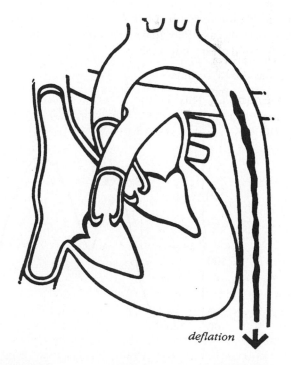

FIGURE 11–3. A properly positioned balloon pump deflating in the descending aorta.

Indications and Contraindications. The indications for IABP use are summarized:

1. Patients with refractory myocardial ischemia
2. Patients with cardiogenic shock
   - myocardial infarction
   - myocarditis
   - cardiomyopathy
   - pharmacologic depression
3. Stabilization of patients before cardiac surgery
   - myocardial infarction
   - postinfarction ventricular septal defect (VSD)
   - mitral regurgitation
   - bridge to cardiac transplantation
4. Support of patients after cardiac surgery
   - reversible LV dysfunction
   - intraoperative myocardial infarction
   - allograft dysfunction after heart transplantation
5. Support of noncardiac surgical patients
   - support during percutaneous coronary angioplasty
   - to maintain coronary artery patency after thrombolytic therapy[21] or angioplasty[24] in the setting of acute myocardial infarction
   - support during noncardiac surgical procedures

There are few absolute contraindications to the use of the IABP. Aortic valve incompetence is a contraindication because balloon inflation in diastole will increase the regurgitant fraction. Aortic dissection and aortic aneurysm are contraindications because balloon inflation could promote frank aortic rupture. Severe peripheral vascular disease may make placement of the IABP via the femoral artery impossible.

Insertion. Most IABP catheters are inserted percutaneously using the Seldinger technique via the femoral artery retrograde into the descending aorta. Surgical cutdown to expose the femoral artery, followed by cannulation of the artery under direct vision using the modified Seldinger technique, is reserved for situations in which location of the femoral artery percutaneously may be difficult, such as with hypotension, lack of pulsatile flow on cardiopulmonary bypass (CPB), obesity, and peripheral vascular disease. The IABP usually is placed through an arterial sheath, but newer models allow placement of the IABP catheter directly into the femoral artery without a sheath. This is a useful alternative for patients with small femoral arteries.

The balloon should be placed so that the proximal tip is distal to the left subclavian artery and the distal end is proximal to the renal arteries. The length of IABP catheter required is estimated by the distance from the femoral artery to the sternomanubrial junction. Final position can be verified with a chest radiograph, fluoroscopy, transesophageal echocardiography,[22] or direct palpation of the descending aorta by the surgeon.

When severe peripheral vascular disease precludes retrograde insertion via the femoral artery, the balloon catheter can be placed antegrade in the descending thoracic aorta via the right subclavian artery, the axillary artery, or the ascending aorta. Placement via the ascending aorta requires a sternotomy. The technique is used only for postcardiotomy patients who cannot otherwise be weaned from cardiopulmonary bypass and necessitates subsequent removal under anesthesia in the operating room.

Complications. The incidence of complications from intra-aortic balloon counterpulsation that are se-

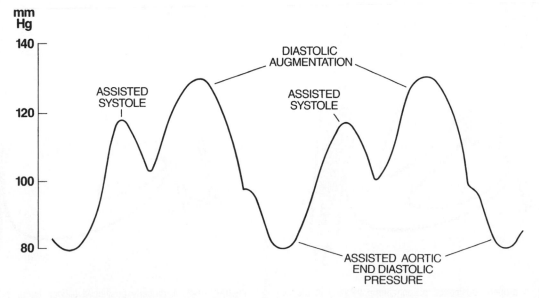

FIGURE 11–4. Arterial pressure trace from a patient receiving 1:1 IABP support with proper timing.

vere enough to require balloon removal or surgical intervention ranges from 17 to 35%.[25] The most common complication is lower limb ischemia. However, there are reports of every major branch of the aorta being occluded by thrombus, embolus, or balloon-induced dissection. Other complications include thrombocytopenia and balloon or console failure.

Management of the IABP.   Optimal performance of the IABP depends on proper triggering and timing.

TRIGGERING.   The microprocessor most commonly makes use of the ECG to trigger the balloon. It uses the R wave as the central timing event and will direct balloon inflation to occur during the T wave (diastole) and balloon deflation immediately before the subsequent QRS complex (onset of systole). The signal to the balloon console can be the ECG transmitted by a cable from the operating room monitor or the ECG derived from a separate set of balloon "skin" leads directly to the console. The former is preferable if the skin leads have not been placed before surgical prepping and draping. Radiofrequency current from the electrocautery used in the operating room can interfere with the ECG trigger. The balloon leads have a special built-in radiofrequency filter that helps alleviate this problem. Alternatively, using the operating room monitor in the more heavily filtered nondiagnostic mode will help filter out some of the noise. Other maneuvers that diminish the effect of radiofrequency current include placing all ECG leads in a single frontal plane, which reduces the potential difference between any of the leads, and using the lowest electrocautery current setting possible, in short bursts.

The balloon pump is not capable of deflating soon enough after detection of the R wave to provide unloading. As a result, most consoles detect the R wave and inflate in diastole after a preset interval that allows completion of mechanical systole. After another preset interval, the balloon deflates in anticipation of the next mechanical systole. Alternate trigger sources are atrial pacer spikes, ventricular or atrial-ventricular pacer spikes, the arterial waveform, and internal (a fixed rate of 40, 60, or 120 cycles per minute used during asystole, CPB, ventricular fibrillation; some models allow a variable internal rate).

TIMING.   Although the ECG is used to trigger balloon inflation and deflation, proper counterpulsation timing is confirmed by examination of an arterial pressure waveform. When the radial artery is transduced, there is a 60-msec delay in waveform transmission from the central aorta. When the femoral artery is used, there is a 120-msec delay in waveform transmission from the central aorta. Inflation using these arterial pressure monitoring sites must be adjusted accordingly. Ideally, balloon inflation occurs at the dicrotic notch in the central aorta. When the radial artery pressure is monitored, inflation should be adjusted to occur 60 msec before the radial artery dicrotic notch. When the femoral artery pressure is monitored, balloon inflation should be adjusted to occur 120 msec before the femoral artery dicrotic notch.

The details of proper timing are illustrated in Figures 11–4 through 11–7. Proper timing requires that the

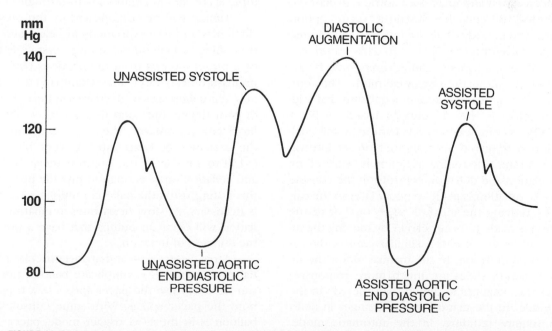

FIGURE 11–5. Arterial pressure trace from a patient receiving 1:2 intra-aortic balloon pump (IABP) support with proper timing.

1. Early Inflation

Inflation of the IAB prior to aortic valve closure

Waveform Characteristics:

- Inflation of IAB prior to dicrotic notch.
- Diastolic augmentation encroaches onto systole (may be unable to distinguish)

Physiologic Effects:

- Potential premature closure of aortic valve
- Potential increase in LVEDV and LVEDP or PCWP
- Increased left ventricular wall stress or afterload
- Aortic Regurgitation
- Increased MVO₂ demand

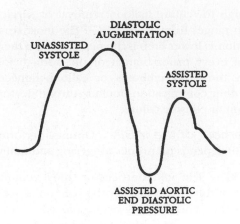

2. Late Inflation

Inflation of the IAB markedly after closure of the aortic valve

Waveform Characteristics:

- Inflation of the IAB after the dicrotic notch.
- Absense of sharp V
- Sub-optimal diastolic augmentation

Physiologic Effects:

- Sub-optimal coronary artery perfusion

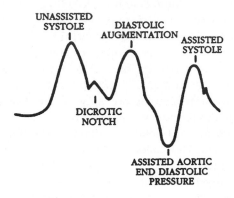

FIGURE 11–6. Arterial waveforms resulting from (1) early balloon inflation and (2) from late balloon inflation. The physiologic consequences of these timing errors are summarized.

IABP be triggered every second or third R wave (1:2 or 1:3). This allows observation of assisted and unassisted systole and of assisted and unassisted aortic end-diastolic pressure. Some IABP consoles contain a "verify" option that highlights the period of balloon inflation in real time on the arterial waveform (*see* Fig. 11–8). This feature is a useful aid in obtaining proper timing. Timing may be accomplished in the automatic or manual mode. The automatic mode uses the R wave and an algorithm that triggers balloon inflation after an interval based on heart rate, which allows completion of mechanical systole. Balloon deflation is triggered after another preset interval based on heart rate. Fine tuning of timing is obtained by use of the inflation and deflation controls on the console (*see* Fig. 11-9). Inflation is made to occur later in the cardiac cycle by moving the inflation slide "out" or to the right. Inflation is made to occur earlier by moving the inflation slide "in" or to the left. A similiar control slide is used to fine tune deflation. In the manual mode, the inflation and deflation slides are much more responsive and cause greater changes in timing than they do in the automatic mode. In the manual mode, changes in heart > 10 bpm require retiming. In the automatic mode, changes in heart rate are adjusted for automatically.

Observation of the balloon pressure waveform also yields useful information about IABP function. This topic is covered in Figures 11-10 through 11-12.

Timing will be complicated by the presence of arrhythmias and large variations in heart rate. Recall that the timing of balloon deflation in systole is determined by a preset interval from the previous QRS. As a result, premature beats rarely are accompanied by proper timing. Acute increases or decreases in heart rate will result in poor timing, but good timing can be obtained when heart rate is constant. The only exception to this is at the extremes of heart rate. At very high heart rates (>130 to 140 bpm), the pump is incapable of inflation and deflation rapid enough to provide proper timing. In this setting, using the balloon pump at a 1:2 ratio usually is necessary. At slow heart rates, premature balloon deflation will occur in pumps that have a preset limit on the duration of inflation.

Atrial, ventricular, and atrioventricular (AV) sequential pacing can also complicate balloon timing. Pumps can be set to use the pacer spikes as a trigger or to ignore the pacer spikes. With some consoles, when the balloon is in the ECG trigger mode, pacer spike rejection is automatic. If the microprocessor has difficulty ig-

3. Early Deflation

Premature deflation of the IAB during the diastolic phase

Waveform Characteristics:

- Deflation of IAB is seen as a sharp drop following diastolic augmentation
- Suboptimal diastolic augmentation
- Assisted aortic end diastolic pressure may be equal to or less than the unassisted aortic end diastolic pressure
- Assisted systolic pressure may rise

Physiologic Effects:

- Sub-optimal coronary perfusion
- Potential for retrograde coronary and cartoid blood flow
- Angina may occur as a result of retrograde coronary blood flow
- Sub-optimal afterload reduction
- Increased MVO_2 demand

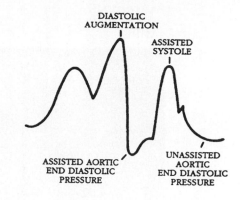

4. Late Deflation

Waveform Characteristics:

- Assisted aortic end-diastolic pressure may be equal to the unassisted aortic end diastolic pressure
- Rate of rise of assisted systole is prolonged
- Diastolic augmentation may appear widened

Physiologic Effects:

- Afterload reduction is essentially absent
- Increased MVO_2 consumption due to the left ventricle ejecting against a greater resistance and a prolonged isovolumetric contraction phase
- IAB may impede left ventricular ejection and increase the afterload

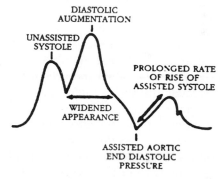

FIGURE 11–7. Arterial waveforms resulting from (1) early balloon deflation and (2) from late balloon deflation. The physiologic consequences of these timing errors are summarized.

noring a pacer spike, the use of bipolar pacing or ECG leads that minimize the pacer spikes may be necessary. Pacer spikes are used as triggers only when an ECG trigger is not effective.

Anticoagulation.   Anticoagulation is necessary both to prevent thrombus formation on the balloon and in the cannulated peripheral vessel. This usually is accomplished with a heparin infusion to maintain a prothrombin time (PTT) 1.5 to 2.0 times control or an activated clotting time (ACT) > 200 seconds. In the post-operative setting, initiation of heparin infusion may be delayed for 12 to 24 hours or until chest tube drainage is minimal. Alternative approaches include aspirin or low-molecular-weight dextran in place of or in addition to heparin.

CardioWest TAH

The CardioWest TAH is the direct descendent of the Symbion (Jarvik) J7-70 TAH. The CardioWest has a 70-mL

stroke volume and can deliver cardiac outputs of 15 L/min. It is a pneumatically driven device and each ventricle has a pneumatic drive line. The drive lines are attached to a drive console on wheels. The drive console is large because it contains four air compressors, two for each driver, and one as a backup (*see* Fig. 11–13).

The prosthetic ventricles are rigid polyurethane, dacron mesh shells divided into a blood and a pneumatic chamber by a four-layer polyurethane diaphragm. The diaphragm is flexible but noncompliant and each layer is separated by a small amount of graphite for lubrication. Unidirectional Medtronic-Hall tilting disc valves are located in the blood chamber. The ventricles are identical, except that the spacing between the inflow and outflow valves in the right ventricle is larger to allow for aortic outflow when the ventricles are attached together with a Velcro patch (*see* Fig. 11–14).

The pneumatic chamber communicates with the pneumatic drive system via the pneumatic driveline. As

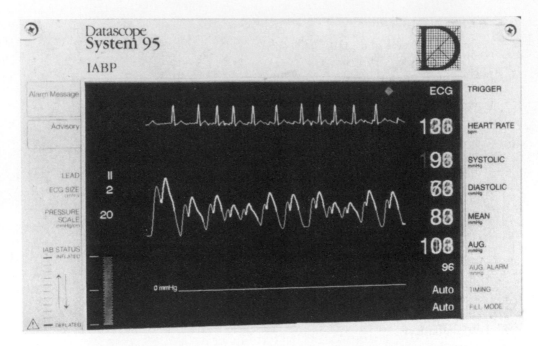

FIGURE 11–8. Use of the "verify" feature highlights the period of balloon inflation in real time on the arterial waveform.

pressurized air is introduced into the pneumatic chamber, the diaphragm moves such that the blood chamber becomes pressurized as well. When the pressure in the blood chamber exceeds the device filling pressure, the inflow valve will close. When pressure in the blood chamber exceeds aortic or pulmonary artery pressure, the outflow valve opens and ejection commences. These processes constitute the isovolemic and ejection phases of systole in the prosthetic ventricle (*see* Fig. 11–15).

At the end of systole, air is vented passively from the pneumatic chamber to the atmosphere and the pressure in the blood chamber falls. This constitutes isovolemic relaxation. When the pressure in the right atrium and left atrium exceeds the pressure in the blood chamber of the corresponding prosthetic ventricle, the inflow valve opens. The diaphragm is free to move in such a manner that virtually the entire volume of the prosthetic ventricle can fill with blood as all the air

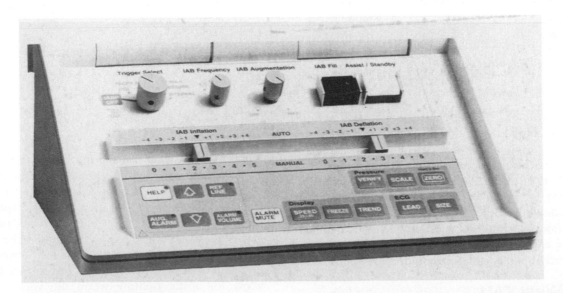

FIGURE 11–9. IABP control console showing the inflation and deflation slides to fine tune balloon timing. The trigger select knob can be seen in the upper right corner of the console. Intra-aortic balloon pump (IABP) frequency selection from 1:1 to 1:3 is the second knob to the right. IABP augmentation is the third knob to the right; this controls the amount of gas in the balloon with variation from minimal volume to full volume.

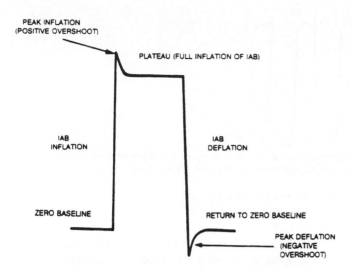

FIGURE 11–10. A normal balloon pressure waveform.

leaves the pneumatic chamber. This constitutes diastole in the prosthetic ventricle (*see* Fig. 11–15).

Indications and Contraindications.
Because implantation of the TAH requires excision of the native ventricles[26] this device is used only as a bridge to cardiac transplantation. Patients who are not suitable candidates for cardiac transplantation are not candidates for the TAH.

Insertion.
Placement of the TAH requires CPB with aortic cross-clamping and bicaval cannulation. The device is placed in the patient's pericardial cavity with the RV and LV pneumatic drive lines exiting through the skin. The patient's native ventricles are excised, leaving a large cuff of right and left atrium. The inflow cuff of each ventricle is anastomosed to the appropriate atrium. End-to-end anastomoses are created between the outflow graft of the prosthetic ventricle and the appropriate great vessel. The TAH has been placed in pa-

tients weighing as little as 50 kg, but the best fit is in patients with weights in the 80-kg range (body surface area > 1.7 m²) with large hearts. Closure of the chest after device implantation in patients who are too small can produce pulmonary and systemic venous obstruction. The inferior vena cava and the left upper and left lower pulmonary veins are at particular risk of obstruction. Venous obstruction limits device output and is ultimately fatal.

Management of the TAH.
The TAH is monitored with the cardiac output monitor and diagnostic unit (COMDU).[27-30] COMDU allows analysis of air exhaust flow during diastole through transduction of a pneumotach. The flow is displayed as a curve with respect to time (*see* Figs. 11–16 and 11–17). Integration of this curve yields the volume of air displaced from the pneumatic chamber during diastole. When averaged over several beats, this is equal to cardiac output. The system allows computation of cardiac output for each ventricle. In addition, transduction of the drive line pressure allows device filling and emptying to be monitored over time, as illustrated in Figures 11–18 and 11–19.

The heart rate and percentage of systole are set by the operator and complete ejection is sought on each cycle. The drive pressures are set just high enough to completely empty the ventricle. The occurrence of a full eject pattern is then seen on the air-pressure waveform. The device is not allowed to fill completely on each beat. This allows automatic adjustment for the difference in volumes pumped by the two ventricles; the LV pumps more than the RV because of the existence of bronchial flow. It also provides for preload reserve. As venous return increases (such as with patient position changes or exercise), stroke volume can increase up to the limit of the 70 mL.

The maximum end-diastolic volume of the prosthetic ventricle may be difficult to achieve when diastole is short (slow ejection rate, high percentage of sys-

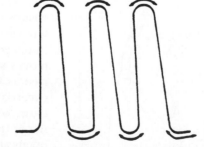

Catheter Kink
Rounded balloon pressure waveform, loss of plateau resulting from kink or obstruction of shuttle gas. This may be caused by kink in catheter tubing, improper IAB catheter position, sheath has not been pulled back to allow inflation of IAB, IAB too large for aorta, IAB is not fully unwrapped, or H_2O condensation in external tubing.

FIGURE 11–11. A balloon pressure waveform from a kinked balloon catheter.

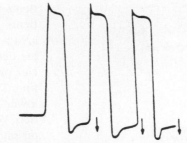

Gas Loss
Leak in the closed
system causing the
balloon pressure
waveform to fall *below*
zero baseline.
This may be due to a
loose connection, leak in IAB Catheter, H₂O condensation in external tubing, or a patient who is
tachycardic and febrile which causes increase gas diffusion through the IAB membrane.

FIGURE 11–12. A balloon pressure waveform from a balloon with a gas leak.

tole) and filling pressure is low. The pneumatic drive system of the CardioWest TAH allows vacuum to be applied to the pneumatic chamber during isovolemic relaxation and diastole to hasten the fall in blood chamber pressure and enhance diastolic filling. To reduce the likelihood of entraining air around anastomotic sites and introducing the risk of air embolism, vacuum generally is not applied until the patient's chest is closed. Normally, −25 to −50 mm Hg of vacuum is applied.

Anticoagulation. Anticoagulation generally is started after protamine reversal of intraoperative heparin and chest tube drainage less than 100 mL/hr for 3 con-

secutive hours. Low-molecular-weight dextran (dextran 40) infused at 25 mL/hr and oral or nasogastric dipyridamole (75 to 100 mg three to four times per day) are started. When chest tube drainage is minimal and serous, the dextran is stopped and a continuous heparin infusion is initiated; the goal is to keep the PTT 1.5 to 2.0 times control. At 1 to 2 weeks postoperatively, the heparin is discontinued and warfarin is started; the goal is an INR of 1.5 to 2.0.[31] Some centers add aspirin (325 to 975 mg/day) as well.

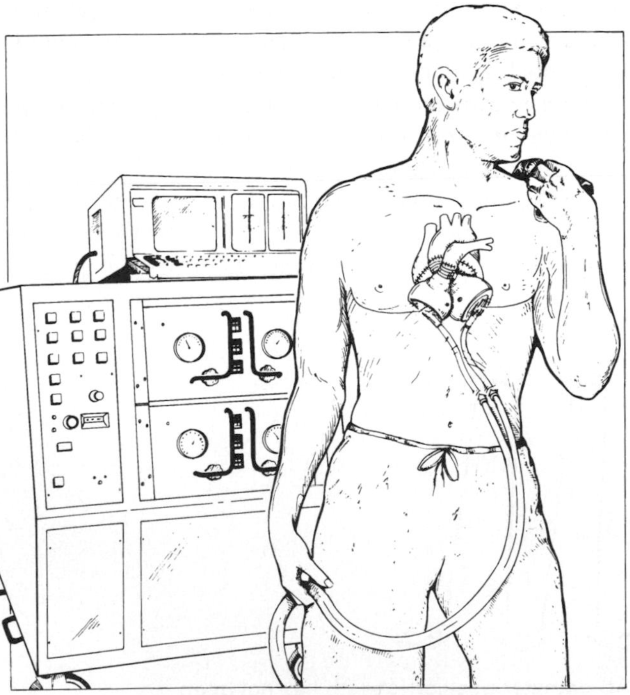

Thoratec VAD System

The Thoratec VAD or Pierce-Donachy VAD (*see* Figs. 11–1 and 11–20) is an extracorporeal, pulsatile BiVAD that can be used in parallel with the RV and in parallel or in series with the LV.[32,33] The device has an effective stroke volume of 65 mL and can deliver a cardiac output of 6.5 L/min. It is a pneumatically driven device and has a pneumatic drive line. The drive line is attached to a drive console on wheels. The drive console is large because it contains four air compressors, two for each driver, and one as a backup.

The prosthetic ventricle is a rigid polysulfone case divided into a blood and a pneumatic chamber by a flexible, noncompliant polyurethane diaphragm. Unidirectional Bjork-Shiley monstrut Derlin inflow and outflow valves are located in the blood chamber. The pneumatic chamber communicates with the pneumatic drive system via the pneumatic driveline. As pressurized air is introduced into the pneumatic chamber, the diaphragm moves such that the blood chamber becomes pressurized as well. When the pressure in the blood chamber exceeds the device filling pressure, the inflow valve will close. When pressure in the blood chamber exceeds aortic or pulmonary artery pressure, the outflow valve opens and ejection commences. These processes constitute the isovolemic and ejection phases of systole in the prosthetic ventricle.

At the end of systole, air is vented passively from the pneumatic chamber to the atomosphere, and the

FIGURE 11–13. Schematic of the CardioWest total artificial heart (TAH) showing the pneumatic drive lines, drive console, and cardiac output monitor and device unit (COMDU).

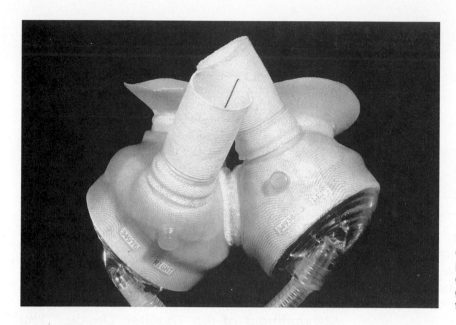

FIGURE 11–14. Close-up of the CardioWest total artificial heart (TAH) prosthetic ventricles joined by a Velcro patch. The atrial inflow cuffs are shown in the background; the dacron outflow grafts are shown in the foreground. The pneumatic drive lines are at the bottom of the picture.

pressure in the blood chamber falls. This constitutes isovolemic relaxation. When the pressure in the chamber filling the prosthetic ventricle (right atrium, left atrium, or left ventricle) exceeds the pressure in the blood chamber, the inflow valve opens. The diaphragm is free to move in such a manner that virtually the entire volume of the prosthetic ventricle can fill with blood as all of the air leaves the pneumatic chamber. This constitutes diastole in the prosthetic ventricle.

Movement of the pump diaphragm is monitored by a Hall sensor built into the rigid case. A small magnet mounted on the diaphragm triggers the Hall sensor when the two come in contact. This information is transmitted to the console via an electrical cable and allows the control console to know when the blood chamber is full. In addition, transduction of the drive line pressure allows device filling and emptying to be monitored over time as described for the CardioWest TAH.

Indications.   The Thoratec VAD is appropriate for intermediate and long-term circulatory support. The device can be used for postcardiotomy support of the LV, RV, or both ventricles. It also can be used as a bridge to transplantation. Use of the Thoratec device in series with the LV is contraindicated in the presence of a mechanical aortic valve or significant aortic insufficiency. Thrombus formation on the mechanical aortic valve can result from the absent or minimal aortic valve opening that oc-

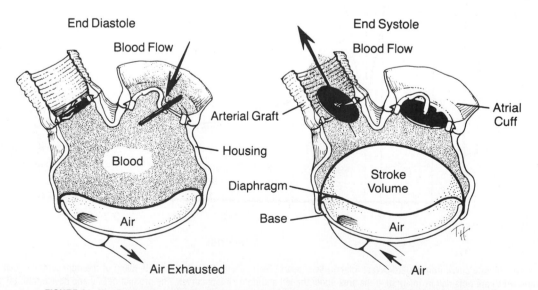

End Diastole
Blood Flow
Arterial Graft
Housing
Blood
Diaphragm
Base
Air
Air Exhausted

End Systole
Blood Flow
Atrial Cuff
Stroke Volume
Air
Air

FIGURE 11–15. Schematic of the CardioWest total artificial heart (TAH) in end diastole and in end systole.

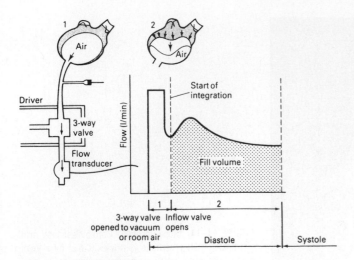

FIGURE 11–16. Schematic of the CardioWest total artificial heart (TAH) pneumotach and the resulting fill-rate curve derived from air flow out of the device in diastole.

curs when the Thoratec, in series with the native LV, is functioning normally. Aortic valve insufficiency will not permit effective or efficient LVAD functioning because a large portion of LVAD ejection will be into the native LV.

Insertion. The device rests on the anterior abdominal wall. Because the device is extracorporeal, it does limit patient mobility. The inflow and outflow conduits are tunneled into the thoracic cavity. For use as an RVAD, the inflow cannula is inserted in the right atrium and the dacron outflow conduit is anastomosed end-to-side to the pulmonary artery. For use as a parallel LVAD, the inflow cannula is inserted in the left atrium and the dacron outflow conduit is anastomosed end-to-side to the aorta. For use as a series LVAD, the inflow conduit is inserted in the LV apex and the dacron outflow conduit is anastomosed end-to-side to the aorta.

Insertion requires a median sternotomy. In the postcardiotomy setting, CPB already is in use because failure to wean from CPB is the indication for placement of the device. Postcardiotomy support is accomplished with atrial cannulation rather than cannulation of the LV apex. This facilitates subsequent weaning of the device. For patients with a bridge to transplantation, CPB is necessary for LV apical cannulation.

Management of the Thoratec Device. Four triggering modes are available: manual, asynchronous, fill-to-empty, and synchronous. In the asynchronous mode, the operator chooses the pumping rate and percentage of systole. In the fill-to-empty mode, the Hall sensor detects a full blood chamber and triggers ejection. The device typically is used in the fill-to-empty mode. In this mode, device output is calculated by the

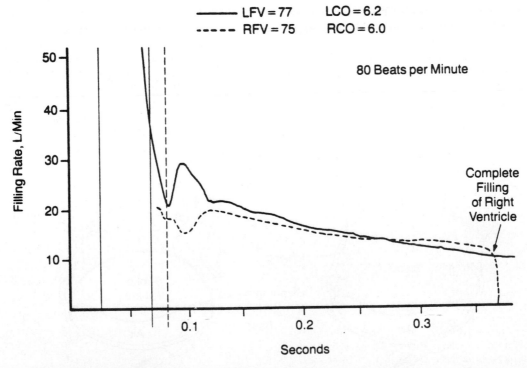

FIGURE 11–17. Actual fill rate curve from a CardioWest total artificial heart (TAH) patient. There is complete filling of the right ventricle. Left fill volume (LFV) and right fill volume (RFV) are obtained by integrating the area under the left and right fill rate curves. The product of LFV and device rate (80 beats per minute) yields the left cardiac output (LCO). The product of RFV and device rate (80 beats per minute) yields the right cardiac output (RCO).

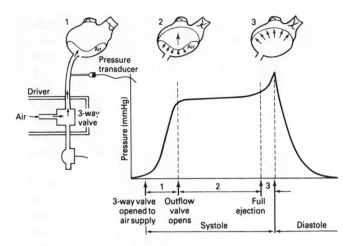

FIGURE 11–18. Schematic of the CardioWest TAH pressure transducer and the resulting pressure waveform in systole and diastole.

console as the product of stroke volume (65 mL) and device rate. Device output, as determined by the console, is accurate only when complete filling occurs.

The drive pressures are set approximately 100 mm Hg higher than systolic pressure (230 to 250 mm Hg for the LVAD and 140 to 160 for the RVAD). The percentage of systole is set to equal one-half the device rate (percentage of systole at 60 bpm = 30%; percentage of systole at

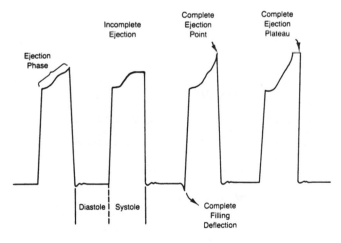

FIGURE 11–19. Actual pressure waveforms from a CardioWest total artificial heart (TAH) patient. The second waveform from the left indicates incomplete ejection of the prosthetic ventricle. This can be rectified either by afterload reduction or by increasing the drive line pressure. The third waveform from the left indicates a drive line pressure just high enough to ensure complete emptying of the prosthetic ventricle. The fourth waveform from the left also indicates complete emptying of the prosthetic ventricle. An excessive plateau is indicative of a drive-line pressure that is higher than necessary. Complete filling of the prosthetic ventricle is indicated by the negative deflection in the pressure waveform during diastole. This is produced by the compliant diaphragm rebounding over the air exhaust port in the ventricular base. In the instance illustrated here, complete filling of the prosthetic ventricle occurs at end diastole.

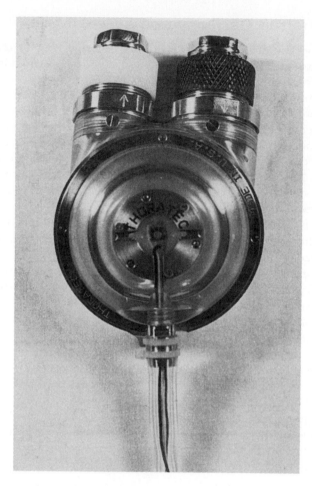

FIGURE 11–20. Thoratec ventricular assist device (VAD). The inflow to the device is on the right and the outflow is on the left. The pneumatic drive line and electrical cable are at the bottom of the device.

80 bpm = 40%). These measures produce complete emptying with an ejection time of 300 msec. The occurrence of a full eject pattern is then seen on the air pressure waveform (*see* Fig. 11-19). Complete device filling also can be seen on the pressure waveform (*see* Fig. 11-19).

The maximum end-diastolic volume of the prosthetic ventricle may be difficult to achieve when diastole is short (slow ejection rate, high percentage of systole) and filling pressure is low. The pneumatic drive systems of the Thoratec VAD allows vacuum to be applied to the pneumatic chamber during isovolemic relaxation and diastole to hasten the fall in blood chamber pressure and enhance diastolic filling. To reduce the likelihood of entraining air around cannulation sites and introducing the risk of air embolism, vacuum should be applied with caution until the patient's chest is closed. Normally, −25 to −50 mm Hg of vacuum is applied, although as much as −100 mm Hg of vacuum is possible.

Anticoagulation.   Anticoagulation is as described for the TAH.

Thermo Cardiosystems HeartMate

The Thermo Cardiosystems (TCI) VAD (*see* Figs. 11–21 through 11–23) is an implantable, pulsatile LVAD used in series with the native heart. The device has a stroke volume of 83 mL and is capable of providing 11 L/min of cardiac output. It is available in pneumatically and electromechanically driven versions. The pneumatic version has an external drive line.[34] The drive line is connected to the pneumatic drive system and system controller, which are on wheels. The pneumatic drive system and system controller are small because there are no air compressors. An electric motor is used to drive a diaphram air pump. The electromechanically driven, vented electric (VE) version has a percutaneous electric and air vent line that attaches to a portable system controller and battery pack that can be worn by the patient.[35] The sealed electric (SE) version under development is totally implantable and has power transduction occurring through transcutaneous induction coils with no percutaneous lines.

The outer shell of the device is titanium; the inner blood-contacting surface of the shell is lined with sintered titanium microspheres. A rigid pusher plate covered by a flexible, biocompatible, polyurethane diaphragm divides the prosthetic ventricle in two. On one side of the pusher plate is the blood chamber; on the other side is the pneumatic or electromechanical pumping mechanism. 25-mm porcine unidirectional inflow

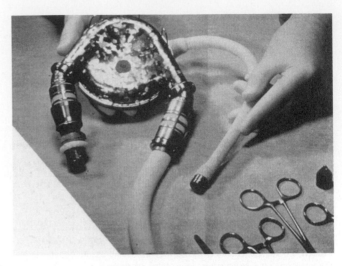

FIGURE 11–22. Photograph of a TCI device. Device inflow is on the left and outflow is on the right. The pneumatic drive line is being held.

and outflow valves are placed in the blood chamber. The textured surfaces are intended to promote formation of a pseudointimal lining after contact with blood.[36]

In the pneumatic version, a preset volume of air is delivered to the blood pump during each beat. Each stroke of the console air pump corresponds to one beat of the blood pump delivered via a piston that drives the pusher plate into the blood chamber. In the electromechanical version, the rotary motion of a low-speed

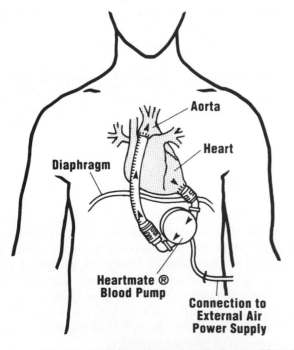

FIGURE 11–21. Schematic of an implanted pneumatically driven TCI device. Cannulation of the LV apex and the end-to-side anastomosis to the aorta are seen. The percutaneous drive line is seen exiting the abdominal wall.

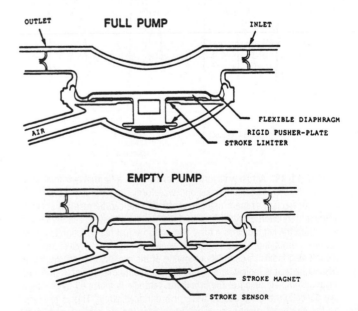

FIGURE 11–23. Schematic cross-section of the pneumatic TCI device. Both systole and diastole are depicted.

torque motor is converted to the linear action of the pusher plate via helical cams. Energy is transferred to a copper coil, creating an intra-LVAD electromagnetic field to actuate rotor assembly rotation. One revolution of the motor is required for complete excursion of the pusher plate. In both instances, the excursion of the pusher plate reduces the volume of and pressurizes the blood chamber. When the pressure in the blood chamber exceeds native LV pressure, the inflow valve closes. When the pressure in the blood chamber exceeds aortic pressure, the outflow valve opens and pumping commences. This represents the isovolemic and ejection phases of device systole.

When the pneumatic piston or the motor is switched off, air is vented to the atmosphere from the pumping chamber and the pusher plate is free to move. When the pressure in the native left ventricle (the chamber filling the prosthetic ventricle) exceeds the pressure in the blood chamber, the inflow valve opens and diastolic filling commences. A Hall sensor in the pneumatic pump detects a full blood chamber and triggers ejection. This allows beat-to-beat stroke volume and device output data to be derived and displayed. In addition, a 6-beat moving average of LVAD output also is displayed.

Indications. The pneumatic version of the TCI device is intended for intermediate to long-term circulatory support as a bridge to transplantation. The electromechanical versions are intended for long-term or permanent implantation as an alternative to heart transplantation. Placement of the device is contraindicated in the presence of a mechanical aortic valve or the existence of significant aortic insufficiency. Thrombus formation on the mechanical aortic valve can result from the combination of minimal anticoagulation and the absent or minimal aortic valve opening that occurs when the TCI LVAD is functioning normally.[37] Aortic valve insufficiency will not permit effective or efficient LVAD functioning because a large portion of LVAD ejection will be into the native LV.[38]

Insertion. The device can be implanted intraperitoneally[39] or in a preperitoneal pocket in the left upper quadrant.[40] The inflow and outflow conduits are tunneled into the thoracic cavity. The inflow conduit is inserted into the LV cavity via the LV apex and the dacron outflow conduit is anastomosed end-to-side to the ascending aorta. Insertion requires a median sternotomy and use of CPB.

Management of the TCI Device. The pneumatic device can function in the asynchronous, fill-to-empty, or synchronous modes. The device usually is operated in the fill-to-empty mode with pump ejection triggered by the transducer when the pump is full. LVAD ejection duration can be set by the operator from

200 to 450 msec to achieve complete emptying of the device without compromising device filling. Because minimal LVAD filling time is 50% of the selected LVAD ejection duration LVAD rate varies inversely with ejection duration. The LVAD rate varies from 89 bpm at an ejection duration of 450 msec to 140 bpm at an ejection duration of 200 msec. The control console monitors device output as the product of device stroke volume and rate on a beat-to-beat basis.

The vented electric version does not use a Hall sensor to measure diaphragm displacement. Ejection duration is constant and LVAD rate varies by automatic changes in LVAD filling time as determined by the pump controller. This is feasible because the device is relatively afterload-insensitive. As preload increases, the pump controller detects a shorter interval between diaphragm and rotor interaction and subsequently shortens LVAD filling time.

Anticoagulation. Formation of the pseudointimal membrane seems to obviate the need for full anticoagulation with heparin or warfarin.[41] Aspirin (81 mg/day) and dipyridamole (75 mg three times per day) have been used as the sole long-term anticoagulants. Coumadin may be added for patients with preexisting thrombus in the native heart.

Abiomed BVS 5000

The Abiomed BVS 5000 (*see* Fig. 11–24) is an extracorporeal pulsatile BiVAD used in parallel with the native ventricles.[42] The device has an effective stroke volume of 80 mL and a cardiac output of 5 L/min. It is a pneumatically driven system and has a pneumatic drive line attached to a computerized control console on wheels.

The device consists of atrial and ventricular chambers arranged vertically in a rigid polycarbonate housing (*see* Fig. 11–25). The atrial and ventricular chambers are polyurethane bladders. The ventricular chamber contains polyurethane unidirectional trileaflet inflow and outflow valves.

The atrial bladder fills continuously by gravity from the patient's native atrium. The ventricular bladder is pressurized by introduction of pressurized air into rigid air chamber around the bladder. When the pressure in the air chamber is atmospheric, atrial bladder pressure exceeds ventricular bladder pressure, the inflow valve opens, and the ventricular bladder fills with blood. This constitutes diastole in the device. When the ventricular bladder is full, the air chamber is pressured. When ventricular bladder pressure exceeds atrial bladder pressure, the inflow valve closes. When pressure in the ventricular bladder exceeds aortic or pulmonary artery pressure, the outflow valve opens and ejection commences. These processes constitute the isovolemic and ejection phases of systole in the prosthetic ventricle (*see* Fig. 11–26).

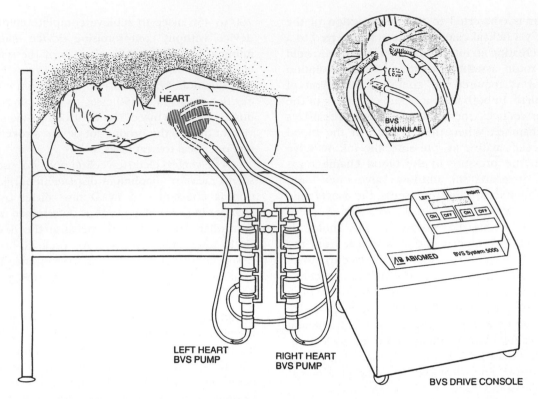

FIGURE 11–24. Schematic of an implanted pneumatically driven Abiomed device used as a biventricular assist device (BiVAD). Cannulation of the left atrium (LA) and the end-to-side anastomosis to the aorta are seen, as are cannulation of the right atrium (RA) and the end-to-side anastomosis to the pulmonary artery. The percutaneous drive lines are seen exiting the abdominal wall. The device is seen to be located below the level of the patient's heart.

Indications. This device is intended for short-term and intermediate circulatory support. It is used primarily for postcardiotomy LV, RV, and biventricular support. In addition, the device has been used as a bridge to transplantation.[43] It has limited application in this role because the device severely limits patient mobility and is gravity-dependent for filling.

Insertion. The device is mounted on IV poles below the level of the patient's heart. Polyvinyl chloride (PVC) tubing brought through the chest wall connects the inflow and outflow cannulae to the device. For use as an RVAD, the inflow cannula is inserted in the right atrium and the dacron outflow conduit is anastomosed end-to-side to the pulmonary artery. For use as an LVAD, the inflow cannula is inserted in the left atrium and the dacron outflow conduit is anastomosed end-to-side to the aorta. Insertion requires a median sternotomy. Although CPB is not absolutely necessary for insertion of the device, it is commonly used. In the postcardiotomy setting, CPB already is in use because failure to wean from CPB is the indication for placement of the device. In the bridge to transplantation setting, femoral venous femoral arterial normothermic CPB has been used to prevent hemodynamic compromise during insertion.[43]

Management of the Abiomed BVS 5000. The pneumatic control console monitors pump function by analysis of air return from the pneumatic drive line. Pump rate and dia-stolic/systolic intervals are determined automatically and the pump functions in the fill-to-empty mode. Device output is monitored and displaced by the control console. A unique feature of this device is that the system is operator-independent. Therefore, engineering and perfusion staff are not necessary during operation of the device.

When the device is used as a BiVAD, differential recovery of the RV and LV function requires careful management due to the limitation of 5 L/min on device output. As RV function recovers, total pulmonary output will be a combination of RVAD output and native RV output. If at the same time there is no LV recovery, systemic output will be determined by LVAD output. If the combined pulmonary output exceeds the maximal output of the LVAD (5 L/min), then LV, LA, and pulmonary venous congestion will occur. The solution is to reduce RVAD output so that pulmonary and systemic outputs are matched. A similar scenario can be described for LV recovery in the absence of RV recovery.

Anticoagulation. Anticoagulation is maintained with a heparin infusion to keep the ACT at 150 to 200 seconds.

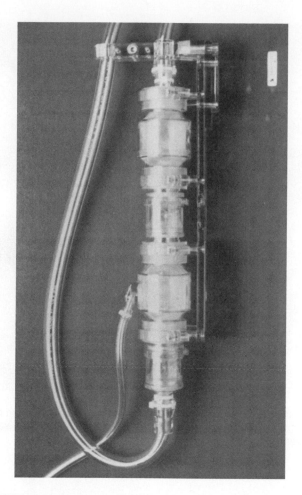

FIGURE 11–25. Photograph of an Abiomed device. Device inflow is on the top, outflow is on the bottom. The pneumatic drive line is seen entering the bottom third of the device from the left.

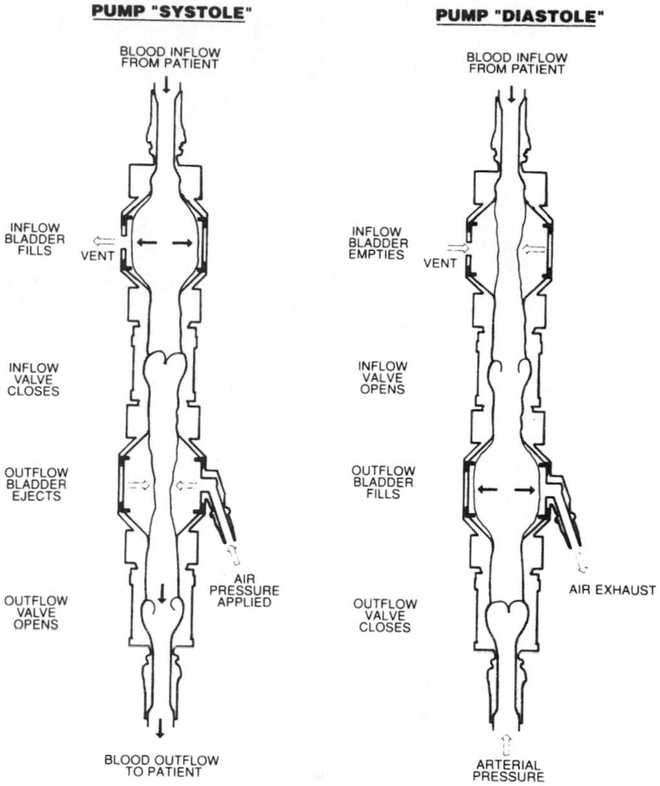

PUMP "SYSTOLE"

BLOOD INFLOW FROM PATIENT

INFLOW BLADDER FILLS — VENT

INFLOW VALVE CLOSES

OUTFLOW BLADDER EJECTS

OUTFLOW VALVE OPENS

AIR PRESSURE APPLIED

BLOOD OUTFLOW TO PATIENT

PUMP "DIASTOLE"

BLOOD INFLOW FROM PATIENT

INFLOW BLADDER EMPTIES — VENT

INFLOW VALVE OPENS

OUTFLOW BLADDER FILLS

OUTFLOW VALVE CLOSES

AIR EXHAUST

ARTERIAL PRESSURE

FIGURE 11–26. Schematic cross section of the Abiomed device. End diastole and end systole are depicted.

Novacor LVAD

The Novacor LVAD (*see* Figs. 11–27 through 11–29) is an implantable pulsatile LVAD used in series with the native heart. The device has a stroke volume of 70 mL and is capable of providing 10 L/min of cardiac output. It is the prototypical pulsatile electromechanical pump, configured to convert electrical energy to the mechanical energy necessary to eject blood from the prosthetic ventricular chamber. One version of the Novacor has a percutaneous electric and air vent line, which attaches to a microprocessor control/monitoring console. A newer version has been developed that features a percutaneous electric and air vent line that attaches to a portable system controller and battery pack that can be worn by the patient.[44]

This prosthetic ventricle consists of a biocompatible sac bonded to symmetrically opposed pusher plates housed in a lightweight shell.[45] 21-mm Carpentier-Edwards porcine unidirectional inflow and outflow valves are placed in the blood chamber. A solenoid en-

ergy converter is used to transfer electrical energy to mechanical energy via preloaded beam springs, which then drive the pusher plates. When the solenoid is open, energy is stored in the beam springs, the pusher plates and blood sac are free to expand, and diastolic filling of the prosthetic ventricle via the left ventricle takes place. When the solenoid is closed, the energy stored in the beam springs is released. The resulting compression of the blood sac between the pusher plates creates the pressure necessary for the isovolemic and ejection phases of systole. Displacement transducers within the solenoid energy converter monitor pusher-plate position. This allows beat-to-beat fill volume, residual volume, and stroke volume to be determined. This information, in combination with device rate, allows device output data to be derived and displayed.

Indications. The original version of the Novacor device is intended for intermediate to long-term circulatory support as a bridge to transplantation. The newer, portable version is intended for long-term or permanent

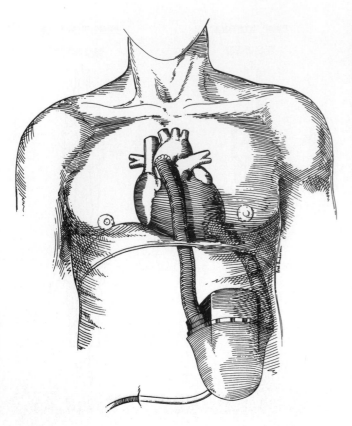

FIGURE 11–27. Schematic of an implanted electromechanically driven Novacor device. Cannulation of the left ventricular (LV) apex and the end-to-side anastomosis to the aorta are seen. The percutaneous drive line is seen exiting the abdominal wall.

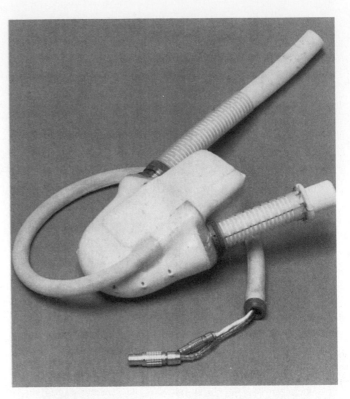

FIGURE 11–28. Photograph of a Novacor device. Device inflow is on the right and outflow is on the left. The electromechanical drive line is seen coiled behind the device.

implantation as an alternative to heart transplantation. Placement of the device is contraindicated in the presence of a mechanical aortic valve or the existence of significant aortic insufficiency. Thrombus formation on the mechanical aortic valve can occur as the result of the absent or minimal aortic valve opening that occurs when the Novacor LVAD is functioning normally. Aortic valve insufficiency will not permit effective or efficient LVAD functioning because a large portion of LVAD ejection will be into the native LV.[38]

Insertion. The device is implanted in the abdominal wall anterior to the posterior rectus sheath. The inflow and outflow conduits are tunneled into the thoracic cavity. The inflow conduit is inserted into the LV cavity via the LV apex and the dacron outflow conduit is anastomosed end-to-side to the ascending aorta. Insertion requires a median sternotomy and use of CPB.

Management of the Novacor. The system was designed to operate in the fill rate trigger mode. This mode was intended to provide operation in synchronization with the LV such that LV ejection produced device filling. This provides counterpulsation and does not allow the aortic valve to open.

In the fill rate trigger mode, the rate at which the pump fills is used to trigger ejection. At the start of device filling, the pump fill rate is high. Toward the end of device filling, the pump fill rate falls. By adjusting the *"end of fill threshold"* setting, the percentage by which the fill rate must fall to trigger device ejection can be set. Usually, this is set at approximately 20%. When left ventricular contractility is poor or preload is reduced, the low *end of fill threshold* necessary to detect small changes in pump fill rate may result in Novacor ejection before completion of ventricular systole. Use of an appropriate amount of *eject delay* corrects this problem by delaying Novacor ejection until the end of ventricular systole. The Novacor also can be operated asynchronously using the fixed-rate trigger or synchronously using the ECG trigger.

In actual clinical practice, filling of the Novacor occurs during LV diastole in some beats and during LV systole in other beats while in the fill-rate trigger mode. This occurs as the result of changes in preload and heart rate with changes in patient activity level. Despite this, the aortic valve rarely opens. Patients who have been discharged from the hospital with the Novacor device have the *end-of-fill threshold* set to 100%. This allows

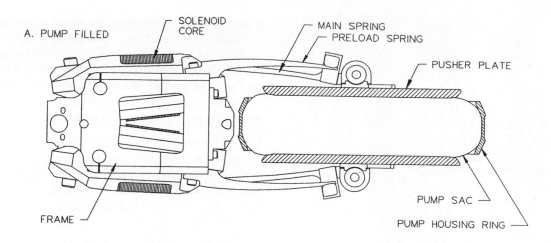

A. PUMP FILLED

SOLENOID CORE

MAIN SPRING
PRELOAD SPRING

PUSHER PLATE

PUMP SAC

PUMP HOUSING RING

FRAME

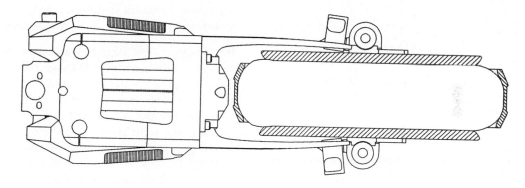

B. SOLENOID CLOSED AND MAGNETICALLY LATCHED; START OF EJECT STROKE

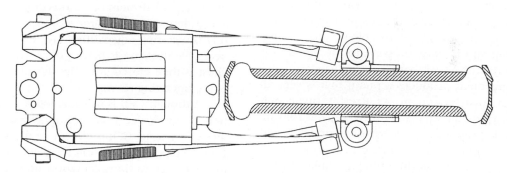

C. END OF EJECT STROKE

FIGURE 11–29. Schematic cross section of the electromechanical Novacor device. **A.** The pump is filled, the solenoid is open. The preload spring limits expansion of the pump sac to 70 mL. **B.** The solenoid is closed and magnetically latched. This constitutes isovolumic contraction. **C.** End of ejection with complete pump ejection.

the device to function as if in a fill-to-empty mode. This allows reliable pump function with no operator intervention.

The control console displays beat-to-beat LVAD output as the product of LVAD stroke volume and rate. Beat-to-beat visualization of the fill-rate curve also is available.

Anticoagulation.   Anticoagulation is as described for the TAH.

Centrifugal Pumps

Centrifugal pumps are extracorporeal, nonpulsatile BiVADs used in parallel with the native ventricles (*see* Fig. 11–30). These devices are capable of providing outputs of 2.0 to 6.0 L/min. Centrifugal pumps use a constrained vortex to impart kinetic energy to fluid in a rotating head. The rotating head consists of a series of concentrically arranged cones or fins contained within a rigid plastic shell (*see* Fig. 10–6). Rotary motion is im-

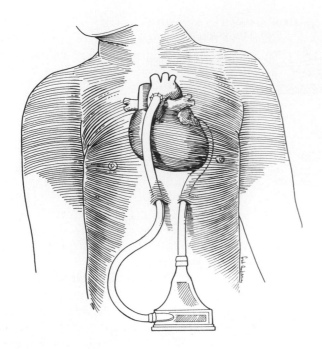

FIGURE 11–30. Schematic of a centrifugal pump used for left ventricular support. Cannulation of the left atrium and the aorta are depicted. The centrifugal pump drive console is not shown.

trifugal pump output requires use of a Doppler or electromagnetic flow probe on the outflow line.

Another possible advantage of centrifugal pumps over occlusive roller pumps is the potential to pump air into the circulation. Inadvertently introduced air tends to remain in the low pressure center of the pump and is not introduced into the circulation.

Indications. Mobilization and exercise are desirable for patients supported long term with circulatory assist devices. Centrifugal pumps seriously limit patient mobility for a number of reasons. The device is extracorporeal, is sensitive to acute fluctuations in preload and afterload, and often is used in settings in which the sternum is left open. As a result, the device is used most commonly for short-term to intermediate LV, RV, or biventricular postcardiotomy support.[46,47] It has been used as a bridge to transplantation, but the inability to mobilize the patient limits its role in this capacity.[48,49]

Insertion. The device is mounted on the drive console. PVC tubing brought through the chest wall or sternotomy connects the inflow and outflow cannulae to the device. Standard CPB arterial and venous cannulae are used. For use as an RVAD, the inflow cannula is inserted in the right atrium and the outflow cannula is inserted into the main pulmonary artery (PA). For use as an LVAD, the inflow cannula is inserted in the left atrium and the outflow cannula is inserted into the ascending aorta. Insertion is accomplished via a median sternotomy. Due to the high incidence of postoperative bleeding, impairment of venous drainage into the device and pulmonary dysfunction in the postcardiotomy setting the sternal edges often are left unopposed and an occlusive dressing is placed over the sternotomy.[47] The chest is then closed after the device has been removed in the operating room.

Although CPB is not absolutely necessary for insertion of the device, it is commonly used. In the postcardiotomy setting, CPB is already in use as failure to wean from CPB is the indication for placement of the device. In the bridge to transplantation setting, CPB generally is not used.

Management of the Centrifugal Pump. The centrifugal pump requires the presence of a perfusionist. Flow is adjusted to meet metabolic demands. If flow does not increase with increases in pump rpm, reduced preload or elevated afterload should be treated. Elevated MAP should be treated by reducing SVR with a vasodilator. Elevated PAP may require treatment with a pulmonary vasodilator. A pulmonary artery catheter will allow assessment of both RVAD preload (CVP) and LVAD preload (peak capillary wedge pressure).

Centrifugal pumps are prone to thrombus formation in the pump head due to heat produced in the

parted to the cones or fins by a drive console. Coupling of the drive console to the pump head is accomplished with magnets in the base of the pump head (*see* Fig. 10–7). Rotation of the cones or fins creates a vortex that is constrained by the rigid plastic housing. This creates lower pressure at the center of the pump than at the periphery. The pressure gradient draws blood into the center of the pump and imparts pressure to the blood as it leaves the pump at the periphery.

This arrangement produces a pump that is very afterload- and preload-dependent. As a result, pump output at a given rpm can vary greatly. At a given rpm increasing outlet pressure or decreasing preload will reduce pump output. Outlet pressure is a combination of the pressure drop across the outlet cannula and the resistance of the recipient vascular bed. For example, at an outlet pressure of 200 mm Hg, a Bio-Medicus pump can generate 4 L/min of flow at 200 rpm. Increasing outlet pressure to 400 mm Hg requires 3000 rpm to maintain 4 L/min of flow.

At the extremes, clamping the inflow or outflow line will result in no pump output despite the fact that the pump head continues to rotate. Because pump output decreases as afterload increases, line pressure in a centrifugal pump can never reach the point at which connections will come apart or the pumping mechanism will fail. This is a major advantage of centrifugal pumps over occlusive roller pumps. Because pump output does not vary directly with rpm, monitoring cen-

bearing housing during rotation. As a result, some manufacturers recommend changing the pump head every 24 to 48 hours. In practice, pump heads often can be used safely for 3 to 5 days. In addition, pump flows lower than 2 L/min are associated with pump head and cannula thrombus formation.

Anticoagulation. A heparin infusion is used to maintain an ACT between 100 and 200 seconds or a PTT between 60 and 80 seconds. The pump head must be monitored for thrombus formation and must be changed if there is evidence of thrombus.

■ ANESTHETIC CONSIDERATIONS

The cardiac anesthesiologist is likely to encounter patients with a circulatory assist device or a TAH in the following circumstances:

- heart transplantation candidates who require placement of a VAD or a TAH as a bridge to transplantation to prevent a deterioration in their medical condition.
- heart transplantation candidates with a VAD or TAH in place who present for cardiac transplantation.
- patients who have undergone a cardiac surgical procedure and require a circulatory assist device or a TAH to allow separation from CPB.
- postcardiotomy shock patients who have had their circulatory assist device weaned and who require operative explanation of the device.
- patients with end-stage cardiomyopathies who undergo permanent implantation of a VAD.

Device Insertion

Induction and maintenance of anesthesia for insertion of a VAD or TAH in a patient with an end-stage cardiomyopathy should be managed as described for patients undergoing heart transplantation (*see* Chapter 7). Implantation of VADs and the TAH requires a median sternotomy and CPB. In addition, placement of the TAH requires bicaval venous cannulation and aortic cross-clamping. Anastomosis of the outflow graft to the side of the ascending aorta for the TCI, Novacor, Abiomed, and Thoratec devices often can be performed off CPB with application of a partially occluding or sidebiting aortic clamp. Application of this clamp may increase impedance to LV ejection and cause LV afterload mismatch with subsequent LV distention. If this technique is chosen, careful monitoring of LV function with TEE is recommended. Placement of the inflow conduit into the apex of the LV for the TCI, Novacor, and Thoratec devices is performed on CPB. Some surgeons place the inflow conduit with the heart fibrillating, whereas others apply an aortic cross-clamp and administer cardioplegia. Centrifugal pumps are used almost exclusively for postcardiotomy support. As a result, they are placed while on CPB as well.

Many of the patients presenting for placement of an mechanical assist are anticoagulated with coumadin because of their dilated cardiomyopathy (*see* Chapter 7). These patients usually require replacement of coagulation factors, particularly when there is dilution of factors on CPB as they already have reduced factor levels. When the PT is markedly elevated, adding fresh frozen plasma to the pump prime in place of a crystalloid solution is warranted. An additional risk for blood loss is the fact that up to 50% of bridge-to-transplant patients have had previous cardiac surgery.

Limiting transfusion of homologous blood products helps reduce the risk of postoperative pulmonary dysfunction, which can seriously impair RV function. In addition, avoidance of homologous blood products limits patient exposure to antibodies, which may make subsequent typing for heart transplantation difficult. Leukocyte filters should be used when administering homologous blood products. Cytomegalovirus (CMV) negative blood must be used in CMV-negative patients.

Use of aprotinin[50] has been shown to reduce blood loss and transfusion requirements for packed cells and components in patients receiving a LVAD. Aprotinin is discussed in detail in Chapter 10. Although the risk of an anaphylactic reaction to aprotinin on the first exposure is small (0.5%), an intravenous test dose of 0.5 or 1.0 mL should be administered; 1.0 mL is equal to 10,000 kallikrein inhibition units (KIU) or 1.4 mg. If there is no reaction after 10 minutes, this is followed by a loading dose of 20,000 KIU/kg over 30 minutes; 20,000 KIU/kg (2.8 mg/kg) is added to the pump prime, and an additional 20,000 KIU/kg (2.8 mg/kg) is infused over 5 hours. The pump prime dose is never added until the test dose and bolus dose are given and no reaction is noted. Initiation of CPB may be necessary to support circulation in the presence of a severe allergic reaction. In bridge-to-transplant patients, aprotinin may be used again to reduce blood loss after the subsequent cardiac transplant. The risk of anaphylaxis upon reexposure is estimated to be as high as 2.8 to 10%.[51-53] There is a 3-fold increase in the risk of an adverse reaction upon reexposure if the previous exposure occurred during the previous 6 months.[52] Reexposure within this interval is not uncommon in patients with a bridge to transplant. For these patients, it is recommended that a skin prick test or intradermal test be performed before administration of a very dilute (<1 μg/mL) intravenous test dose.[54] Patients with previous exposure may benefit from pretreatment with steroids and a histamine H_1/H_2 receptor antagonist. In addition, some recommend delaying injection of the bolus dose until the surgeon is ready to commence CPB so that circulatory support can be initiated immediately in case of a reaction.

The existence of a patent foramen ovale (PFO) or any site for intracardiac shunting must be excluded before placement of any mechanical assist device that is capable of reducing LA pressure below RA pressure. Decompression of the LV and reduction in LA pressure below RA pressure will produce right-to-left intracardiac shunting and hypoxemia. This is particularily likely in the setting in which RA pressure is elevated, such as when there is concomitant RV dysfunction or elevated PA pressure. In addition, it introduces the possibility of producing systemic air emboli from bubbles introduced into the RA by intravenous lines. All of the devices described in this chapter, except the IABP, are capable of producing such shunting.[55,56] Either surgical examination or transesophageal echocardiography (TEE) can be used to determine whether a PFO exists. Two-dimensional echocardiographic views of the intra-atrial septum in conjunction with color flow imaging may be sufficient to detect a PFO. However, because most patients receiving mechanical assist devices have elevated LA pressures, the presence of a PFO by TEE should not be ruled out without the use of provocative measures to reduce LAP below RAP. Release of a Valsalva maneuver (actually release of positive end-expiratory pressure) will transiently reduce LAP below RAP. When this is used in conjunction with agitated saline contrast, two-dimensional echocardiographic imaging of the RA, LA, and intra-atrial septum detection of a PFO is reliable.[57] Agitated saline contrast two-dimensional echocardiography is described in detail in Chapter 3.

Meticulous deairing of the native cardiac chambers and the assist device is necessary to prevent systemic air emboli. The patient usually is kept in steep Trendelenberg position until deairing is completed. TEE is useful in detecting intracardiac air and in guiding the deairing process.[58]

Management of Patients With Devices in Place. Postdevice implantation management is tailored to the patient, the specific device, and the setting. The following issues must be considered:

FUNCTION OF THE NONASSISTED VENTRICLE. Proper functioning of an LVAD requires an RV that functions well enough to match the combined output of the LV and the LVAD. An RV that is capable of delivering only 3 L/min to the pulmonary circulation and LA will severely compromise optimal functioning of an LVAD that can deliver 6 L/min. Because many patients requiring LVAD implantation have concomitant RV dysfunction, there may be a need for inotropic/vasodilator or mechanical support of the RV after LVAD implantation. Preoperative prediction of which patients will need inotropic sup-

port of the RV after LVAD implantation and which patients will require an RVAD can be difficult. Preoperative clinical factors that may be useful in predicting the need for inotopic or mechanical support of the RV after LVAD implantation are:[59]

- low mixed venous saturation (<40%)
- impairment of mental status
- high inotrope need and a low ratio of RV ejection fraction to inotrope need

The effects of LVAD implantation on RV function are complex and are summarized:

- Contractility — complete pressure unloading of the LV with an LVAD shifts the intraventricular septum to the left and reduces the LV contribution to RV contraction. Systolic ventricular interdependence is such that LV contraction may account for most RV-developed pressure and volume outflow.[60] In addition, there may be loss of RV contraction in the areas adjacent to the leftward-shifted intraventricular septum.[61] As a result, LVAD insertion generally results in impairment of RV systolic function.
- Afterload — insertion of an LVAD generally produces a reduction in RV afterload.[60,62] Insertion of an LVAD results in reduction of LA pressures by reducing LV distention. Reduction in LA pressures results in reduced pulmonary venous congestion and a reduction in pulmonary vascular resistance (PVR) and PA pressures despite the increase in cardiac output and pulmonary blood flow that accompanies implantation. Reduction of RV afterload improves RV function through enhanced shortening of the RV free wall. Not all patients have immediate normalization of PVR and PA pressures. Patients with longstanding pulmonary venous congestion may have an additional component of pulmonary hypertension that may take days or weeks to resolve. In addition, although PA pressures decrease routinely after LVAD implantation, the transpulmonary gradient (TPG) (mean peak arterial pressure–left atrial pressure) routinely increases slightly postimplantation but falls by 24 hours postoperatively. This is most likely due to the residual pulmonary edema, and the effects of cardiopulmonary bypass and blood product administration on the pulmonary vascular bed.[60]
- Preload — LVAD insertion increases RV preload. Because LVAD insertion improves RV compliance, RV end-diastolic volume (EDV) increases while RV end-diastolic pressure (EDP) decreases. As a result, LVAD implantation may acutely decrease mitral regurgitation while worsening tricuspid re-

gurgitation (TR) both acutely[63] and chronically.[64] This is presumably secondary to a leftward shift of the intraventricular septum, increased RV compliance, and an increasing volume load to the RV with increased cardiac output.

- Coronary perfusion — LVAD insertion may improve RV function by increasing aortic blood pressure and improving RV coronary blood flow.

On balance, LVAD insertion results in global impairment of RV systolic function, which is offset by increased RV preload and reduced RV afterload such that RV output is maintained or increased.[60,65] 20 to 30% of patients receiving an LVAD will require placement of an RVAD for RV failure, which persists despite aggressive pharmacologic therapy to improve RV function.[60] These patients usually have (1) a component of pulmonary vascular resistance that is not immediately reduced by decompression of the LV, and (2) underlying RV contractile dysfunction particularily of the intraventricular septum.[65] Septal dysfunction causes the intraventricular septum to move away from the RV free wall during systole. The RV free wall cannot compensate for this movement, even in the setting of reduced afterload and RV stroke volume falls.[65]

Treatment of RV dysfunction and TR with pulmonary vasodilators and inotropes will be necessary for patients who manifest severe RV dysfunction after LVAD implantation. Severe RV dysfunction will produce a low LVAD output in conjunction with a high CVP and TEE detected TR with RV distention and hypokinesis. Management of RV dysfunction with inotropes and vasodilators is discussed in detail in Chapter 7. TEE is valuable in guiding therapy to reduce TR and improve RV function.

PRELOAD TO THE DEVICE.   Proper functioning of all assist devices excluding the IABP are dependent on delivery of adequate volume to the device. TEE is useful in determining the etiology of poor preload to a device. The following causes should be considered:

- hypovolemia
- poor positioning/obstruction of the inflow cannula. This is particularly important in RVADs and LVADs, which operate in parallel with the native heart (Abiomed, Thoratec, centrifugal pumps) as cannulae placed in the RA or LA. TEE is used to ensure unobstructed inflow to the device.[66] Care must be taken to ensure that atrial cannula do not cross the AV valve or impinge on the intraatrial septum. For devices in series with the native heart (Thoratec, TCI, Novacor), the ventricular cannula must not impinge on the ventricular free wall, septum, or papillary muscles.[67] No substantial pressure gradient should exist across the inflow conduit.

- inferior vena cava (IVC), superior vena cava (SVC), or pulmonary venous obstruction in TAH patients. In TAH patients, TEE is used to ensure that there is no obstruction of the SVC, IVC, or pulmonary veins.
- impaired RV function with delivery of inadequate volumes of blood across the pulmonary circulation to a LVAD. This was discussed previously in this chapter.

AFTERLOAD PRESENTED TO THE DEVICE.   The performance of both pulsatile and nonpulsatile assist devices are influenced by afterload. As addressed previously, centrifugal pumps have reduced performance as vascular resistance increases.

At very high afterload, pulsatile pumps will develop increasing residual volumes as they fail to empty completely. This is analogous to an increasing end-systolic volume in the native ventricle with the end result being a reduced stroke volume. By increasing driveline pressure, pneumatic pumps such as the Thoratec and CardioWest TAH can be made to empty completely at higher afterloads. The result will be elevated MAP or PAP and the potential for more hemolysis. A more practical solution is reduction of afterload with vasodilators.

At systolic pressures in excess of 160 mm Hg, the Novacor device begins to have increased residual volume and also begins to overheat. As SVR increases in patients with the pneumatic TCI and Abiomed devices, the ejection time necessary to completely empty the device increases.[68] This, in turn, reduces maximal pump rate per minute because minimal LVAD filling time is a fixed proportion of the selected LVAD ejection duration. In all of these circumstances, afterload reduction is warranted.

Another source of device malfunction related to afterload is obstruction to outflow. TEE is used to ensure that there is no significant pressure gradient distal to the outflow cannulae or conduits in the great vessels.

CARDIAC OUTPUT DETERMINATION

- *TAH* — cardiac output is displayed by the COMDU of the Cardiowest TAH. A thermodilution pulmonary artery catheter is not necessary and, in fact, must be removed before device implantation.
- *LVADs* — device output is equal to systemic cardiac output as long as the aortic valve remains closed. TEE will readily determine if this is true. This situation is likely for devices in series with the LV and less likely for devices in parallel with the LV. If there is ejection from the native LV in conjunction with device output, then thermodilution cardiac output can be used as an accurate measure of the combined native ventricular and device output. Patients with LVADs require pul-

monary catheters to aid in management of concomitant RV dysfunction.

- *RVADs* — device output is equal to pulmonic output as long as the pulmonic valve remains closed. TEE will readily determine if this is true. Because RVADs are placed in series with the RV, the total pulmonic output is more likely to be a combination of native RV output and RVAD output. In this setting, thermodilution cardiac outputs will not be accurate because the transit times of blood and saline through the native RV and the RVAD will be different. This will interfere with the thermodilution technique.

EFFECTS OF VENTILATION.   Positive-pressure ventilation may adversely affect RV function by mechanically compressing the pulmonary vasculature if peak airway pressures are high. This can reduce native RV output and delivery of blood to an LV assist device.

The TAH ventricle functions as an extrathoracic chamber surrounded by atmospheric pressure in diastole and connected to an atrium and great vessel that are surrounded by intrathoracic pressure.[69] Because there is no compliant intraventricular septum, there is no ventricular interdependence. Increases in intrathoracic pressure will reduce filling of the native atria from the systemic and pulmonary veins but will enhance filling of the prosthetic ventricles. Despite this, respiratory variation of systemic blood pressure will occur in the setting of hypovolemia or dilation of venous capacitance vessels.

EFFECTS OF INDUCTION AND MAINTENANCE AGENTS. Induction and maintenance of anesthesia in the patient with an assist device or TAH should take into account the hemodynamic effects of the chosen anesthetic agents. The effect of induction agents on myocardial contractility must be taken into account. Although the effects of agents on myocardial contractility are not important in TAH patients, the effects of agents on the peripheral vasculature do influence hemodynamics.[70,71]

DEVICE WEANING.   Devices are weaned by gradually withdrawing support while assessing ventricular function and hemodynamics. This usually requires the presence of a PA catheter and arterial line. The IABP is weaned by decreasing the pump rate from 1:1 to 1:2 to 1:3. Centrifugal pumps are weaned by decreasing the pump flow rate. The risk of thrombus formation is enhanced when the pump flow rate is at or less than 2 L/min. Therefore, adequate anticoagulation should be maintained and the pump should be withdrawn promptly after weaning down to this level. Weaning of the Abiomed and Thoratec devices involves adjustment of the device to operate at a decreased fixed rate. TEE has proved to be very valuable in guiding weaning of circulatory assist devices because

it allows on-line assessment of RV and LV function during the weaning process.[72]

■ REFERENCES

1. Pennington DG, Swartz M, Codd JE, et al: Intra-aortic balloon pumping in cardiac surgical patients: A nine-year experience. *Ann Thorac Surg* 1983; **36:**125-131.
2. Ott RA, Mills TC, Eugene J: Current concepts in the use of ventricular assist devices. *Cardiac Surgery: State of the Art Reviews* 1989; **3:**521-543.
3. Pennington DG, Samuels LD, Williams G, et al: Experience with the Pierce-Donachy ventricular assist device in postcardiotomy patients with cardiogenic shock. *World J Surg* 1985; **9:**37-46.
4. Pennington DG: Circulatory support at the turn of the decade. A clinician's view. *ASAIO Trans* 1990; **36:**M126-131.
5. Pae WE: Ventricular assist devices and total artificial hearts: A combined registry experience. *Ann Thorac Surg* 1992; **55:**295-298.
6. Pennington DG, McBride LR, Kanter KR, et al: Effect of perioperative myocardial infarction on survival of postcardiotomy patients supported with ventricular-assist devices. *Circulation* 1988; **78**(suppl 3):110-115.
7. Pennington DG, Bernhard WF, Golding LR, et al: Long-term followup of postcardiotomy patients with profound cardiogenic shock treated with ventricular assist devices. *Circulation* 1985; **72**(suppl 2):216-226.
8. Kanter KR, Ruzevich SA, Pennington DG, et al: Follow-up of survivors of mechanical circulatory support. *J Thorac Cardiovasc Surg* 1988; **96:**72-80.
9. Evans RW, Manninen DL, Garrison LP, Maier AM: Donor availability as the primary determinant of the future of heart transplantation. *JAMA* 1986; **255:**1892-1898.
10. Copeland JG, Emery RW, Levinson MM, Copeland J, McAleer MJ, Riley JE: The role of mechanical support and transplantation in treatment of patients with end stage cardiomyopathy. *Circulation* 1985; **72**(suppl 2):7-12.
11. Starnes VA, Oyer PE, Portner PM, et al: Isolated left ventricular assist as bridge to cardiac transplantation. *J Thorac Cardiovasc Surg* 1988; **96:**62-71.
12. Hill JD, Farrar DJ, Hershon JJ, et al: Use of a prosthetic ventricle as a bridge to cardiac transplantation for postinfarction cardiogenic shock. *N Engl J Med* 1986; **314:**626-628.
13. Copeland JG, Levinson MM, Smith R, et al: The total artificial heart as a bridge to transplantation: A report on two cases. *JAMA* 1986; **256:**2991-2995.
14. Mehta SM, Aufiero TX, Pae WE, et al: Combined registry for the clinical use of mechanical ventricular assist pumps and the total artificial heart in conjunction with heart transplantation: Sixth official report — 1994. *J Heart Lung Transplant* 1995; **14:**585-593.
15. Copeland JG, Pavie A, Duveau D, et al: Bridge to transplantation with the CardioWest total artificial heart: The international experience 1993 to 1995. *J Heart Lung Transplant* 1996; **15:**94-99.
16. Didisheim P, Olsen DB, Farrar DJ: Infections and thromboembolism with implantable cardiovascular devices. *ASAIO Trans* 1989; **35:**54-70.
17. Pennington DG, McBride LR, Swartz MT, et al: Use of the Pierce-Donachy ventricular assist device in patients with cardiogenic shock after cardiac operations. *Ann Thorac Surg* 1989; **47:**130-135.
18. Jaski BE, Branch KR, Adamson R, et al: Excerise hemodynamics during long-term implantation of a left ventricular assist device in patients awaiting heart transplantation. *J Am Coll Cardiol* 1993; **22:**1574-1580.

19. Levinson MM, Copeland JG, Smith RG, et al: Indexes of hemolysis in human recipients of the Jarvik-7 total artificial heart: A cooperative report of fifteen cases. *J Heart Transplant* 1986; **3**:236-248.

20. Kern MJ, Aguirre F, Bach R, et al: Augmentation of coronary blood flow by intraaortic balloon pumping in patients after coronary angioplasty. *Circulation* 1993; **87**:500-511.

21. Gurbel PA, Anderson RD, MacCord CS, et al: Arterial diastolic pressure augmentation by intraaortic balloon counterpulsation enhances the onset of coronary reperfusion by thrombolytic therapy. *Circulation* 1994; **89**:361-365.

22. Katz ES, Tunick PA, Kronzon I: Observations of coronary blood flow augmentation and balloon function during intraaortic balloon counterpulsation using transesophageal echocardiography. *Am J Cardiol* 1992; **69**:1635-1639.

23. Cheung AT, Savino JS, Weiss SJ: Beat-to-beat augmentation of left ventricular function by intraaortic counterpulsation. *Anesthesiology* 1996; **84**:545-554.

24. Ohman EM, George BS, White CJ: Use of aortic counterpulsation to improve sustained coronary artery patency during acute myocardial infarction. Results of a randomized trial. *Circulation* 1994; **90**:792-799.

25. Gottlieb SO, Brinker JA, Borken AM, et al: Identification of patients at high risk for complications of intra-aortic balloon counterpulsation: A multivariate risk factor analysis. *Am J Cardiol* 1984; **53**:1135-1139.

26. DeVries WC, Anderson JL, Joyce LD, et al: Clinical use of the total artificial heart. *N Engl J Med* 1984; **310**:273-278.

27. Mays JB, Hastings W, Williams MA, et al: Drive system management of emergency conditions in three permanent total artificial heart patients. *ASAIO Trans* 1986; **32**:221-225.

28. Willshaw P, Neilsen SD, Nanas J, et al: A cardiac output monitor and diagnostic unit for pneumatically driven artificial hearts. *Artif Organs* 1984; **8**:215-219.

29. Mays JB, Williams MA, Barker LE, et al: Clinical management of total artificial heart drive systems. *JAMA* 1988; **259**:881-885.

30. Shaw WJ, Pantalos GM, Everett S, et al: Factors influencing the accuracy of the cardiac output monitoring and diagnostic unit for pneumatic artificial hearts. *ASAIO Trans* 1990; **36**:M264-268.

31. Szukalski EA, Reedy JE, Pennington DG, et al: Oral anticoagulation in patients with ventricular assist devices. *ASAIO Trans* 1990; **36**:M700-703.

32. Farrar DJ, Hill JD, Gray LA, et al: Heterotopic prosthetic ventricles as a bridge to cardiac transplantation. A multicenter study in 29 patients. *N Engl J Med* 1988; **318**:333-340.

33. Ganzel BL, Gray LA, Slater AD, Mavroudis C: Surgical techniques for the implantation of heterotopic prosthetic ventricles. *Ann Thorac Surg* 1989; **47**:113-120.

34. McCarthy PM, James KB, Savage RM, et al: Implantable left ventricular assist device. Approaching an alternative for end-stage heart failure. *Circulation* 1994; **90**(suppl II): II-83-II-86.

35. Frazier OH: First use of an untethered, vented electric left ventricular assist device for long-term support. *Circulation* 1994; **89**:2908-2914.

36. Burton NA, Lefrak EA, Macmanus Q, et al: A reliable bridge to cardiac transplantation: The TCI left ventricular assist device. *Ann Thorac Surg* 1993; **55**:1425-14312.

37. Frazier OH, Rose EA, Macmanus Q, et al: Multicenter clinical evaluation of the HeartMate 1000 IP left ventricular assist device. *Ann Thorac Surg* 1992; **53**:1080-1090.

38. Oz MC, Rose EA, Levin HR: Selection criteria for placement of left ventricular assist devices. *Am Heart J* 1995; **129**:173-177.

39. Portner PM, Baumgartner WA, Cabrol C, et al: Internal pulsatile circulatory support. *Ann Thorac Surg* 1993; **55**:261-265.

40. McCarthy PM, Wang N, Vargo R: Preperitoneal insertion of the HeartMate 1000 IP implantable left ventricular assist device. *Ann Thorac Surg* 1994; **57**:634-638.

41. Rose EA, Levin HR, Oz MC, et al: Artificial circulatory support with textured interior surfaces. A counterintuitive approach to minimizing thromboembolism. *Circulation* 1994; **90**:II-87-II-91.

42. Jett GK: Abiomed BVS 5000: Experience and potential advantages. *Ann Thorac Surg* 1996; **61**:301-304.

43. Champsaur G, Ninet J, Vigneron M, et al: Use of the Abiomed BVS System 5000 as a bridge to cardiac transplantation. *J Thorac Cardiovasc Surg* 1990; **100**:122-128.

44. Vetter HO, Kaulbach HG, Schmitz C, et al: Experience with the Novacor left ventricular assist system as a bridge to cardiac transplantation, including the new wearable system. *J Thorac Cardiovasc Surg* 1995; **109**:74-80.

45. Portner PM, Oyer PE, Jassawalla JS, et al: An alternative in end-stage heart disease: Long-term ventricular assistance. *Heart Transplant* 1983; **3**:47-59.

46. Noon GP, Ball JW, Short HD: Bio-Medicus centrifugal ventricular support for postcardiotomy cardiac failure: A review of 129 cases. *Ann Thorac Surg* 1996; **61**:291-295.

47. Curtis JJ, Walls JT, Schmaltz RA, et al: Use of centrifugal pumps for postcardiotomy ventricular failure: Technique and anticoagulation. *Ann Thorac Surg* 1996; **61**:296-300.

48. Bolman RM, Cox JL, Marshall W, et al: Circulatory support with a centrifugal pump as a bridge to cardiac transplantation. *Ann Thorac Surg* 1989; **47**:108-112.

49. Bolman RM, Spray TL, Cox JL: Heart transplantation in patients requiring preoperative mechanical support. *J Heart Transplant* 1987; **6**:273-280.

50. Goldstein DJ, Seldomridge A, Chen JM: Use of aprotinin in LVAD recipients reduces blood loss, blood use, and perioperative mortality. *Ann Thorac Surg* 1995; **59**:1063-1068.

51. Diefenbach C, Abel M, Limpers B, et al: Fatal anaphylactic shock after aprotinin reexposure in cardiac surgery. *Anesth Analg* 1995; **80**:830-831.

52. Dietrich W, Spath P, Ebell A, et al: Prevalence of anaphylactic reactions to aprotinin: Analysis of two hundred forty-eight reexposures to aprotinin in heart operations. *J Cardiovasc Thorac Surg* 1997; **113**:194-201.

53. Goldstein DJ, Oz MC, Smith CR, et al: Safety of repeat aprotinin administration for LVAD recipients undergoing cardiac transplantation. *Ann Thorac Surg* 1996; **61**:692-695.

54. Levy JH: Antibody formation after drug administration during cardiac surgery: Parameters for aprotinin use. *J Heart Lung Transplant* 1993; **12**:S26-32.

55. Baldwin RT, Duncan JM, Frazier OH, et al: Patent foramen ovale: A cause of hypoxemia in patients on left ventricular support. *Ann Thorac Surg* 1991; **52**:865-867.

56. Shapiro GC, Leibowitz, Oz MC, et al: Diagnosis of patient foramen ovale with transesophageal echocardiography in a patient supported with a left ventricular assist device. *J Heart Lung Transplant* 1995; **14**:594-597.

57. Konstadt SN, Louie EK, Black S, et al: Intraoperative detection of patent foramen ovale by transesophageal echocardiography. *Anesthesiology* 1991; **74**:21-216.

58. Orihashi K, Matsuura Y, Hamamaka Y, et al: Retained intracardiac air in open heart operations examined by transesophageal echocardiography. *Ann Thorac Surg* 1993; **55**:1467-1471.

59. Kormos RL, Gaisor TA, Kawai A, et al: Transplant candidate's clinical status rather than right ventricular function defines need for univentricular versus biventricular support. *J Thorac Cardiovasc Surg* 1996; **111**:773-783.

60. Pavie A, Leger P: Physiology of univentricular versus biventricular support. *Ann Thorac Surg* 1996; **61**:347-349.

61. Morita S, Kormos RL, Mandarino WA, et al: Right ventricular/arterial coupling in the patient with left ventricular assistance. *Circulation* 1992; **86**(suppl 2): II-316-II-325.

62. McCarthy PM, Savage RM, Fraser CD, et al: Hemodynamic and physiologic changes during support with an implantable left ventricular assist device. *J Thorac Cardiovasc Surg* 1995; **109:**409-418.

63. Holman WL, Bourge RC, Fan P, et al: Influence of left ventricular assist on valvular regurgitation. *Circulation* 1993; **88:**309-318.

64. Holman WL, Bourge RC, Fan P, et al: Influence of longer term left ventricular assist device support on valvular regurgitation. *ASAIO J* 1994; **40:**M454-M459.

65. Santamore WP, Gray LA: Left ventricular contributions to right ventricular systolic function during LVAD support. *Ann Thorac Surg* 1996; **61:**350-356.

66. Faggian G, Dan M, Bortolotti U, et al: Implantation of an external biventricular assist device: Role of transesophageal two-dimensional echocardiography. *J Heart Transplant* 1990; **9:**441-443.

67. Savage RM, McCarthy PM, Stewart WJ, et al: Intraoperative transesophageal echocardiographic evaluation of the implantable left ventricular assist device. *Video J Echo* 1992; **2:**125-136.

68. Branch KR, Dembitsky WP, Peterson KL, et al: Physiology of the native heart and thermo Cardiosystems left ventricular assist device complex at rest and during exercise: Implications for chronic support. *J Heart Lung Transplant* 1994; **13:**641-651.

69. Robotham JL, Mays JB, Williams MA, DeVries WC: Cardiorespiratory interactions in patients with an artificial heart. *Anesthesiology* 1990; **73:**599-609.

70. Rouby J-J, Leger P, Andreev A, et al: Peripheral vascular effects of halothane and isoflurane in humans with an artificial heart. *Anesthesiology* 1990; **72:**462-469.

71. Rouby J-J, Leger P, Andreev A, et al: Peripheral vascular effects of thiopental and propofol in humans with artificial hearts. *Anesthesiology* 1991; **75:**32-42.

72. Barzilai B, Davila-Roman VG, Eaton M, et al: Transesophageal echocardiography predicts successful withdrawal of ventricular assist devices. *J Thorac Cardiovasc Surg* 1992; **104:**1410-1416.

12

Myocardial Preservation

James A. DiNardo

Early efforts in cardiac surgery were hindered by the failure to appreciate that postoperative myocardial failure after technically successful operative procedures was not due to compromised preoperative function but to extensive damage sustained during the operative procedure. Eventually, it was understood that myocardial necrosis was common in patients dying after cardiac surgery and that the necrosis was linked to events occurring during cardiopulmonary bypass (CPB).[1,2] Later, it was appreciated that postoperative myocardial function (cardiac index) and the probability of survival were inversely related to the extent of myocardial necrosis (creatine phosphokinase [CPK]-MB elevations).[3] Such work led to efforts to improve protection of the myocardium during cardiac surgery.

Initially, surgeons attempted to operate on both normothermic and hypothermic empty, beating, or fibrillating hearts. These conditions provided poor operative exposure and, for the reasons discussed in Chapter 10, resulted in myocardial necrosis. Eventually, aortic cross-clamping evolved as the method of choice for providing surgical exposure. Recall that the aortic cross-clamp is a completely occlusive clamp placed across the aorta between the aortic perfuser and the aortic valve/coronary ostia. This clamp isolates the heart from direct perfusion during CPB and helps provide an immobile, bloodless field for the surgeon.

Myocardial preservation must involve optimal protection of the heart during the entire operative procedure and not just during the period of aortic cross-clamping. The principles of myocardial protection during the pre-CPB period are dealt with extensively in Chapters 4, 5, 6, and 7. Protection on CPB prior to aortic cross-clamping is dealt with in Chapter 10. This chapter will deal with myocardial preservation during aortic cross-clamping and in the reperfusion period that follows removal of the aortic cross-clamp.

■ CONSEQUENCES OF AORTIC CROSS-CLAMPING

Myocardial ischemia occurs as the result of severely compromised or absent myocardial perfusion. Hypoxia, on the other hand, refers to a reduction in substrate delivery with maintained perfusion. Because aortic cross-clamping isolates the coronary circulation from perfusion, global myocardial ischemia will result unless protective measures are taken. To understand the nature of these protective measures, it is necessary to examine the consequences of global myocardial ischemia.

Cessation of Oxidative Phosphorylation. This is the first metabolic derangement to occur. The

349

electron transport chain is interrupted and the Kreb's cycle is inhibited. This occurs within minutes of cross-clamping and results in termination of high-energy phosphate production in the form of adenosine triphosphate (ATP) and creatine phosphate (CP).[4]

Depletion of ATP and CP Stores. ATP supplies energy directly to the myocardium, whereas CP acts as an intermediate energy source to resupply ATP.[5] CP stores are depleted first. Within 15 minutes, ATP stores are reduced by one-half and CP stores are essentially depleted.[6]

Anaerobic Metabolism. Glucose is the only substrate available for anaerobic metabolism in the myocardium. To provide substrate for glycolysis, glycogenolysis must occur. Large glycogen stores may provide ample substrate for anaerobic production of ATP, but unless there is adequate washout of the hydrogen ions and lactate produced from anaerobic glycolysis, further glycolysis will be inhibited by sufficiently high concentrations of these metabolites. Generally, anaerobic production of ATP ends a few minutes after it starts in the globally ischemic myocardium.[7]

Inhibition of Free Fatty Acid Oxidation. Normally, free fatty acids are the major energy source for the myocardium in the postabsorptive state. Ischemia interferes with free fatty acid oxidation and with fatty acid uptake and transfer into the myocardium.[8]

Depletion of the Adenine Nucleotide Pool. After 30 to 40 minutes of global ischemia, the progressive degradation of ATP to adenosine 5´-diphosphate (ADP), ADP to adenosine monophosphate (AMP), and AMP to inosine and hypoxanthine depletes the myocardium of its adenine sources. Therefore, reperfusion of energy sources to replenish ATP levels will be fruitless at this time unless the adenine precursors to form ATP are provided as well.[9,10]

Impairment of Calcium Homeostasis. The consequences of impaired calcium homeostasis are summarized in Figure 12-1. Homeostasis of intracellular calcium is dependent on two ATP-dependent processes: sequestration of calcium into the sarcoplasmic reticulum and extrusion of calcium across the sarcolemma. At 30 minutes of global ischemia, the myocardium's ability to regulate intracellular calcium is impaired by depletion of ATP stores. Loss of calcium homeostasis results in sustained myocardial contracture because sequestration of calcium is necessary to break the actin–myosin cross-bridges that allow diastolic relaxation to occur.[11] In addition, high intracellular calcium levels cause further depletion of ATP stores through activation of myosin ATPase.

Disruption of Cellular Architecture. By 30 minutes of global ischemia, there is swelling of mitochondria and sarcoplasmic reticulum due to increased osmolarity

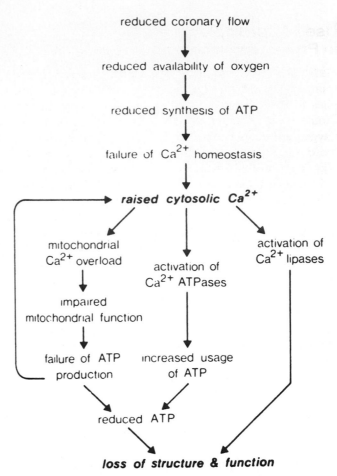

FIGURE 12–1. Consequences of impaired calcium homeostasis secondary to reduced coronary blood flow. *(From: Nayler WG: The role of calcium in the ischemic myocardium. Am J Pathol 1981; 102:263.)*

generated by the metabolites of anaerobic metabolism.[12] After 30 minutes, there is progressive accumulation of the products of membrane degradation. Ischemia-induced reduction of free radical scavengers results in continued lipid peroxidation and membrane destruction via oxygen-free radicals.[13] After 60 minutes, there is destruction of the cell membrane such that cell death occurs.

■ CARDIOPLEGIA

Administration of cardioplegic solution is the most commonly used method of preventing ischemic myocardial damage during aortic cross-clamping. The current composition and mode of administration of cardioplegic solutions to prevent ischemia has evolved since its introduction in 1955 by Melrose and associates.[14] More recently, cardioplegia solutions have been used to replenish energy stores in ischemic hearts before further ischemia is induced and to avoid and reverse the reperfusion injuries that occur after cross-clamp removal.[15]

Use of Cardioplegia in Preventing Ischemia

Rationale. As discussed previously, aortic cross-clamping drastically reduces oxygen and substrate supplies to the myocardium. Ideally, cardioplegia solutions should be formulated to promptly reduce myocardial oxygen consumption and to provide substrates to meet these reduced energy demands so that preischemic energy stores are not depleted.[16] It is therefore logical to reduce myocardial oxygen consumption as much as possible. Cardioplegia solutions are formulated to induce electromechanical arrest of the heart in diastole. Because electromechanical work constitutes 95% of total myocardial oxygen consumption, the arrested heart will have very low energy requirements. In the arrested state, only basal energy requirements (those required to keep cellular metabolic processes intact) must be met. Figure 10–2 illustrates the very low oxygen consumption associated with induced arrest. Aerobic and anaerobic metabolism can provide enough energy to meet basal energy requirements as long as there is periodic replenishment of substrates and washout of metabolites.

Composition. There is considerable variability in the composition of cardioplegia solutions used in different institutions. As yet, there is no "ideal" cardioplegia solution.[17] In 1980, it was estimated that it would take one million controlled experiments to fully study all of the possible combinations of then-available cardioplegia constituents.[18] Despite this uncertainty regarding the composition of the ideal cardioplegia solution, it is clear that an effective cardioplegia solution must:

- induce prompt arrest of the heart in diastole to reduce myocardial oxygen consumption.
- induce hypothermia to further reduce myocardial oxygen consumption.
- provide sufficient substrates to meet the metabolic demands of the arrested heart.
- provide buffering to counteract the acidosis that accompanies ischemia.
- provide increased osmolarity to prevent the cellular edema that accompanies ischemia.
- provide membrane stabilization with additives or avoidance of hypocalcemia.
- have no adverse effects of its own.
- have a composition suitable for delivery to all areas of the myocardium.[19]

To fulfill these requirements, a typical cardioplegia solution contains the components described in the following sections.

POTASSIUM. Increasing extracellular potassium concentration is the primary method used to induce electromechanical arrest in most cardioplegia solutions.

Extracellular hyperkalemia results in depolarization of the cell membrane and sustained diastole. The potassium concentration necessary to induce prompt arrest varies from solution to solution. For example, myocardial hypothermia reduces the extracellular potassium concentration required to induce arrest. Likewise, crystalloid cardioplegia solutions require lower extracellular potassium concentrations to induce arrest than do blood cardioplegia solutions.

Nonetheless, cardioplegia solutions generally have a potassium concentration of 15 to 30 mEq/L. This concentration produces prompt electromechanical arrest, usually within minutes. Concentrations of potassium higher than 40 mEq/L have been shown to be detrimental because they increase calcium influx by increasing calcium conductance.[20] Recall that increased intracellular calcium will increase wall tension and myocardial oxygen consumption. In addition, increasing calcium conductance while ischemia-induced loss of calcium homeostasis is occurring will exacerbate ischemic damage.

HYPOTHERMIA. Hypothermia is an important component of cardioplegia solutions because it:

- reduces myocardial oxygen consumption even in the arrested heart (*see* Fig. 12–2).
- reduces the degree of extracellular hyperkalemia needed to cause electromechanical arrest.[19]
- is additive with potassium-induced arrest in preventing ischemic damage.[21-23]

Generally, cardioplegia solutions are cooled to approximately 4 to 10°C. Despite delivery of these cold solutions into the coronary arteries, it often is difficult to cool the myocardium to less than 15°C for several reasons:

- The presence of coronary stenoses may prevent homogenous delivery of the cold cardioplegia solutions.[24]
- Noncoronary collaterals perfuse the heart with blood at the temperature of the systemic perfusate. This results in rewarming of the heart.
- Systemic venous return rewarms the septal areas of the heart unless the vena cavae are individually cannulated and isolated from the heart with tourniquets.

CALCIUM. As discussed previously, loss of calcium homeostasis has been implicated in causing cell dysfunction and death after ischemia. For this reason, it might be assumed that the addition of calcium to cardioplegia solutions is detrimental. In fact, a small amount of calcium (more than 50 mM) is necessary to prevent the calcium paradox[25] and to allow functional recovery after aortic cross-clamp removal. Calcium paradox is the massive cellular destruction that occurs when the my-

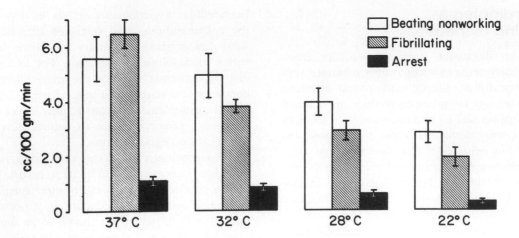

FIGURE 12–2. Left ventricular oxygen consumption during three functional states (beating empty, fibrillating, and arrested) and at four temperatures. Hypothermia clearly reduces myocardial oxygen consumption for any of the functional states. Below 37°C, the beating, empty heart consumes the most oxygen, followed in decreasing order by the fibrillating and the arrested heart. *(From: Buckberg GD: Studies of the effects of hypothermia on regional myocardial blood flow and metabolism during cardiopulmonary bypass. J Thorac Cardiovasc Surg 1977; 73:89.)*

ocardium is reperfused with a calcium-containing solution after a period of calcium-free perfusion.[26] Calcium paradox is due to washout of calcium from the sarcolemma with subsequent inability of the sarcolemma to limit calcium influx when presented with a calcium load. Calcium paradox seems particularly likely to occur if the cardioplegia solution is very alkalotic.[27,28]

Despite this risk, most crystalloid cardioplegia solutions do not have calcium added to them. Calcium paradox is prevented by delivery of an adequate concentration of calcium via the systemic perfusate from noncoronary collaterals and by the presence of hypothermia.[29] Blood cardioplegia solutions deliver varying concentrations of calcium to the myocardium. The exact concentration depends on how extensively the blood solution is diluted before it is used as a medium for cardioplegia.[30]

SODIUM. The optimal sodium concentration is unknown, but most cardioplegia solutions avoid extreme hypo- or hypernatremia relative to intracellular sodium concentration for the following reasons:

1. Perfusion of the heart with a hyponatremic solution may predispose accumulation of intracellular calcium with subsequent increases in wall tension and myocardial oxygen consumption.[31]
2. Perfusion of the heart with a hypernatremic solution results in accumulation of intracellular sodium. This may result in cellular edema. It also may result in an accumulation of intracellular calcium as the sodium–calcium exchange pump pumps sodium out of and calcium into the cell.

For these reasons, most cardioplegia solutions have sodium concentrations in the range of 100 to 120 mEq/L.

BUFFERING. Recall that the anaerobic metabolism that accompanies ischemia results in cellular acidosis and that the accumulation of acids results in inhibition of further anaerobic metabolism. Buffering will allow anaerobic metabolism to continue and will thus reduce ATP depletion in the ischemic myocardium. As discussed in detail in Chapter 10, as myocardial temperature decreases the appropriate uncorrected pH becomes more alkalotic. Therefore, the buffers chosen must be effective at the alkalotic pH that is appropriate in the hypothermic myocardium. Tromethamine (THAM), bicarbonate, phosphate, and histidine are all used as buffers in cardioplegia solutions.

Histidine may be a superior buffer because:

1. It shifts its pKa into the alkaline range as temperature decreases and therefore is an effective buffer over a wide variety of temperatures and pHs.
2. It provides crystalloid cardioplegia solutions with greater buffering capacity than crystalloid cardioplegia solutions buffered with standard concentrations of either bicarbonate or THAM.[32,33] Blood cardioplegia has been shown to provide better myocardial buffering than crystalloid cardioplegia buffered with bicarbonate due to the presence of the histidine buffering system in blood.[33,34] Histidine added to crystalloid cardioplegia can provide a buffering capacity similar to that of blood cardioplegia.[32,33]

OSMOLARITY. Because myocardial edema accompanies ischemia, cardioplegia solutions must be formulated to minimize further accumulation of intracellular fluid. Cardioplegia solutions with osmolarities greater than 400 mosm have been demonstrated to result in an exacerbation of myocardial edema,[35] probably by inducing increases in intracellular sodium.[36] On the other hand, solutions with a low osmolarity will result in accumulation of intracellular water and further edema. The ideal osmolarity remains undetermined but probably is approximately 370 mosm.[37] Mannitol and albumin are the additives commonly used to manipulate osmolarity in cardioplegia solutions.

SUBSTRATES. Energy production during anaerobic metabolism requires provision of a substrate. Glucose and insulin as components of a cardioplegia solution allow uptake of glucose into the myocardium for use during anaerobic metabolism. Anaerobic metabolism results in the production of lactic acid and nicotinamide adenine dinucleotide (NADH). Accumulation of these metabolites leads to the eventual shutdown of further anaerobic metabolism. Substrate provision is useful only if there is periodic washout of the metabolites that inhibit anaerobic metabolism.[38] In fact, in the absence of periodic washout of metabolites, substrate enhancement has been demonstrated to be deleterious to myocardial recovery after aortic cross-clamping.[39] In clinical practice, this washout occurs through noncoronary collateral flow or through intermittent reinfusion of a cardioplegia solution.

The use of glucose and insulin before aortic cross-clamping may result in improved postcross-clamp myocardial function.[40] Infusion of insulin and glucose before aortic cross-clamping results in a shift from oxidative lipolysis to glycolysis as well as an increase in glycogen stores. This preischemic accumulation of glycogen stores and the early shift to anaerobic metabolism may have a protective effect during ischemia.

Glucose and insulin concentrations in cardioplegia solutions vary greatly from institution to institution. In fact, some institutions do not add either entity to their solutions. Some glucose is present in blood cardioplegia and, therefore, little or no glucose must be added when blood is used as a cardioplegia vehicle.

CRYSTALLOID VERSUS BLOOD SOLUTIONS. The necessary constituents of an effective cardioplegia solution can be delivered in either a crystalloid or a blood medium. There are important differences between the two formulations.

PREPARATION. Crystalloid solutions generally are prepared by the hospital pharmacy in containers that are delivered to the perfusionist. Blood solutions are prepared by drawing off oxygenated blood from the CPB circuit into a separate reservoir. Potassium and other additives are then added to the blood in the sufficient amounts to obtain the desired concentration.

HYPOTHERMIA. Crystalloid solutions generally are cooled to 4°C before delivery. Initial fears that aggressive cooling of blood cardioplegia solutions would lead to sludging in the coronary capillaries has not materialized in clinical practice. Blood cardioplegia solutions with hematocrits in the range of 10 to 15% delivered at temperatures between 4° and 10°C currently are being used successfully.[15,41]

OXYGENATION. Blood cardioplegia solutions are routinely oxygenated because the solution is formulated using oxygenated blood from the CPB circuit. The amount of oxygen that can be delivered to the myocardium by a blood cardioplegia solution is only a fraction of the solution's total oxygen content. The fraction of total oxygen content available for delivery is dependent on the solution's temperature and the hematocrit. The lower the temperature and the higher the hematocrit, the less oxygen will be available for delivery to the myocardium.[42] The hypothermia-induced leftward shift of the oxyhemoglobin dissociation curve increases hemoglobin's affinity for oxygen and decreases oxygen availability to the myocardium. The delivery of oxygen carried in the dissolved state is unaffected by changes in hemoglobin's affinity for oxygen. For this reason, solutions with high hematocrits, in which the quantity of oxygen carried dissolved in plasma is reduced, will have a reduced oxygen-delivery capacity at low temperatures.

Crystalloid cardioplegia solutions are not routinely oxygenated. Oxygenation of crystalloid solutions is accomplished easily by bubbling gas into the solution before delivery. Aeration of a bicarbonate containing crystalloid cardioplegia solution with 100% oxygen drives off carbon dioxide and results in severe alkalosis. For this reason, aeration with a 95 to 98% oxygen and 2 to 5% carbon dioxide mixture is recommended.[30,43]

An increase in the total oxygen content of a crystalloid solution occurs with decreasing temperature due to the enhanced solubility of oxygen in crystalloid at low temperatures. Crystalloid cardioplegia solutions are capable of delivering their entire oxygen content to the myocardium because all oxygen is carried in the dissolved state. Therefore, as the temperature of a crystalloid cardioplegia solution decreases, the quantity of oxygen it delivers to the myocardium increases.[44]

EFFICACY. Blood cardioplegia solutions offer several potential advantages over crystalloid solutions:[45]

- Improved capillary perfusion due to the presence of red cells.[46]
- More homogenous delivery of blood cardioplegia in the presence[47] and absence of coronary stenoses.[30]
- Improved buffering due to the presence of the histidine buffering system present in red cells.[32-34]
- Reduced myocardial edema due to the onconicity of blood.[48]

- Reduced risk of calcium paradox and improved functional recovery after ischemia due to the physiologic calcium concentration provided by blood.[27,30]
- Presence of red cell enzyme catalase to scavenge free radicals produced by ischemia.[49]

Whether these differences between sanguineous and asanguineous cardioplegia solutions offer any clear clinical advantage remains less clear-cut. Extensive work in both animals and humans has been conducted.

WORK IN ANIMALS.   Oxygenated blood cardioplegia solutions have been demonstrated to provide better preservation of myocardial high-energy phosphate stores, ultrastructure, and function than nonoxygenated crystalloid cardioplegia solutions in animals. Likewise, animal work demonstrates that oxygenated crystalloid cardioplegia provides better myocardial preservation than does nonoxygenated crystalloid cardioplegia.[44,50] When differences in calcium concentration have been accounted for, the evidence demonstrates that oxygenated blood cardioplegia and oxygenated crystalloid cardioplegia provide comparable degrees of left ventricular functional recovery and ATP preservation.[30]

WORK IN HUMANS.   Comparison of blood and crystalloid cardioplegia solutions within a study and between different studies is complicated by several factors:

- The lack of controlled, randomized trials.
- Differences in the compositions and temperatures of the various solutions.
- Differences in delivery of the cardioplegia solutions (multidose or intermittent delivery for one solution versus continuous infusion for the other).
- Differences in the criteria used to determine the success of myocardial preservation.
- Differences in the preoperative systolic function of study patients.

Despite these problems, several statements can be made with certainty. For patients with preserved left ventricular function undergoing coronary artery bypass surgery, intermittent delivery of oxygenated blood cardioplegia solution has been shown to provide protection from ischemic injury and preservation of left ventricular performance in the early postoperative period equal[51-53] or superior[54-59] to intermittent delivery of nonoxygenated crystalloid cardioplegia solution.

For patients with compromised preoperative left ventricular function, the evidence suggests that oxygenated blood cardioplegia provides superior preservation of postoperative left ventricular function compared with nonoxygenated crystalloid cardioplegia.[53,55]

A recent comparison of antegrade blood cardioplegia, antegrade crystalloid cardioplegia, and combined antegrade/retrograde blood cardioplegia revealed little difference in myocardial infarction, stroke, and respiratory and wound infections between antegrade crystalloid and blood cardioplegia.[60] Combined use of antegrade and retrograde blood cardioplegia was associated with a lower complication rate than antegrade crystalloid cardioplegia, primarily due to its beneficial effects in the subset of reoperation patients.[60] Therefore, for the reoperation patients, it is conceivable that the advantage seen is due more to the route of cardioplegia delivery than the crystalloid or blood composition.

Adjuvant Agents

There has been recent interest in the use of additional agents in cardioplegia solutions.

CALCIUM CHANNEL BLOCKERS.   Because loss of calcium homeostasis is a major factor in causing ischemia-induced myocardial damage, the use of calcium channel blockers in cardioplegia solutions has gained attention. Calcium channel blockers may exert their principal beneficial effect by preventing calcium influx and subsequent high-energy phosphate hydrolysis during cardioplegic arrest[61] and by preventing calcium influx during reperfusion. Animal studies have demonstrated improved preservation of myocardial function with the addition of calcium channel blockers to crystalloid[62,63] and blood[64] cardioplegia solutions.

The addition of calcium channel blockers (nifedipine, verapamil, diltiazem) to cardioplegia solutions has been studied in humans. A controlled, randomized clinical trial testing the addition of nifedipine to cold crystalloid potassium cardioplegia demonstrated improved postoperative left ventricular function in high-risk patients undergoing either coronary bypass or valve replacement surgery.[65,66] This study demonstrated no difference in the extent of myocardial injury as determined by CPK–MB between the control and treatment groups. It was observed that patients in the nifedipine cardioplegia group often required temporary pacing for atrioventricular (AV) nodal block after cross-clamp removal. The addition of nifedipine to cold crystalloid magnesium cardioplegia resulted in more effective sparing of high-energy phosphate stores only in patients undergoing procedures in which myocardial temperatures were higher than 15°C (aortic valve replacement).[67] However, no improvement in clinical outcome was noted.

A clinical trial of verapamil added to cold crystalloid cardioplegia demonstrated no advantage over standard cold crystalloid cardioplegia in the preservation of ventricular function.[68] Furthermore, significant negative inotropic effects and AV nodal dysfunction were associated with the use of verapamil cardioplegia. This study has been criticized because it studied only low-risk patients undergoing procedures with short aortic cross-clamp times.[69] Better preservation of myocardial function might have been noted in patients at higher risk for ischemic-induced ventricular dysfunction.

Clinical trials of diltiazem added to crystalloid[70] and blood[71] cardioplegia have been performed in patients undergoing elective coronary artery bypass surgery with preserved ventricular function. Both studies demonstrate lower levels of myocardial injury as determined by CPK–MB levels and an increased incidence of AV nodal dysfunction compared with control. After diltiazem cardioplegia, improved myocardial metabolism (decreased lactate production) but depressed postoperative systolic function was observed in one study,[70] whereas postoperative systolic function remained unchanged in the other.[71]

Clinical study differences in the composition of cardioplegia solutions, in the dosages of calcium channel blockers added to the cardioplegia solutions, in the operative procedures, and in the extent of preoperative ventricular dysfunction make it difficult to draw any firm conclusions about the efficacy of calcium channel blockers added to cardioplegia solutions. The issue of whether their routine use is justified is unresolved, but the data suggest that their addition will be of greatest use for patients at highest risk for calcium-induced ischemic damage. This must be tempered with the knowledge that negative inotropism and AV nodal dysfunction may accompany use of these agents in cardioplegia solutions.

ALLOPURINOL.   Allopurinol is a competitive inhibitor of xanthine oxidase, whereas its chief metabolite, alloxanthine, is a noncompetitive inhibitor. Xanthine oxidase is an important enzyme in the generation of the free radicals that have been implicated in causing myocardial damage when oxygen is reintroduced into the ischemic myocardium.[13] Allopurinol added to cold blood[72] and crystalloid[73] cardioplegia has been shown to improve myocardial protection in the severely ischemic animal ventricle. It has been suggested that pretreatment with allopurinol 24 hours before an ischemic event would allow buildup of alloxanthine and might provide superior protection to allopurinol administered in cardioplegia.[72]

FREE RADICAL SCAVENGERS.   An alternative to inhibition of free radical production is supplementation with agents capable of scavenging free radicals. Animal studies have demonstrated improved myocardial protection in the ischemic myocardium after use of crystalloid cardioplegic supplemented with the free radical scavengers superoxide dismutase (SOD), catalase, deferoxamine, and mannitol.[73-77]

ADENINE NUCLEOTIDES.   Myocardial ischemia promotes production of adenosine. Adenosine added to cardioplegia mitigates postischemic ventricular function in animals.[78] Acadesine, a purine nucleoside analog, raises adenosine levels in ischemic myocardium but not in nonischemic myocardium. Acadesine selectively augments adenosine production in ischemic myocardium without increasing production in nonischemic myocardium.[79] Although the mechanism of action is unclear, the action of acadesine seems to be mediated through adenosine A_1 and A_2 receptors and may act through activation of the ATP-sensitive potassium channel.[80] Acadesine added to cold cardioplegia improves postischemic ventricular function in animal models.[79]

NITRIC OXIDE.   There may be a role for nitric oxide (NO) or NO donors in cardioplegia solutions because it has been demonstrated that failure to preserve NO-mediated vasodilation during reperfusion results in decreased postreperfusion myocardial blood flow.[81]

Use of Cardioplegia in Preventing Reperfusion Injury and in Resuscitating Ischemic Myocardium

Rationale.   Reperfusion injury is defined as the functional, metabolic, and structural alterations caused by reperfusion after a period of temporary ischemia such as that induced by aortic cross-clamping.[15,82] Although cardioplegia is used to minimize the ischemic insult associated with aortic cross-clamping, the potential for reperfusion injury exists in cardiac surgical procedure after removal of the aortic cross-clamp and reperfusion of the heart with the systemic perfusate.

Reperfusion injury is characterized by (1) intracellular calcium accumulation, (2) cellular swelling leading to a no-reflow phenomenon and reduced ventricular compliance, and (3) inability of the myocardium to use oxygen, even in the presence of adequate coronary blood flow and oxygen content.

Reperfusion solutions are infused into the myocardium after completion of the surgical procedure and before removal of the aortic cross-clamp. They are formulated to prevent or minimize the reperfusion injury that accompanies reperfusion of the heart with systemic blood.

Extensive experimental work in animals[15,82] and anecdotal experience in humans[15,82] has shown these solutions to be effective in improving ventricular function after aortic cross-clamping. To date, controlled clinical trials of reperfusion solutions in humans are limited.[83-85] Most of the animal and human work to date has involved use of blood perfusates, although crystalloid perfusates have been shown to be effective in both animals[86] and humans.[85] Both improved[83,85] and unchanged[84] ventricular function has been demonstrated after the use of reperfusion solutions in humans. Differences in the composition, temperature, and delivery of the solutions used, and in the operative procedures performed, make it difficult to draw any firm conclusions regarding the efficacy of reperfusion solutions in humans.

Despite this, there is support for use of reperfusion solutions in patients with preexisting poor ventricular function and in those who require long cross-clamp times.[87]

Resuscitation of ischemic myocardium can be accomplished through warm induction of cardioplegic arrest. The goal is to resuscitate ischemic areas while optimizing preservation of the nonischemic areas. Warm induction of cardioplegic arrest after aortic cross-clamping and combined with rapid ventricular decompression on CPB seems to improve repletion of myocardial energy stores and improve myocardial recovery after an acute ischemic event and in patients with hypertrophy.[88-90] In the present era of rapid intervention in evolving myocardial infarction with angioplasty and thrombolytic agents, this strategy may be even more effective.

Composition. As with cardioplegia solutions used to prevent ischemia, there is no consensus on the composition of the ideal reperfusion/resuscitation solution. Nonetheless, it would seem to be desirable that the solution should:

- Maintain arrest of the heart in diastole to reduce myocardial oxygen consumption.
- Induce normothermia to optimize the rate of metabolic recovery.
- Initiate aerobic metabolism with an oxygenated solution.
- Provide buffering to counteract acidosis and optimize enzymatic and metabolic recovery.
- Provide increased osmolarity to minimize reperfusion edema.
- Provide sufficient substrate to allow aerobic energy production.
- Temporarily reduce calcium ion availability.
- Provide substrate to scavenge free radicals.

The attributes of a typical reperfusion solution that fulfills these requirements are described in the following sections.

POTASSIUM. For reperfusion solutions, sufficient potassium to maintain arrest in diastole is required. This is accomplished clinically using 8 to 10 mEq/L in a blood medium.[15] For warm induction solutions, 25 mEq/L of potassium in a blood medium is required.

NORMOTHERMIA. Hypothermia delays the repair of damaged enzyme systems[91,92] because the repair process is temperature-dependent. Clinically, use of a normothermic (37°C) reperfusion solution has been shown to result in improved functional recovery.[15,83]

SUBSTRATES. Glutamate and aspartate are amino acids that serve to replenish Kreb's cycle intermediates that are depleted during ischemia[93] and which enhance aerobic metabolism and reparative processes. Reperfusion and warm induction with an L-glutamine- and asparatate-containing solution has been shown to result in the return of oxidative metabolism, enhanced oxygen uptake, improved ATP repletion, and better preservation of systolic function after ischemic insult.[94-96]

BUFFERING. As previously discussed in detail, maintenance of temperature-appropriate pH is essential to ongoing cellular metabolic processes. Because acidosis accompanies ischemia, any reperfusion solution should be formulated to counteract acidosis and normalize pH. THAM has been used with clinical success as a buffer in blood reperfusion solutions.[82] Additional buffering capacity is available in the form of histidine when a blood reperfusate is used. The glutamic acid–sodium hydroxide buffer system has been used with clinical success in crystalloid reperfusate.[85]

OSMOLARITY. As with cardioplegia solutions used to prevent ischemia, reperfusion solutions must be formulated to prevent progression of the edema that accompanies ischemia. Maintenance of an osmolarity of 360 mosm and avoidance of perfusion pressures greater than 60 mm Hg have been shown to be effective in this regard.[82]

CALCIUM HOMEOSTASIS. Because loss of calcium homeostasis is the major determinant of reperfusion injury, careful control of calcium concentration in the reperfusate is essential. The optimal concentration of calcium in reperfusate is unknown, but it seems to be in the range of 0.15 to 0.25 mmol/L with a blood medium[15,97] and in the normal serum range of 1.0 mmol/L with a crystalloid medium.[85] Clinically, the desired calcium concentration in a blood reperfusate is obtained by using citrate–phosphate–dextrose (CPD) to chelate excess calcium before its administration.[15]

FREE RADICAL SCAVENGERS. Because free-radical-induced damage occurs when ischemic myocardium is reperfused with an oxygen-containing solution, modification of the reperfusate with free radical scavengers seems appropriate. In fact, the free radical scavengers superoxide dismutase,[98] catalase,[97] and mannitol[99] added to reperfusion solutions have been shown to be effective in reducing free-radical-induced reperfusion injury in animals.

■ DELIVERY OF CARDIOPLEGIA

For any cardioplegia solution to be effective, the delivery must be optimized.

Delivery System. Cardioplegia is delivered under pressure to the heart via either a pressurized bag or roller pump system. The roller pump system offers several advantages: easy incorporation of a continuous cooling system to maintain cardioplegia hypothermia, easy incorporation of the mixing apparatus necessary for blood cardioplegia systems, and second-to-second control of cardioplegia infusion pressure and flow rates. The delivery system should have a 0.8-mm filter to prevent particular contaminants from reaching the coronary circulation and inducing coronary vasospasm.[100]

Delivery Pressure. It is necessary to have a means of monitoring infusion pressure because it has been demonstrated that excessive infusion pressures can result in myocardial edema and ventricular dysfunction.[101] Infusion pressure can be monitored in the cardioplegia line itself or directly at the site of administration. As will be discussed, safe delivery pressure will be dictated by the site of administration.

Delivery Frequency. It generally is agreed that during the period of aortic cross-clamping, cardioplegia should be reinfused at least every 20 minutes. This strategy allows washout of metabolites and replacement of the cardioplegia solution components that may have been depleted or washed out by noncoronary collateral flow. If ECG or visual evidence of myocardial contraction is present, reinfusion of cardioplegia is necessary immediately, regardless of the time elapsed since the previous infusion.

Volume of Delivery. The optimal cardioplegia infusion volume is unknown. In general, 10 to 20 mL/kg/min of cardioplegia is delivered during the initial infusion with the larger volumes being reserved for hypertrophied ventricles.[102]

Subsequent infusion usually is 10 to 15 mL/kg. With this method, the rate of infusion will be limited by the infusion site and the safe maximal delivery pressure.

Some centers are more concerned with the duration of cardioplegia delivery than the volume infused and prefer to deliver cardioplegia by controlling infusion pressure and delivering cardioplegia over a time interval of 1.5 to 3 minutes for initial arrest and 1 to 1.5 minutes for subsequent infusions.

Composition of Subsequent Infusions. It has been demonstrated that after diastolic arrest has been obtained with hyperkalemic, hypothermia cardioplegia, diastolic arrest can be maintained with a hypothermic solution containing a lower potassium concentration.[103] Patients receiving cold crystalloid high-potassium (20 or 27 mEq/L) cardioplegia in both the initial and subsequent infusions had a higher incidence of postoperative high-grade ventricular ectopy[104] and AV nodal dissociation dysrhythmias[105] than patients receiving an initial infusion of cold crystalloid high-potassium cardioplegia followed by subsequent infusions of cold crystalloid low-potassium (5 or 7 mEq/L) cardioplegia. No differences in postoperative ventricular function could be detected between the two groups in either of these studies.

Site of Administration. Optimal delivery of cardioplegia must be tailored to the operative procedure and operative technique. Several methods are available for cardioplegia delivery. Delivery may be via the arterial system (antegrade) or via the venous system (retrograde).

INFUSION INTO THE AORTIC ROOT. This method is accomplished by placement of a cannula (14 to 16 gauge) into the aorta root between the aortic cross-clamp and the aortic valve/coronary ostia. Placement of a cannula with two lumens — one for cardioplegia delivery and the other for venting or pressure monitoring — is popular and allows measurement of aortic root pressure during cardioplegia delivery. A double-lumen cannula is illustrated in Figure 12–3.

For this method to be effective, a competent aortic valve must be present. Otherwise, the cardioplegia solution will flow into the left ventricle with resultant ventricular distension and inadequate delivery of cardioplegia to the coronary ostia.

When coronary artery stenoses are present and revascularization is planned, cardioplegia delivery distal to stenoses will be enhanced by infusion of cardioplegia into the aortic root after completion of each of the proximal (aortic-saphenous vein) and distal (saphenous-coronary artery) anastomoses. Ideally, with this method, the proximal anastomoses are completed before placement of the aortic cross-clamp. Because cross-clamping is required for exposure during creation of the distal but not the proximal anastomoses, cross-clamp time can be minimized with this strategy.

INFUSION INTO THE GRAFTS. In revascularization procedures, cardioplegia can be infused down the free end of each saphenous vein after completion of the distal anastomosis with the proximal anastomoses completed after cross-clamp removal. For cardioplegia to be delivered down each completed graft, this method requires a manifold that allows simultaneous infusion of cardioplegia down the free ends of several saphenous veins at the same time.

INFUSION DIRECTLY INTO THE CORONARY OSTIA. This method is used for procedures in which the aortic valve is incompetent and cardioplegia cannot be delivered into the aortic root or for procedures in which the aortic root must be opened (aortic valve replacement). For this method to work effectively, the surgeon must identify the coronary ostia and cannulate them with specially designed catheters through which cardioplegia is infused. Figure 12–3 illustrates one of these catheters. The catheters come in a variety of sizes to allow proper placement without damage to the ostia.

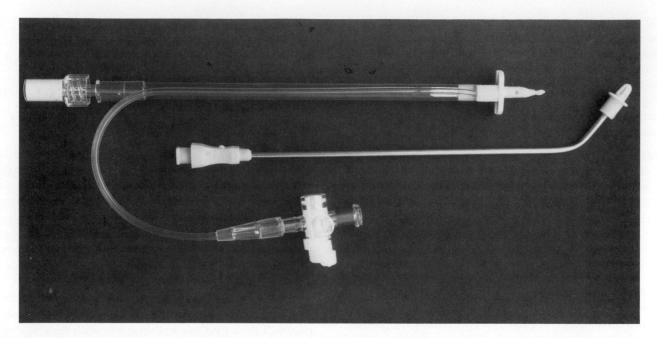

FIGURE 12–3. Bottom. Specially designed cannula used to directly cannulate coronary ostia for delivery of cardioplegia solution. **Top.** Double-lumen catheter used for delivery of cardioplegia into the aortic root. Lumen connected to a stopcock can be used for venting via aortic root or for measurement of aortic root pressure. Catheter is placed in aortic root with use of purse-string suture and needle-tipped stylet shown in place here. After catheter has been placed in the aorta, the stylet is removed and the central lumen is used for cardioplegia infusion.

Delivery of cardioplegia with this method can be complicated in several ways. The tip of the catheter may extend past the bifurcation of the left main coronary artery such that the catheter may only perfuse either the left anterior descending or the circumflex artery. This is particularly true in patients with bicuspid aortic valves because the left main coronary artery is shorter than normal. In 50% of patients, the conus artery to the right ventricle arises separately from the aortic sinus and will not be perfused by cannulation of the right coronary ostium. Finally, damage to the ostia with late stenosis can occur with direct cannulation.[3]

For all three of these antegrade delivery sites, the infusion pressure should not exceed 150 mm Hg.[106]

RETROGRADE CORONARY SINUS PERFUSION. Retrograde coronary sinus perfusion (RCSP) involves infusion of cardioplegia into the coronary sinus retrograde into the great and small cardiac veins. There is a large venous network free of atherosclerotic disease that allows adequate retrograde perfusion of the entire myocardium via this route.

This method requires placement of a purse-string suture in the right atrium (RA) and creation of a small atriotomy. A specially designed coronary sinus catheter is placed in the coronary sinus by the surgeon via the atriotomy. This usually can be accomplished before initiation of CPB. TEE is useful to confirm positioning because the coronary sinus is visualized easily. After the catheter is in position, the purse-string suture is cinched

up. In addition, a self-inflating balloon at the tip of the catheter helps keep it secured. Delivery of cardioplegia commences after aortic cross-clamping. Most of the retrograde perfusion drains via the thebesian veins, but the aortic root usually is vented during cardioplegia infusion to allow egress of the solution. Most coronary sinus catheters have a pressure-monitoring lumen that is transduced during cardioplegia infusion. To prevent disruption of the venous network and intramyocardial hemorrhage, retrograde perfusion should occur at a pressure of 30 to 50 mm Hg.

The retrograde route of cardioplegia administration has been shown to be particularly useful in certain clinical settings and may be advantageous in several others as well:

- RCSP has gained popularity for use in aortic valve replacement so that the difficulties in direct cannulation of the coronary ostia can be avoided.[107]
- Due to the unpredictable efficacy of aortic root infusion of cardioplegia in which aortic incompetence exists, retrograde perfusion may be superior to aortic root perfusion when mild aortic incompetence exists and no valve replacement is planned.
- RCSP has been shown to result in more homogeneous distribution of cardioplegia than antegrade delivery in animals[108] and humans[109] with coronary stenoses. This is believed to be secondary to

the fact that the large venous network is free of atherosclerotic disease. Better preservation of ventricular function with retrograde infusion has been demonstrated in animals with coronary stenoses.[110] Nonetheless, a clinical trial comparing retrograde and aortic root cardioplegia delivery failed to demonstrate any differences in postoperative CPK-MB or lactate dehydrogenas (LDH) fractions, right or left ventricular stroke work, or regional wall motion in patients undergoing elective revascularization.[111]

- Retrograde perfusion is useful in reoperative procedures in patients with patent IMA grafts. Retrograde perfusion during internal mammary artery (IMA) occlusion will provide cardioplegia delivery to the myocardium distal to the patent graft.
- RCSP provides poor protection of the RV and posterior septum probably as a result of venovenous shunting through arteriosinusoidal and thesbesian vessels directly into the RV.[112,113] As a result only 30% to 70% of delivered retrograde cardioplegia reaches myocardial tissue.[114] As a result some centers use RCSP in conjunction with antegrade perfusion either in an alternating fashion[115] or simultaneously[116] in patients with coronary artery disease.

■ ADJUNCTS TO PRESERVATION WITH CARDIOPLEGIA

Myocardial preservation is influenced by factors other than the efficient delivery of cold cardioplegia solution. The most important of these factors are discussed in the sections that follow.

Topical Hypothermia. Experimentally, 4° to 6°C is the temperature range for optimal myocardial preservation.[117] As discussed previously, it is difficult to achieve this degree of hypothermia in clinical practice. It is possible, with the use of cold cardioplegia solution and topical saline slush or ice chips, to achieve and maintain temperatures lower than 15°C. Unfortunately, the use of saline slush and ice chips has been associated with problems. Myocardial damage due to freezing has been demonstrated in hearts exposed to slush or ice for more than 30 minutes.[118] Phrenic nerve paresis due to freezing has been reported in 60 to 80% of cases in which slush or ice is used.[117,119] For these reasons, many centers use either intermittent or continuous infusions of saline at 4°C into the pericardial well to obtain topical cooling.

Control of Noncoronary and Bronchial Collateral Blood Flow. Excessive bronchial collateral blood flow results in rewarming of the heart by distend-

ing it with blood at the temperature of the systemic perfusate. Excessive noncoronary collateral flow results not only in distension and rewarming of the heart but in the washout of cardioplegia solutions as well. Systemic hypothermia on CPB is effective in reducing rewarming, but careful control of systemic flow and pressure on CPB is necessary to reduce the magnitude of collateralized flow (*see* Chapter 10).

Decompression of the Heart. Distension of the heart has two deleterious consequences: it results in poor distribution of cardioplegia solution to the subendocardium due to the high intracavitary pressures, and it results in rewarming of the heart due to distension of the heart with blood at body temperature. For these reasons, venting of the heart may be necessary (*see* Chapter 10).

Preventing Rewarming of the Posterior Surface of the Heart. Because the posterior surface of the heart lies on top of the mediastinum, which is at systemic temperature, it is at high risk of rewarming during aortic cross-clamping. To prevent this, many surgeons place a pad soaked in iced saline behind the heart in the pericardium to shield it from the mediastinal structures. This may help prevent mitral valve dysfunction secondary to posterior papillary muscle ischemia. "Freezing" the TEE probe during CPB also will reduce rewarming by terminating ultrasound transmission.

Normothermic Cardioplegia and CPB. Currently, there is interest in warm heart surgery, specifically normothermic blood cardioplegia (retrograde or antegrade) combined with normothermic CPB.[120] To date, randomized trials have shown little benefit of this approach in terms of myocardial preservation as compared with traditional hypothermic methods.[120] In addition, normothermic CPB may be associated with a higher risk of neurologic complications (*see* Chapters 10 and 13).[121-123]

■ SPECIAL CONSIDERATIONS IN NEONATES, INFANTS, AND CHILDREN

Despite advances in the surgical correction of congenital cardiac lesions, postoperative low cardiac output leading to long-term ventricular dysfunction or death continues to be a concern.[124] This has focused attention on the effectiveness of current myocardial protection techniques in the repair of congenital heart disease. Most work to date on myocardial preservation has involved adult humans or adult animal preparations. Unfortunately, the existence of major structural, metabolic, and functional differences between infant and adult hearts makes extrapolation of these studies to neonates and infants difficult. These differences are summarized in the following sections.

Calcium Homeostasis. Neonatal hearts have a poorly developed sarcoplasmic reticulum, T-tubule system, and calcium-pumping mechanism. This results in a greater reliance on extracellular calcium to provide excitation–contraction coupling and is a factor in the diminished tension development capabilities of the neonatal myocardium.

ATPase Activity. Fetal light-chain myosin has a diminished ability to hydrolyse ATP, which contributes to the diminished tension-development capability of neonatal hearts. This light-chain myosin remains in patients with congenital heart disease.

Capacity for Anaerobic Metabolism. The neonatal heart has an enhanced capacity for anaerobic metabolism compared with the adult heart secondary to its large glycogen stores. For this reason, the neonatal heart tolerates longer periods of hypoxia.[125,126] Hypoxia (reduced substrate delivery with maintained perfusion) allows the products of anaerobic metabolism that inhibit further anaerobic metabolism and cause tissue damage to be washed out. This permits glycogen to be used for sustained anaerobic energy production.

Tolerance for Ischemia. The neonatal heart seems to possess greater tolerance for ischemia (severely reduced or absent perfusion) than adult hearts due to enhanced glycogen stores, better maintenance of ischemic calcium exchange, higher levels of ATP substrates, and increased amino acid use.[127] Prolonged periods of ischemia may be more poorly tolerated than in adults.[128,129] In the absence of perfusion, the enhanced capacity for anaerobic metabolism of the immature myocardium leads to a rapid accumulation of the products of anaerobic metabolism such as lactate. Therefore, in contrast to hypoxia or short periods of ischemia, prolonged ischemia results in severe acidosis and tissue damage and in the rapid inhibition of further production of high-energy phosphates in the neonatal myocardium. Cyanosis further increases the vulnerability of the neonatal heart to ischemia.[130]

Tension Development. In comparison to the adult heart, the neonatal heart contains a reduced number of poorly organized contractile units.[131] In the immature myocardium, a larger proportion of the myocyte is devoted to the protein synthetic processes needed for cell growth. In addition to the factors already addressed, this accounts for the reduced tension development capabilities of the neonatal heart. This reduced tension development capability makes the neonate very susceptible to any depression of systolic function after cardiac surgery.

Work done both in animals and in humans suggests that improved myocardial preservation can be obtained in neonates, infants, and children by tailoring myocardial preservation efforts to the specific needs of the immature myocardium:

- Delivery of cardioplegia to neonates, infants, and small children requires some modifications. 30 to 30 mL/kg of cardioplegia may be necessary to induce arrest. The pressure of antegrade delivery must be modified such that, in the neonate, infusion pressure is no more than 40 to 50 mm Hg to avoid myocardial edema. Retrograde cardioplegia delivery currently is being investigated for pediatric cases and specially designed catheters are now available.[132]

- Topical cooling is much more effective in the neonate than in the adult due to the smaller cardiac mass and greater surface area: wall thickness ratio in neonates.[133-135]

- A commonly used adult crystalloid cardioplegia solution has been shown to result in inadequate preservation of postischemic hemodynamic function in immature hearts.[136-138] Improved postischemic functional recovery has been demonstrated with use of hypothermic blood potassium cardioplegia with a normal serum calcium concentration.[134]

- Infants younger than 3 months of age and infants with preoperative heart failure have an increased susceptibility to ultrastructural myocardial injury despite the use of cold crystalloid cardioplegia and topical hypothermia.[139]

- Children undergoing repair of tetralogy of Fallot are at particular risk for inadequate myocardial preservation. Poor functional recovery of ventricular function and depletion of ATP stores have been demonstrated in patients undergoing repair using moderate systemic hypothermia combined with cardioplegia arrest.[140,141] This may be due to a defect in oxidative metabolism in the chronically hypertrophied right ventricle of these cyanotic children[138] or to the difficulty in obtaining adequate myocardial protection in the presence of the voluminous bronchial and noncoronary collateral blood flow seen in these patients.[137] Recall that noncoronary collateral flow will wash out cardioplegia and that bronchial return will result in warming of the heart. This collateral blood flow can be eliminated through the use of circulatory arrest. In fact, improved recovery of right ventricular function, reduced need for post-CPB inotropic support, and less evidence of myocardial necrosis, as indicated by CPK-MB levels, have been demonstrated in patients undergoing tetralogy of Fallot repair with systemic deep hypothermic arrest in addition to cardioplegic protection.[140]

■ REFERENCES

1. Najafi H, Henson DE, Dye WS: Left ventricular hemorrhagic necrosis. *Ann Thorac Surg* 1969; **7**:550-561.

2. Taber RE, Morales AR, Fine G: Myocardial necrosis and the postoperative low-cardiac-output syndrome. *Ann Thorac Surg* 1967; **4**:12-28.

3. Kirklin JW, Conti VR, Blackstone EH: Prevention of myocardial damage during cardiac operations. *N Engl J Med* 1979; **301**:135-141.

4. Kubler W, Spieckermann PG: Regulation of glycolysis in the ischemic and the anoxic myocardium. *J Mol Cell Cardiol* 1970; **1**:350-377.

5. Levitsky S, Feinberg H: Protection of the myocardium with high energy solutions. *Ann Thorac Surg* 1975; **20**:86-90.

6. Foker JE, Einzig S, Wang T, Anderson RW: Adenosine metabolism and myocardial preservation. Consequences of adenosine catabolism on myocardial high-energy compounds and tissue blood flow. *J Thorac Cardiovasc Surg* 1980; **80**:506-516.

7. Mochizuki S, Neely JR: Control of glyceralderhyde-3-phosphate dehydrogenase in cardiac muscle. *J Mol Cell Cardiol* 1979; **11**:221-236.

8. Opie LH: Effects of regional ischemia on metabolism of glucose and fatty acids: Relative rates of aerobic and anaerobic energy production during myocardial infarction and comparison with effects of anoxia. *Circ Res* 1976; **38**:52-74.

9. Jennings RB, Reimer KA, Hill ML, Mayer SE: Total ischemia in dog hearts, in vitro. I. Comparison of high energy phosphate production, utilization, and depletion, and of adenine nucleotide catabolism in total ischemia in vitro vs severe ischemia in vivo. *Circ Res* 1981; **49**:892.

10. Reimer KA, Hill MA, Jennings RB: Prolonged depletion of ATP and the adenine nucleotide pool due to delayed resynthesis of adenine nucleotides following reversible myocardial ischemic injury in dogs. *J Mol Cell Cardiol* 1981; **13**:229-239.

11. Braunwald EB: Mechanism of action of calcium-channel-blocking agents. *N Engl J Med* 1982; **307**:1618-1627.

12. Nayler WG, Elz JS: Reperfusion injury: Laboratory artifact or clinical dilemma? *Circulation* 1986; **74**:215-221.

13. McCord JM: Oxygen-derived free radicals in postischemic tissue injury. *N Engl J Med* 1985; **312**:159-163.

14. Melrose DG, Dreyer B, Bentall HH, Baker JBE: Elective cardiac arrest. *Lancet* 1955; **2**:21-22.

15. Buckberg GD: Strategies and logic of cardioplegic delivery to prevent, avoid, and reverse ischemic and reperfusion damage. *J Thorac Cardiovasc Surg* 1987; **93**:127-139.

16. Tabayashi K, McKeown PP, Miyamoto M, et al: Ischemic myocardial protection. Comparison of nonoxygenated crystalloid, oxygenated crystalloid, and oxygenated flurocarbon cardioplegia solutions. *J Thorac Cardiovasc Surg* 1988; **95**:239-246.

17. McGoon DC: The ongoing quest for ideal myocardial protection. A catalog of the recent English literature. *J Thorac Cardiovasc Surg* 1985; **89**:639-653.

18. McGoon DC: The quest for ideal myocardial protection. *J Thorac Cardiovasc Surg* 1980; **79**:150.

19. Buckberg GD: A proposed "solution" to the cardioplegic controversy. *J Thorac Cardiovasc Surg* 1979; **77**:803-815.

20. Rich TL, Brady AJ: Potassium contracture and utilization of high energy phosphates in rabbit heart. *Am J Physiol* 1974; **226**:105-113.

21. Kay HR, Levine FH, Fallon JT, et al: Effect of cross-clamp time, temperature, and cardioplegic agents on myocardial function after induced arrest. *J Thorac Cardiovasc Surg* 1978; **76**:590-603.

22. Engelman RM, Rousou JH, Longo F, et al: The time course of myocardial high-energy phosphate degradation during potassium cardioplegic arrest. *Surgery* 1979; **86**:138-147.

23. Hess ML, Krause SM, Greenfield LJ: Assessment of hypothermic, cardioplegic protection of the global ischemic canine myocardium. *J Thorac Cardiovasc Surg* 1980; **80**:293-301.

24. Daggett WM, Jacobs MA, Coleman WS, et al: Myocardial temperature mapping: Improved intraoperative myocardial preservation. *J Thorac Cardiovasc Surg* 1981; **82**:883-888.

25. Jynge P: Protection of the ischemic myocardium: Calcium-free cardioplegia infusates and the additive effects of coronary infusion and ischemia in the induction of the calcium paradox. *J Thorac Cardiovasc Surg* 1980; **28**:303.

26. Zimmerman ANE, Hulsmann HC: Paradoxical influence of calcium ions on the permeability of the cell membranes of the isolated rat heart. *Nature* 1966; **211**:646-647.

27. Hendren WG, Geffin GA, Love TR, et al: Oxygenation of cardioplegia solutions. Potential for the calcium paradox. *J Thorac Cardiovasc Surg* 1987; **94**:614-625.

28. Bielecki K: The influence of changes in pH of the perfusion fluid on the occurrence of the calcium paradox in the isolated rat heart. *Cardiovasc Res* 1969; **3**:268.

29. Rich TL, Langer GA: Calcium depletion in rabbit myocardium: Calcium paradox protection by hypothermia and cation substitution. *Circ Res* 1982; **51**:131-141.

30. Heitmiller RF, DeBoer LWV, Geffin GA, et al: Myocardial recovery after hypothermic arrest: A comparison of oxygenated crystalloid to blood cardioplegia. The role of calcium. *Circulation* 1985; **72**(suppl 2):241-253.

31. Renlund DG, Lakaytta EG, Mellits ED, Gerstenbleth G: Calcium dependent enhancement of myocardial diastolic tone and energy utilization dissociates systolic work and oxygen consumption during low sodium perfusion. *Circ Res* 1985; **57**:876-888.

32. Del Nido PJ, Wilson GJ, Mickle DAG: The role of cardioplegic solution buffering in myocardial protection: A biochemical and histopathologic assessment. *J Thorac Cardiovasc Surg* 1985; **89**:689-699.

33. Tait GA, Booker PD, Wilson GJ, et al: Effect of multidose cardioplegia and cardioplegic solution buffering on myocardial tissue acidosis. *J Thorac Cardiovasc Surg* 1982; **83**:824-829.

34. Warner KG, Josa M, Bulter MD, et al: Regional changes in myocardial acid production during ischemic arrest: A comparison of sanguineous and asanguineous cardioplegia. *Ann Thorac Surg* 1988; **45**:75-81.

35. Wildenthal K, Mierzwiak DS, Mitchell JH: Acute effects of increased serum osmolality on left ventricular performance. *Am J Physiol* 1969; **219**:898.

36. Lado MG, Sheu SS, Fozzard HA: Effects of tonicity on tension and intracellular sodium and calcium activities in sheep. *Circ Res* 1984; **54**:576-585.

37. Follette DM, Fey K, Mulder DM, et al: Prolonged safe aortic cross-clamping by combining membrane stabilization, multidose cardioplegia, and physiologic reperfusion. *J Thorac Cardiovasc Surg* 1977; **74**:682-694.

38. Hewitt RL, Lolley DM, Adrouny GA: Protective effect of glycogen and glucose on the anoxic arrested heart. *Surgery* 1974; **75**:1.

39. Hearse DJ, Stewart DA, Braimbridge MV: Myocardial protection during ischemic cardiac arrest. Possible deleterious effects of glucose and mannitol in coronary infusates. *J Thorac Cardiovasc Surg* 1978; **76**:16-27.

40. Haider W, Eckersberger F, Wolner E: Preventive insulin administration for myocardial protection in cardiac surgery. *Anesthesiology* 1984; **60**:422-429.

41. Lazar HL, Roberts AJ: Recent advances in cardiopulmonary bypass and the clinical application of myocardial protection. *Surg Clin North Am* 1985; **65:**455-476.

42. Digerness SB, Vanin V, Wideman FE: In vitro comparison of oxygen availability from asanguineous and sanguineous cardioplegic solutions. *Circulation* 1981; **64:**80-83.

43. Boggs BR, Torchiana DF, Geffin GA: Optimal myocardial preservation with an acalcemic crystalloid cardioplegia solution. *J Thorac Cardiovasc Surg* 1987; **93:**838-846.

44. Guyton RA, Dorsey LMA, Craver JM, et al: Improved myocardial recovery after cardioplegic arrest with an oxygenated crystalloid solution. *J Thorac Cardiovasc Surg* 1985; **89:**877-887.

45. Daggett WM, Randolph JD, Jacobs M, et al: The superiority of cold oxygenated dilute blood cardioplegia. *Ann Thorac Surg* 1987; **43:**397-402.

46. Suaudeau J, Shaffer B, Daggett WM: Role of procaine and washed cells in the isolated dog heart perfused at 5°C. *J Thorac Cardiovasc Surg* 1982; **84:**886-896.

47. Robertson JM, Buckberg GD, Vinten-Johansen J, Leaf JD: Comparison of distribution beyond coronary stenoses of blood and asanguineous cardioplegia solution. *J Thorac Cardiovasc Surg* 1983; **86:**80-86.

48. Foglia RP, Steed DL, Follette DM, et al: Iatrogenic myocardial edema with potassium cardioplegia. *J Thorac Cardiovasc Surg* 1979; **78:**217-222.

49. Casak AS, Bulkley GB, Bulkley BH: Oxygen-free-radical scavengers protect the arrested globally ischemic heart upon reperfusion. *Surg Forum* 1980; **31:**313-316.

50. Tabayashi K, McKeown PP, Miyamoto M, et al: Ischemic myocardial protection. Comparison of nonoxygenated crystalloid, oxygenated crystalloid, and oxygenated fluorocarbon cardioplegia solutions. *J Thorac Cardiovasc Surg* 1988; **95:**239-246.

51. Shapira N, Kirsh M, Jochim K, Behrendt DM: Comparison of the effect of blood cardioplegia to crystalloid on myocardial contractility in man. *J Thorac Cardiovasc Surg* 1980; **80:**647-655.

52. Engleman RM, Rousou JH, Lemeshow S, Dobbs WA: The metabolic consequences of blood and crystalloid cardioplegia. *Circulation* 1981; **64**(suppl 2):67-74.

53. Roberts AJ, Moran JM, Sanders JH, et al: Clinical evaluation of the relative effectiveness of multidose crystalloid and cold blood cardioplegia in coronary artery bypass graft surgery: A nonrandomized matched-pair analysis. *Ann Thorac Surg* 1982; **33:**421- 433.

54. Singh AK, Farrugia R, Teplitz C, Karlson KE: Electrolyte versus blood cardioplegia: Randomized clinical and myocardial ultrastructural study. *Ann Thorac Surg* 1982; **33:**218-227.

55. Fremes SE, Christakis GT, Weisel RD, et al: A clinical trial of blood and crystalloid cardioplegia. *J Thorac Cardiovasc Surg* 1984; **88:**726-741.

56. Mullen JC, Christakis GT, Weisel RD, et al: Late postoperative ventricular function after blood and crystalloid cardioplegia. *Circulation* 1986; **74**(suppl 3):89-98.

57. Codd JE, Barner HB, Pennington DG, et al: Intraoperative myocardial protection: A comparison of blood and asanguineous cardioplegia. *Ann Thorac Surg* 1985; **39:**125-133.

58. Catinella FP, Cunningham JN Jr, Spencer FL: Myocardial protection during prolonged aortic cross-clamping. Comparison of blood and crystalloid cardioplegia. *J Thorac Cardiovasc Surg* 1984; **88:**411-423.

59. Daggett WM, Randolph JD, Jacobs M, et al: The superiority of cold oxygenated dilute blood cardioplegia. *Ann Thorac Surg* 1987; **43:**397-402.

60. Loop FD, Higins TL, Panda R, et al: Myocardial protection during cardiac operations. Decreased morbidity and lower cost with blood cardioplegia and coronary sinus perfusion. *J Thorac Cardiovasc Surg* 1992; **104:**608-618.

61. Boe SL, Dixon CM, Tamara A, et al: The control of myocardial CA^{++} sequestration with nifedipine cardioplegia. *J Thorac Cardiovasc Surg* 1982; **84:**678-684.

62. Magovern GJ, Dixon CM, Burkholder JA: Improved myocardial protection with nifedipine and potassium based cardioplegia. *J Thorac Cardiovasc Surg* 1981; **82:**239-244.

63. Pinsky WW, Lewis RW, McMillin-Wood JB, et al: Myocardial protection from ischemic arrest. Potassium and verapamil cardioplegia. *Am J Physiol* 1981; **9:**H326-335.

64. Standeven JW, Jellinek M, Menz IJ, et al: Cold blood diltiazem cardioplegia. *J Thorac Cardiovasc Surg* 1984; **87:**201-212.

65. Clark RE, Christlieb IY, Ferguson TB, et al: The first American clinical trial of nifedipine in cardioplegia. A report of the first 12 month experience. *J Thorac Cardiovasc Surg* 1981; **82:**848-859.

66. Clark RE, Magovern GJ, Christlieb IY, Boe S: Nifedipine cardioplegia experience: Results of a 3-year cooperative clinical study. *Ann Thorac Surg* 1983; **36:**654-666.

67. Flameng W, De Meyere R, Daenen W, et al: Nifedipine as an adjunct to St. Thomas' Hospital cardioplegia. A double-blind, placebo-controlled, randomized clinical trial. *J Thorac Cardiovasc Surg* 1986; **91:**723-731.

68. Guffin A, Kates RA, Holbrook GW, et al: Verapamil and myocardial preservation in patients undergoing coronary artery bypass surgery. *Ann Thorac Surg* 1986; **41:**589-591.

69. Clark RE: Verapamil, cardioplegia, and coronary artery bypass grafting. *Ann Thorac Surg* 1986; **41:**585-586.

70. Christakis GT, Fremes SE, Weisel RD, et al: Diltiazem cardioplegia. A balance of risk and benefit. *J Thorac Cardiovasc Surg* 1986; **91:**647-661.

71. Barner HB, Swartz MT, Devine JE, et al: Diltiazem as an adjunct to cold blood potassium cardioplegia: A clinical assessment of dose and prospective randomization. *Ann Thorac Surg* 1987; **43:** 191-197.

72. Vinten-Johansen J, Chiantella V, Faust KB, et al: Myocardial protection with blood cardioplegia in ischemically injured hearts: Reduction of reoxygenation injury with allopurinol. *Ann Thorac Surg* 1988; **45:**319-326.

73. Myers CL, Weiss SJ, Kirsh MM, et al: Effects of supplementing hypothermic crystalloid cardioplegic solution with catalase, super oxide dimutase, allopurinol, or deferoxamine on functional recovery of globally ischemic and reperfused isolated hearts. *J Thorac Cardiovasc Surg* 1986; **91:**281-289.

74. Stewart JH, Blackwell WH, Crute SL, et al: Inhibition of surgically induced ischemia/reperfusion injury by oxygen-free radical scavengers. *J Thorac Cardiovasc Surg* 1983; **86:**262-272.

75. Otani H, Engelman RM, Rousou JA, et al: Cardiac performance during reperfusion improved by pretreatment with oxygen free-radical scavengers. *J Thorac Cardiovasc Surg* 1986; **91:**290-295.

76. Menasche P, Grousset C, Gauduel Y, et al: Enhancement of cardioplegic protection with the free radical scavenger peroxidase. *Circulation* 1986; **74**(suppl 3):138-144.

77. Menasche P, Grousset C, Gauduel Y, et al: Prevention of hydroxyl radical formation: A critical concept for improving cardioplegia. Protective effect of deferoxamine. *Circulation* 1987; **76**(suppl 5):180-185.

78. Hudspeth DA, Nakanishi K, Vinten-Johansen J, et al: Adenosine in blood cardioplegia prevents postischemic dysfunction in ischemically injured heart. *Ann Thorac Surg* 1994; **58:**1637-1644.

79. The Multicenter Study of Perioperative Ischemia (McSPI) Research Group: Effects of Acadesine on the incidence of myocardial infarction and adverse cardiac outcomes after coronary artery bypass graft surgery. *Anesthesiology* 1995; **83:**658-673.

80. Rosenkranz ER: Substrate enhancement of cardioplegic solution: Experimental studies and clinical evaluation. *Ann Thorac Surg* 1995; **60:**797-800.

81. Pearl JM, Laks H, Drinkwater DC, et al: Loss of endothelium-dependent vasodilation and nitric oxide release after myocardial protection with University of Wisconsin solution. *J Thorac Cardiovasc Surg* 1994; **107:**257-264.

82. Rosenkranz ER, Buckberg GD: Myocardial protection during surgical coronary reperfusion. *J Am Coll Cardiol* 1983; **1:**1235-1246.

83. Teoh KH, Christakis GT, Fermes SE, et al: Accelerated myocardial metabolic recovery with terminal warm blood cardioplegia (hot shot). *Surg Forum* 1985; **36:**272-275.

84. Roberts AJ, Woodhall DD, Knauf DG, Alexander JA: Coronary artery bypass graft surgery: Clinical comparison of cold blood cardioplegia, warm cardioplegic induction, and secondary cardioplegia. *Ann Thorac Surg* 1985; **40:**483-487.

85. Menasche P, Dunica S, Kural S, et al: An asanguine reperfusion solution: An effective adjunct to cardioplegic protection in high-risk valve operations. *J Thorac Cardiovasc Surg* 1984; **88:**278-286.

86. Menasche P, Grousset C, de Boccard G, Piwnica A: Protective effect of an asanguineous reperfusion solution on myocardial performance following cardioplegic arrest. *Ann Thorac Surg* 1984; **37:**222-228.

87. Buckberg GD: Update on current techniques of myocardial protection. *Ann Thorac Surg* 1995; **60:**805-814.

88. Cleveland JC, Meldrum DR, Rowland RT, et al: Optimal myocardial preservation: Cooling, cardioplegia, and conditioning. *Ann Thorac Surg* 1996; **61:**760-768.

89. Allen BS, Buckberg GD, Schwaiger M, et al: Studies of controlled reperfusion after ischemic. XVI. Early recovery of regional wall motion in patients following surgical revascularization after 8 hours of coronary occlusion. *J Thorac Cardiovasc Surg* 1986; **92:**632-640.

90. Hanafy HM, Allen BS, Winkelman JW, et al: Warm blood cardioplegia induction: an underused modality. *Ann Thorac Surg* 1994; **58:**1589-1594.

91. Lazar HL, Buckberg GD, Manganaro A, et al: Limitations imposed by hypothermia during recovery from ischemia. *Surg Forum* 1980; **31:**312-315.

92. Metzdorff MT, Grunkemeier GL, Starr A: Effect of initial reperfusion temperature on myocardial preservation. *J Thorac Cardiovasc Surg* 1986; **91:**545-550.

93. Svedjeholm R, Ekroth R, Joachimsson PO, et al: Myocardial uptake of amino acids and other substrates in relation to myocardial oxygen consumption four hours after cardiac operations. *J Thorac Cardiovasc Surg* 1990; **101:**688-694.

94. Rosenkranz ER, Okamoto F, Buckberg GD, et al: Safety of prolonged aortic clamping with blood cardioplegia. II. Glutamate enrichment in energy depleted hearts. *J Thorac Cardiovasc Surg* 1984; **88:**402-410.

95. Rosenkranz ER, Okamoto F, Buckberg GD, et al: Safety of prolonged aortic clamping with blood cardioplegia. III. Aspartate enrichment of glumamate-blood cardioplegia in energy-depleted hearts after ischemic and repersion injury. *J Thorac Cardiovasc Surg* 1986; **91:**428-435.

96. Rosenkranz ER, Buckberg GD, Laks H, et al: Warm induction of cardioplegia with glutamate-enriched blood in coronary patients with cardiogenic shock who are dependent on inotropic drugs and intra-aortic balloon support. Initial experience and operative strategy. *J Thorac Cardiovasc Surg* 1983; **86:**507-518.

97. Allen BS, Okamoto F, Buckberg GD, et al: Studies of controlled reperfusion after ischemia. IX. Reperfusion composition: Benefits of marked hypocalcemia and diltiazem on regional recovery. *J Thorac Cardiovasc Surg* 1986; **92:**564-572.

98. Chambers DJ, Braimbridge MV, Hearse DJ: Prevention of production, or scavenging of free radicals enhances myocardial protection with cardioplegic arrest. *Circulation* 1985; **72**(suppl 3):376.

99. Ouriel K, Gensberg ME, Patti CS: Preservation of myocardial function with mannitol reperfusate. *Circulation* 1985; **72**(suppl 2):254-258.

100. Robinson LA, Braimbridge MV, Hearse DJ: The potential hazard of particulate contamination of cardioplegia solutions. *J Thorac Cardiovasc Surg* 1984; **87:**48-58.

101. Johnson RE, Dorsey LM, Moye SE: Cardioplegia infusion: The safe limits of pressure and temperature. *J Thorac Cardiovasc Surg* 1982; **83:**813-823.

102. Matasuda H, Maeda S, Hirose H: Optimum dose of cold potassium cardioplegia for patients with chronic aortic valve disease: Determination by left ventricular mass. *Ann Thorac Surg* 1986; **41:**22-26.

103. Ellis RJ, Mangano DT, Van Dyke DC, Ebert PA: Protection of myocardial function not enhanced by high concentrations of potassium during cardioplegic arrest. *J Thorac Cardiovasc Surg* 1979; **78:**698-707.

104. Dewar M, Rosengarten MD, Samson R, Chiu RCJ: Is high potassium solution necessary for reinfusions in "multidose" cold cardioplegia? A randomized prospective study using computerized holter system. *Ann Thorac Surg* 1987; **43:**409-415.

105. Ellis RJ, Mavroudis C, Gardner C, et al: Relationship between atrioventricular arrhythmias and the concentration of K$^+$ ion in cardioplegic solution. *J Thorac Cardiovasc Surg* 1980; **80:**517-526.

106. Johnson RE, Dorsey LM, Moye SJ, et al: Cardioplegic infusion. The safe limits of pressure and temperature. *J Thorac Cardiovasc Surg* 1982; **83:**813-823.

107. Menasche P, Kural S, Fauchet M, et al: Retrograde coronary sinus perfusion: a safe alternative for ensuring cardioplegia delivery in aortic valve surgery. *Ann Thorac Surg* 1982; **34:**647.

108. Gundy SR, Kirsh MN: A comparison of retrograde cardioplegia versus antegrade cardioplegia in the presence of coronary artery obstruction. *Ann Thorac Surg* 1984; **38:**124-127.

109. Shapira N, Lemole GM, Spagna PM, et al: Antegrade and retrograde infusion of cardioplegia: Assessment by thermovision. *Ann Thorac Surg* 1987; **43:**92-97.

110. Mori F, Ivey TD, Tabayashi K, et al: Regional myocardial protection by retrograde coronary sinus infusion of cardioplegic solution. *Circulation* 1986; **74**(suppl 3):116-124.

111. Guiraudon GM, Campbell CS, McLellan DG, et al: Retrograde coronary sinus versus aortic root perfusion with cold cardioplegia: Randomized study of levels of cardiac enzymes in 40 patients. *Circulation* 1986; **74**(suppl 3):105-115.

112. Partington MT, Acar C, Buckberg CD, et al: Studies of retrograde cardioplegia. I. Capillary blood flow districution to myocardium supplied by open and occluded arteries. *J Thorac Cardiovasc Surg* 1989; **97:**605-612.

113. Aronson S, Lee BK, Liddicoat JR, et al: Assessment of retrograde cardioplegia distribution using contrast echocardiography. *Ann Thorac Surg* 1992; **52:**810-814.

114. Ikonomidis JS, Yau TM, Weisel RD, et al: Optimal flow rates for retrograde warm cardioplegia. *J Thorac Cardiovasc Surg* 1994; **107:**510-519.

115. Partington MT, Acar C, Buckberg CD, et al: Studies of retrograde cardioplegia. II. Advantages of antegrade/retrograde cardioplegia to optimize distribution in jeopardized myocardium. *J Thorac Cardiovasc Surg* 1989; **97:**613-622.

116. Ihnken K, Morita K, Buckberg GD, et al: The safety of simultaneous arterial and coronary sinus perfusion: experimental background and initial clinical results. *J Thorac Cardiac Surg* 1994; **9:**15-25.

117. Daily PO, Pfeffer TA, Wisniewski JB, et al: Clinical comparisons of methods of myocardial protection. *J Thorac Cardiovasc Surg* 1987; **93:**324-336.

118. Speicher CE, Ferrigan L, Wolfson SK, et al: Cold injury of myocardium and pericardium in cardiac hypothermia. *Surg Gynecol Obstet* 1962; **114:**659-665.

119. Wheeler WE, Rubis LJ, Jones CW, Harrah JD: Etiology and prevention of topical cardiac hypothermia-induced phrenic nerve injury and left lower lobe atelectasis during cardiac surgery. *Chest* 1985; **88:**680-683.

120. Birdi I, Izzat MB, Bryan A, et al: Normothermic techniques during open heart operations. *Ann Thorac Surg* 1996; **61:**1573–1580.

121. Martin TD, Craver JM, Gott JP, et al: Prospective, randomized trial of retrograde warm blood cardioplegia: myocardial benefit and neurologic threat. *Ann Thorac Surg* 1994; **57:**298–304.

122. Mora CT, Henson MB, Weintraub WS, et al: The effect of temperature management during cardiopulmonary bypass on neurologic and neuropsychologic outcomes in patients undergoing coronary revascularization. *J Cardiovasc Thorac Surg* 1996; **112:**514–522.

123. The Warm Heart Investigators: Randomized trial of normothermic versus hypothermic coronary bypass surgery. *Lancet* 1994; **343:**559–563.

124. Bull C, Cooper J, Stark J: Cardioplegic protection of the child's heart. *J Thorac Cardiovasc Surg* 1984; **88:**287–293.

125. Jarmakani JM, Nagatomo T, Nakazawa M, Langer GA: Effect of hypoxia on myocardial high-energy phosphates in the neonatal mammalian heart. *Am J Physiol* 1978; **235:**H475–481.

126. Young HH, Tatsuo S, Kenya N, et al: Effect of hypoxia and reoxygenation on mitochondrial function in the neonatal myocardium. *Am J Physiol* 1983; **245:**H998–1006.

127. Hammon JW: Myocardial protection in the immature heart. *Ann Thorac Surg* 1995; **60:**839–842.

128. Chiu RC-J, Bindon W: Why are newborn hearts vulnerable to global ischemia? The lactate hypothesis. *Circulation* 1987; **76** (suppl 5):146–149.

129. Wittnich C, Peniston C, Ianuzzo D, Abel JG, Salerno TA: Relative vulnerability of neonatal and adult hearts to ischemic injury. *Circulation* 1987; **76**(suppl 5):156–160.

130. Fujiwara T, Kurtis T, Anderson W, et al: Myocardial protection in cyanotic neonatal lambs. *J Thorac Cardiovasc Surg* 1988; **96:**700–710.

131. Friedman WF: Intrinsic physiological properties of the developing heart. *Prog Cardiovasc Dis* 1972; **57:**87–111.

132. Drinkwater DC, Cushen CK, Laks, et al: The use of combined antegrade-retrograde infusions of blood cardioplegic solutions in pediatric patients undergoing heart operations. *J Thorac Cardiovasc Surg* 1992; **104:**1349–1355.

133. Lamberti JJ, Cohn LH, Laks H, et al: Local cardiac hypothermia for myocardial protection during correction of congenital heart disease. *Ann Thorac Surg* 1975; **20:**446–454.

134. Corno AF, Bethencourt DM, Laks H, et al: Myocardial protection in the neonatal heart. A comparison of topical hypothermia and crystalloid and blood cardioplegic solutions. *J Thorac Cardiovasc Surg* 1987; **93:**163–172.

135. Ganzel BL, Katzmark SL, Mavroudis C: Myocardial preservation in the neonate. Beneficial effects of cardioplegia and systemic hypothermia on piglets undergoing cardiopulmonary bypass and myocardial ischemia. *J Thorac Cardiovasc Surg* 1988; **96:**414–422.

136. Watanabe H, Yokosawa T, Eguchi S, Imai S: Functional and metabolic protection of the neonatal myocardium from ischemia. Insufficient protection by cardioplegia. *J Thorac Cardiovasc Surg* 1989; **97:**50–58.

137. Magovern JA, Pae WE, Miller CA, Waldhausen JA: The immature and mature myocardium. Responses to multidose crystalloid cardioplegia. *J Thorac Cardiovasc Surg* 1988; **95:**618–624.

138. Baker JE, Boerboom LE, Olinger GN: Age-related changes in the ability of hypothermia and cardioplegia to protect ischemic rabbit myocardium. *J Thorac Cardiovasc Surg* 1988; **96:**717–724.

139. Sawa Y, Matsuda H, Shimazaki Y, et al: Ultrastructural assessment of the infant myocardium receiving crystalloid cardioplegia. *Circulation* 1987; **76**(suppl 5):141–145.

140. Yamaguchi M, Imai M, Ohashi H, et al: Enhanced myocardial protection by systemic deep hypothermia in children undergoing total correction of tetralogy of Fallot. *Ann Thorac Surg* 1986; **41:**639–646.

141. Del Nido PJ, Mickle DAG, Wilson GJ, et al: Inadequate myocardial protection with cold cardioplegic arrest during repair of tetralogy of Fallot. *J Thorac Cardiovasc Surg* 1988; **95:**223–229.

13

Cardiac Surgery and the Central Nervous System

Bradley J. Hindman

■ INCIDENCE AND OUTCOME

Neurologic injuries occurring in association with cardiac surgery can diminish the quality of life after otherwise successful operations. In addition, neurologic injuries constitute a major cause of perioperative mortality.[1] Despite a vast amount of literature, most reports concerning the incidence and outcome of these complications are not reliable, primarily because of retrospective design. In 1983, Sotaniemi prospectively examined 100 patients before and after valve replacement.[2] Postoperatively, 35 of 96 survivors (36%) had some new neurologic abnormality. Seven patients had deficits that the author considered "obvious." Nevertheless, only four of these seven deficits (57%) were noted by other physicians. Postoperative detection of all new neurologic signs with routine ward observation was only 4 of 35 (11%). Failure to employ formal prospective testing continues. For example, in 1994, the Warm Heart Surgery Investigators reported a perioperative stroke rate of 1.6% in 1732 patients randomized to undergo cardiac surgery with either normothermic or hypothermic cardiopulmonary bypass (CPB).[3] Neurologic outcome was assessed using routine clinical observation. However, in a subset of these patients in whom prospective examinations were performed (*n* = 155), the stroke rate was reported to be 3.9%.[4] Also in 1994, Martin et al. reported an overall perioperative stroke rate of 2.0% in a study of 1001 patients randomized to

normothermic or hypothermic CPB.[5] Stroke incidence was assessed by retrospective chart review (routine postoperative observation). In a subset of these patients in whom prospective assessments were made (*n* = 138), Mora et al. reported an overall stroke rate of 5.1%.[6] Therefore, studies that do not employ formal prospective neurologic testing (which constitutes most of the literature) report only 30 to 50% of the overt strokes and much lower percentage of more subtle neurologic abnormalities. Therefore, conclusions drawn from retrospective studies regarding incidence, pathogenesis, and outcome are questionable.

Another difficulty in interpreting incidence and outcome data arises from inconsistencies in methods used to evaluate neurologic status. Some studies employ clinical neurologic examinations, others neuropsychological testing,[4,7-11] and still others biochemical parameters,[12] electroencephalography,[13,14] and, more recently, magnetic resonance imaging (MRI).[15-18] Currently, it is not possible to know how an abnormality detected with one modality relates to another or how a given abnormality affects patients' functional status. Furthermore, only a few reports describe temporal aspects of neurologic injury — specifically, its onset and resolution over time. This limitation is important because studies now indicate 20 to 40% of perioperative neurologic deficits have their onset days after surgery.[19-26] The pathophysiology and management of these "delayed" events may differ considerably from those occurring intraoperatively. Nevertheless, delayed neurologic events have not been specifically studied.

Of available prospective reports, only a handful have complete descriptions of operative, anesthetic and CPB management, or have any substantive follow-up. Therefore, from most reports, it is impossible to discern: (1) when neurologic deficits were first noted; (2) what may have contributed to their occurrence; and (3) to what extent patients recovered or were disabled. Also, as operative, anesthetic, and CPB techniques have changed (as have the demographics of patients undergoing cardiac surgery[27]), reports from the 1960s, 1970s, and possibly even the 1980s may be only marginally relevant to current practice (the 1990s). Finally, to identify neurologic complications that are unique to cardiac surgery patients and to provide insight into their mechanisms, comparisons between cardiac and noncardiac surgery patients are necessary. Therefore, ideally, incidence and outcome studies should include a matched noncardiac surgery control group.

With the above considerations in mind, the following will focus on a series of reports by Shaw et al. concerning the incidence and outcome of neurologic injuries occurring in association with coronary artery bypass grafting (CABG).[19,28-32] Arguably, these reports are probably the best existing literature because of their large study population, prospective design, trained examiners, standard evaluative procedures, detailed reporting, long-term follow-up, and inclusion of a noncardiac surgery control group. Although derived from patients undergoing CABG only, findings are in general agreement with those that include other types of adult cardiac surgery.

Clinical Neurologic Findings

Shaw (a neurologist) and colleagues examined 312 patients before CABG.[19,28-31] Follow-up neurologic examinations were performed 7 days after surgery and 6 months later. Anesthesia was maintained with fentanyl, droperidol, and nitrous oxide, supplemented with a "volatile agent." "Moderate hemodilution" and hypothermia (28°C) were employed during CPB (1.6 to 2.4 L·min^{-1}·m^{-2}), and both membrane and bubble oxygenators without arterial filtration, and both pulsatile and nonpulsatile CPB were used. There is no description of arterial pressure or acid–base management during CPB. Preoperatively, 109 of 312 (35%) patients had neurologic abnormalities, most often peripheral nerve lesions, abnormal tendon reflexes, or primitive reflexes. Although this seems like an extraordinarily high incidence of pre-existing neurologic abnormalities, other prospective studies report comparable incidences (13-73%).[11,21,33,34] The control group consisted of 50 patients undergoing major vascular surgery (abdominal aortic aneurysm repair, aortofemoral bypass). The control group was well matched to the CABG group in terms of age, history of heart disease, hypertension, pre-existing neurologic symptoms, type of anesthesia, operative duration, intensive care unit (ICU) duration, and postoperative inotrope use.[30] New neurologic abnormalities developed in 191 of 308 (62%) patients surviving CABG versus 9 of 49 (18%) patients surviving vascular surgery (see Table 13-1). Most notably, of 308 patients surviving CABG, one suffered a fatal hypotensive global ischemic event (0.3%) and definite stroke occurred in 15 patients (5%). Possible mild strokes occurred in nine additional patients (3%). In stark contrast, new neurologic findings in vascular surgery patients were limited almost exclusively to peripheral neuropathies.

Of CABG patients suffering a definite stroke, 58% still had a deficit 6 months postoperatively, leaving more than half with a "significant functional disability." Possible minor strokes, noted initially in nine patients, uniformly resolved by 6 months. New visual field defects, present in eight patients (3%) at 7 days postoperatively,

TABLE 13–1. NEUROLOGIC STATUS 7 DAYS POSTOPERATIVELY

New Neurologic Findings	CABG (n = 308)	Peripheral Vascular (n = 49)
Fatal cerebral injury	1/308 (0.3%)	0
Depressed consciousness >24 hours	10/308 (3%)	0
Stroke	15/308 (5%)	0
Reversible ischemic deficit	9/308 (3%)	0
Ophthalmological abnormalities[a]	78/308 (25%)	0
Primitive reflexes	123/308 (39%)	2/49 (4%)
Psychosis	4/308 (1%)	0
Peripheral neuropathy	37/308 (12%)	7/49 (14%)

[a] Ophthalmological disorders include: visual field defects, retinal infarction, retinal emboli, reduced acuity.

CABG = coronary artery bypass graft.

*(Data from: Shaw P, Bates D, Cartlidge NEF, et al: Early neurological complications of coronary artery bypass surgery. BMJ 1985; **291**:1384–1376; and Shaw PJ, Bates D, Cartlidge NEF, et al: Neurologic and neuropsychological morbidity following major surgery: Comparison of coronary artery bypass and peripheral vascular surgery. Stroke 1987; **18**:700–707.)*

were still present in 57% at 6 months. New primitive reflexes, considered to indicate diffuse cortical injury, and noted in 123 patients at 7 days postoperatively (39%), persisted in approximately 50% of patients at 6 months. At 6 months, 10 patients (4% of those evaluable) had functionally important deficits, preventing return to work in 4 (2%). Therefore, it is clear that patients with CABG had a much greater incidence, severity, and diversity of neurologic injury when compared with noncardiac surgery patients and, although there was improvement over time, 2 to 4% were permanently and significantly disabled.

Neuropsychologic Alterations

Impairment of cognition, memory, and psychomotor coordination commonly is noted postoperatively;[8,11,35,36] often in patients who would, on cursory examination, seem normal. For example, Slogoff et al. reported that 25% of patients who appeared neurologically normal after cardiac surgery had impaired neuropsychologic performance.[37] Studies indicate that standard neurologic examinations can, at times, be remarkably insensitive to cerebral injuries. For example, Sellman et al., comparing pre- and post-CABG MRI images found new (large) cerebral infarctions in 2 of 29 (7%) patients who were, nonetheless, without any overt sign of neurologic injury.[15] The current consensus is that marked impairment of neuropsychologic performance after cardiac surgery is probably due to subclinical brain injury, probably occurring during surgery and/or CPB. Nevertheless, as will be discussed, the relationship between specific perioperative events and long-term neuropsychologic dysfunction has not yet been established.

One of the major difficulties in neuropsychologic testing is controlling for the numerous determinants of performance. To what degree is a change in performance due to practice, motivation, illness, drugs,[38] mood,[39,40] etc., and how much is due to actual brain dysfunction? More importantly, and even more difficult to determine, is the degree to which, in a given patient, a performance change is "significant." For example, a slight decrease in motor skill might be inconsequential to most patients but might be disabling to a musician. For this reason, studies of neuropsychologic performance are, preferably, based on individual performance, rather than on group performance. In the study by Shaw et al., 10 neuropsychologic tests were administered preoperatively and at follow-up examinations.[29,31] A change in an individual's performance was considered significant if the change exceeded the standard deviation of the group performance. Although arbitrary,[36] this change is probably "significant," in that an individual's performance would have to change his/her percentile rank ~33%. As shown in Table 13–2, at 7 days postoperatively,

patients with CABG had markedly greater incidence and severity of deterioration in neuropsychologic performance relative to their preoperative baseline as compared with vascular surgery patients.

Approximately 79% of patients with CABG had a decrement in at least 1 of 10 tests, and 24% had a decrement in at least three tests. In contrast, 69% of the vascular surgery patients had no significant decrement in any test, and no patient had a decrement in more than two tests. Cognitive abilities that deteriorated most greatly were psychomotor speed, attention and concentration, new learning ability, and auditory short-term memory. Nearly 1 out of every 12 patients with CABG (8%) was so intellectually impaired as to be overtly disabled in routine postoperative hospital activities. Therefore, as was the case with standard neurologic signs, patients with CABG had a far greater incidence and severity of acute neuropsychologic deterioration than did comparable surgical patients.

The results of 6-month follow-up testing in patients with CABG are shown in Table 13–3. One group of patients (20% of the cohort) had no significant decrement in neuropsychologic performance relative to their preoperative baseline at 7 days after surgery. Therefore, there was no evidence of brain injury due to CABG. An-

TABLE 13–2. NEUROPSYCHOLOGIC STATUS COMPARED WITH PREOPERATIVE PERFORMANCE AT 7 DAYS POSTOPERATIVELY

Severity of Deterioration	CABG ($n = 298$)	Control ($n = 48$)
None	21%	69%
Mild (1–2/10 tests)	55%	31%
Moderate (3–4/10 tests)	19%	0%
Severe (≥5/10 tests)	5%	0%
Symptomatic	30%	0%
Disabled	8%	0%

CABG = coronary artery bypass graft.

*(Data from: Shaw PJ, Bates D, Cartlidge NEF, et al: Neurologic and neuropsychological morbidity following major surgery: Comparison of coronary artery bypass and peripheral vascular surgery. Stroke 1987; **18**:700–707.)*

TABLE 13–3. POSTOPERATIVE NEUROPSYCHOLOGIC PERFORMANCE COMPARED WITH PREOPERATIVE BASELINE IN 252 PATIENTS TESTED AT BOTH 7 DAYS AND 6 MONTHS

7 days	6 months	n (%)
Normal	Impaired	19 (8%)
Normal	Normal	31 (12%)
Impaired	Normal	78 (31%)
Impaired	Impaired (different tests)	43 (17%)
Impaired	Impaired (same tests)	81 (32%)

*(Data from: Shaw PJ, Bates D, Cartlidge NEF, et al: Long-term intellectual dysfunction following coronary artery bypass graft surgery: A six month follow-up study. Q J Med 1987; **62**:259–268.)*

other group of patients (31% of the cohort), who had significant decrements in performance 7 days after operation, either returned to or exceeded preoperative performance 6 months postoperatively. Therefore, whatever caused early neuropsychologic impairment had apparently resolved. Another group of patients (17% of the cohort) had impaired performance relative to preoperative baseline at first follow-up, and had impairment 6 months postoperatively, although on different tests (in other words, impaired in tests A, B, C at 7 days, impaired on tests D, E, F at 6 months). Although declining in their neuropsychologic status, it is difficult to confidently conclude that cardiac surgery was directly causative. A fourth group of patients (32% of the cohort) had impaired performance at 7 days compared with their preoperative baseline, and continued impairment in the same tests 6 months later, although usually not to the same degree (impaired in tests A, B, C at 7 days, and still impaired in tests A, B, C at 6 months). Almost certainly, this group, nearly one-third of the evaluable patients, sustained some form of subtle neurologic injury that originated in the perioperative period.

Of all patients having measurable decrements in neuropsychologic performances at 6 months (~50% of the total cohort), most had, in fact, improved over time. Only approximately one-third of these patients (~15% of the cohort) reported any noticeable symptoms — usually problems with memory and concentration. Only three of the evaluable patients (~1%) had seriously disabling cognitive impairment at 6 months (all of whom had had major perioperative strokes). Although the work of Shaw et al. clearly indicated that cardiac surgery patients are uniquely at risk of neuropsychologic deterioration, not all studies confirm this finding. In a report from England, Treasure et al. did *not* detect differences in neuropsychologic status between patients undergoing cardiac and noncardiac surgery.[38] In this study, the incidence of neuropsychologic deterioration in cardiac surgery patients was comparable to that reported by Shaw et al.,[29,31] but in contrast, noncardiac surgery patients had equally severe and sustained neuropsychologic deterioration. A recent prospective study from Canada made similar observations. Murkin et al. compared neurologic and neuropsychologic outcomes among 316 patients undergoing CABG and a group of 40 patients undergoing major vascular or thoracic operations.[11] Study findings are summarized in Table 13–4. Patients undergoing CABG had greater acute and long-term incidences of new neurologic abnormalities detectable by standard neurologic testing. Acutely, CABG patients also had a greater incidence of cognitive abnormalities. However, by 2 months after operation, the incidence of cognitive abnormalities was comparable between groups. What cannot be determined from this study is whether long-term cognitive dysfunction ob-

TABLE 13–4. NEUROLOGIC AND COGNITIVE ABNORMALITIES AFTER CARDIAC AND NONCARDIAC SURGERY

Time After Surgery	New Abnormality	Group	
		CABG	Control
7 Days	Neurologic	30%	17%[a]
	Cognitive	78%	56%[b]
2 Months	Neurologic	17%	3%[c]
	Cognitive	33%	42%

[a] $P = 0.085$.
[b] $P = 0.003$.
[c] $P = 0.050$.

(Data from: Murkin JM, Martzke JS, Buchan AM, Bentley C, Wong CJ: A randomized study of the influence of perfusion technique and pH management strategy in 316 patients undergoing coronary artery bypass surgery II. Neurologic and cognitive outcomes. J Thorac Cardiovasc Surg 1995; **110**:349–362.)

served in both surgical groups was due to the same or different causes. Is it possible that surgery and anesthesia per se (not strictly cardiac surgery and CPB) may lead to long-term cognitive dysfunction in a certain fraction of patients? Indeed, it has been suggested that certain patients may be predisposed to perioperative neurologic/cognitive deterioration by possessing genes associated with Alzheimer's disease.[11,41] Therefore, neuropsychologic impairment after cardiac surgery certainly is *not* exclusively due to brain injury specific to cardiac surgery and CPB.[35] Nevertheless, because numerous studies find associations between early neuropsychologic impairment and perioperative factors, there probably is some component of these injuries that is related to acute perioperative brain injury. For example, investigations have found that CPB duration,[11,21,38,42,43] multiple valve replacement,[42,44] age,[9,11,21,38] and hypotension during CPB[38] are associated with early neuropsychologic impairment. In Shaw's study, moderate and severe deterioration in neuropsychologic performance at 7 days (*see* Table 13–3) was correlated with: (1) a preoperative history of stroke/transient ischemic attack (TIA); (2) postoperative hypotension; (3) a large decrease in hemoglobin; (4) the presence of peripheral vascular disease; and (5) ICU duration.[32] In contrast, three recent studies have been unable to identify any perioperative factor as being associated with longer-term (2 to 6 months) neuropsychologic outcome.[11,32,38] If long-term neuropsychologic changes due to organic brain injury were occurring during surgery and CPB, one would expect some association with some perioperative factor. Shaw et al. found only a preoperative history of congestive heart failure and poor ejection fraction to be associated with long-term impairment in neuropsychologic function.[32] Murkin et al. found cognitive impairment at 2 months to be related only to age.[11] No other perioperative factor, including CPB duration, glucose, acid–base management, arterial pressure, pulsation etc., had an independent effect. Therefore, although clinical intuition suggests that sustained deterioration of neuropsychologic performance after cardiac surgery is the result of some subtle form of perioperative brain injury, a firm association between perioperative events specific to cardiac surgery and its occurrence are lacking.

Summary

Prospective reports from the 1990s indicate that 2.5% to 5% of adult cardiac surgery patients sustain unequivocal focal neurologic injury (stroke) in the perioperative period.[1,4,6,11,35,45,46] Tuman et al. reported that patients with CABG having neurologic complications had three times longer ICU stays (9 ± 11 days versus 3 ± 3 days) and nine times greater perioperative mortality (36% versus 4%) than patients free of neurologic injury.[1] Similarly, patients having neurologic complications after CABG have significantly longer hospital stay than those who do not (21 ± 18 versus 9 ± 10 days, respectively).[47] Although patients with focal deficits often (~ 75%) make a good functional recovery,[1,28,33,34] 20 to 30% of those having a stroke have permanent neurologic disability.[28,33,34] Patients who fail to regain consciousness after surgery have a very poor prognosis.[1,19,33]

In the first postoperative week, subtle neurologic abnormalities and/or neuropsychologic deterioration are noted in 30 to 60% of adult cardiac surgery patients.[4,6,8,11,19,21,29,35,36,48] Although improving over time, approximately 30 to 50% of patients have measurable decrements in neuropsychologic performance 2 to 6 months postoperatively,[11,31,35,39,48] although only approximately 10 to 15% report any change in mental abilities. Therefore, there is significant neurologic morbidity associated with cardiac surgery, with increased perioperative mortality, length of ICU and hospital stay and, in a substantive fraction of patients, long-term neurologic and cognitive impairment.

■ RISK FACTORS AND MECHANISMS OF INJURY

Ascending Aortic Atherosclerosis

To explore possible mechanisms of injury, Shaw et al. used multivariate analysis, correlating clinical variables with the occurrence of new neurologic signs.[32] The results are shown in Table 13–5. Signs of systemic arteriosclerosis stood out as the single most consistent risk factors for the development of neurologic abnormalities in association with cardiac surgery.

Transcranial Doppler (TCD) studies demonstrate that cerebral embolization commonly occurs during car-

TABLE 13–5. RISK FACTORS FOR DEVELOPMENT OF NEW POSTOPERATIVE NEUROLOGIC SIGNS

Finding	Risk Factors
Depressed consciousness >24 hours	Subclavian bruit, prior TIA, difficulty terminating CPB, large decrease in hemoglobin
Definite stroke	Peripheral vascular disease, preoperative CHF
Retinal emboli	Pressure difference between arms, prior stroke
New palmomental reflex	Large decrease in hemoglobin
New snout reflex	Subclavian bruits, mean arterial pressure <40 mm Hg
Severe neuropsychologic change	Peripheral vascular disease, large decrease in hemoglobin

CHF = congestive heart failure; CPB = cardiopulmonary bypass; TIA = transient ischemic attack.

(Data from: Shaw PJ, Bates D, Cartlidge NEF, et al: An analysis of factors predisposing to neurological injury in patients undergoing coronary bypass operations. Q J Med 1989; 72:633–646.)

diac surgery but most especially with aortic manipulation.[45,49-54] Whenever the aorta is cannulated and clamped, atheromatous material can be dislodged and embolized to the brain. Recently, work of Barbut et al.[53,54] and Clark et al.[52] indicate that most cerebral emboli occurring during cardiac surgery result from aortic manipulation. In these latter studies, postoperative neurologic impairment correlated with the number of cerebral emboli. Atheromas also can be "sand-blasted" off the aortic lumen by the high shear forces of perfusate exiting the aortic perfusion cannula.[55] It is, therefore, not surprising that moderate to severe atherosclerosis of the ascending aorta (present in 10 to 30% of adult cardiac surgery patients)[55-62] has emerged as the principal risk factor for the development of focal neurologic injury (stroke) in adult cardiac surgery patients (*see* Fig. 13–1).[23,46,55,63-68]

In an autopsy series of 221 adults who have died in the hospital after cardiac surgery, Blauth et al. found atheroemboli in 37% of patients who had severe atherosclerosis of the ascending aorta versus 2% in patients free of significant ascending aortic disease ($P < 0.001$).[69] Brain was the organ most frequently embolized. Multivariate risk factors for ascending aortic atherosclerosis were: (1) concomitant peripheral vascular disease; (2) increasing age; and (3) hypertension. These risk factors are strikingly similar to risk factors identified by Shaw et al. (subclavian bruits, peripheral vascular disease, and blood pressure asymmetries) for the development of stroke, retinal emboli, primitive reflexes, and severe neuropsychologic deficits after CABG.[32] Recently, Mills and Everson observed a 79% incidence of concomitant carotid disease in patients having severe ascending aortic calcification.[64] Likewise, Katz et al. found a strong association between carotid bruits and severe atheromatous disease of the aortic arch.[55] Therefore, the presence

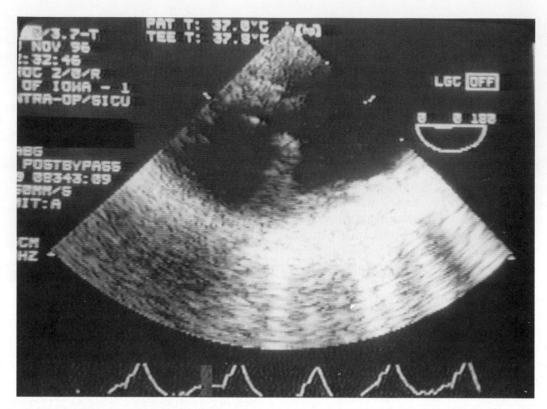

FIGURE 13–1. Transesophageal echocardiographic image of a large mobile atherosclerotic plaque in the transverse aorta. *(Photo courtesy of Intraoperative Echocardiography Service, Department of Anesthesia, University of Iowa College of Medicine.)*

of carotid disease may serve as a marker of aortic disease (more below).

There are only few reports of the consequences of routine cannulation and clamping of aortas recognized as being severely diseased. Stroke incidence in each report was 50%.[55,56,64] An important advance was described by Wareing et al., wherein intraoperative ultrasound (epiaortic scanning) was used to locate ascending aortic abnormalities.[57] Moderate or severe ascending aortic disease was identified in 60 of 500 (14%) adults undergoing cardiac operation. Aortic palpation alone identified only one-third of these patients. When significant disease was identified, the procedure was modified to avoid manipulation, cannulation, or clamping the atherosclerotic segment. Using these techniques, these investigators and other groups[55,59,62] report perioperative neurologic complications that seem to be no more frequent in patients with ascending aortic atherosclerosis than in those free of aortic disease (~1.5%). Other methods now being used to minimize aortic plaque disruption include single-clamp techniques,[70] long aortic cannulas that direct perfusate into the descending aorta,[71] and alternative cannulation sites (descending aorta or axillary artery).[72] With severe atheromatous disease or circumferential calcification, more aggressive techniques such as aortic endarterectomy or aortic replacement are advocated by some.[55,56,58]

Transesophageal echocardiography (TEE) may be a useful tool to localize ascending aortic irregularities. Using this technique, Katz et al. identified severe atheromatous disease in the aortic arch in 18% of patients aged 65 years or older.[55] In agreement with other studies, palpation alone did not identify these high-risk patients. However, Konstadt et al. have shown that TEE is insensitive when compared with epiaortic scanning.[60] Because of the tracheal air shadow, much of the ascending aorta cannot be visualized with TEE, and aortic cannulation sites can only rarely be visualized. In the Konstadt et al. study, aortic disease identified by epiaortic scanning was often missed by TEE. Subsequent work by this group indicates, however, that TEE may serve as an excellent screening tool.[61] Patients who, on TEE examination, had no sign of atheromatous disease in either the arch or ascending or descending aorta, had an extremely low incidence of atheromatous disease in the ascending aorta when sought by epiaortic scanning. In contrast, TEE evidence of atheromatous disease was associated with a high likelihood (34% positive predictive value) of significant disease in the regions assessable by epiaortic scanning.[61]

Cerebrovascular Disease

The role of coexisting cerebrovascular disease (CVD) in the development of perioperative neurologic injury has been a longstanding concern. Carotid artery atherosclerosis is present in 5 to 15% of adult cardiac surgery patients[22,26,58,73-79] and is considered by many to increase the risk of neurologic complications.[22,77,80,81]

Prospective studies of cardiac surgery patients report an incidence of asymptomatic carotid *bruits* of 6 to 16%.[73-75,82,83] When evaluated as a risk factor for the development of perioperative stroke, asymptomatic carotid bruits have consistently failed to be a reliable predictor.[74,75,82,83] The most likely reason for this is that carotid bruits are neither a sensitive nor specific sign of CVD. Studies of Balderman et al.,[73] Barnes et al.,[74] and Ivey et al.[82] each show only 25 to 35% of carotid bruits associated with a significant carotid stenosis. Conversely, when Barnes et al. prospectively identified 40 cardiac surgery patients as having carotid obstruction using Doppler screening (12% of the cohort), only 27% of these patients had an audible bruit.[74] Therefore, the presence or absence of a carotid bruit correlates poorly with the presence or absence of carotid stenosis. Reed et al. reported the presence of carotid bruits increased perioperative stroke risk almost 400%.[20] However, strokes did not correlate with the side of the bruit. In light of the fact that carotid bruits are not reliable indicators of hemodynamically significant carotid stenoses, this finding suggests that carotid bruits may act as a marker for other processes contributing to perioperative stroke (i.e., ascending aortic atherosclerosis, see above).

Controversy surrounds the management of cardiac surgery patients with known carotid stenoses. A principal concern has been that carotid stenoses will limit cerebral blood flow (CBF) during CPB and that stroke will be the result. Therefore, the principal justification for carotid endarterectomy (CEA) in these patients has been the presumption that CEA would protect the brain from hypoperfusion during CPB and thereby reduce stroke incidence. On one hand, some studies indicate that asymptomatic carotid stenoses do not either: (1) limit CBF during CPB[84-86]; or (2) confer increased risk for acute perioperative stroke.[74,76,87-89] On the other hand, there are sufficient reports indicating that carotid stenoses *are* a risk factor for stroke with cardiac surgery[26,78,79] and that the possibility cannot be dismissed. A key question to be asked is the following: in the presence of known carotid stenoses, is the incidence of stroke after cardiac surgery less in those patients who have undergone CEA (either before or during the cardiac surgery) as compared with patients who have not undergone CEA? In other words, is CEA protective?

An interesting study, albeit retrospective and non-randomized, is that of Brener et al.[77] Over a 7-year period, the author's practice changed. Initially, all patients with asymptomatic carotid stenoses had combined CEA/cardiac surgery. Over time, the authors phased out this practice. Eventually, no patient with asymptomatic

TABLE 13–6. POSTOPERATIVE STROKE/TIA IN CARDIAC SURGERY PATIENTS WITH ASYMPTOMATIC CAROTID STENOSIS

Carotid Disease	Perioperative Stroke/TIA
Normal Carotids	74/3894 = 2%
Unilateral stenosis	
Simultaneous CEA:	2/35 = 6%
No CEA:	3/49 = 6%
Bilateral stenosis	
Simultaneous CEA:	0/15 = 0%
No CEA:	0/10 = 0%
Stenosis/occlusion	
Simultaneous CEA:	3/7 = 43%
No CEA:	1/5 = 20%

CEA = carotid endarterectomy; TIA = transient ischemic attack.

(Data from: Brener BJ, Brief DK, Alpert J, Goldenkranz RJ, Parsonnet V: The risk of stroke in patients with asymptomatic carotid stenosis undergoing cardiac surgery: A follow-up study. J Vasc Surg 1987; 5:269–279.)

carotid disease had CEA before or during cardiac surgery. The results of their retrospective review are shown in Table 13–6. Although the presence the carotid disease significantly increased the risk of perioperative stroke/TIA as compared with patients with normal carotids (5-fold), CEA did not seem to reduce the risk of acute perioperative stroke. A similar conclusion can be drawn from the report of Hertzer et al., concerning 274 patients with CABG who had at least one carotid stenosis (≥70% diameter reduction).[80] Acute perioperative stroke after CABG occurred in 9 of 193 (5%) patients undergoing CEA before or simultaneous with CABG (i.e., "protected") versus 6 of 81 patients (7%) undergoing CABG without CEA (i.e., "unprotected"). Therefore, CEA did not convincingly provide neurologic protection in this series. Finally, a meta-analysis of reports through 1992 found the overall incidence of acute perioperative stroke after cardiac surgery in patients with known carotid stenoses to be ~5.6% (range, 0 to 10%) in those who underwent combined carotid and coronary revascularization (i.e., "protected") versus ~5.2% (range, 0 to 17%) in patients undergoing CABG only (i.e., "unprotected").[81] Therefore, there is little evidence, especially in the absence of symptoms, that CEA protects patients from acute perioperative stroke in association with cardiac surgery. The association between carotid disease and ascending aortic atherosclerosis[55,64] may explain why "prophylactic" CEA does not seem to reduce the incidence of acute perioperative stroke in patients with carotid stenoses. Quite simply, stroke after heart surgery in patients with asymptomatic carotid bruits/stenoses is more likely the result of cerebral emboli from an atherosclerotic aorta than from hemispheric hypoperfusion.

However, several studies indicate that in the days,[22] weeks,[90] and months[88] after CABG, patients with significant carotid stenoses are at much greater risk of new neurologic symptoms than patients without cerebrovascular disease (and possibly those who underwent CEA at time of CABG.[88]) This is consistent with the findings of Roederer et al. who found a dramatic increase in neurologic symptoms when previously asymptomatic carotid stenoses (first detected as carotid bruits) exceeded 80% reduction in luminal diameter.[91] Therefore, all patients, including cardiac surgery patients, having significant carotid stenosis must be considered at high risk of neurologic symptoms (TIA/stroke). Two recent studies reported that long-term neurologic outcome was superior in patients with asymptomatic carotid stenosis ≥50 to 60% who underwent "prophylactic" CEA versus medical therapy.[92,93] Therefore, the unanswered question is whether overall long-term neurologic morbidity would be reduced in patients with coexisting (but asymptomatic) carotid disease and symptomatic coronary disease by performance of simultaneous CABG/CEA or whether better outcome will result from staged procedures. Currently, the answer is not known, but there is plenty of (conflicting) opinion.[25,94]

With rare exception,[95,96] studies agree that prior neurologic symptoms (stroke/TIA) markedly increase the risk of neurologic complications with heart surgery.[1,20,23,26,32,63,67,89,97] A recent prospective case control study by Redmond et al. noted that patients with prior stroke who underwent cardiac surgery (7% of the total cohort) had much greater perioperative neurologic morbidity than patients without prior stroke (44% versus 1.4%, respectively).[24] In patients with prior stroke: (1) new strokes occurred in 9% (66% mortality); and (2) old deficits either reappeared or worsened in 36%. The time between prior stroke and cardiac surgery did not seem to matter. Patients with prior stroke took three times as long to emerge from anesthesia, had three times longer ICU and hospital stays, and had 10 times greater 30-day mortality. Clearly, patients with prior or ongoing neurologic symptoms are a high-risk group. Presumably, neurologically symptomatic patients have either more severe cerebral and/or aortic atherosclerosis, and/or brain regions with impaired autoregulation, and/or poor collateral perfusion, rendering them more susceptible to cerebral ischemia. It is also probable that patients with prior stroke have less "functional" reserve, such that comparatively minor disturbances of neurologic function cannot be compensated for and, therefore, are more clinically apparent.

It is now established that CEA improves long-term neurologic outcome in symptomatic patients with carotid stenoses ≥70%.[98,99] Therefore, neurologically symptomatic patients scheduled for nonemergent heart surgery deserve carotid examination and, if significant carotid disease exists, they should be considered candidates for CEA. Decisions regarding simultaneous versus staged procedures should be decided individually, based on the acuity/severity of both the carotid and cardiac disease. There are, as yet, no definitive studies regarding which approach results in the best overall morbidity and mortality.

Other Patient-Related Risk Factors

Advancing age is a consistent risk factor for the development of neurologic and neuropsychologic complications, although exactly why this is remains unknown.[1,8,9,10,11,35,67] Because incidences of aortic and carotid disease increase with age, perhaps older patients receive a greater number of cerebral emboli during surgery. Alternatively, perhaps the older brain has less functional reserve, such that insults are simply more apparent.

Studies indicate that poor preoperative ventricular function also is a risk factor for the development of neurologic and/or neuropsychologic complications.[20,32,31,95,100] Presumably, poor ventricular function is associated with low postoperative systemic pressure and perfusion, factors that are linked with worse neurologic outcome.[1,23,32,34,95,100]

Left ventricular thrombi are recognized as a potential source of cerebral emboli.[23,101] Breuer et al. reported 15 perioperative strokes in 155 cardiac surgery patients in whom left ventricular thrombi were seen on preoperative cardiac catheterization.[102] The perioperative stroke rate in this group (10%) exceeded that of a comparable group of 421 patients (2 to 5%) who had no left ventricular thrombi.[102] Therefore, although only a small percentage of patients presenting for cardiac surgery will have intracardiac thrombi, disruption or mobilization of thrombi during surgery will place these patients at risk of embolic stroke.

The CPB Circuit

Prolonged CPB continues to be associated with poor neurologic and/or neuropsychologic outcome, presumably because of progressive cerebral embolization.[11] CPB may introduce a wide variety of materials into the systemic circulation. Material may include microscopic or macroscopic air, antifoaming agents,[103-106] fat,[107,108] fibers[109] and plastic chips,[110] and aggregates of leukocytes,[111] platelets,[112] and fibrin.[113-116] The suspicion that microemboli created by CPB systems cause perioperative neurologic injury has dominated the literature since the earliest days of its use. Controversies have centered on which CPB and oxygenator systems create the fewest microemboli, the utility of filtration in removing emboli, and whether neurologic outcome is improved when microparticle embolization is decreased.

Studies have repeatedly shown membrane oxygenators produce fewer numbers of microscopic gas emboli than bubble oxygenators.[117-122] Some studies suggest membrane oxygenators produce fewer platelet and fibrin emboli as well.[113,115,123] Microbubbles produced by bubble oxygenators range from 70 to 150 μm in diameter.[111,120,124,125,126] Membrane oxygenators produce emboli that are rarely larger than 50 μm.[113,120] Factors that increase microbubble release from bubble oxygenators include: (1) increasing the gas flow to blood flow ratio[120,124-127]; (2) low blood levels in the oxygenator[124,125,127]; and (3) agitation of the oxygenator.[124,125,127]

Using fluroescein angiography, Blauth et al. observed retinal vascular occlusions in 21 of 21 patients undergoing CPB with a bubble oxygenator.[128] Occlusions occurred in 50 μm vessels (arterioles) and 4 of 21 (19%) had focal fluorescein leakage during CPB, indicating loss of vascular integrity. (Companion studies in dogs showed the occlusions to be due to platelet-fibrin microaggregates 20-70 μm in diameter.) Although there seemed to be partial reperfusion 30 minutes after CPB in ~80% of cases, 2 of 16 (13%) patients had persistently occluded retinal vessels 8 days postoperatively. New cotton wool spots, indicative of focal retinal ischemia, were seen in 2 of 21 (10%) patients. It is reasonable to think that a similar process occurs in the cerebral vasculature, resulting in diffuse multifocal microinfarcts. Based on TCD studies, which can detect particles at least in the 30 to 50 μm range,[49,126] there is no doubt that membrane oxygenation and/or arterial filtration reduce the embolic challenge to the brain during CPB.[49,50,126,129,130] Therefore, it would seem that a decrease in pump-related microemboli might lead to a decrease in neuropsychologic deterioration. This was confirmed in a report in 1994 by Pugsley et al.[129] One hundred patients undergoing CPB (28°C) with a bubble oxygenator were randomized to inline arterial filtration or its absence. Eight weeks after surgery, patients in the filtered group had a lesser incidence of neuropsychologic deterioration than nonfiltered patients (8% versus 27%, respectively, $P < 0.03$). Furthermore, neuropsychologic impairment correlated directly with the number of cerebral emboli occurring during CPB (*see* Fig. 13-2). Therefore, gas microemboli created by bubble oxygenators cause dose-dependent neurologic injury. Thus, it is reasonable to take steps to reduce microemboli generation (membrane oxygenation) and delivery (arterial filters, α-stat management [see below]) during CPB. Nevertheless, the efficacy of such steps to reduce perioperative neurologic impairment has only partial verification.

The Operative Field

Although membrane oxygenators and/or arterial line filters can nearly eliminate microscopic gas emboli from the CPB circuit, they cannot eliminate the other major source of arterial gas emboli during cardiac surgery,

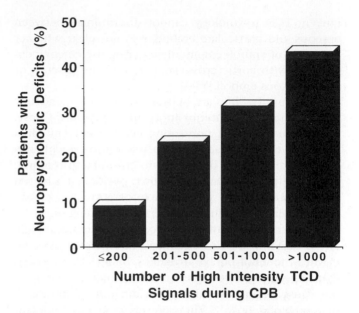

FIGURE 13–2. Relationship between number of high intensity TCD signals (HITS) during cardiac surgery and incidence of postoperative neuropsychologic abnormalities. *(Data from: Pugsley W, Klinger L, Paschalis C, Treasure T, Harrison M, Newman S: The impact of microemboli during cardiopulmonary bypass on neuropsychological functioning. Stroke 1994; 25:1393–1399.)*

namely those originating from the operative field. Echocardiographic studies have repeatedly demonstrated that, despite deairing techniques, left ventricular (LV) air (macroscopic or microscopic) is present in virtually 100% of patients undergoing open-chamber procedures.[131-135] Even in closed-chamber procedures, 15 to 50% of patients have intracavitary air.[131,132,135] With aortic cross-clamp removal and resumption of LV ejection, air enters the systemic and cerebral[54,135] circulations. Using TCD, van der Linden et al. demonstrated that in patients undergoing open-chamber procedures, the period of greatest cerebral embolization was *not* during CPB but, rather, was with resumption of left ventricular ejection.[51] Other investigators have made comparable observations.[126] For this reason, some authors advocate using TEE as a means to monitor and document clearance of macroscopic and microscopic air before resumption of ejection, presuming this will decrease neurologic injuries. However, Topal et al. found that although valve replacement patients had a much greater incidence and severity of intracardiac microbubbles compared with patients with CABG, neurologic outcome was indistinguishable between groups.[136] Therefore, at least in Topal's study, intracardiac microbubbles, as detected by TEE, did not clearly affect neurologic outcome. Therefore, although microbubbles produced by bubble oxygenators are associated with neuropsychologic dysfunction, the extent to which air (microscopic or macroscopic) from the field contributes to perioperative neurologic injury is currently uncertain. Because current TCD technology cannot discriminate between gaseous and particulate emboli, it is not clear whether the bolus of emboli commonly entering the cerebral circulation with aortic cross-clamp release are gaseous or atheromatous emboli.[45,53,54]

Because bubbles are buoyant, they have a tendency to float "upward" (anterior in a supine patient). Consequently, in hopes of preventing cerebral air emboli, a common clinical practice is to place the patient in a head-down position before aortic cross-clamp removal. When the patient is in a head-down position, it is hoped microbubbles in the left ventricle or aorta will either: (1) exit via a vent in the anterior ascending aorta; or (2) preferentially flow away from the brachiocephalic circulation into the descending aorta. However, using an in vitro model of bubble dynamics, Butler et al. showed that dependent flow angles (even as much as $-90°$) did not cause bubbles to move in a direction opposite to that of blood flow.[137] The only effect of a dependent flow angle was to decrease net forward bubble velocity, at most (at $-90°$) 21%. Therefore, even when the patient is in a head-down position, microbubbles can still be expected to travel in the direction of arterial blood flow, although at lesser velocity.

The literature is fairly evenly divided regarding whether or not open procedures (e.g., valve, ventricular aneurysm) have a greater incidence of neurologic complications versus closed procedures (e.g., CABG), although recent work cannot detect a difference.[39,95] A retrospective study from Japan indicates that now, perhaps due to increasing age and incidence of vascular disease in patients with CABG, neurologic complications may occur more frequently in patients with CABG as compared with valve patients.[97]

■ CONTROVERSIES IN PERIOPERATIVE MANAGEMENT

In addition to primary prevention (of cerebral emboli), a parallel approach to the problem of perioperative neurologic injury has been to establish anesthetic and CPB techniques that optimally maintain cerebral physiology and/or minimize damage secondary to an cerebral ischemic insult.

Glucose Management

Hyperglycemia during CPB is commonplace. At issue is whether hyperglycemia during CPB affects neurologic outcome. Using a dog model of CPB, Feerick et al. showed hyperglycemic CPB resulted in increased brain lactate concentration when compared to normoglycemic CPB.[138] Nevertheless, CBF, cerebral metabolic rate for oxygen (CMR_{O_2}), brain water content and high-energy phosphate concentrations, and cerebrospinal fluid pH did not differ between normoglycemic and hyperglycemic animals. Therefore, there is little evidence that hyperglycemia during CPB is primarily injurious to the brain. Instead, the concern associated with hyperglycemia relates to the extent to which hyperglycemia may secondarily exacerbate neurologic injuries resulting from temporary or permanent ischemic insults occurring during surgery.[139]

The literature uniformly and unequivocally demonstrates that hyperglycemia exacerbates neurologic injuries whenever neurologic insults, either focal[140-142] or global,[143-145] have an associated reperfusion phase. Hyperglycemia, by providing more substrate for anaerobic glycolysis, results in a greater degree of intracellular lactic acidosis in ischemic tissue.[146-150] Ischemic intracellular acidosis is associated with loss of neuronal ion and volume control, lactate clearance, and mitochondrial ATP generation.[151] In addition, intracellular acidosis damages endothelial and glial cells such that postischemic blood–brain barrier disruption is made worse by hyperglycemia.[152] Therefore, in cardiac surgical procedures in which temporary cerebral ischemia is planned, such as circulatory arrest, avoidance of hyperglycemia is prudent and well justified.

However, most neurologic injuries associated with cardiac surgery probably result from permanent focal cerebral emboli, either atheroemboli from the ascending aorta or microemboli from the CPB pump (see above). Although permanent focal lesions have no reperfusion phase, they often have associated zones of marginal viability ("ischemic penumbra") that depend on residual collateral blood flow and other compensatory mechanisms (increased oxygen extraction, anaerobic adenosine triphosphate [ATP] generation) to maintain viability.[153] The literature is inconsistent regarding whether hyperglycemia has a beneficial[154,155] or detrimental[156,157] effect on penumbral neurons and the final extent of infarction. The effect of glucose on penumbral neurons probably depends both on the level of residual blood flow[142] and time. If penumbral blood flow reductions are not too extreme, hyperglycemia can aid penumbral neurons by providing additional substrate for anaerobic ATP generation.[147,150] Viability is maintained as long as critical intracellular acidosis does not occur.[146-148] Hyperglycemia also seems to inhibit recurrent membrane depolarization in the penumbra.[158] Such depolarizations increase neuronal metabolic demand,[158] further worsening energy depletion,[159] and result in a more extensive infarction.[160,161] Therefore, when assessed in the first few hours after the onset of permanent focal ischemia, animal studies find that hyperglycemia seems to provide some neurologic protection.[154,155] Unfortunately, that protection is not sustained. Neuronal tolerance to intracellular acidosis diminishes over time (2 to 6 hours).[162] Although intracellular acidosis may be tolerated for a while, especially if ATP is generated, acidotic penumbral tissue eventually will progress to infarction. Furthermore, neuronal death secondary to intracellular acidosis has a latency period as long as 48 hours.[162] Only with long-term evaluation (>48 hours) can the final effect of glucose on neurologic outcome be assessed accurately. In studies in which animals have been recovered for longer periods (14 days) after permanent focal ischemia, the adverse effect of hyperglycemia has been marked and unequivocal.[156,157]

Nevertheless, current clinical studies challenge the supposition that hyperglycemia during CPB should adversely affect neurologic outcome. In a famous study by Metz and Keats, 107 nondiabetic patients undergoing elective CABG were randomized to receive either lactated Ringer's (LR) solution or, alternatively, D_5LR as priming and maintenance fluid during surgery.[163] During CPB, the D_5LR group had glucose concentrations ranging from 600 to 800 mg/dL, whereas the LR group had glucose concentrations from 200 to 250 mg/dL. During CPB, D_5LR patients had greater urine output than LR patients (937 ± 481 versus 537 ± 370 mL, respectively) and required less fluid to maintain reservoir volume (144 ± 270 versus 1147 ± 1149 mL, respectively). As a result, net intraoperative fluid gain was less in the D_5LR group than in the LR group (+2821 ± 805 versus +4336 ± 1278 mL, respectively). On postoperative day 5, D_5LR patients had lost 1 ± 3 kg relative to their preoperative weight, whereas LR patients had a weight gain of 1 ± 3 kg. Dramatically, Metz and Keats reported no neurologic injury in 54 patients undergoing CABG managed with D_5LR versus one stroke and one case of encephalopathy in 53 patients in whom glucose was avoided. They suggested hyperglycemic CPB did no harm and might even have neurologic benefit. Nevertheless, in this author's opinion, these findings and conclusions should be viewed with skepticism. Considering a 3 to 5% stroke rate in current prospective studies (see above), the stroke rate reported by Metz and Keats (1 of 107) seems inappropriately low. Likewise, considering the current incidence of acute neuropsychologic abnormalities of 30 to 40%, an encephalopathy rate <1% also seems inappropriately low. In this author's opinion, the low rate of neurologic complications reported in this study probably was caused by insensitive/inadequate detection methods and, as a result, its conclusions are not reliable.

To date, reports concerning the effect of glucose on neuropsychologic outcome after cardiac surgery have been published only in abstract form.[164,165] Frasco et al. performed neurologic examinations and psychometric tests before and after cardiac surgery in 60 adults.[164] During CPB, blood glucose concentrations varied between 103 to 379 mg/dL, and glucose concentra-

tions >250 mg/dL were treated with insulin. Postoperative test scores indicated significant new cognitive dysfunction was present in the study population. Nevertheless, in 11 of 12 tests, there was no correlation between mean glucose during CPB and postoperative neuropsychologic performance. Shevde et al. randomized 59 adults to either "tight" control of glucose during surgery and CPB ($n = 27$; mean glucose, 189 mg/dL) or minimal control ($n = 28$; mean glucose, 269 mg/dL).[165] Although there was evidence of acute cognitive/neuropsychologic dysfunction on postoperative day 3, there was no difference between groups. Therefore, even when sensitive tests of neurologic function have been employed, hyperglycemia during CPB has not seemed to adversely affect neurologic outcome.

How is one to reconcile the apparent discordance between the animal literature and the human literature? In the human studies cited above, CPB was conducted with moderate hypothermia. Lundgren et al. showed that even mild hypothermia (32° to 33°C) markedly attenuates the detrimental effects (both neurologic and histologic) of hyperglycemia in rats undergoing 10 to 15 minutes of cerebral ischemia.[166] Similarly, Dietrich et al. have shown that hypothermia (30°C) limits hyperglycemic exacerbation of blood–brain barrier disruption after an ischemic insult,[152] and Nedergaard et al. showed that delayed neuronal necrosis secondary to acidosis could be prevented by a period of hypothermia (32°C).[162] Therefore, the lack of a detrimental effect of hyperglycemia on neurologic outcome in human CPB studies might possibly be ascribed to the use of hypothermia. The findings of a recent large clinical trial are consistent with that possibility.

Martin et al. observed a greater incidence of neurologic complications (4.5%) in a group of 493 patients randomized to warm (≥35°C) surgery/CPB as compared with a group of 508 patients randomized to a hypothermic (≤28°C) technique (1.4%)[5] (see below for more on this study). In their discussion, the authors noted that normothermic patients had greater blood glucose concentrations during CPB than hypothermic patients but did not report the values. In a subsequent report composed of a subset of these patients, Mora et al. reported that glucose during CPB equaled 276 ± 100 mg/dL in the warm group ($n = 68$) versus 152 ± 66 in the hypothermic group ($n = 70$).[6] No hypothermic patient had a new central neurologic deficit versus 7 of 68 (10%) normothermic patients ($P = 0.006$). Interestingly, in the study by Mora et al., the incidence of neuropsychologic deficits did *not* differ between groups. From the Martin and Mora reports, it is impossible to know whether worse neurologic outcome in the normothermic group was caused by warmer brain temperatures, greater blood glucose, or the combination of the two. Nevertheless, the implication is clear. During cardiac surgery, the normothermic brain may be more sensitive to the adverse effects of hyperglycemia than the hypothermic brain.

Considering what is known, it would seem prudent to correct hyperglycemia whenever the brain is warm and at risk of neurologic injury. Admittedly, however, there currently are no clinical outcome data to support this recommendation, only a large body of animal data.

Mild and Moderate Hypothermia

Hypothermia has long been considered to provide a measure of "cerebral protection" during CPB. However, starting in the early 1990s, there has been great interest in the use of normothermic ("warm") cardioplegia and normothermic bypass.[167,168] At issue is whether neurologic outcome might be worse with "warm bypass" as compared with traditional moderately hypothermic (27° to 29°C) bypass.

Mechanisms of Protection. Within limits, as temperature decreases, the brain's tolerance to ischemia increases. By reducing cerebral metabolic rate, hypothermia slows the rate of high-energy phosphate depletion[169-172] and the development of intracellular acido-

sis during cerebral ischemia.[170-172] In this way, hypothermia is thought to delay or prevent neuronal energy failure and terminal membrane depolarization during an ischemic period.[173] Therefore, traditionally, brain protection has been considered to be solely related to the degree of cerebral metabolic suppression afforded by hypothermia.

Croughwell et al., studying 41 adults during CPB at 27°C, found CMR_{O_2} was reduced to a value ~36% of the normothermic value (1.4 ± 0.3 versus 0.5 ± 0.2 mL•100 g^{-1}•min^{-1}).[174] In this and comparable adult studies, the CMR_{O_2} ratio over a 10°C interval, referred to as Q_{10}, ranges from 2.4 to 2.8.[175-177] The effect of hypothermia to decrease CMR_{O_2} may be somewhat greater in children than in adults. Greeley et al., studying brain blood flow and metabolism in 46 children during CPB, found CMR_{O_2} to decrease logarithmically with decreasing temperature to values ~36% and ~12% of normothermic values at 28°C and 19°C, respectively (*see* Fig. 13–3).[178] In this study, Q_{10} ranged between 3.3 and 3.6. Based on these Q_{10} values, one would predict that: (1) at 27°C, the brain would tolerate ischemia approximately three times longer than it would at 37°C (9 to 15 minutes);

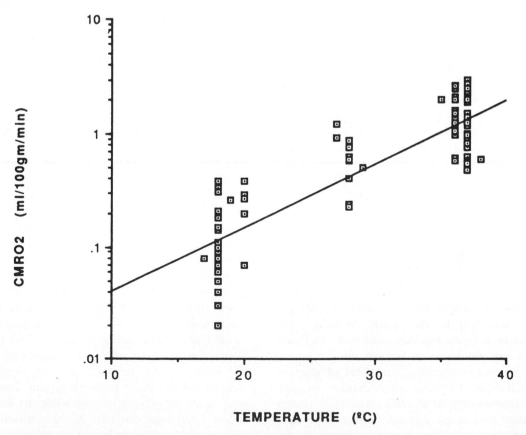

FIGURE 13–3. Temperature dependence of CMR_{O_2} during cardiopulmonary bypass in children. *(Reproduced with permission from: Greeley WJ, Kern FH, Ungerleider RM, et al: The effect of hypthermic cardiopulmonary bypass and total circulatory arrest on cerebral metabolism in neonates, infants and children. J Thorac Cardiovasc Surg 1991; 101:783–794.)*

and (2) at 17°C, the brain would tolerate ischemia 3×3 (9) times longer than it would at 37°C (27 to 45 minutes). Although these times are consistent with times required to exhaust ATP reserves at these temperatures, in general, tolerable ischemic durations exceed these intervals. Clearly, hypothermia does more.[179]

New evidence indicates that hypothermia confers cerebral protection even when cellular energy failure occurs[169,180-182] via modulation of intra- and postischemic phenomena.[183] Notable is the discovery that even mild hypothermia attenuates peri-ischemic excitatory neurotransmitter release.[184-187] Release of excitatory amino acids (e.g., glutamate, aspartate) is thought to contribute to neuronal injury by, among other actions, activation of N-methyl-D-aspartate (NMDA) receptor-gated calcium channels, which result in a massive increase in intracellular calcium concentration.[188] Increased intracellular calcium triggers a pathological cascade that includes free-fatty-acid release, free radical production, and the uncoupling of mitochondrial oxidative metabolism.[188] Hypothermia, by limiting or preventing glutamate release, lessens or prevents neurologic injury. Hypothermia also has been shown to attenuate postischemic free radical,[189] edema, and leukotriene formation.[190] The neuroprotective effect of mild-to-moderate hypothermia (30° to 35°C) seems to be mediated primarily via attenuation of these intra- and postischemic phenomena and *not* by metabolic reduction.[179,183]

Although mild-to-moderate hypothermia clearly provides a measure of neurologic protection in the face of temporary cerebral ischemia,[180,182,191] it is less clear how much hypothermia protects brain in the presence of a permanent lesion (e.g., atherosclerotic embolus). Using non-CPB rat models of permanent focal cerebral ischemia, Ridenour et al. found mild hypothermia (2 hours at 33°C) did not reduce the extent of cerebral infarction,[192] whereas Onesti et al. found deep hypothermia (~1 hour at 24°C) did.[193] Using similar models, Kader et al. reported moderate hypothermia (30° to 34°C) significantly reduced infarct volumes after permanent focal ischemia in rats,[194] whereas Morikawa et al. did not achieve statistical significance at 30°C.[195] Therefore, laboratory evidence suggests moderately hypothermic CPB (27° to 30°C) might provide some measure of brain protection when compared with normothermic CPB, even for permanent lesions (e.g., atheroemboli).

Hypothermic versus Normothermic Heart Surgery. Recent studies reach what seem, at first, to be opposing conclusions regarding the neurologic safety of warm CPB. The Warm Heart Surgery Investigators (WHSI) found no difference in perioperative stroke incidence (1.6%) in 1732 patients randomized to undergo CABG under either "normothermic" (33° to 37°C)

or hypothermic (25° to 30°C) CPB.[3] Notably, most patients in the "warm" group were allowed to cool spontaneously during CPB, resulting in mild hypothermia. As mentioned earlier, prospective neurologic testing was not used for the entire cohort. However, in a subset of patients in whom prospective testing was conducted (n = 155), McLean et al. still found no difference between groups in either acute or long-term neuropsychologic outcome.[4] In contrast, Martin et al. reported a greater incidence of neurologic complications in 493 patients randomized to warm surgery/CPB as compared with 508 patients randomized to a hypothermic technique, 4.5% versus 1.4%, respectively.[5] This study differed from the WHSI/McLean study in that warm patients were actively warmed throughout CPB. The heater/cooler bath temperature was kept at 39° to 40°C and bladder temperatures ranged between 35° to 37°C.[6] Considering that brain temperature usually is closer to perfusate temperature than bladder temperature,[196] it seems possible that a substantial fraction of the "warm" patients in the Martin and Mora study may have been slightly hyperthermic (i.e., brain temperatures >37°C). As discussed below, even mild hyperthermia worsens the effect of cerebral ischemic insults. Warm patients in the Martin and Mora study also had greater blood glucose concentrations during CPB than did hypothermic patients, ~275 versus ~150 mg/dL, respectively.[6] Because hyperglycemia may exacerbate neurologic injury, particularly during normothermia (see above), it is impossible to know whether the worse neurologic outcome in the Martin and Mora normothermic group was due to slight cerebral hyperthermia, greater blood glucose, or the combination of the two. Finally, in the Martin and Mora study, patients in the warm group received continuous retrograde normothermic cardioplegia, whereas the hypothermic group received intermittent antegrade cardioplegia. A recent TCD study indicates greater cerebral embolization occurs with cross-clamp release when a retrograde cardioplegia technique is used compared with antegrade techniques.[45] Therefore, in the Martin and Mora study, patients randomized to warm CPB were: (1) definitely hyperglycemic; (2) probably hyperthermic; and (3) possibly received more emboli. These three factors may account for worse neurologic outcome in the warm group. Interestingly, however, in the subgroup of patients undergoing prospective neuropsychologic examinations, reported by Mora et al., outcomes did not differ between temperature groups.[6] Therefore, both the McLean et al. and Mora et al. studies indicate that neuropsychologic outcomes do *not* seem to be markedly affected by temperature management.

Because hypothermia during CPB does not seem to confer clear-cut neurologic/neuropsychologic benefit, it would seem that most neurologic insults are (1) of a type not greatly affected by hypothermia (e.g., permanent emboli); and/or (2) principally occur during normothermic periods of the procedure (aortic cannulation, aortic cross-clamp removal, emergence from CPB). Alternatively, neurologic benefits afforded by hypothermia may somehow be negated by a counterbalancing adverse effect. Accordingly, considerable attention recently has been given to the rewarming phase of CPB.

Rewarming: Jugular Venous Desaturation and Hyperthermic Overshoot.

Jugular bulb blood is (usually) representative of mixed cerebral venous blood.[197] As such, jugular bulb oxyhemoglobin saturation provides a rough index of the relationship between global brain oxygen delivery and consumption. A normal (normothermic) jugular venous saturation is approximately 60%. During hypothermic CPB (with α-stat management [see below]), jugular venous saturation usually is approximately 75%.[174,198-200] A number of groups have reported marked decreases in jugular venous saturation during CPB rewarming, with jugular venous saturation less than 50% occurring in 25 to 50% of patients.[8,9,198-202] In some studies, the degree of jugular desaturation seemed to be related to rewarming rate. Nakajima et al.[200] and van der Linden et al.[201] both noted that jugular venous desaturation was greater with greater rewarming rates. Importantly, jugular venous desaturation may be associated with adverse neurologic outcome. Croughwell et al.[8] and Newman et al.[9] reported an association between the magnitude of rewarming-induced jugular venous desaturation and the severity of postoperative neuropsychologic dysfunction. These authors suggested jugular venous desaturation indicated a clinically significant "mismatch" between cerebral oxygen delivery and consumption during the rewarming phase of CPB, resulting in some degree of inadequate brain oxygenation. At issue, therefore, was whether rapid rewarming on CPB might cause greater jugular venous desaturation and greater neuropsychologic injury. Of note, in both the Croughwell et al. and Newman et al. studies, which included many of the same patients, patients who had the greatest degree of rewarming-induced jugular venous hemoglobin desaturation could, in general, be identified *before* rewarming was initiated. Patients having greater jugular desaturation with rewarming had lesser CBF, greater CMR_{O_2}, and greater oxygen extraction during steady-state hypothermic CPB than patients in whom jugular venous desaturation did not occur. This suggests that patients having the greatest degree of rewarming-induced cerebral venous hemoglobin desaturation may have had some preexisting cerebrovascular abnormality. Therefore, increased neuropsychologic impairment in patients with marked cerebral venous hemoglobin desaturation may have been caused by abnormalities in flow/metabolism

coupling (and/or brain injury) that were present before rewarming, rather than to rewarming-induced jugular venous hemoglobin desaturation per se. Indeed, a recent study by Newman et al. reported that the rewarming rate had no independent effect on postoperative neuropsychologic outcome.[10] Similarly, jugular venous desaturation had only a minor independent effect on neuropsychologic outcome. The principal determinants of neuropsychologic outcome were patient-related: age, preoperative neuropsychologic status, and years of education (the latter being protective). Therefore, currently, it does not seem that jugular venous desaturation per se has a large effect on neurologic outcome. Instead, the degree of desaturation that occurs with rewarming is largely determined by the characteristics of the patients themselves.

With the appreciation that even mild hypothermia confers marked cerebral protection came the realization that mild hyperthermia is very detrimental to the injured brain. Animal studies indicate that brain temperatures only 2°C greater than normal markedly exacerbate injury resulting from an ischemic insult.[203,204] Recent prospective studies in nonsurgical stroke patients indicate even mild hyperthermia (>1°C greater than normal) is independently associated with poor outcomes.[205,206] The effect of hyperthermia to worsen outcome occurs at all levels of initial stroke severity.[205] A common practice to speed rewarming is to increase arterial perfusate temperature to 40°C or greater. Because the brain is well perfused, it warms more quickly than the rest of the body.[196] Therefore, commonly used temperature monitors (esophageal, rectal, bladder, and even nasopharyngeal) usually underestimate brain temperature during rewarming.[196] Therefore, recent reports suggest brain temperatures of 38° to 39°C probably frequently occur because of aggressive rewarming and inaccurate temperature monitoring ("hyperthermic overshoot").[10,207-209] At issue is whether rewarming-induced cerebral hyperthermia could exacerbate neurologic injuries, negating the benefits of hypothermia. Reexamining the data from the McLean et al. study (a subgroup of the WHSI study), Buss et al. reported that 44% of patients were rewarmed to nasopharyngeal temperatures ≥38°C.[207] Neuropsychologic outcome did not seem to be significantly worse in these patients as compared with those rewarmed to lesser temperature. The authors suggested that the duration of cerebral hyperthermia during rewarming may not be long enough to adversely affect outcome. Indeed, the duration of hyperthermia may be the key. Birdi et al. reported that patients who were actively warmed to maintain nasopharyngeal temperatures of 37°C throughout CPB (just like in the Martin et al. study, see above) had much worse neuropsychologic outcomes than patients maintained at 32° or 28°C.[210] Therefore, current evidence suggests that sustained normothermia during CPB is associated with less favorable outcomes. Whether transient hyperthermic overshoot during rewarming from hypothermic CPB has adverse effects is unclear. On the other hand, because it cannot help and may hurt, it would seem prudent to avoid it whenever possible.

Hypothermic Acid–Base Management During Moderate Hypothermia: α-stat versus pH-stat

Poikilotherms and hibernators tend to use two very different acid–base strategies under hypothermic conditions, α-stat and pH-stat, respectively (see below). Because humans are neither poikilotherms nor hibernators, and normally do not become hypothermic, it has been unclear which hypothermic acid–base strategy might be most appropriate for humans during hypothermic CPB. To date, the α-stat versus pH-stat controversy has focused on the brain because, as will be discussed, hypothermic acid–base management has been shown to influence cerebral physiology during CPB. At issue is whether hypothermic acid–base management affects neurologic outcome.

Before discussing the clinical aspects of α-stat and pH-stat management, a review of the underlying physiology is helpful. Electrochemical neutrality is defined as the point where [H$^+$] equals [OH$^-$]. At 37°C, the [H$^+$] at neutrality = 1.58×10^{-7} mole/L, giving a neutral pH (pN) = 6.80.[211] Although we tend to think of "neutral" pH (pN) = 7.00, this is true only at 25°C, where [H$^+$] = [OH$^-$] = 1×10^{-7} mole/L. When aqueous solutions are cooled, both [H$^+$] and [OH$^-$] decrease because of a reduction in the spontaneous dissociation of water. For example, at 17°C, the [H$^+$] at neutrality ≈ 0.7×10^{-7} mole/L; giving a pN = 7.14. Therefore, with anaerobic cooling of aqueous solutions (including blood) pN spontaneously increases, following the relationship: $\Delta pN/\Delta T \approx -0.017$ pH units/°C.[212] With some exceptions,[212,213] poikilotherms tend to maintain intracellular pH near pN over a wide range of body temperatures. Simultaneously, they maintain extracellular pH at more alkalotic values, keeping a fairly constant intra- to extracellular pH gradient of 0.5 to 0.7 pH units.[211] Therefore, at 37°C, intracellular pH ≈ 6.8 and extracellular (blood) pH ≈ 7.4. As poikilotherms cool, both intra- and extracellular pH increase in a manner virtually identical to the anaerobic cooling of water: $\Delta pH/\Delta T \approx -0.017$ pH units/°C.[214] Reeves observed the pK of the histidine imidazole group also varies with temperature in a fashion almost identical to that of water: $\Delta pK/\Delta T \approx -0.016$ pK units/°C.[215] By maintaining intracellular pH near pN, poikilotherms maintain the ionization state of histidine imidazole (called α) at a constant level, despite changing body temperature, hence the name "α-stat." The α-stat hypothesis contends

that the histidine imidazole ionization state is the primary determinant of both the charge state and pH-dependent function of many of the body's key functional proteins.[212] Therefore, during hypothermia under α-stat conditions, changing body temperature does not alter histidine ionization. Consequently, protein charge state, structure, and function remain more nearly normal, and poikilotherms can remain active over a wide range of body temperatures.

Poikilotherms achieve this by appearing to anaerobically cool their blood. As poikilotherms cool, both intracellular and extracellular (blood) pH increase as described above. Simultaneously, because gas solubility increases with decreasing temperature, the partial pressure of carbon dioxide (CO$_2$) decreases, although total blood CO$_2$ content does not change. (Henry's law states the amount of a gas in solution is proportional to its partial pressure. Therefore, [CO$_2$] = P$_{CO_2}$ × α, where [CO$_2$] = concentration of CO$_2$ in solution [mmol/L], α = temperature-dependent solubility coefficient of CO$_2$ in aqueous solution (mmol•L^{-1}•mm Hg^{-1}), P$_{CO_2}$ = partial pressure of CO$_2$ [mm Hg]. This can be rewritten as P$_{CO_2}$ = ([CO$_2$]/α). With hypothermia, α increases; therefore, P$_{CO_2}$ decreases.) Therefore, poikilotherms establish what seems to be a respiratory alkalosis when blood gases are corrected to actual in vivo temperature, "worsening" with deepening hypothermia relative to normothermic blood gas values. α-stat management is approximated during human hypothermic CPB by maintaining pH$_a$ = 7.40 and P$_a$CO$_2$ = 40 mm Hg as measured at 37°C, regardless of the patient's actual in vivo temperature (blood gases are not temperature-corrected). When corrected to in vivo temperature, this technique is seen to result in a respiratory alkalosis (low P$_a$CO$_2$, high pH$_a$), a consequence of the spontaneous shift of pH and P$_{CO_2}$ with decreasing temperature; *see* Table 13–7.[216] α-stat proponents suggest that in humans, as in poikilotherms, this respiratory alkalosis is, in fact, physiologically appropriate and will better preserve intracellular electrochemical neutrality and "normal" cellular structure and function. This assumes, of course, that the key functional group in all human tissues (including brain) is histidine imidazole (it may not be).

The other hypothermic acid–base strategy, referred to as "pH stat," approximates that of hibernators. In contrast to poikilotherms, hibernators become extremely inactive when cold. pH-stat management maintains pH$_a$ = 7.40 and P$_a$CO$_2$ = 40 mm Hg as measured at, or corrected to, the subjects actual in vivo temperature (i.e., blood gases are temperature-corrected). As discussed above, anaerobic cooling of blood results in a shift of pH to more alkaline values and a reduction of P$_a$CO$_2$. To maintain fixed (temperature-corrected) values of pH$_a$ and P$_a$CO$_2$ during cooling, H$^+$ (CO$_2$) must be added. Therefore, with pH stat management, it is necessary to increase the total

TABLE 13–7. α-STAT VERSUS pH-STAT ACID–BASE MANAGEMENT[a]

In vivo Temperature	Measured and Reported at 37°C				Corrected to in vivo Temperature			
	pH		P_{CO_2} (mm Hg)		pH		P_{CO_2} (mm Hg)	
	α-stat	pH-stat	α-stat	pH-stat	α-stat	pH-stat	α-stat	pH-stat
37°C	7.40	7.40	40	40	7.40	7.40	40	40
33°C	7.40	7.34	40	47	7.44	7.40	35	40
30°C	7.40	7.30	40	54	7.50	7.40	29	40
27°C	7.40	7.26	40	62	7.55	7.40	26	40
23°C	7.40	7.21	40	74	7.60	7.40	22	40
20°C	7.40	7.18	40	84	7.65	7.40	19	40
17°C	7.40	7.14	40	96	7.69	7.40	17	40

[a] Corrections for temperature taken from Andritsch RF, Muravchick S, Gold MI: Temperature correction of arterial blood-gas parameters: A comparative review of methodology. Anesthesiology 1981; **55:**311–316.

CO_2 content of blood as temperature is reduced. As shown in Table 13–7, pH-stat management produces relative hypercarbia and acidemia compared with α-stat management, increasing in magnitude as temperature decreases. Most enzyme reaction rates are pH-dependent, and many enzymes have pH optima that follow the predictions of α-stat theory.[217,218] Because pH-stat management creates a relatively acidic intracellular environment, this would be expected to decrease enzyme reaction rates, adenosine triphosphate (ATP) consumption, and, consequently, metabolic rate (CMR_{O_2}). In fact, this process has been proposed as the mechanism by which hibernating species, which follow pH-stat acid–base strategy, reduce oxygen consumption in nonessential organs to lowest possible values (*see Profound Hypothermia and Circulatory Arrest* below).[218-220]

There has been considerable work regarding whether hypothermic blood gas management (α-stat versus pH-stat) influences cerebral metabolism during hypothermic CPB. The existing human data are limited to adults during moderate hypothermia and are somewhat contradictory. Prough et al. measured CMR_{O_2} in 25 adults during CPB at 27°C over a P_aCO_2 range that encompassed both α-stat and pH-stat conditions.[221] These investigators found that CMR_{O_2} decreased with increasing P_aCO_2. CMR_{O_2} values under pH-stat conditions were ~50% that of α-stat values (0.2 ± 0.1 versus 0.4 ± 0.1 mL•100 g^{-1}•min^{-1}, respectively). Rogers et al. measured CMR_{O_2} in adults during CPB at 27°C, finding pH-stat patients to have CMR_{O_2} values ~20% less than α-stat patients.[222] In contrast, Murkin et al.[176] and Stephan et al.[223] reported CMR_{O_2} values in patients having α-stat or pH-stat management (~27°C) that were indistinguishable. In agreement with the latter authors, we found no apparent difference in CMR_{O_2} between α-stat and pH-stat management in our rabbit model of CPB at 27°C.[224,225] Therefore, at moderate hypothermia (≥27°C), the weight of current evidence indicates that CMR_{O_2} is minimally affected by choice of blood gas management. Inspection of Table 13–7 suggests pH_a and P_aCO_2 differences between α-stat and pH-

stat are modest at temperatures ≥27°C and would seem unlikely to greatly affect CMR_{O_2}.

CBF, like CMR_{O_2}, also decreases during hypothermic CPB. Nevertheless, the cerebral vasculature retains its responsiveness to changing P_aCO_2.[226-229] Consequently, the relative hypercarbia of pH-stat management results in: (1) greater CBF relative to α-stat patients and (2) impairment of cerebral autoregulation. A highly illustrative study was that of Murkin et al., wherein 38 adults underwent CPB at ~26°C under either α-stat or pH-stat management.[176] As shown in Figure 13–4, CBF seemed to be independent of perfusion pressure under α-stat conditions, i.e., cerebral autoregulation was intact. In contrast, under pH-stat conditions, CBF seemed to vary with perfusion pressure, i.e., cerebral autoregulation was absent.

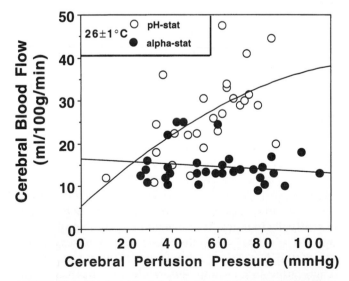

FIGURE 13–4. Cerebral blood flow versus cerebral perfusion pressure (mean arterial pressure minus central venous pressure) in adults undergoing cardiopulmonary bypass under α-stat and pH-stat conditions. *(Modified and reproduced with permission from: Murkin JM, Farrar JK, Tweed A, McKenzie FN, Guíraudon G: Cerebral autoregulation and flow/metabolism coupling during cardiopulmonary bypass: The influence of PaCO2. Anesth Analg 1987; **66:**825–832.)*

Other studies in adults during moderately hypothermic CPB have been consistent with these findings.[230-235] Because in Murkin's study CMR_{O_2} did not differ between α-stat or pH-stat patients, it was clear pH-stat management resulted in a greater CBF/CMR_{O_2} ratio than did α-stat management.[176] At issue was whether the increased cerebral perfusion afforded by pH-stat management: (1) provided some margin of safety during hypotensive periods during CPB (potentially good); or (2) alternatively, resulted in unnecessary cerebral hyperperfusion (potentially bad by increasing the number of emboli).

As can be seen in Figure 13–4, as cerebral perfusion pressure decreases, CBF differences between α-stat and pH-stat diminish. In the range of perfusion pressures often used during cardiopulmonary bypass (~50 to 70 mm Hg), CBF differences between α-stat and pH-stat often are fairly small. As arterial pressure decreases even more, the curves converge. Lundar et al., using TCD to measure CBF velocity in humans during hypothermic CPB, found the cerebral vasodilatory effect of CO_2 depended on arterial pressure. CBF responses to CO_2 decreased when MAP was less than ~60 mm Hg.[252] There comes a point (~30 mm Hg at 27°C) at which autoregulatory cerebral vasodilation (afforded by α-stat management) is roughly equal to CO_2-induced cerebral vasodilation (afforded by pH-stat management). Therefore, if perfusion pressure falls below this level, CBF will decrease with either technique. Consequently, pH-stat management would seem incapable of providing substantively greater CBF than α-stat management in the presence of hypotension during CPB.[236]

At moderate hypothermia (~27°C), CMR_{O_2} differences between α-stat and pH-stat management seem minimal. Likewise, over a fairly broad range of cerebral perfusion pressure, CBF differences also are fairly small. Because of the small differences in CBF and CMR_{O_2} between techniques, one might anticipate that neurologic outcome would be minimally affected, if at all, by choice of blood gas management. The first study to address this issue supported this hypothesis. Bashein et al. randomized 86 adults undergoing cardiac surgery to either α-stat or pH-stat management.[7] CPB was conducted at ~30°C with an unfiltered bubble oxygenator with mean arterial pressure ranging from 50 to 60 mm Hg. Neuropsychologic testing was conducted preoperatively, and at 7 days and 6 months postoperatively. In this study, CBF and CMR_{O_2} were not measured. Both short- and long-term neuropsychologic status were unaffected by choice of hypothermic acid–base management. However, three subsequent studies indicate a modest benefit to α-stat management. Stephan et al. randomized 65 adults to α-stat or pH-stat management during CPB at 26°C.[223] These investigators used a filtered membrane oxygenator with arterial pressure ranging from 55 to 85 mm Hg. As expected at these higher perfusion pressures, CBF was greater in pH-stat patients as compared with α-stat patients (CMR_{O_2} did not differ between groups). New neurologic deficits were more common in pH-stat patients (10 of 35) as compared with α-stat patients (2 of 30), $P = 0.04$. Patel et al. randomized 70 adults to either α-stat or pH-stat management (28°C) and found a greater incidence of neuropsychologic abnormalities at 6 weeks after surgery in pH-stat patients (49% versus 20%, $P = 0.02$).[237] Most recently, Murkin et al. randomized 316 patients to either α-stat or pH-stat management (26° to 28°C).[11] CPB was conducted with a membrane oxygenator and arterial filtration, and patients also were randomized to pulsatile or nonpulsatile perfusion. Over all, there was no difference in neurologic or neuropsychologic outcome between groups. However, in patients undergoing CPB for ≥90 minutes, those managed with α-stat had a lesser incidence of neuropsychologic abnormalities at 2 months postoperatively than did those managed with pH-stat (27% versus 44%, respectively; $P = 0.05$). Therefore, over all, there seems to be no neurologic disadvantage to α-stat management during continuous CPB at moderate hypothermia, and probably a slight advantage. Presumably, the benefit of α-stat management is due to the lesser CBF of this technique, resulting in less cerebral embolization during CPB. However, because CBF differences between techniques often are small and cerebral embolization during CPB with membrane oxygenation and arterial filtration is low, neurologic outcome differences between α-stat and pH-stat are not detectable until CPB durations are prolonged.

Systemic Arterial Pressure

Cerebral metabolic demands are decreased during CPB by use of hypothermia and anesthetics. At the same time, however, cerebral oxygen delivery is reduced by hemodilution and hypothermia-induced CBF reduction. Therefore, the safe lower limit of arterial pressure required to adequately support CBF and CMR_{O_2} during CPB have been a matter of sustained interest and controversy.

A classic and often cited study is that of Stockard et al., in which perioperative neurologic outcome was suggested to correlate with changes in intraoperative blood pressure and electroencephalography.[238] In this study, hypothermia (28° to 32°C) was not consistently induced during CPB but rather was "employed during lengthy procedures." The report did not state whether P_aCO_2 was corrected for temperature nor the degree to which hemodilution was employed. During CPB, systemic flow was maintained at 2.2 L·min⁻¹·m⁻², irrespective of arterial pressure. The authors proposed an index of hypotension, referred to as the tm_{50}, as a predictor of perioperative neurologic dysfunction:

$$tm_{50} = \int [50 - MAP(mm\ Hg)] \cdot \delta t(min)$$

Six of seven patients with a tm_{50} >100 mm Hg•min had abnormal intraoperative electroencephalogram (EEG) patterns and "generalized" postoperative neurologic deficits. Presumably, patients with a tm_{50} > 100 mm Hg•min had cerebral hypoperfusion. Only two of 16 patients with tm_{50} < 100 mm Hg•min had transient postoperative deficits that could be attributable to intraoperative events. None of these 16 patients had intraoperative EEG abnormalities. The authors proposed: (1) mean arterial pressure (MAP) should be at least 50 mm Hg during bypass; and (2) a tm_{50} > 100 mm Hg•min was predictive of irreversible EEG changes and postoperative neurologic dysfunction, presumably on an ischemic basis.

Stockard's findings can be criticized because patients having neurologic deficits were significantly older and had longer CPB durations than patients who had no deficits (both independent risk factors). Furthermore, and more importantly, it is not clear which patients were hypothermic and which were normothermic (the paper suggests that most were normothermic), so the recommendations made by Stockard et al. may not apply to hypothermic CPB. Nevertheless, the concept behind tm_{50} is attractive and consistent with clinical intuition — a little hypotension for a little while is better tolerated than marked hypotension for a long time.

In the 25 years since Stockard's report, most studies examining the issue have not found an association between arterial pressure and/or tm_{50} during CPB and postoperative neurologic or neuropsychologic dysfunction. During moderately hypothermic CPB (26° to 28°C), Govier et al.[230] and Murkin et al.[176] found CBF to be independent of MAP between ~30 and 100 mm Hg. More recent work by Newman et al. has demonstrated that CBF is, in fact, slightly MAP-dependent during moderately hypothermic CPB.[9] However, increasing MAP from ~50 to ~75 mm Hg increased CBF only ~15%. Furthermore, even when low MAP results in decreased CBF, increased brain oxygen extraction often may be sufficient to maintain brain oxygenation. Feddersen et al. found that although CBF decreased at MAPs ≤ 30 mm Hg during hypothermic CPB, increased brain oxygen extraction preserved cerebral metabolism at normotensive levels.[175] Therefore, overall, during moderately hypothermic CPB (α-stat), cerebral autoregulation and oxygen extraction seem sufficient to maintain adequate cerebral perfusion and oxygenation.

This conclusion is supported by most recent reports wherein no correlation between neurologic impairment and tm_{50} during CPB, either as a continuous or dichotomous variable, could be demonstrated.[7,10,95] Only one contemporary report suggests that arterial pressure during CPB may influence neurologic outcome. Gold et al. randomized 248 patients undergoing elective CABG to either "low" (52 ± 5 mm Hg) or "high"

(69 ± 7 mm Hg) arterial pressure during moderately hypothermic (28° to 30°C) CPB.[239] Patients were prospectively examined preoperatively and 1 day, 2 days, 7 days, and 6 months after operation. At 6 months after operation, (1) the cumulative incidence of stroke was 7.2% (low pressure) versus 2.4% (high pressure) (P = 0.13); and (2) the cumulative incidence of TIA was 3.2% (low pressure) versus 0.8% (high pressure). Interestingly, the incidence of neuropsychologic deterioration (12%) did not differ between groups. This study is difficult to interpret because it did not state when the strokes or TIAs occurred during the 6-month postoperative period. However, Hartman et al. reported stroke incidence 7 days after surgery in a subset of these patients who also had intraoperative TEE rating of descending aortic atherosclerosis (n = 189).[46] The overall incidence of stroke at 7 days was 4.8% (*see* Table 13–8). Patients with high-grade atherosclerosis (III, IV, V) had fewer strokes when maintained at high pressure (2 of 30; 7%) than when maintained at low pressure (7 of 36; 19%) during CPB; P = 0.14. Although the Gold and Hartman studies suggest that increasing arterial pressure during CPB might reduce stroke, they do not achieve statistical significance. That, coupled with the fact that long-term neuropsychologic status did not differ between groups, indicates that if frank hypotension is avoided, MAP during CPB probably does not have a large affect on neurologic outcome. However, high-risk patients (i.e., those with severe aortic atherosclerosis) *may* have better outcomes when maintained at higher perfusion pressures. These patients are at high risk of cerebral embolization of atheromatous debris. In the setting of permanent focal ischemia, animal studies indicate that infarct volumes are reduced by induction of moderate hypertension. Increased arterial pressure increases collateral perfusion to ischemic territories.[240] Therefore, whenever in a "high-risk" circumstance (advanced age, prior stroke, marked carotid or aortic atherosclerosis), it seems only prudent to attempt to maintain perfusion pressures on the "higher" rather than on the "lower" side.

TABLE 13–8. INCIDENCE OF PERIOPERATIVE STROKE ACCORDING TO ATHEROMA GRADE AND ARTERIAL PRESSURE MANAGEMENT DURING CPB

Group	Atheroma Grade[a]				
	I	II	III	IV	V
Low	0/17	0/35	1/16 (6%)	2/14 (14%)	4/6 (67%)
High	0/26	0/45	1/20 (5%)	0/5 (5%)	1/5 (20%)

[a] Atheroma grade: I: normal to mild intimal thickening; II: severe intimal thickening without protruding atheroma; III: atheroma protruding <5 mm; IV: atheroma protruding ≥5 mm; V: atheroma of any size with mobile components.

(Data from: Hartman GS, Yao F-S, Bruefach M, et al: Severity of aortic atheromatous disease diagnosed by transesophageal echocardiography predicts stroke and other outcomes associated with coronary artery surgery: A prospective study. Anesth Analg 1996; **83**:701–708.)

This may be particularly true during normothermic CPB. Hypotension (systolic blood pressure < 80 mm Hg), low cardiac output, and the need for hemodynamic support in the weaning, post-CPB, and ICU phases is clearly associated with adverse neurologic outcome.[1,23,32,34,67,95] Tranmer et al. recently showed, in monkeys undergoing middle cerebral artery occlusion, that CBF in the ischemic region, in contrast to the nonischemic region, was exquisitely sensitive to changes in cardiac output.[241] Ischemic brain regions have impaired autoregulation.[242] Increasing arterial pressure increases CBF and may preserve viability of a region that would have died otherwise. Therefore, it makes perfect sense that hemodynamic instability post-CPB should contribute to neurologic morbidity.

Barbiturates

Traditionally, barbiturates have been considered to be "cerebral protective" agents. There has been interest in whether barbiturate administration during cardiac surgery and/or CPB might reduce neurologic injury. To put existing studies into perspective, a brief overview of barbiturate protection is helpful.

Anesthetic barbiturates cause a dose-dependent reduction of spontaneous neuronal synaptic activity and cerebral metabolism. At maximal effect, barbiturates produce a flat (isoelectric) EEG. With an isoelectric EEG, cerebral metabolic demands are approximately halved. Residual metabolic demands are due to processes that are vital to neuronal viability, such as maintenance of transmembrane ion gradients, protein synthesis, and other basal homeostatic processes. These latter processes are unaffected by barbiturates.[173,243-245] It has long been postulated that barbiturate-induced cerebral metabolic suppression might increase the tolerable duration of cerebral ischemia. By eliminating the synaptic component of cerebral metabolic rate, neuronal ATP stores could go toward maintenance of basal homeostatic processes. However, under conditions of ischemia severe enough to induce a flat EEG, barbiturates do not affect cerebral metabolic rate (derived from basal requirements). In this circumstance, there is no possible metabolic or energetic benefit in barbiturate administration. After ATP stores have been exhausted and/or CBF decreases below that needed to maintain homeostatic metabolisms, neurons depolarize and die, unaffected by the presence of barbiturates.[173,246] Thus, at best, barbiturate-induced metabolic suppression can only buy some time. Usually, that time is short.

In "no-flow" or "low-flow" states, animal studies indicate that metabolic suppression delays onset of neuronal depolarization by only 1 to 2 minutes.[179,247] Therefore, one can imagine that in clinical settings in which there is severe ischemia (profound hypotension, cardiac arrest, circulatory arrest), this rather small amount of "protection" easily could be rendered inconsequential. In fact, in models of global cerebral ischemia in dogs[248] and primates,[249] neither pentobarbital[248] nor thiopental[249] confer neurologic benefit. Similarly, use of thiopental after cardiac arrest in humans (a global ischemic insult) also has been found to be without neurologic benefit.[250] In contrast to these disappointing results, barbiturates have been found to be effective in decreasing (not eliminating) neurologic injury in animal models of temporary focal cerebral ischemia.[251-256] In these studies, large doses of barbiturates were administered to maximally suppress the EEG and cerebral metabolism. Indeed, EEG suppression has been the endpoint used in virtually all studies to achieve maximal barbiturate effect. However, recent work by Warner et al., in a rat model of temporary focal ischemia, indicates that, contrary to previous belief, lower doses of barbiturates (which do not suppress the EEG nor reduce metabolism as greatly) may be as effective as the larger (EEG-flattening) doses.[257] This is a potentially important observation because large doses of barbiturates are associated with prolonged emergence and adverse hemodynamic sequellae (see below). However, the mechanism of barbiturate cerebral protection in the setting of temporary focal ischemia is unclear. In light of Warner's recent findings, metabolic reduction seems much less likely as the mechanism. Just exactly how barbiturates provide cerebral protection is not currently understood.

In a famous and often cited study, Nussmeier et al. randomized 182 patients undergoing open cardiac procedures to receive either standard anesthetic/surgical management or thiopental in addition to standard management.[258] Thiopental was given by constant infusion in the pre- and intra-CPB period at doses sufficient to maintain a flat EEG (40 ± 8 mg/kg). Perfusion pressure was maintained equally in both groups. CPB was maintained near normothermia (≥34°C) with a bubble oxygenator without arterial filtration. At 10 days postoperatively, patients receiving thiopental had a lower incidence of neuropsychiatric abnormalities (0 of 89, 0%) than those who had not received thiopental (7 of 89, 7.5%) ($P < 0.025$). In stark contrast, in a subsequent study, Zaidan et al. found no evidence of neurologic benefit with thiopental in 300 patients undergoing CABG.[259] Similar to the Nussmeier study, thiopental was given to maintain EEG burst suppression throughout the procedure (30 ± 11 mg/kg). Zaidan's study differed from Nussmeier's in that a membrane oxygenator, in-line arterial filtration, and systemic hypothermia (28°C) were used during CPB. Strokes occurred in 5 of 149 (3%) of patients receiving thiopental versus 2 of 151 (1.3%) receiving placebo. Although thiopental did not improve neurologic outcome, patients receiving thiopental had an 80% greater need for inotropes after CPB, required 50% longer to regain consciousness, and required postoperative ventilation ~30% longer.[259] Marked differences between these two studies probably account for their very different outcomes.

Because Nussmeier's patients underwent procedures (1) with an open ventricle, (2) at normothermia ($\geq34°C$), and (3) with an unfiltered bubble oxygenator, they almost certainly received numerous cerebral gas microemboli both during CPB and with resumption of ejection. By decreasing CBF,[260] thiopental probably decreased the number of gas emboli received by the brain. In addition, to the extent that microbubbles may act as temporary focal lesions before being cleared,[261] thiopental also may have provided some primary neurologic protection. In contrast, Zaidan's patients underwent (1) closed cardiac procedures, (2) with hypothermia (28°C), and (3) with a filtered membrane oxygenator. Zaidan's patients were at low risk of air embolism during CPB and already had hypothermic brain protection, to which thiopental would add little. Patients suffering stroke in Zaidan's study had documented focal lesions on computed tomography (CT) scan, suggestive of a permanent focal lesion (atheromatous plaque) in which short-term barbiturate therapy is ineffective. Under "usual" CPB conditions in which cerebral embolization is low grade (membrane oxygenator, and/or arterial filter) and/or hypothermic protection is already present, barbiturates are very unlikely to provide substantive brain protection. Therefore, the effectiveness of thiopental in reducing neurologic and neuropsychologic abnormalities after cardiac surgery must be seriously questioned and its use must be balanced against some clear disadvantages, specifically cardiac depression and prolonged emergence and ventilatory requirements. The most rational (but unproved) use of thiopental (or etomidate or propofol[262]) might be those settings in which, under normothermia, a shower of emboli is anticipated (such as resumption of ejection after an open-chamber procedure). By decreasing CBF during the shower, the number of emboli received by the brain might be reduced. Reduction of the number of emboli should result in better outcome, but that is unproved.

Pulsatile Perfusion

A longstanding question in CPB management has been whether conventional nonpulsatile flow may, in some way, compromise cerebral perfusion and contribute to neurologic injury occurring during cardiac surgery.

Animal studies in the 1970s and 1980s indicated that nonpulsatile flow unfavorably influenced cerebral perfusion. In normothermic dogs, nonpulsatile perfusion resulted in (1) cerebral capillary collapse, intravascular sludging, and venodilation[263]; (2) histopathology consistent with ischemia in arterial boundary zones[264]; and (3) an approximately 20% decrease in CBF.[265,266] Collec-

tively, these studies suggested that brain blood flow and oxygenation might be better maintained with pulsatile CPB. Consequently, some cardiac surgery groups routinely employ pulsatile CPB or use it when patients are considered to be at special risk of neurologic complications.

There are several theories regarding how pulsatile perfusion might produce different circulatory effects as compared with equivalent mean flow achieved with nonpulsatile perfusion. However, the extent to which these mechanisms apply to the cerebral circulation, if at all, is unknown. Some authors propose that the greater peak hydraulic power of pulsatile flow recruits capillary beds that would otherwise be closed under nonpulsatile conditions.[267,268] By so doing, pulsatile perfusion is believed to decrease vascular resistance,[267-270] increase the uniformity of tissue perfusion,[271] decrease oxygen diffusion distances, and improve tissue oxygenation.[267,269,272] The greater peak sheer stress of pulsatile flow also may inhibit red blood cell aggregation and flow stagnation[263] and/or promote release of endothelial-derived vasodilators such as prostacyclin[273] and nitric oxide.[274] However, another proposal is that baroreceptor reflexes, which depend on arterial pulse rate, pulse pressure, and dP/dt,[275-277] play an important role in blood flow regulation. In the absence of pulsatile flow, reflex mechanisms mediated via the carotid sinus, brain stem cardiovascular centers, and the autonomic nervous system[277] increase arterial and venous smooth muscle tone.[277-279] In this way, vascular resistance, and perhaps blood flow distribution as well, can be influenced by pulsatility.

Despite these theoretical differences, numerous studies do not find systemic hemodynamic[280-284] blood flow or metabolic[280,281,285,286] differences between pulsatile and nonpulsatile perfusion. A criticism of studies that find no difference between pulsatile and nonpulsatile CPB is that the artificial pressure waveform may not have adequately reproduced the essential features of the native waveform.[287] This criticism is easy to make and difficult to refute because the critical features of pulsatile flow (dP/dt, pulse rate, pulse pressure, systolic/diastolic ratio, etc.) are not known. Therefore, choosing any one descriptor of arterial pressure waveform characteristics (pulse pressure, dP/dt, systolic/diastolic ratio) as defining "pulsatility" is arbitrary and subject to error. Some authors advocate the use of energy indices to quantitate pulsatile perfusion.[267,288] These indices require measurement of arterial flow waveforms, as opposed to, or in addition to, pressure waveforms. Nevertheless, energy indices do not always distinguish pulsatile from nonpulsatile flow.[267] Furthermore, as Grossi et al. observed, pulse shape and pulse rate distinguish pulsatile and nonpulsatile flow and not energy indices per se.[288]

Recently, using our rabbit model of CPB, our laboratory tested whether CBF and CMR_{O_2} differed between pulsatile and nonpulsatile CPB. A wide range of pulsatile waveforms were tested, both at normothermia (37°C)[289] and moderate hypothermia (27°C).[290] Artificial pulse waveforms were produced that were virtually indistinguishable from native waveforms. Nevertheless, neither under hypothermic or normothermic conditions, neither CBF nor CMR_{O_2} were affected by pulsation. At least in the normal brain, nonpulsatile CPB does not seem to be disadvantageous in terms of maintaining bulk brain blood flow or metabolism. Our findings are in contrast the earlier animal work and may be due to advances in perfusion technology and differences in experimental design.[289]

There is, to date, no clinical evidence of superior neurologic outcome with pulsatile perfusion. In the Shaw et al. study of patients undergoing CABG, there was no difference in neurologic outcome between patients undergoing pulsatile ($n = 134$) or nonpulsatile ($n = 178$) CPB.[32] Unfortunately, perfusion technique was not randomized and criteria for assigning patients to pulsatile versus nonpulsatile perfusion were not stated. Therefore, it is possible that selection bias may have masked neurologic outcome differences between perfusion techniques. In a much smaller study, Henze et al. assigned patients undergoing CABG to pulsatile ($n = 8$) versus nonpulsatile ($n = 14$) CPB.[291] Consistent with our laboratory's findings, CBF and CMR_{O_2} during CPB did not differ between groups. Also, there were no neurologic outcome differences between groups. However, the sample size of this study is too small relative to the occurrence rate (one case of arm paresis in each group) to provide adequate statistical power by which to conclude that pulsatile perfusion was without neurologic benefit. Most recently, Murkin et al. randomized 316 patients undergoing CABG to pulsatile versus nonpulsatile CPB (patients also were randomized to α-stat versus pH management).[11,292] Although pulsation significantly improved overall mortality,[292] it had no affect on either neurologic or neuropsychologic outcomes in survivors.[11] Notably, in this study, pulse pressure during CPB was only 17 ± 6 mm Hg and pulse waveforms were not shown. As discussed above, it is possible that the degree of pulsation achieved was simply not "pulsatile enough" to affect the brain. Nevertheless, it is doubtful that native arterial waveforms can be produced during human CPB. This is because the relatively small aortic cannulas used in human CPB result in marked damping of pulsatile waveforms.[267,271,288] As practically achievable, it seems that pulsatile CPB has little effect on the brain or the processes resulting in brain injury during cardiac surgery.

Profound Hypothermia and Circulatory Arrest

Profound hypothermia (14° to 19°C) is the principal means of neurologic protection during surgical procedures requiring markedly reduced systemic perfusion and/or circulatory arrest. Such procedures include repair of congential heart defects in children and some forms of aortic disease in adults. Animal studies show, at 13° to 20°C, hypothermic circulatory arrest (HCA) is tolerated for 60 to 75 minutes without subsequent histologic or behavioral evidence of neurologic injury.[293-296] Nevertheless, clinically, hypothermic brain protection seems to be less effective. Clinical studies report that 10 to 30% of children[297-301] and an equal percentage of adults[302-305] have some form of acute perioperative neurologic injury after HCA. (Choreoathetosis is a rare [1 to 2%], but potentially catastrophic, complication of profound hypothermia and HCA that seems to be unique to children.[300,307-310] In adults undergoing HCA for aortic atheromatous disease, a substantive fraction of neurologic injuries seem to result from cerebral emboli.[305]) It is now quite clear, both in children[301,306] and adults,[305] that the incidence of neurologic abnormalities correlates directly with HCA duration. As a consequence, there has been intense interest in improving brain protection during deep hypothermia.

Hypothermic brain protection is graded, with increasing protection as brain temperature decreases.[311,312] Therefore, achievement of desired brain temperature before HCA is a critical determinant of the effectiveness of the technique. Recent studies suggest that brain cooling may, in fact, often be incomplete. Using retrospective data, Bellinger et al. reported infants cooled on CPB for less than 20 minutes had worse postoperative developmental scores than children who, undergoing equivalent periods of HCA, had greater durations of pre-HCA cooling.[313] The authors suggested that despite achievement of desired rectal temperatures, brain cooling may have been incomplete in infants with shorter cooling periods. In support of that conclusion, Greeley et al. found 4 of 23 (17%) of children cooled on CPB for ≥15 minutes to have comparatively low jugular bulb saturation just before HCA.[178] Kern et al. found 6 of 17 (35%) children, cooled on bypass for only 7 to 10 minutes, to have comparatively low jugular bulb saturations before HCA.[314] Both authors interpreted their findings as indicating that, despite attaining target nasopharyngeal or tympanic temperatures, brain cooling probably was incomplete in a significant portion of children. Recently, Stone et al. demonstrated surrogate temperature monitors (tympanic, nasopharyngeal, etc.) commonly *under*estimate true brain temperature by as much as 4-5°C prior to HCA (in other words, the brain is often warmer than indicated) (*see* Fig. 13–5).[196] Therefore, a key issue in the application of HCA is the duration of cooling needed to ensure brain temperature equilibration.

To address this issue, our group developed a mathematical model of human brain heat transport.[315] The model allowed us to determine factors that have the

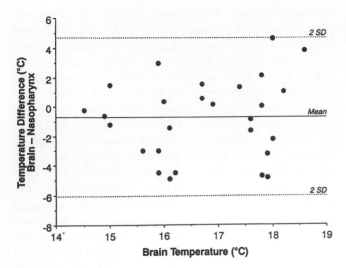

FIGURE 13–5. Difference between brain temperature and nasopharyngeal temperature in adults just before hypothermic circulatory arrest. *(Reproduced with permission Stone JG, Young WL, Smith CR, et al: Do standard monitoring sites reflect true brain temperature when profound hypothermia is rapidly induced and reversed? Anesthesiology 1995; 82:344–351.)*

greatest effect on the rate, and the completeness, of brain cooling during CPB. Using this model, a computer simulation of cooling the infant brain from 37° to 17°C indicated that 22 to 26 minutes may be required before brain temperature equilibration is complete. This prediction is consistent with the findings of the above studies and suggests that, often, inadequate time is provided for brain cooling before HCA. The model also indicated that packing the head in ice will increase the rate of brain cooling, although more in children than in adults. Given the inaccuracy of indirect brain temperature monitors, the time dependence of cooling, and results of clinical studies, it seems advisable to maintain perfusion cooling for 5 to 10 minutes after attaining target temperature to increase the likelihood of truly achieving desired brain temperature.

Using retrospective data, Jonas et al. reported that postoperative developmental outcome in children undergoing HCA seemed to be better in those who were managed with the pH-stat technique as compared with those who received α-stat management (*see Hypothermic Acid–Base Management During Moderate Hypothermia, above*).[316] The authors noted that the prearrest cooling duration in their population was somewhat short, 14.5 ± 6.2 minutes. They hypothesized that the better postoperative developmental outcome in the (hypercarbic) pH-stat patients was due to greater CBF during prearrest cooling, resulting in more complete brain cooling. α-stat patients were proposed as having lesser CBF and, consequently, to have had incomplete brain cooling before arrest. Indeed, some animal studies suggest ventilatory gas mixtures containing 7 to 10% CO_2

may increase the rate of brain cooling during CPB, presumably because of increased CBF.[317,318] On this basis, many groups in the 1970s and 1980s added CO_2 to their ventilatory gas mixtures during cooling (achieving concentrations of 2.5 to 10%).[297,300] Nevertheless, numerous studies do not support this practice. Using a rabbit model of CPB, our group found no difference in the rate of brain cooling from 37° to 17°C between groups managed with either α-stat or pH-stat strategies.[319] Watanabe et al., ventilating dogs with either 5% CO_2/95% O_2 (pH-stat conditions) or 100% O_2 (α-stat conditions), observed no difference in the rate of brain cooling to 20°C.[318] Aoki et al.,[320] and Kirshbom et al.,[321] cooling piglets to 18°C, also found no difference in the rate of brain cooling between α-stat and pH-stat management. Likewise, in human infants, Burrows et al. found no difference in cerebral perfusion between α-stat and pH-stat when brain temperatures were <25°C.[322] Despite differences in P_aCO_2 between α-stat and pH-stat management, CBF differences often may not be sufficiently great to substantively affect the rate of brain cooling.

An alternative explanation for the developmental outcome differences observed by Jonas et al.[316] is that pH-stat management might have some "neuroprotective" effect. Using our rabbit model of CPB, we demonstrated, at 17°C, that pH-stat management reduced CMR_{O_2} ~ 40% below that achieved with α-stat management.[319] A similar observation was made by Skaryak et al. in pigs.[323] pH-stat-induced CMR_{O_2} reduction may be due to suppression of cerebral metabolism by the greater P_aCO_2 of pH-stat management. As discussed above (*see* section on *Hypothermic Acid–Base Management During Hypothermia*), most enzyme reaction rates are pH-dependent, and many enzymes have pH optima that follow the predictions of α-stat theory. Because pH-stat management creates a relatively acidic intracellular environment, this would be expected to decrease enzyme reaction rates, ATP consumption, and, consequently, CMR_{O_2}. It is possible the additional CMR reduction of pH-stat management may significantly increase the allowable duration of HCA before onset of terminal membrane depolarization and, thereby, provide an extra measure of brain protection.

It is very important to note, however, that although membrane depolarization is the first step in the ischemic cascade, it is not the sole determinant of neurologic outcome. When depolarization occurs, many subsequent events and processes (calcium influx, excitatory neurotransmitter release, reperfusion injury) play critical roles in determining the final extent of neurologic injury.[179,183,324] How, or if, hypothermic acid–base management affects each of these processes and, consequently, net neurologic outcome in the setting of complete global cerebral ischemia (i.e., HCA) currently is unknown. The existing literature is contradictory. Watanabe et al. showed recovery of brain Po_2 and brain pH after HCA was more complete in animals receiving α-stat management as compared to pH-stat management.[318] In contrast, Aoki et al.[320] and Hiramatsu et al.[325] observed more rapid normalization of brain pH and ATP after HCA with pH-stat management. Kirshbom et al. observed no differences in recovery of CBF and CMR_{O_2} after HCA between α-stat and pH-stat management in piglets.[321] However, in this latter study, in animals with systemic-pulmonary collaterals, recovery was slightly better in pH-stat animals. It has been suggested that systemic-pulmonary collaterals, which are common in children with cyanotic heart disease, may increase the risk of perioperative neurologic injury.[326] Such shunts are proposed to divert blood away from the cerebral circulation during pre-HCA cooling and result in impaired brain cooling.[326] The hypercarbia of pH-stat management may tend to simultaneously dilate the cerebral vasculature and constrict the pulmonic vasculature. In theory, this will increase CBF and improve brain cooling. The findings of Kirshbom et al. are consistent with that hypothesis. Nevertheless, currently, it is unknown which hypothermic acid–base strategy (α-stat versus pH-stat, if either) provides optimal neurologic outcome for patients requiring HCA.

In a series of reports, Greeley et al. demonstrated that HCA alters CBF and CMR_{O_2} in the post-HCA period. Children undergoing cardiac surgery with *continuous* CPB, with either moderate (28°C) or profound (18°C) hypothermia, had restoration of CBF and CMR_{O_2} to pre-bypass levels upon warming and separation from CPB.[178,327,328] In contrast, children undergoing HCA at 18°C (39 ± 17 minutes) were found to have significantly decreased CMR_{O_2}, brain oxygen extraction, and CBF in the warming and post-CPB periods. Greeley's work clearly showed, even when the duration of HCA is well within the clinically "safe" period, that brain physiology is disordered for some time afterward. Subsequent clinical studies, using TCD to observe CBF velocity patterns, have been consistent with Greeley's findings.[329-331]

Animal studies by Swain et al., using ^{31}P nuclear magnetic resonance techniques, show that during HCA, progressive intracellular acidosis develops in the brain, along with ATP and creatine phosphate depletion.[332] Although these biochemical changes could be prevented by maintaining systemic flow at only 10 mL•kg^{-1}•min^{-1}, 5 mL•kg^{-1}•min^{-1} was not adequate. HCA with an intermittent period of reperfusion, sometimes used when prolonged HCA is necessary, did not support brain biochemistry as well as continuous low-flow CPB. These investigators also found that intermittent perfusion of the cerebral circulation with a cold (4°C) crystalloid solution ("cerebroplegia") during HCA maintained intracellular pH and energy state far better than HCA alone, with a shorter latency to EEG recovery upon rewarming (36 ± 6

minutes versus 117 ± 23 minutes, respectively; $P < 0.05$).[333] Animals receiving cerebroplegia were found to have better neurologic outcome after 2 hours of HCA than a group undergoing HCA alone.[334] Notably, neurologic outcome also was significantly improved in a group that simply had their heads packed in ice during the arrest period (the HCA-alone group did not). Therefore, much of the beneficial effect of "cerebroplegia" simply may have been by maintaining cerebral hypothermia during the arrest interval. Indeed, many studies show that, during HCA, brain temperature drifts toward ambient room temperature. By decreasing skull temperature, packing the head in ice reduces the temperature gradient for conductive heat gain[315] and helps maintain cerebral hypothermia during HCA. In animals models, simply packing the head in ice significantly improves neurologic tolerance to HCA.[334,335]

Until recently, delayed recovery of CBF, CMR_{O_2}, and electrophysiology after HCA was not clearly associated with poor clinical neurologic outcome. Indeed, in Greeley's studies, neurologic outcome in the HCA and continuous flow groups were indistinguishable. However, a randomized prospective trial of HCA versus low-flow CPB (50 mL•kg^{-1}•min^{-1}) in 171 children undergoing repair of D-transposition indicates that neurologic outcome is superior with low-flow CPB.[301,306] In this study, patients undergoing HCA were more likely to have postoperative seizures, as defined clinically or electroencephalographically, and had a greater release of brain isoenzyme of creatine kinase (CK-BB). The incidence of seizures and magnitude of CK-BB release both correlated with HCA duration. Overall, neurologic outcome did not differ between groups at discharge. However, at 1 year follow-up, infants assigned to HCA, as compared with those assigned to low-flow CPB, had a lower mean developmental scores ($P = 0.01$) and a higher proportion of scores ≥2 standard deviations below the population mean (27% versus 12% percent, $P = 0.02$).[306] Both developmental impairment and neurologic abnormalities were related to HCA duration.

The work of Swain and others show that a critical level of systemic flow is necessary to prevent brain biochemical deterioration during profound hypothermia, and yet, what that value is clinically is unknown. In fact, the critical perfusion level probably varies from patient to patient. TCD studies indicate that, in children, when systemic flows are less than 50 mL•kg^{-1}•min^{-1} that cerebral perfusion is, at times, so low as to be undetectable[330] and that CBF patterns may be distinctly abnormal in 30 to 40% of patients upon restoration of full flow and rewarming.[330,336] There are instances when low flow seems physiologically equivalent to no flow. Therefore, TCD may be useful as a monitor whereby systemic pressure and flow during low-flow CPB can be maintained at a level that maintains cerebral perfusion.

However, many cardiac procedures are not amenable to low-flow techniques. Consequently, there also is interest in methods of maintaining cerebral perfusion either via selective cerebral perfusion or retrograde cerebral perfusion. In general, retrograde cerebral perfusion seems to be clinically effective,[337-340] but a prospective clinical trial versus HCA alone has not yet been performed.

During the last 10 years, there has been a great deal of work documenting CPB results in an increase in inflammatory mediators, such as tumor necrosis factor, complement, and various interleukins. Whether inflammatory upregulation has primary or secondary adverse effects on the brain is currently unknown. However, there is some evidence that inflammatory upregulation adversely affects post-CPB pulmonary[341] and cardiac[342,343] function. Consequently, there has been interest in reducing or inhibiting these inflammatory mediators. One technique being investigated is modified ultrafiltration (MUF), which is used to decrease whole body water content and increase hemoglobin concentration.[344] MUF also seems to decrease circulating concentrations of inflammatory mediators.[345-348] In two reports, Journos et al. demonstrated improved systemic oxygenation and lesser periods of postoperative ventilation in children who received MUF after cardiac surgery.[347,348] Neither study addressed neurologic outcome. A provocative recent animal study by Skaryak et al. indicated that MUF increased post-HCA CMRo$_2$.[349] The mechanism by which MUF increased CMRo$_2$ was not addressed. Nevertheless, it suggests that post-HCA inflammatory processes might influence neurologic outcomes. This is likely to be an area of intensive future investigation.

Hemodilution and Postoperative Anemia

Hemodilution is used during CPB to compensate for hypothermia-induced increases in blood viscosity, to reduce blood utilization, and supposedly, to improve tissue oxygen delivery. Both human and animal studies indicate brain oxygenation is adequate with hematocrit (Hct) levels in the mid-20s during CPB at 27°C. Many centers, in an attempt to avoid transfusion, accept Hct levels in the 20s in the early postoperative period. At issue is whether marked anemia during the first few postoperative days could adversely affect neurologic outcome in patients who sustain a neurologic insult before or during CPB.

Hemodilution increases CBF in areas of cerebral ischemia, presumably via reduction of blood viscosity.[350,351] For this reason, hemodilution has been investigated as a possible treatment modality for stroke. In animal studies, hemodilution to a Hct of 30% seems to provide a moderate degree of neurologic bene-

fit,[350,352,353] although in one study, reduction in infarct size was critically dependent on maintenance of normal arterial pressure.[350] Similarly, in a few small studies of human stroke patients, hemodilution to a Hct level in the low 30s also seems to confer modest neurologic benefit.[354,355] Despite these encouraging reports, four other trials have failed to demonstrate any neurologic benefit with hemodilution in nonsurgical human stroke patients (Hct decreased from ~43% to ~36%).[356-359]

The normal cerebrovascular response to hemodilution is to increase both CBF and oxygen extraction. In this way, brain oxygen delivery and consumption are maintained at essentially normal levels.[360] For hemodilution to confer neurologic benefit in ischemic tissue, Hct must be reduced to a level at which increases in blood flow more than compensate for decreased arterial oxygen content, such that net cerebral oxygen delivery in the ischemic region actually increases. This is a delicate balance. Inadequate hemodilution is unlikely to confer benefit (perhaps the case in the human multicenter trials), and conversely, excessive hemodilution could be detrimental. In normal brain, increased CBF and oxygen extraction seem to be able to perserve brain oxygen consumption down to hemoglobin concentrations of ~6 g/dL.[360] However, because hemodilution-induced increases in CBF in penumbral tissue are not as great as those of normal brain[351] one would predict that penumbral tissue might not be as tolerant to marked hemodilution and that marked postoperative anemia could adversely affect neurologic outcome. Evidence is accumulating that this could be the case.

In 1982, Savageau et al. reported that neuropsychologic impairment 9 days after cardiac surgery was associated with Hct levels less than 30% in the first 12 hours after surgery.[100] In 1989, Shaw et al. reported that acute neurologic and neuropsychologic outcome was significantly worse in cardiac surgery patients hvaing the greatest perioperative reductions in Hct.[32] Using a middle cerebral artery occlusion model in dogs, Lee et al. found that although infarction volumes decreased with hemodilution to a hemoglobin concentration of 10 g/dL, infarction volumes increased with greater levels of hemodilution.[361] Similarly, using an embolic stroke model in rabbits, our group observed larger infarctions in animals randomized to a hemoglobin concentration of 6 g/dL versus those randomized to a hemoglobin concentration of 11 g/dL.[362] Collectively, these studies suggest that acute anemia can exert a detrimental effect on neurologic outcome, especially when hemoglobin concentrations are less than 10 g/dL (i.e., Hct < 30%).

Postoperatively, Hct levels in the low 30s, with maintenance of blood pressure and cardiac output, would seem unlikely to be detrimental and possibly may be beneficial to patients sustaining neurologic injury during surgery or CPB. On the other hand, there is reason to believe that postoperative Hct levels in the 20s may have an adverse effect on neurologic outcome. Recently, an American Society of Anesthesiologists task force formulated guidelines for blood component therapy.[363] The task force stated that "transfusion is rarely indicated when the hemoglobin concentration is greater than 10 g/dL and is almost always indicated when it is less than 6 g/dL, especially when the anemia is acute." It went on to state, "the determination of whether intermediate hemoglobin concentrations (6–10 g/dL) justify or require RBC transfusion should be based on the patient's risk for complications of inadequate oxygenation. . . ." In this author's opinion, transfusion is justified for patients who have an acute neurologic deficit and who are acutely and markedly anemic (i.e., those with Hct < 30%, Hgb < 10 g/dL). Use of oxygen-carrying hemodilutants, such as cross-linked or recombinant hemoglobins, hold real promise in the future treatment and management of acute cerebral ischemia.[352] These agents soon may be in our armamentarium.

■ REFERENCES

1. Tuman KJ, McCarthy RJ, Najafi H, Ivankovich AD: Differential effects of advanced age on neurologic and cardiac risks of coronary artery operations. *J Thorac Cardiovasc Surg* 1992; **104:**1510-1517.

2. Sotaniemi KA: Cerebral outcome after extracorporeal circulation. Comparison between prospective and retrospective evaluations. *Arch Neurol* 1983; **40:**75-77.

3. The Warm Heart Investigators: Randomised trial of normothermic versus hypothermic coronary bypass surgery. *Lancet* 1994; **343:**559-563.

4. McLean RF, Wong BI, Naylor CD, et al: Cardiopulmonary bypass, temperature, and central nervous system dysfunction. *Circulation* 1994; **90**(part 2):II-250-II-255.

5. Martin TD, Craver JM, Gott JP, et al: Prospective, randomized trial of retrograde warm blood cardioplegia: Myocardial benefit and neurologic threat. *Ann Thorac Surg* 1994; **57:**298-304.

6. Mora CT, Henson MB, Weintraub WS, et al: The effect of temperature management during cardiopulmonary bypass on neurologic and neuropsychologic outcomes in patients undergoing coronary revascularization. *J Thorac Cardiovasc Surg* 1996; **112:**514- 522.

7. Bashein G, Townes BD, Nessly ML, et al: A randomized study of carbon dioxide management during hypothermic cardiopulmonary bypass. *Anesthesiology* 1990; **72:**7-15.

8. Croughwell ND, Newman MF, Blumenthal JA, et al: Jugular bulb saturation and cognitive dysfunction after cardiopulmonary bypass. *Ann Thorac Surg* 1994; **58:**1702-1708.

9. Newman MF, Croughwell ND, Blumenthal JA, et al: Effect of aging on cerebral autoregulation during cardiopulmonary bypass. Association with postoperative cognitive dysfunction. *Circulation* 1994; **90**(part 2):II-243-II-249.

10. Newman MF, Kramer D, Croughwell ND, et al: Differential age effects of mean arterial pressure and rewarming on cognitive dysfunction after cardiac surgery. *Anesth Analg* 1995; **81:**236-242.

11. Murkin JM, Martzke JS, Buchan AM, Bentley C, Wong CJ: A randomized study of the influence of perfusion technique and pH management strategy in 316 patients undergoing coronary

12. artery bypass surgery. II. Neurologic and cognitive outcomes. *J Thorac Cardiovasc Surg* 1995; **110:**349-362.

12. Westaby S, Johnsson P, Parry AJ, et al: Serum S100 protein: A potential marker for cerebral events during cardiopulmonary bypass. *Ann Thorac Surg* 1996; **61:**88-92.

13. Edmonds HL, Griffiths LK, van der Laken J, Slater AD, Shields CB: Quantitative electroencephalographic monitoring during myocardial revascularization predicts postoperative disorientation and improves outcome. *J Thorac Cardiovasc Surg* 1992; **103:**555-563.

14. Bashein G, Nessly ML, Bledsoe SW, et al: Electroencephalography during surgery with cardiopulmonary bypass and hypothermia. *Anesthesiology* 1992; **76:**878-891.

15. Sellman M, Hindmarsh T, Ivert T, Semb BKH: Magnetic resonance imaging of the brain before and after open heart operations. *Ann Thorac Surg* 1992; **53:**807-812.

16. McConnell JR, Fleming WH, Chu WK, et al: Magnetic resonance imaging of the brain in infants and children before and after cardiac surgery. *Am J Dis Child* 1990; **144:**374-378.

17. Schmidt R, Fazekas F, Offenbacher H, et al: Brain magnetic resonance imaging in coronary artery bypass grafts: A pre- and postoperative assessment. *Neurology* 1993; **43:**775-778.

18. Simonson TM, Yuh WTC, Hindman BJ, Embrey RP, Halloran JI, Behrendt DM: Contrast MR imaging of the brain after high perfusion cardiopulmonary bypass. *Am J Neuroradiol* 1994; **15:**3-7.

19. Shaw P, Bates D, Cartlidge NEF, Heaviside D, Julian DG, Shaw DA: Early neurological complications of coronary artery bypass surgery. *BMJ* 1985; **291:**1384-1387.

20. Reed GL, Singer DE, Picard EH, DeSanctis RW: Stroke following coronary-artery bypass surgery. *N Engl J Med* 1988; **319:**1246-1250.

21. Carella F, Travaini G, Contri P, et al: Cerebral complications of coronary bypass surgery. A prospective study. *Acta Neurol Scand* 1988; **77:**158-163.

22. Faggioli GL, Curl GR, Ricotta JJ: The role of carotid screening before coronary artery bypass. *J Vasc Surg* 1990; **12:**724-731.

23. Lynn GM, Stefanko K, Reed JF, Gee W, Nicholas G: Risk factors for stroke after coronary artery bypass. *J Thorac Cardiovasc Surg* 1992; **104:**1518-1523.

24. Redmond JM, Greene PS, Goldsborough MA, et al: Neurologic injury in cardiac surgical patients with a history of stroke. *Ann Thorac Surg* 1996; **61:**42-47.

25. Akins CW, Moncure AC, Daggett WM, et al: Safety and efficacy of concomitant carotid and coronary artery operations. *Ann Thorac Surg* 1995; **60:**311-318.

26. Ricotta JJ, Faggioli GL, Castilone A, Hassett JM: Risk factors for stroke after cardiac surgery: Buffalo cardiac-cerebral study group. *J Vasc Surg* 1995; **21:**359-364.

27. Disch DL, O'Connor GT, Birkmeyer JD, Olmstead EM, Levy DG, Plume SK: Changes in patients undergoing coronary artery bypass grafting: 1987-1990. *Ann Thorac Surg* 1994; **57:**416-423.

28. Shaw PJ, Bates D, Cartlidge NEF, et al: Neurological complications of coronary artery bypass graft surgery: Six month follow-up study. *BMJ* 1986; **293:**165-167.

29. Shaw PJ, Bates D, Cartlidge NEF, et al: Early intellectual dysfunction following coronary bypass surgery. *Q J Med* 1986; **58:**59-68.

30. Shaw PJ, Bates D, Cartlidge NEF, et al: Neurologic and neuropsychological morbidity following major surgery: Comparison of coronary artery bypass and peripheral vascular surgery. *Stroke* 1987; **18:**700-707.

31. Shaw PJ, Bates D, Cartlidge NEF, et al: Long-term intellectual dysfunction following coronary artery bypass graft surgery: A six month follow-up study. *Q J Med* 1987; **62:**259-268.

32. Shaw PJ, Bates D, Cartlidge NEF, et al: An analysis of factors predisposing to neurological injury in patients undergoing coronary bypass operations. *Q J Med* 1989; **72:**633-646.

33. Sotaniemi KA: Brain damage and neurological outcome after open-heart surgery. *J Neurol Neurosurg Psychol* 1980; **43:**127-135.

34. Breuer AC, Furlan AJ, Hanson MR, et al: Central nervous system complications of coronary artery bypass graft surgery: Prospective analysis of 421 patients. *Stroke* 1983; **14:**682-687.

35. Heyer EJ, Delphin E, Adams DC, et al: Cerebral dysfunction after cardiac operations in elderly patients. *Ann Thorac Surg* 1995; **60:**1716-1722.

36. Mahanna EP, Blumenthal JA, White WD, et al: Defining neuropsychological dysfunction after coronary artery bypass grafting. *Ann Thorac Surg* 1996; **61:**1342-1347.

37. Slogoff S, Girgis KZ, Keats AS: Etiologic factors in neuropsychiatric complications associated with cardiopulmonary bypass. *Anesth Analg* 1982; **61:**903-911.

38. Treasure T, Smith PLC, Newman S, et al: Impairment of cerebral function following cardiac and other major surgery. *Eur J Cardiothorac Surg* 1989; **3:**216-221.

39. Townes BD, Bashein G, Hornbein TF, et al: Neurobehavioral outcomes in cardiac operations. A prospective controlled study. *J Thorac Cardiovasc Surg* 1989; **98:**774-782.

40. Newman S, Klinger L, Venn G, Smith P, Harrison M, Treasure T: Subjective reports of cognition in relation to assessed cognitive performance following coronary artery bypass surgery. *J Psychosomat Res* 1989; **33:**227-233.

41. Newman MF, Croughwell ND, Blumenthal JA, et al: Predictors of cognitive decline after cardiac operation. *Ann Thorac Surg* 1995; **59:**1326-1330.

42. Åberg T, Kihlgren M: Cerebral protection during open-heart surgery. *Thorax* 1977; **32:**525-533.

43. Smith PLC, Newman SP, Ell PJ, et al: Cerebral consequences of cardiopulmonary bypass. *Lancet* 1986; **1:**823-825.

44. Åberg T, Åhlund P, Kihlgren M: Intellectual function late after open-heart operation. *Ann Thorac Surg* 1983; **36:**680-683.

45. Baker AJ, Naser B, Benaroia M, Mazer CD: Cerebral microemboli during coronary artery bypass using different cardioplegia techniques. *Ann Thorac Surg* 1995; **59:**1187-1191.

46. Hartman GS, Yao F-S, Bruefach M, et al: Severity of aortic atheromatous disease diagnosed by transesophageal echocardiography predicts stroke and other outcomes associated with coronary artery surgery: A prospective study. *Anesth Analg* 1996; **83:**701-708.

47. Weintraub WS, Jones EL, Craver J, Guyton R, Cohen C: Determinants of prolonged length of hospital stay after coronary bypass surgery. *Circulation* 1989; **80:**276-284.

48. Sotaniemi KA, Juolasmaa A, Hokkanen ET: Neuropsychologic outcome after open-heart surgery. *Arch Neurol* 1981; **38:**2-8.

49. Pugsley W, Klinger L, Paschalis C, et al: Microemboli and cerebral impairment during cardiac surgery. *Vasc Surg* 1990; **24:**34-43.

50. Padayachee TS, Parsons S, Theobold R, Linley J, Gosling RG, Deverall PB: The detection of microemboli in the middle cerebral artery during cardiopulmonary bypass: A transcranial Doppler ultrasound investigation using membrane and bubble oxygenators. *Ann Thorac Surg* 1987; **44:**298-302.

51. van der Linden J, Casimir-Ahn H: When do cerebral emboli appear during open heart operations? A transcranial Doppler study. *Ann Thorac Surg* 1991; **51:**237-241.

52. Clark RE, Brillman J, Davis DA, Lovell MR, Price TRP, Magovern GJ: Microemboli during coronary artery bypass grafting. Genesis and effect on outcome. *J Thorac Cardiovasc Surg* 1995; **109:**249-258.

53. Barbut D, Hinton RB, Szatrowski TP, et al: Cerebral emboli detected during bypass surgery are associated with clamp removal. *Stroke* 1994; **25:**2398-2402.

54. Barbut D, Yao FS, Hager DN, Kavanaugh P, Trifiletti RR, Gold JP: Comparison of transcranial Doppler ultrasonography and transesophageal echocardiography to monitor emboli during coronary artery bypass surgery. *Stroke* 1996; **27:**87-90.

55. Katz ES, Tunick PA, Rusinek H, Ribakove G, Spencer FC, Kronzon I: Protruding aortic atheromas predict stroke in elderly patients undergoing cardiopulmonary bypass: Experience with intraoperative transesophageal echocardiography. *J Am Coll Cardiol* 1992; **20:**70-77.

56. Ribakove GH, Katz ES, Galloway AC, et al: Surgical implications of transesophageal echocardiography to grade the atheromatous aortic arch. *Ann Thorac Surg* 1992; **53:**758-763.

57. Wareing TH, Davila-Roman VG, Barzilai B, Murphy SF, Kouchoukos NT: Management of the severely atherosclerotic ascending aorta during cardiac operations. A strategy for detection and treatment. *J Thorac Cardiovasc Surg* 1992; **103:**453-462.

58. Wareing TH, Davila-Roman VG, Baily BB, et al: Strategy for the reduction of stroke incidence in cardiac surgical patients. *Ann Thorac Surg* 1993; **55:**1400-1408.

59. Bar-El Y, Goor DA: Clamping of the atherosclerotic ascending aorta during coronary artery bypass operations. Its cost in strokes. *J Thorac Cardiovasc Surg* 1992; **104:**469-474.

60. Konstadt SN, Reich DL, Quintana C, Levy M: The ascending aorta: How much does transesophageal echocardiography see? *Anesth Analg* 1994; **78:**240-244.

61. Konstadt SN, Reich DL, Kahn R, Viggiani RF: Transesophageal echocardiography can be used to screen for ascending aortic atherosclerosis. *Anesth Analg* 1995; **81:**225-228.

62. Duda AM, Letwin LB, Sutter FP, Goldman SM: Does routine use of aortic ultrasonography decrease the stroke rate in coronary artery bypass surgery? *J Vasc Surg* 1995; **21:**98-109.

63. Gardner TJ, Horneffer PJ, Manolio TA, Hoff SJ, Pearson TA: Major stroke after coronary artery bypass surgery: Changing magnitude of the problem. *J Vasc Surg* 1986; **3:**684-687.

64. Mills NL, Everson CT: Atherosclerosis of the ascending aorta and coronary artery bypass. *J Thorac Cardiovasc Surg* 1991; **102:**546-553.

65. McKibbin DW, Bulkley BH, Green WR, Gott VL, Hutchins GM: Fatal cerebral atheromatous embolization after cardiopulmonary bypass. *J Thorac Cardiovasc Surg* 1976; **71:**741-745.

66. Parker FB, Marvasti MA, Bove EL: Neurologic complications following coronary artery bypass. The role of atherosclerotic emboli. *J Thorac Cardiovasc Surg* 1985; **33:**207-209.

67. Singh AK, Bert AA, Feng WC, Rotenberg FA: Stroke during coronary artery bypass grafting using hypothermic versus normothermic perfusion. *Ann Thorac Surg* 1995; **59:**84-89.

68. Marschall K, Kanchuger M, Kessler K, et al: Superiority of transesophageal echocardiography in detecting aortic arch atheromatous disease: Identification of patients at increased risk of stroke during cardiac surgery. *J Cardiothorac Vasc Anesth* 1994; **8:**5-13.

69. Blauth CI, Cosgrove DM, Webb BW, et al: Atheroembolism from the ascending aorta. An emerging problem in cardiac surgery. *J Thorac Cardiovasc Surg* 1992; **103:**1104-1112.

70. Aranki SF, Rizzo RJ, Adams DH, et al: Single-clamp technique: An important adjunct to myocardial and cerebral protection in coronary operations. *Ann Thorac Surg* 1994; **58:**296-303.

71. Grossi EA, Kanchuger MS, Schwartz DS, et al: Effect of cannula length on aortic arch flow: Protection of the atheromatous aortic arch. *Ann Thorac Surg* 1995; **59:**710-712.

72. Sabik JF, Lytle BW, McCarthy PM, Cosgrove DM: Axillary artery: An alternative site of arterial cannulation for patients with extensive aortic and peripheral vascular disease. *J Thorac Cardiovasc Surg* 1995; **109:**885-891.

73. Balderman SC, Gutierrez IZ, Makula P, Bhayana JN, Gage AA: Noninvasive screening for asymptomatic carotid artery disease prior to cardiac operation. *J Thorac Cardiovasc Surg* 1983; **85:**427-433.

74. Barnes RW, Liebman PR, Marszalek PB, Kirk CL, Goldman MH: The natural history of asymptomatic carotid disease in patients undergoing cardiovascular surgery. *Surgery* 1981; **90:**1075-1083.

75. Turnipseed WD, Berkoff HA, Belzer FO: Postoperative stroke in cardiac and peripheral vascular disease. *Ann Surg* 1980; **192:** 365-368.

76. Breslau PJ, Fell G, Ivey TD, Bailey WW, Miller DW, Strandness DE: Carotid arterial disease in patients undergoing coronary artery bypass operations. *J Thorac Cardiovasc Surg* 1981; **82:**765-767.

77. Brener BJ, Brief DK, Alpert J, Goldenkranz RJ, Parsonnet V: The risk of stroke in patients with asymptomatic carotid stenosis undergoing cardiac surgery: A follow-up study. *J Vasc Surg* 1987; **5:**269-279.

78. Salasidis GC, Latter DA, Steinmetz OK, Blair J-F, Graham AM: Carotid artery duplex scanning in preoperative assessment for coronary artery revascularization: The association between peripheral vascular disease, carotid artery stenosis, and stroke. *J Vasc Surg* 1995; **21:**154-162.

79. Schwartz LB, Bridgman AH, Kieffer RW, et al: Asymptomatic carotid artery stenosis and stroke in patients undergoing cardiopulmonary bypass. *J Vasc Surg* 1995; **21:**146-153.

80. Hertzer NR, Loop FD, Beven EG, O'Hara PJ, Krajewski LP: Surgical staging for simultaneous coronary and carotid disease: A study including prospective randomization. *J Vasc Surg* 1989; **9:**455-463.

81. Rizzo RJ, Whittemore AD, Couper GS, et al: Combined carotid and coronary revascularization: The preferred approach to the severe vasculopath. *Ann Thorac Surg* 1992; **54:**1099-1109.

82. Ivey TD, Strandness DE, Williams DB, Langlois Y, Misbach GA, Kruse AP: Management of patients with carotid bruit undergoing cardiopulmonary bypass. *J Thorac Cardiovasc Surg* 1984; **87:** 183-189.

83. Ropper AH, Wechsler LR, Wilson LS: Carotid bruit and the risk of stroke in elective surgery. *N Engl J Med* 1982; **307:**1388-1390.

84. von Reutern GM, Hetzel A, Birnbaum D, Schlosser V: Transcranial Doppler ultrasonography during cardiopulmonary bypass in patients with severe carotid stenosis or occlusion. *Stroke* 1988; **19:**674-680.

85. Gravlee GP, Roy RC, Stump DA, Hudspeth AS, Rogers AT, Prough DS: Regional cerebrovascular reactivity to carbon dioxide during cardiopulmonary bypass in patients with cerebrovascular disease. *J Thorac Cardiovasc Surg* 1990; **99:**1022-1029.

86. Johnsson P, Algotsson L, Ryding E, Ståhl E, Messeter K: Cardiopulmonary perfusion and cerebral blood flow in bilateral carotid artery disease. *Ann Thorac Surg* 1991; **51:**579-584.

87. Furlan AJ, Craciun AR: Risk of stroke during coronary artery bypass graft surgery in patients with internal carotid artery disease documented by angiography. *Stroke* 1985; **15:**797-799.

88. Schultz RD, Sterpetti AV, Feldhaus RJ: Early and late results in patients with carotid disease undergoing myocardial revascularization. *Ann Thorac Surg* 1988; **45:**603-609.

89. Gerraty RP, Gates PC, Doyle JC: Carotid stenosis and perioperative stroke risk in symptomatic and asymptomatic patients undergoing vascular or coronary surgery. *Stroke* 1993; **24:**1115-1118.

90. Barnes RW, Nix ML, Sansonetti B, Turley DG, Goldman MR: Late outcome of untreated asymptomatic carotid disease following cardiovascular operations. *J Vasc Surg* 1985; **2:**843-849.

91. Roederer GO, Langlois YE, Jager KA, et al: The natural history of carotid arterial disease in asymptomatic patients with cervical bruits. *Stroke* 1984; **15:**605-613.

92. Hobson RW II, Weiss DG, Fields WS, et al: Efficacy of carotid endarterectomy for asymptomatic carotid stenosis. *N Engl J Med* 1993; **328:**221-227.

93. Executive Committee for the Asymptomatic Carotid Atherosclerosis Study: Endarterectomy for asymptomatic carotid artery stenosis. *JAMA* 1995; **273:**1421-1428.

94. Mackey WC, Khabbaz K, Bojar R, O'Donnell TF: Simultaneous carotid endarterectomy and coronary bypass: Perioperative risk and long-term survival. *J Vasc Surg* 1996; **24:**58-64.

95. Slogoff S, Reul GJ, Keats AS, et al: Role of perfusion pressure and flow in major organ dysfunction after cardiopulmonary bypass. *Ann Thorac Surg* 1990; **50:**911-918.

96. Beall AC, Jones JW, Guinn GA, Svensson LG, Nahas C: Cardiopulmonary bypass in patients with previously completed stroke. *Ann Thorac Surg* 1993; **55:**1383-1385.

97. Kuroda Y, Uchimoto R, Kaieda R, et al: Central nervous system complications after cardiac surgery: A comparison between coronary artery bypass grafting and valve surgery. *Anesth Analg* 1993; **76:**222-227.

98. Mayberg MR, Wilson SE, Yatsu F, et al: Carotid endarterectomy and prevention of cerebral ischemia in symptomatic carotid stenosis. *JAMA* 1991; **266:**3289-3294.

99. NASCE Trial Collaborators: Beneficial effect of carotid endarterectomy in symptomatic patients with high-grade carotid stenosis. *N Engl J Med* 1991; **325:**445-453.

100. Savageau JA, Stanton BA, Jenkins CD, Klein MD: Neuropsychological dysfunction following elective cardiac operation. I. Early assessment. *J Thorac Cardiovasc Surg* 1982; **84:**585-594.

101. Hartman RB, Harrison EE, Pupello DF, Vijayanagar R, Sbar SS: Characteristics of left ventricular thrombus resulting in perioperative embolism. *J Thorac Cardiovasc Surg* 1983; **86:**706-709.

102. Breuer AC, Franco I, Marzewski D, Soto-Velasco J: Left ventricular thrombi seen by ventriculography are a significant risk factor for stroke in open-heart surgery (abstract). *Ann Neurol* 1981; **10:**103-104.

103. Ehrenhaft JL, Claman MA, Layton JM, Zimmerman GR: Cerebral complications of open-heart surgery: further observations. *J Thorac Cardiovasc Surg* 1961; **42:**514-526.

104. Lindberg DAB, Lucas FV, Sheagren J, Malm JR: Silicone embolization during clinical and experimental heart surgery employing a bubble oxygenator. *Am J Pathol* 1961; **39:**129-144.

105. Brierly JB: Neuropathological findings in patients dying after open-heart surgery. *Thorax* 1963; **18:**291-304.

106. Orenstein JM, Sato N, Aaron B, Buchholz B, Bloom S: Microemboli observed in deaths following cardiopulmonary bypass surgery: silicone antifoam agents and polyvinyl chloride tubing as sources of emboli. *Hum Pathol* 1982; **13:**1082-1090.

107. Solis RT, Noon GP, Beall AC, DeBakey ME: Particulate microembolism during cardiac operation. *Ann Thorac Surg* 1974; **17:** 332-344.

108. Clark RE, Margraf HW, Beauchamp RA: Fat and solid filtration in clinical perfusions. *Surgery* 1975; **77:**216-224.

109. Dimmick JE, Bove KE, McAdams AJ, Benzing G: Fiber embolization — A hazard of cardiac surgery and catheterization. *N Engl J Med* 1975; **292:**685-687.

110. Reed CC, Romagnoli A, Taylor DE, Clark DK: Particulate matter in bubble oxygenators. *J Thorac Cardiovasc Surg* 1974; **68:**971-974.

111. Dutton RC, Edmunds LH: Measurement of emboli in extracorporeal perfusion systems. *J Thorac Cardiovasc Surg* 1973; **65:** 523-530.

112. Guidoin RG, Awad JA, Laperche Y, Morin PJ, Haggis GH: Nature of deposits in a tubular membrane oxygenator after prolonged extracorporeal circulation. *J Thorac Cardiovasc Surg* 1975; **69:** 479-491.

113. Dutton RC, Edmunds LH, Hutchinson JC, Roe BB: Platelet aggregate emboli produced in patients during cardiopulmonary bypass with membrane and bubble oxygenators and blood filters. *J Thorac Cardiovasc Surg* 1974; **67:**258-265.

114. Allardyce DB, Yoshida SH, Ashmore PG: The importance of microembolism in the pathogenesis of organ dysfunction caused by prolonged use of the pump oxygenator. *J Thorac Cardiovasc Surg* 1966; **52:**706-715.

115. Ashmore PG, Svitek V, Ambrose P: The incidence and effects of particulate aggregation and microembolism in pump-oxygenator systems. *J Thorac Cardiovasc Surg* 1968; **55:**691-697.

116. Hill JD, Aguilar MJ, Baranco A, de Lanerolle P, Gerbode F: Neuropathological manifestations of cardiac surgery. *Ann Thorac Surg* 1969; **7:**409-419.

117. Carlson RG, Lande AJ, Ivey LA, et al: The Lande-Edwards membrane oxygenator for total cardiopulmonary support in 110 patients during heart surgery. *Surgery* 1972; **72:**913-919.

118. Carlson RG, Lande AJ, Landis B, et al: The Lande-Edwards membrane oxygenator during heart surgery. *J Thorac Cardiovasc Surg* 1973; **66:**894-905.

119. Kessler J, Patterson RH: The production of microemboli by various blood oxygenators. *Ann Thorac Surg* 1970; **9:**221-228.

120. Abts LR, Beyer RT, Galletti PM, et al: Computerized discrimination of microemboli in extracorporeal circuits. *Am J Surg* 1978; **135:**535-538.

121. Yost G: The bubble oxygenator as a source of gaseous microemboli. *Med Instrum* 1985; **19:**67-69.

122. Liu JF, Su ZK, Ding WX: Quantitation of particulate microemboli during cardiopulmonary bypass: Experimental and clinical studies. *Ann Thorac Surg* 1992; **54:**1196-1202.

123. Solis RT, Kennedy PS, Beall AC, Noon GP, DeBakey ME: Cardiopulmonary bypass. Microembolization and platelet aggregation. *Circulation* 1975; **52:**103-108.

124. Patterson RH, Kessler J: Microemboli during cardiopulmonary bypass detected by ultrasound. *Surg Gynecol Obstet* 1969; **129:**505-510.

125. Gallagher EG, Pearson DT: Ultrasonic identification of sources of gaseous microemboli during open heart surgery. *Thorax* 1973; **28:**295-305.

126. Padayachee TS, Parsons S, Theobold R, Linley J, Gosling RG, Deverall PB: The effect of arterial filtration on reduction of gaseous microemboli in the middle cerebral artery during cardiopulmonary bypass. *Ann Thorac Surg* 1988; **45:**647-649.

127. Loop FD, Szabo J, Rowlinson RD, Urbanek K: Events related to microembolism during extracorporeal perfusion in man: Effectiveness of in-line filtration recorded by ultrasound. *Ann Thorac Surg* 1976; **21:**412-420.

128. Blauth CI, Arnold JV, Schulenberg WE, McCartney AC, Taylor KM, Loop FD: Cerebral microembolism during cardiopulmonary bypass. *J Thorac Cardiovasc Surg* 1988; **95:**668-676.

129. Pugsley W, Klinger L, Paschalis C, Treasure T, Harrison M, Newman S: The impact of microemboli during cardiopulmonary bypass on neuropsychological functioning. *Stroke* 1994; **25:**1393-1399.

130. Blauth CI, Smith P, Newman S, et al: Retinal microembolism and neuropsychological deficit following clinical cardiopulmonary bypass: Comparison of a membrane and a bubble oxygenator. *Eur J Cardiothorac Surg* 1989; **3:**135-139.

131. Oka Y, Moriwaki KM, Hong Y, et al: Detection of air emboli in the left heart by M-mode transesophageal echocardiography following cardiopulmonary bypass. *Anesthesiology* 1985; **63:**109-113.

132. Oka Y, Inoue T, Hong Y, Sisto DA, Strom JA, Frater RWM: Retained intracardiac air. Transesophageal echocardiography for definition of incidence and monitoring removal by improved techniques. *J Thorac Cardiovasc Surg* 1986; **91:**329-338.

133. Orihashi K, Matsuura Y, Hamanaka Y, et al: Retained intracardiac air in open heart operations examined by transesophageal echocardiography. *Ann Thorac Surg* 1993; **55:**1467-1471.

134. Orihashi K, Matsuura Y, Sueda T, Shikata H, Mitsui N, Sueshiro M: Pooled air in open heart operations examined by transesophageal echocardiography. *Ann Thorac Surg* 1996; **61:**1377-1380.

135. Tingleff J, Joyce FS, Pettersson G: Intraoperative echocardiographic study of air embolism during cardiac operations. *Ann Thorac Surg* 1995; **60:**673-677.

136. Topol EJ, Humphrey LS, Borkon AM, et al: Value of intraoperative left ventricular microbubbles detected by transesophageal two-dimensional echocardiography in predicting neurologic outcome after cardiac operations. *Am J Cardiol* 1985; **56:**773-775.

137. Butler BD, Laine GA, Leiman BC, et al: Effect of the Trendelenburg position on the distribution of arterial air emboli in dogs. *Ann Thorac Surg* 1988; **45:**198-202.

138. Feerick AE, Johnston WE, Jenkins LW, Lin CY, Mackay JH, Prough DS: Hyperglycemia during hypothermic canine cardiopulmonary bypass increases cerebral lactate. *Anesthesiology* 1995; **82:**512-520.

139. Lanier WL: Glucose management during cardiopulmonary bypass: Cardiovascular and neurologic implications (editorial). *Anesth Analg* 1991; **72:**423-427.

140. de Courten-Myers GM, Kleinholz M, Wagner KR, Myers RE: Fatal strokes in hyperglycemic cats. *Stroke* 1989; **20:**1707-1715.

141. Nedergaard M: Transient focal ischemia in hyperglycemia rats is associated with increased cerebral infarction. *Brain Res* 1987; **408:**79-85.

142. Prado R, Ginsberg MD, Dietrich WD, Watson BD, Busto R: Hyperglycemia increases infarct size in collaterally perfused but not end-arterial vascular territories. *J Cereb Blood Flow Metab* 1988; **8:**186-192.

143. Lanier WL, Stangland KJ, Scheithauer BW, Milde JH, Michenfelder JD: The effects of dextrose infusion and head position on neurologic outcome after complete cerebral ischemia in primates: Examination of a model. *Anesthesiology* 1987; **66:**39-48.

144. Nakakimura K, Fleisher JE, Drummond JC, et al: Glucose administration before cardiac arrest worsens neurologic outcome in cats. *Anesthesiology* 1990; **72:**1005-1011.

145. Warner DS, Gionet TX, Todd MM, McAllister AM: Insulin-induced normoglycemia improves ischemic outcome in hyperglycemic rats. *Stroke* 1992; **23:**1775-1781.

146. Combs DJ, Dempsey RJ, Maley M, Donaldson D, Smith C: Relationship between plasma glucose, brain lactate, and intracellular pH during cerebral ischemia in gerbils. *Stroke* 1990; **21:**936-942.

147. Folbergrová J, Memezawa H, Smith M-L, Siesjö BK: Focal and perifocal changes in tissue energy state during middle cerebral artery occlusion in normo- and hyperglycemic rats. *J Cereb Blood Flow Metab* 1992; **12:**25-33.

148. Wagner KR, Kleinholz M, de Courten-Myers GM, Myers RE: Hyperglycemic versus normoglycemic stroke: Topography of brain metabolites, intracellular pH, and infarct size. *J Cereb Blood Flow Metab* 1992; **12:**213-222.

149. Anderson RV, Siegman MG, Balaban RS, Ceckler TL, Swain JA: Hyperglycemia increases cerebral intracellular acidosis during circulatory arrest. *Ann Thorac Surg* 1992; **54:**1126-1130.

150. Wagner SR, Lanier WL: Metabolism of glucose, glycogen, and high-energy phosphates during complete cerebral ischemia: A comparison of normoglycemic, chronically hyperglycemic diabetic, and acutely hyperglycemic nondiabetic rats. *Anesthesiology* 1994; **81:**1516-1526.

151. Siesjö BK: Pathophysiology and treatment of focal cerebral ischemia. Part II: Mechanisms of damage and treatment. *J Neurosurg* 1992; **77:**337-354.

152. Dietrich WD, Alonso O, Busto R: Moderate hyperglycemia worsens acute blood-brain barrier injury after forebrain ischemia in rats. *Stroke* 1993; **24:**111-116.

153. Siesjö BK: Pathophysiology and treatment of focal cerebral ischemia. Part I: Pathophysiology. *J Neurosurg* 1992; **77:**169-184.

154. Zasslow MA, Pearl RG, Shuer LM, Steinberg GK, Lieberson RE, Larson CP: Hyperglycemia decreases acute neuronal ischemic changes after middle cerebral artery occlusion in cats. *Stroke* 1989; **20:**519-523.

155. Kraft SA, Larson C, Shuer LM, Steinberg GK, Benson GV, Pearl RG: Effect of hyperglycemia on neuronal changes in a rabbit model of focal cerebral ischemia. *Stroke* 1990; **21:**447-450.

156. de Courten-Myers G, Myers RE, Schoolfield L: Hyperglycemia enlarges infarct size in cerebrovascular occlusion in cats. *Stroke* 1988; **19:**623–630.

157. de Courten-Myers GM, Kleinholz M, Wagner KR, Myers RE: Normoglycemia (not hypoglycemia) optimizes outcome from middle cerebral artery occlusion. *J Cereb Blood Flow Metab* 1994; **14:** 227–236.

158. Nedergaard M, Astrup J: Infarct rim: Effect of hyperglycemia on direct current potential and [14C]2-deoxyglucose phosphorylation. *J Cereb Blood Flow Metab* 1986; **6:**607–615.

159. Back T, Kohno K, Hossmann KA: Cortical negative DC deflections following middle cerebral artery occlusion and KCl-induced spreading depression: Effect on blood flow, tissue oxygenation, and electroencephalogram. *J Cereb Blood Flow Metab* 1994; **14:**12–19.

160. Gill R, Andine P, Hillered L, Persson L, Hagberg H: The effect of MK-801 on cortical spreading depression in the penumbral zone following focal ischaemia in the rat. *J Cereb Blood Flow Metab* 1992; **12:**371–379.

161. Chen Q, Chopp M, Bodzin G, Chen H: Temperature modulation of cerebral depolarization during focal cerebral ischemia in rats: Correlation with ischemic injury. *J Cereb Blood Flow Metab* 1993; **13:**389–394.

162. Nedergaard M, Goldman SA, Desai S, Pulsinelli WA: Acid-induced death in neurons and glia. *J Neurosci* 1991; **11:**2489–2497.

163. Metz S, Keats AS: Benefits of a glucose-containing priming solution for cardiopulmonary bypass. *Anesth Analg* 1991; **72:**428.

164. Frasco P, Croughwell N, Blumenthal J, et al: Association between blood glucose level during cardiopulmonary bypass and neuropsychiatric outcome (abstract). *Anesthesiology* 1991; **75:**A55.

165. Shevde K, Kharode S, Harigopal P: Neuropsychological dysfunction following cardiac surgery. The role of intraoperative plasma glucose (abstract). *Anesthesiology* 1994; **81:**A222.

166. Lundgren J, Smith ML, Siesjö BK: Influence of moderate hypothermia on ischemic brain damage incurred under hyperglycemic conditions. *Exp Brain Res* 1991; **84:**91–101.

167. Lichtenstein SV, Ashe KA, El Dalati H, Cusimano RJ, Panos A, Slutsky AS: Warm heart surgery. *J Thorac Cardiovasc Surg* 1991; **101:**269–274.

168. Christakis GT, Koch JP, Deenar KA, et al: A randomized study of the systemic effects of warm heart surgery. *Ann Thorac Surg* 1992; **54:**449–457.

169. Sutton LN, Clark BJ, Norwood CR, Woodford EJ, Welsh FA: Global cerebral ischemia in piglets under conditions of mild and deep hypothermia. *Stroke* 1991; **22:**1567–1573.

170. Berntman L, Welsh FA, Harp JR: Cerebral protective effect of low-grade hypothermia. *Anesthesiology* 1981; **55:**495–498.

171. Chopp M, Knight R, Tidwell CD, Helpern JA, Brown E, Welch KMA: The metabolic effects of mild hypothermia on global cerebral ischemia and recirculation in the cat: Comparison to normothermia and hyperthermia. *J Cerebral Blood Flow Metab* 1989; **9:**141–148.

172. Michenfelder JD, Theye RA: The effects of anesthesia and hypothermia on canine cerebral ATP and lactate during anoxia produced by decapitation. *Anesthesiology* 1970; **33:**430–439.

173. Astrup J, Skovsted P, Gjerris F, Sorensen HR: Increase in extracellular potassium in the brain during circulatory arrest: Effects of hypothermia, lidocaine, and thiopental. *Anesthesiology* 1981; **55:**256–262.

174. Croughwell N, Smith LR, Quill T, et al: The effect of temperature on cerebral metabolism and blood flow in adults during cardiopulmonary bypass. *J Thorac Cardiovasc Surg* 1992; **103:**549–554.

175. Feddersen K, Aren C, Nilsson NJ, Radegran K: Cerebral blood flow and metabolism during cardiopulmonary bypass with special reference to effects of hypotension induced by prostacyclin. *Ann Thorac Surg* 1986; **41:**395–400.

176. Murkin JM, Farrar JK, Tweed A, McKenzie FN, Guiraudon G: Cerebral autoregulation and flow/metabolism coupling during cardiopulmonary bypass: The influence of P_aCO_2. *Anesth Analg* 1987; **66:**825–832.

177. Stephan H, Sonntag H, Lange H, Rieke H: Cerebral effects of anaesthesia and hypothermia. *Anaesthesia* 1989; **44:**310–316.

178. Greeley WJ, Kern FH, Ungerleider RM, et al: The effect of hypothermic cardiopulmonary bypass and total circulatory arrest on cerebral metabolism in neonates, infants and children. *J Thorac Cardiovasc Surg* 1991; **101:**783–794.

179. Todd MM, Warner DS: A comfortable hypothesis reevaluated. Cerebral metabolic depression and brain protection during ischemia (editorial). *Anesthesiology* 1992; **76:**161–164.

180. Busto R, Dietrich WD, Globus MYT, Valdes I, Scheinberg P, Ginsberg MD: Small differences in intraischemic brain temperature critically determine the extent of ischemic neuronal injury. *J Cereb Blood Flow Metab* 1987; **7:**729–738.

181. Natale JE, D'Alecy LG: Protection from cerebral ischemia by brain cooling without reduced lactate accumulation in dogs. *Stroke* 1989; **20:**770–777.

182. Welsh FA, Sims RE, Harris VA: Mild hypothermia prevents ischemic injury in gerbil hippocampus. *J Cereb Blood Flow Metab* 1990; **10:**557–563.

183. Ginsberg MD, Sternau LL, Globus MYT, Dietrich WD, Busto R: Therapeutic modulation of brain temperature: Relevance to ischemic brain injury. *Cerebrovasc Brain Metab Rev* 1992; **4:**189–225.

184. Globus MYT, Busto R, Dietrich WD, Martinez E, Valdes I, Ginsberg MD: Effect on ischemia on the in vivo release of striatal dopamine, glutamate, and gamma-aminobutyric acid studied by intracerebral microdialysis. *J Neurochem* 1988; **51:**1455–1464.

185. Globus MYT, Busto R, Dietrich WD, Martinez E, Valdes I, Ginsberg MD: Intra-ischemic extracellular release of dopamine and glutamate is associated with striatal vulnerability to ischemia. *Neurosci Lett* 1988; **91:**36–40.

186. Busto R, Globus MYT, Dietrich WD, Martinez E, Valdes I, Ginsberg MD: Effect of mild hypothermia on ischemia-induced release of neurotransmitter and free fatty acid in rat brain. *Stroke* 1989; **20:**904–910.

187. Baker AJ, Zornow MH, Grafe MR, et al: Hypothermia prevents ischemia-induced increases in hippocampal glycine concentrations in rabbits. *Stroke* 1991; **22:**666–673.

188. Siesjö BK: Pathophysiology and treatment of focal cerebral ischemia. Part I: Pathophysiology. *J Neurosurg* 1992; **77:**169–184.

189. Baiping L, Xiujuan T, Hongwei C, Qiming X, Quling G: Effect of moderate hypothermia on lipid peroxidation in canine brain tissue after cardiac arrest and resuscitation. *Stroke* 1994; **25:** 147–152.

190. Dempsey RJ, Combs DJ, Maley ME, Cowen DE, Roy MW, Donaldson DL: Moderate hypothermia reduces postischemic edema development and leukotriene production. *Neurosurgery* 1987; **21:**177–181.

191. Sano T, Drummond JC, Patel PM, Grafe MR, Watson JC, Cole DJ: A comparison of the cerebral protective effects of isoflurane and mild hypothermia in a model of incomplete forebrain ischemia in the rat. *Anesthesiology* 1992; **76:**221–228.

192. Ridenour TR, Warner DS, Todd MM, McAllister AM: Mild hypothermia reduces infarct size resulting from temporary but not permanent focal ischemia in rats. *Stroke* 1992; **23:**733–738.

193. Onesti ST, Baker CJ, Sun PP, Solomon RA: Transient hypothermia reduces focal ischemic brain injury in the rat. *Neurosurgery* 1991; **29:**369–373.

194. Kader A, Brisman MH, Maraire N, Huh JT, Solomon RA: The effect of mild hypothermia on permanent focal ischemia in the rat. *Neurosurgery* 1992; **31:**1056–1061.

195. Morikawa E, Ginsberg MD, Dietrich WD, et al: The significance of brain temperature in focal cerebral ischemia: Histopathological

consequences of middle cerebral artery occlusion in the rat. *J Cereb Blood Flow Metab* 1992; **12**:380-389.

196. Stone JG, Young WL, Smith CR, et al: Do standard monitoring sites reflect true brain temperature when profound hypothermia is rapidly induced and reversed? *Anesthesiology* 1995; **82**:344-351.

197. Stocchetti N, Paparella A, Bridelli F, Bacchi M, Piazza P, Zuccoli P: Cerebral venous oxygen saturation studied with bilateral samples in the internal jugular veins. *Neurosurgery* 1994; **34**:38-44.

198. Cook DJ, Oliver WC, Orszulak TA, Daly RC: A prospective, randomized comparison of cerebral venous oxygen saturation during normothermic and hypothermic cardiopulmonary bypass. *J Thorac Cardiovasc Surg* 1994; **107**:1020-1029.

199. Endoh H, Shimoji K: Changes in blood flow velocity in the middle cerebral artery during nonpulsatile hypothermic cardiopulmonary bypass. *Stroke* 1994; **25**:403-407.

200. Nakajima T, Kuro M, Hayaski Y, Kitaguchi K, Uchida O, Takaki O: Clinical evaluation of cerebral oxygen balance during cardiopulmonary bypass: On-line continuous monitoring of jugular venous oxyhemoglobin saturation. *Anesth Analg* 1992; **74**:630-635.

201. van der Linden J, Ekroth R, Lincoln C, Pugsley W, Scallan M, Tyden H: Is cerebral blood flow/metabolic mismatch during rewarming a risk factor after profound hypothermic procedures in small children? *Eur J Cardiothorac Surg* 1989; **3**:209-215.

202. Croughwell ND, Frasco P, Blumenthal JA, Leone BJ, White WD, Reves JG: Warming during cardiopulmonary bypass is associated with jugular bulb desaturation. *Ann Thorac Surg* 1992; **53**:827-832.

203. Minamisawa H, Smith M-L, Siesjo BK: The effect of mild hyperthermia and hypothermia on brain damage following 5, 10, and 15 minutes of forebrain ischemia. *Ann Neurol* 1990; **28**:26-33.

204. Dietrich WD, Busto R, Valdes I, Loor Y: Effects of normothermic versus mild hyperthermic forebrain ischemia in rats. *Stroke* 1990; **21**:1318-1325.

205. Reith J, Jørgensen HS, Pedersen PM, et al: Body temperature in acute stroke: Relation to stroke severity, infarct size, mortality, and outcome. *Lancet* 1996; **347**:422-425.

206. Azzimondi G, Bassein L, Nonino F, et al: Fever in acute stroke worsens prognosis. A prospective study. *Stroke* 1995; **26**:2040-2043.

207. Buss MI, McLean RF, Wong BI, et al: Cardiopulmonary bypass, rewarming, and central nervous system dysfunction. *Ann Thorac Surg* 1996; **61**:1423-1427.

208. Nathan HJ, Lavallee G: The management of temperature during hypothermic cardiopulmonary bypass: I — Canadian survey. *Can J Anaesth* 1995; **42**:669-671.

209. Cook DJ, Orszulak TA, Daly RC, Buda DA: Cerebral hyperthermia during cardiopulmonary bypass in adults. *J Thorac Cardiovasc Surg* 1996; **111**:268-269.

210. Birdi I, Regragui IA, Izzat MB, Bryan AJ, Angelini GD: Effects of cardiopulmonary perfusion temperature: A randomized, controlled trial (letter). *Ann Thorac Surg* 1996; **60**:744-751.

211. Rahn H, Reeves RB, Howell BJ: Hydrogen ion regulation, temperature, and evolution. *Am Rev Respir Dis* 1975; **112**:165-172.

212. Nattie EE: The alphastat hypothesis in respiratory control and acid-base balance. *J Appl Physiol* 1990; **69**:1201-1207.

213. Hickey PR, Hansen DD: Temperature and blood gases: The clinical dilemma of acid-base management for hypothermic cardiopulmonary bypass, in Tinker JH (ed): *Cardiopulmonary Bypass: Current Concepts and Controversies*. Philadelphia, WB Saunders Co, 1989, pp 1-20.

214. Malan A, Wilson TL, Reeves RB: Intracellular pH in cold-blooded vertebrates as a function of body temperature. *Respir Physiol* 1976; **28**:29-47.

215. Reeves RB: An imidazole alphastat hypothesis for vertebrate acid-base regulation: Tissue carbon dioxide content and body temperature in bullfrogs. *Respir Physiol* 1972; **14**:219-236.

216. Andritsch RF, Muravchick S, Gold MI: Temperature correction of arterial blood-gas parameters: A comparative review of methodology. *Anesthesiology* 1981; **55**:311-316.

217. Somero GN, White FN: Enzymatic consequences under alphastat regulation, in Rahn H, Prakash O (eds): *Acid-Base Regulation and Body Temperature*. Boston, Martinus Nijhoff Publishers, 1985, pp 35-80.

218. Somero GN: Protons, osmolytes, and fitness of internal milieu for protein function. *Am J Physiol* 1986: **251**:R197-213.

219. Malan A: Acid-base regulation during hibernation, in Rahn H, Prakash O (eds): *Acid-Base Regulation and Body Temperature*. Boston, Martinus Hijhoff Publishers, 1985, pp 33-53.

220. Malan A, Mioskowski E: pH-temperature interactions on protein function and hibernation: GDP binding to brown adipose tissue mitochondria. *J Comp Physiol B* 1988; **158**:487-493.

221. Prough DS, Rogers AT, Stump DA, Mills SA, Gravlee GP, Taylor C: Hypercarbia depresses cerebral oxygen consumption during cardiopulmonary bypass. *Stroke* 1990; **21**:1162-1166.

222. Rogers AT, Prough DS, Roy RC, et al: Cerebrovascular and cerebral metabolic effects of alterations in perfusion flow rate during hypothermic cardiopulmonary bypass in man. *J Thorac Cardiovasc Surg* 1992; **103**:363-368.

223. Stephan H, Weyland A, Kazmaier S, Henze T, Menck S, Sonntag H: Acid-base management during hypothermic cardiopulmonary bypass does not affect cerebral metabolism but does affect blood flow and neurological outcome. *Br J Anaesth* 1992; **69**:51-57.

224. Hindman BJ, Dexter F, Cutkomp J, Smith T, Todd MM, Tinker JH: Cerebral blood flow and metabolism do not decrease at stable brain temperature during cardiopulmonary bypass in rabbits. *Anesthesiology* 1992; **77**:342-350.

225. Hindman BJ, Dexter F, Cutkomp J, Smith T, Tinker JH: Hypothermic acid-base management does not affect cerebral metabolic rate for oxygen (CMR_{O_2}) at 27°C. A study during cardiopulmonary bypass in rabbits. *Anesthesiology* 1993; **79**:580-587.

226. Prough DS, Stump DA, Roy RC, et al: Response of cerebral blood flow to changes in carbon dioxide tension during hypothermic cardiopulmonary bypass. *Anesthesiology* 1986; **64**:576-581.

227. Johnsson P, Messeter K, Ryding E, Kugelberg J, Stahl E: Cerebral vasoreactivity to carbon dioxide during cardiopulmonary perfusion at normothermia and hypothermia. *Ann Thorac Surg* 1989; **48**:769-775.

228. Kern FH, Underleider RM, Quill TJ, et al: Cerebral blood flow response to changes in arterial carbon dioxide tension during hypothermic cardiopulmonary bypass in children. *J Thorac Cardiovasc Surg* 1991; **101**:618-622.

229. Hindman BJ, Funatsu N, Harrington J, Cutkomp J, Todd MM, Tinker JH: Cerebral blood flow response to $PaCO_2$ during hypothermic cardiopulmonary bypass in rabbits. *Anesthesiology* 1991; **75**:662-668.

230. Govier AV, Reves JG, McKay RD, et al: Factors and their influence on regional cerebral blood flow during nonpulsatile cardiopulmonary bypass. *Ann Thorac Surg* 1984; **38**:592-600.

231. Lundar T, Lindegaard KF, Froysaker T, Aaslid R, Grip A, Nornes H: Dissociation between cerebral autoregulation and carbon dioxide reactivity during nonpulsatile cardiopulmonary bypass. *Ann Thorac Surg* 1985; **40**:582-587.

232. Lundar T, Lindegaard KF, Froysaker T, et al: Cerebral carbon dioxide reactivity during nonpulsatile cardiopulmonary bypass. *Ann Thorac Surg* 1986; **41**:525-530.

233. Johnsson P, Messeter K, Ryding E, Nordstrom L, Stahl E: Cerebral blood flow and autoregulation during hypothermic cardiopulmonary bypass. *Ann Thorac Surg* 1987; **43**:386-390.

234. Rogers AT, Stump DA, Gravlee GP, et al: Response of cerebral blood flow to phenylephrine infusion during hypothermic cardiopulmonary bypass: Influence of $PaCO_2$ management. *Anesthesiology* 1988; **69**:547-551.

235. Brusino FG, Reves JG, Smith LR, Prough DS, Stump DA, McIntyre RW: The effect of age on cerebral blood flow during hypothermic cardiopulmonary bypass. *J Thorac Cardiovasc Surg* 1989; **97:**541-547.

236. Hindman BJ, Funatsu N, Harrington J, et al: Differences in cerebral blood flow between alpha-stat and pH-stat management are eliminated during periods of decreased systemic flow and pressure. *Anesthesiology* 1991; **74:**1096-1102.

237. Patel RL, Turtle MRJ, Chambers DJ, Newman S, Venn GE: Hyperperfusion and cerebral dysfunction. Effect of differing acid-base management during cardiopulmonary bypass. *Eur J Cardiothorac Surg* 1993; **7:**457-464.

238. Stockard JJ, Bickford RG, Schauble JF: Pressure-dependent cerebral ischemia during cardiopulmonary bypass. *Neurology* 1973; **23:**521-529.

239. Gold JP, Charlson ME, Williams-Russo P, et al: Improvement of outcomes after coronary artery bypass. A randomized trial comparing intraoperative high versus low mean arterial pressure. *J Thorac Cardiovasc Surg* 1995; **110:**1302-1314.

240. Cole DJ, Drummond JC, Osborne TN, Matsumura J: Hypertension and hemodilution during cerebral ischemia reduce brain injury and edema. *Am J Physiol* 1990; **259:**H211-H217.

241. Tranmer BI, Keller TS, Kindt GW, Archer D: Loss of cerebral regulation during cardiac output variations in focal cerebral ischemia. *J Neurosurg* 1992; **77:**253-259.

242. Dirnagl U, Pulsinelli W: Autoregulation of cerebral blood flow in experimental focal brain ischemia. *J Cereb Blood Flow Metab* 1990; **10:**327-336.

243. Astrup J, Sorensen PM, Sorensen HR: Inhibition of cerebral oxygen and glucose consumption in the dog by hypothermia, pentobarbital, and lidocaine. *Anesthesiology* 1981; **55:**263-268.

244. Astrup J, Sorensen PM, Sorensen HR: Oxygen and glucose consumption related to Na$^+$-K$^+$ transport in canine brain. *Stroke* 1981; **12:**726-730.

245. Michenfelder JD: The interdependency of cerebral functional and metabolic effects following massive doses of thiopental in the dog. *Anesthesiology* 1974; **41:**231-236.

246. Branston NM, Hope T, Symon L: Barbiturates in focal ischemia of primate cortex: Effects on blood flow distribution, evoked potential and extracellular potassium. *Stroke* 1979; **10:**647-653.

247. Verhaegen MJ, Todd MM, Warner DS: A comparison of cerebral ischemic flow thresholds during halothane/N$_2$O and Isoflurane/N$_2$O anesthesia in rats. *Anesthesiology* 1992; **76:**743-754.

248. Steen PA, Milde JH, Michenfelder JD: No barbiturate protection in a dog model of complete cerebral ischemia. *Ann Neurol* 1979; **5:**343-349.

249. Gisvold SE, Safar P, Hendrickx HHL, Rao G, Moossy J, Alexander J: Thiopental treatment after global brain ischemia in pigtailed monkeys. *Anesthesiology* 1984; **60:**88-96.

250. Brain Resuscitation Clinical Trial I Study Group: Randomized clinical study of thiopental loading in comatose survivors of cardiac arrest. *N Engl J Med* 1986; **314:**397-403.

251. Hoff JT, Smith AL, Hankinson HL, Nielsen SL: Barbiturate protection from cerebral infarction in primates. *Stroke* 1975; **6:**28-33.

252. Michenfelder JD, Milde JH: Influence of anesthetics on metabolic, functional and pathological responses to regional cerebral ischemia. *Stroke* 1975; **6:**405-410.

253. Michenfelder JD, Milde JH, Sundt TM: Cerebral protection by barbiturate anesthesia. *Arch Neurol* 1976; **33:**345-350.

254. Moseley J, Laurent JP, Molinari GF: Barbiturate attenuation of the clinical course and pathologic lesions in a primate stroke model. *Neurology* 1975; **25:**870-874.

255. Selman WR, Spetzler RF, Roessmann UR, Rosenblatt JI, Crumrine RC: Barbiturate-induced coma therapy for focal cerebral ischemia: Effect after temporary and permanent MCA occlusion. *J Neurosurg* 1981; **55:**220-226.

256. Warner DS, Zhou J, Ramani R, Todd MM: Reversible focal ischemia in the rat: Effects of halothane, isoflurane, and methohexital anesthesia. *J Cereb Blood Flow Metab* 1991; **11:**794-802.

257. Warner DS, Takaoka S, Wu B, et al: Electroencephalographic burst suppression is not required to elicit maximal neuroprotection from pentobarbital in a rat model of focal cerebral ischemia. *Anesthesiology* 1996; **84:**1475-1484.

258. Nussmeier NA, Arlund C, Slogoff SL: Neuropsychiatric complications after cardiopulmonary bypass: Cerebral protection by a barbiturate. *Anesthesiology* 1986; **64:**165-170.

259. Zaidan JR, Klochany AI, Martin WM, Ziegler JS, Harless DM, Andrews RB: Effect of thiopental on neurologic outcome following coronary artery bypass grafting. *Anesthesiology* 1991; **74:**406-411.

260. Woodcock TE, Murkin JM, Farrar JK, Tweed WA, Guivaudon GM, McKenzie N: Pharmacologic EEG suppression during cardiopulmonary bypass: Cerebral hemodynamic and metabolic effects of thiopental or isoflurane during hypothermia and normothermia. *Anesthesiology* 1987; **67:**218-224.

261. Helps SC, Meyer-Witting M, Reilly PL, Gorman DF: Increasing doses of intracarotid air and cerebral blood flow in rabbits. *Stroke* 1990; **21:**1340-1345.

262. Newman MF, Murkin JM, Roach G, et al: Cerebral physiologic effects of burst suppression doses of propofol during nonpulsatile cardiopulmonary bypass. *Anesth Analg* 1995; **81:**452-457.

263. Matsumoto T, Wolferth CC, Perlman MH: Effects of pulsatile and nonpulsatile perfusion upon cerebral and conjunctival microcirculation in dogs. *Am Surg* 1971; **37:**61-64.

264. Sanderson JM, Wright G, Sims FW: Brain damage in dogs immediately following pulsatile and non-pulsatile blood flow in extracorporeal circulation. *Thorax* 1972; **27:**275-286.

265. Dernevik L, Arvidsson S, William-Olsson G: Cerebral perfusion in dogs during pulsatile and nonpulsatile extracorporeal circulation. *J Cardiovasc Surg* 1985; **26:**32-35.

266. Tranmer BI, Gross CE, Kindt GW, Adey GR: Pulsatile versus nonpulsatile blood flow in the treatment of acute cerebral ischemia. *Neurosurgery* 1986; **19:**724-731.

267. Shepard RB, Kirklin JW: Relation of pulsatile flow to oxygen consumption and other variables during cardiopulmonary bypass. *J Thorac Cardiovasc Surg* 1969; **58:**694-702.

268. Raj JU, Kaapa P, Anderson J: Effect of pulsatile flow on microvascular resistance in adult rabbit lungs. *J Appl Physiol* 1992; **72:**73-81.

269. Jacobs LA, Klopp EH, Seamone W, Topaz SR, Gott VL: Improved organ function during cardiac bypass with a roller pump modified to deliver pulsatile flow. *J Thorac Cardiovasc Surg* 1969; **58:**703-712.

270. Minami K, Korner MM, Vyska K, Kleesiek K, Knobl H, Korfer R: Effects of pulsatile perfusion on plasma catecholamine levels and hemodynamics during and after cardiac operations with cardiopulmonary bypass. *J Thorac Cardiovasc Surg* 1990; **99:**82-91.

271. Williams GD, Seifen AB, Lawson NW, et al: Pulsatile perfusion versus conventional high-flow nonpulsatile perfusion for rapid core cooling and rewarming of infants for circulatory arrest in cardiac operation. *J Thorac Cardiovasc Surg* 1979; **78:**667-677.

272. Dunn J, Kirsh MM, Harness J, Carroll M, Straker J, Solan H: Hemodynamic, metabolic, and hematologic effects of pulsatile cardiopulmonary bypass. *J Thorac Cardiovasc Surg* 1974; **68:**138-147.

273. Watkins WD, Peterson MB, Kong DL, et al: Thromboxane and prostacyclin changes during cardiopulmonary bypass with and without pulsatile flow. *J Thorac Cardiovasc Surg* 1982; **84:**250-256.

274. Hutcheson IR, Griffith TM: Release of endothelium-derived relaxing factor is modulated both by frequency and amplitude of pulsatile flow. *Am J Physiol* 1991; **261:**H257-H262.

275. Angell James JE: The effects of altering mean pressure, pulse pressure and pulse frequency on the impulse activity in baroreceptor fibres from the aortic arch and right subclavian artery in the rabbit. *J Physiol (Lond)* 1971; **214**:65-88.

276. Chapleau MW, Abboud FM: Determinants of sensitization of carotid baroreceptors by pulsatile pressure in dogs. *Circ Res* 1989; **65**:566-577.

277. Chapleau MW, Hajduczok G, Abboud FM: Pulsatile activation of baroreceptors causes central facilitation of baroreflex. *Am J Physiol* 1989; **256**:H1735-H1741.

278. Nakayama K, Tamiya T, Yamamoto K, et al: High-amplitude pulsatile pump in extracorporeal circulation with particular reference to hemodynamics. *Surgery* 1963; **54**:798-809.

279. Minami K, Vyska K, Korfer R: Role of the carotid sinus in response of integrated venous system to pulsatile and nonpulsatile perfusion. *J Thorac Cardiovasc Surg* 1992; **104**:1639-1646.

280. Louagie YA, Gonzalez M, Collard E, et al: Does flow character of cardiopulmonary bypass make a difference? *J Thorac Cardiovasc Surg* 1992; **104**:1628-1638.

281. Dapper F, Neppl H, Wozniak G, et al: Effects of pulsatile and nonpulsatile perfusion mode during extracorporeal circulation — A comparative clinical study. *J Thorac Cardiovasc Surg* 1992; **40**:345-351.

282. Kono K, Philbin DM, Coggins CH, et al: Adrenocortical hormone levels during cardiopulmonary bypass with and without pulsatile flow. *J Thorac Cardiovasc Surg* 1983; **85**:129-133.

283. Frater RWM, Wakayama S, Oka Y, et al: Pulsatile cardiopulmonary bypass: Failure to influence hemodynamics or hormones. *Circulation* 1980; **62**(Suppl I):I-19-I-25.

284. Alston RP, Murray L, McLaren AD: Changes in hemodynamic variables during hypothermic cardiopulmonary bypass. Effects of flow rate, flow character, and arterial pH. *J Thorac Cardiovasc Surg* 1990; **100**:134-144.

285. Driessen JJ, Fransen G, Rondelez L, Schelstraete E, Gevaert L: Comparison of the standard roller pump and a pulsatile centrifugal pump for extracorporeal circulation during routine coronary artery bypass grafting. *Perfusion* 1991; **6**:303-311.

286. Alston RP, Singh M, McLaren AD: Systemic oxygen uptake during hypothermic cardiopulmonary bypass. Effects of flow rate, flow character, and arterial pH. *J Thorac Cardiovasc Surg* 1989; **98**:757-768.

287. Runge TM, Trinkle JK: Does flow character of cardiopulmonary bypass make a difference? (letter). *J Thorac Cardiovasc Surg* 1994; **107**:642-644.

288. Grossi EA, Connolly MW, Krieger KH, et al: Quantification of pulsatile flow during cardiopulmonary bypass to permit direct comparison of the effectiveness of various types of "pulsatile" and "nonpulsatile" flow. *Surgery* 1985; **98**:547-554.

289. Hindman BJ, Dexter F, Smith T, Cutkomp J: Pulsatile versus nonpulsatile flow. No difference in cerebral blood flow or metabolism during normothermic cardiopulmonary bypass in rabbits. *Anesthesiology* 1995; **82**:241-250.

290. Hindman BJ, Dexter F, Ryu KH, Smith T, Cutkomp J: Pulsatile versus nonpulsatile cardiopulmonary bypass: No difference in brain blood flow or metabolism at 27° C. *Anesthesiology* 1994; **80**:1137-1147.

291. Henze T, Stephan H, Sonntag H: Cerebral dysfunction following extracorporeal circulation for aortocoronary bypass surgery: No differences in neuropsychological outcome after pulsatile versus nonpulsatile flow. *J Thorac Cardiovasc Surg* 1990; **38**:65-68.

292. Murkin JM, Martzke JS, Buchan AM, Bentley C, Wong CJ: A randomized study of the influence of perfusion technique and pH management strategy in 316 patients undergoing coronary artery bypass surgery. I. Mortality and cardiovascular morbidity. *J Thorac Cardiovasc Surg* 1995; **110**:340-348.

293. O'Connor JV, Wilding T, Farmer P, Sher J, Ergin MA, Griepp RB: The protective effect of profound hypothermia on the canine central nervous system during one hour of circulatory arrest. *Ann Thorac Surg* 1986; **41**:255-259.

294. Mujsce DJ, Towfighi J, Vannucci RC: Physiologic and neuropathologic aspects of hypothermic circulatory arrest in newborn dogs. *Pediatr Res* 1990; **28**:354-360.

295. Fessatidis IT, Thomas VL, Shore DF, Sedgwick ME, Hunt RH, Weller RO: Brain damage after profoundly hypothermic circulatory arrest: Correlations between neurophysiologic and neuropathologic findings. An experimental study in vertebrates. *J Thorac Cardiovasc Surg* 1993; **106**:32-41.

296. Mezrow CK, Sadeghi AM, Gandsas A, et al: Cerebral blood flow and metabolism in hypothermic circulatory arrest. *Ann Thorac Surg* 1992; **54**:609-616.

297. Tharion J, Johnson DC, Celermajer JM, Hawker RM, Cartmill TB, Overton JH: Profound hypothermia with circulatory arrest. Nine years' clinical experience. *J Thorac Cardiovasc Surg* 1982; **84**:66-72.

298. Ferry PC: Neurologic sequelae of cardiac surgery in children. *Am J Dis Child* 1987; **141**:309-312.

299. Ferry PC: Neurologic sequelae of open-heart surgery in children. An "irritating question." *Am J Dis Child* 1990; **144**:369-373.

300. Brunberg JA, Reilly E, Doty DB: Central nervous system consequences in infants of cardiac surgery using deep hypothermia and circulatory arrest. *Circulation* 1974; **49**(suppl II):II-60-II-68.

301. Newberger JW, Jonas RA, Wernovsky G, et al: A comparison on the perioperative neurologic effects of hypothermic circulatory arrest versus low-flow cardiopulmonary bypass in infant heart surgery. *N Engl J Med* 1993; **329**:1057-1064.

302. Davis EA, Gillinov AM, Cameron DE, Reitz BA: Hypothermic circulatory arrest as a surgical adjunct: A 5-year experience with 60 adult patients. *Ann Thorac Surg* 1992; **53**:402-407.

303. Griepp RB, Ergin MA, Lansman SL, Galla JD, Pogo G: The physiology of hypothermic circulatory arrest. *Semin Thorac Cardiovasc Surg* 1991; **3**:188-193.

304. Svensson LG, Crawford ES, Hess KR, et al: Deep hypothermia with circulatory arrest. Determinants of stroke and early mortality in 656 patients. *J Thorac Cardiovasc Surg* 1993; **106**:19-31.

305. Ergin MA, Galla JD, Lansman SL, Quintana C, Bodian C, Griepp RB: Hypothermic circulatory arrest in operations on the thoracic aorta. Determinants of operative mortality and neurologic outcome. *J Thorac Cardiovasc Surg* 1994; **107**:788-799.

306. Bellinger DC, Jonas RA, Rappaport LA, et al: Developmental and neurologic status of children after heart surgery with hypothermic circulatory arrest or low-flow cardiopulmonary bypass. *N Engl J Med* 1995; **332**:549-555.

307. DeLeon S, Ilbawi M, Arcilla R, et al: Choreoathetosis after deep hypothermia without circulatory arrest. *Ann Thorac Surg* 1990; **50**:714-719.

308. Wical BS, Tomasi LG: A distinctive neurologic syndrome after induced profound hypothermia. *Pediatr Neurol* 1990; **6**:202-205.

309. Robinson RO, Samuels M, Pohl KRE: Choreic syndrome after cardiac surgery. *Arch Dis Child* 1988; **63**:1466-1469.

310. Medlock MD, Cruse RS, Winek SJ, et al: A 10-year experience with postpump chorea. *Ann Neurol* 1993; **34**:820-826.

311. Gillinov AM, Redmond JM, Zehr KJ, et al: Superior cerebral protection with profound hypothermia during circulatory arrest. *Ann Thorac Surg* 1993; **55**:1432-1439.

312. Mujsce DJ, Towfighi J, Heitjan DF, Vannucci RC: Differences in intraischemic temperature influence neurological outcome after deep hypothermic circulatory arrest in newborn dogs. *Stroke* 1994; **25**:1433-1442.

313. Bellinger DC, Wernovsky G, Rappaport LA, et al: Cognitive development of children following early repair of transposition of the

great arteries using deep hypothermic circulatory arrest. *Pediatrics* 1991; **87**:701-707.

314. Kern FH, Jonas RA, Mayer JE, Hanley FL, Castaneda AR, Hickey PR: Temperature monitoring during CPB in infants: Does it predict efficient brain cooling? *Ann Thorac Surg* 1992; **54**:749-754.

315. Dexter F, Hindman BJ: Computer simulation of brain cooling during cardiopulmonary bypass. *Ann Thorac Surg* 1994; **57**:1171-1179.

316. Jonas RA, Bellinger DC, Rappaport LA, et al: Relation of pH strategy and developmental outcome after hypothermic circulatory arrest. *J Thorac Cardiovasc Surg* 1993; **106**:362-368.

317. Payne WS, Theye RA, Kirklin JW: Effect of carbon dioxide on rate of brain cooling during induction of hypothermia by direct blood cooling. *J Surg Res* 1963; **3**:54-57.

318. Watanabe T, Miura M, Inui K, et al: Blood and brain tissue gaseous strategy for profoundly hypothermic total circulatory arrest. *J Thorac Cardiovasc Surg* 1991; **102**:497-504.

319. Hindman BJ, Dexter F, Cutkomp J, Smith T: pH-stat management reduces cerebral metabolic rate for oxygen CMR_{O_2} during profound hypothermia ($17°C$). A study during cardiopulmonary bypass in rabbits. *Anesthesiology* 1995; **82**:983-995.

320. Aoki M, Nomura F, Stromski ME, et al: Effects of pH on brain energetics after hypothermic circulatory arrest. *Ann Thorac Surg* 1993; **55**:1093-1103.

321. Kirshbom PM, Skaryak LR, DeBernardo LR, et al: pH-stat cooling improves cerebral metabolic recovery after circulatory arrest in a piglet model of aortopulmonary collaterals. *J Thorac Cardiovasc Surg* 1996; **111**:147-157.

322. Burrows FA, Jonas RA, Hickey PR: Acid-base management alters cerebral perfusion during cardiopulmonary bypass (abstract). *Anesthesiology* 1994; **81**:A1398.

323. Skaryak LA, Chai PJ, Kern FH, Greeley WJ, Ungerleider RM: Blood gas management and degree of cooling: Effects on cerebral metabolism before and after circulatory arrest. *J Thorac Cardiovasc Surg* 1995; **110**:1649-1657.

324. White BC, Grossman LI, Krause GS: Brain injury by global ischemia and reperfusion: A theoretical perspective on membrane damage and repair. *Neurology* 1993; **43**:1656-1665.

325. Hiramatsu T, Miura T, Forbess JM, et al: pH strategies and cerebral energetics before and after circulatory arrest. *J Thorac Cardiovasc Surg* 1995; **109**:948-958.

326. Wong PC, Barlow CF, Hickey PR, et al: Factors associated with choreoathetosis after cardiopulmonary bypass in children with congenital heart disease. *Circulation* 1992; **86**(suppl II): II-118-II-126.

327. Greeley WJ, Ungerleider RM, Smith LR, Reves JG: The effects of deep hypothermic cardiopulmonary bypass and total circulatory arrest on cerebral blood flow in infants and children. *J Thorac Cardiovasc Surg* 1989; **97**:737-745.

328. Greeley WJ, Ungerleider RM, Kern FH, Brusino FG, Smith LR, Reves JG: Effects of cardiopulmonary bypass on cerebral blood flow in neonates, infants, and children. *Circulation* 1989; **80**(suppl I):I-209-I-215.

329. Astudillo R, van der Linden J, Ekroth R, et al: Absent diastolic cerebral blood flow velocity after circulatory arrest but not after low flow in infants. *Ann Thorac Surg* 1993; **56**:515-519.

330. Burrows FA, Bissonnette B: Cerebral blood flow velocity patterns during cardiac surgery utilizing profound hypothermia with low-flow cardiopulmonary bypass or circulatory arrest in neonates and infants. *Can J Anaesth* 1993; **40**:298-307.

331. O'Hare B, Bissonnette B, Bohn D, Cox P, Williams W: Persistent low cerebral blood flow velocity following profound hypothermic circulatory arrest in infants. *Can J Anaesth* 1995; **42**:964-971.

332. Swain JA, McDonald TJ, Griffith PK, et al: Low-flow hypothermic cardiopulmonary bypass protects the brain. *J Thorac Cardiovasc Surg* 1991; **102**:76-84.

333. Robbins RC, Balaban RS, Swain JA, McDonald TJ, Schneider B, Groom RC: Intermittent hypothermic asanguineous cerebral perfusion (cerebroplegia) protects the brain during prolonged circulatory arrest. A phosphorus 31 nuclear magnetic resonance study. *J Thorac Cardiovasc Surg* 1990; **99**:878-884.

334. Crittenden MD, Roberts CS, Rose L, et al: Brain protection during circulatory arrest. *Ann Thorac Surg* 1991; **51**:942-947.

335. Mault JR, Ohtake S, Klingensmith ME, Heinle JS, Greeley WJ, Ungerleider RM: Cerebral metabolism and circulatory arrest: Effects of duration and strategies for protection. *Ann Thorac Surg* 1993; **55**:57-64.

336. Jonassen AE, Quaegebeur JM, Young WL: Cerebral blood flow velocity in pediatric patients is reduced after cardiopulmonary bypass with profound hypothermia. *J Thorac Cardiovasc Surg* 1995; **110**:934-943.

337. Safi HJ, Brien HW, Winter JN, et al: Brain protection via cerebral retrograde perfusion during aortic arch aneurysm repair. *Ann Thorac Surg* 1993; **56**:270-276.

338. Yasuura K, Okamoto H, Ogawa Y, et al: Resection of aortic aneurysms without aortic clamp technique with the aid of hypothermic total body retrograde perfusion. *J Thorac Cardiovasc Surg* 1994; **107**:1237-1243.

339. Deeb GM, Jenkins E, Bolling SF, et al: Retrograde cerebral perfusion during hypothermic circulatory arrest reduces neurologic morbidity. *J Thorac Cardiovasc Surg* 1995; **109**:259-268.

340. Pagano D, Carey JA, Patel RL, et al: Retrograde cerebral perfusion: Clinical experience in emergency and elective aortic operations. *Ann Thorac Surg* 1995; **59**:393-397.

341. Tönz M, Mihaljevic T, von Swgesser LK, Fehr J, Schmid ER, Turine MI: Acute lung injury during cardiopulmonary bypass. Are the neutrophils responsible? *Chest* 1995; **108**:1551-1556.

342. Sawa Y, Shimazaki Y, Kadoba K, et al: Attenuation of cardiopulmonary bypass-derived inflammatory reactions reduces myocardial reperfusion injury in cardiac operations. *J Thorac Cardiovasc Surg* 1996; **111**:29-35.

343. Hennein HA, Ebba H, Rodriguez JL, et al: Relationship of the proinflammatory cytokines to myocardial ischemia and dysfunction after uncomplicated coronary revascularization. *J Thorac Cardiovasc Surg* 1994; **108**:626-635.

344. Elliott MJ: Ultrafiltration and modified ultrafiltration in pediatric open heart operations. *Ann Thorac Surg* 1993; **56**:1518-1522.

345. Andreasson S, Göthberg S, Berggren H, Bengtsson A, Eriksson E, Risberg B: Hemofiltration modifies complement activation after extracorporeal circulation in infants. *Ann Thorac Surg* 1993; **56**:1515-1517.

346. Millar AB, Armstrong L, van der Linden J, et al: Cytokine production and hemofiltration in children undergoing cardiopulmonary bypass. *Ann Thorac Surg* 1993; **56**:1499-1502.

347. Journois D, Pouard P, Greeley WJ, Mauriat P, Vouhé P, Safran D: Hemofiltration during cardiopulmonary bypass in pediatric cardiac surgery. Effects on hemostasis, cytokines, and complement components. *Anesthesiology* 1994; **81**:1181-1189.

348. Journois D, Israel-Biet D, Pouard P, et al: High-volume, zero-balanced hemofiltration to reduce delayed inflammatory response to cardiopulmonary bypass in children. *Anesthesiology* 1996; **85**:965-976.

349. Skaryak LA, Kirshbom PM, DiBernardo LR, et al: Modified ultrafiltration improves cerebral metabolic recovery after circulatory arrest. *J Thorac Cardiovasc Surg* 1995; **109**:744-752.

350. Cole DJ, Drummond JC, Shapiro HM, Hertzog RE, Brauer FS: The effect of hypervolemic hemodilution with and without hypertension on cerebral blood flow following middle cerebral artery occlusion in rats anesthetized with isoflurane. *Anesthesiology* 1989; **71**:580-585.

351. Korosue K, Heros RC: Mechanism of cerebral blood flow augmentation by hemodilution in rabbits. *Stroke* 1992; **23**:1487-1493.

352. Cole DJ, Schell RM, Drummond JC, Reynolds L: Focal cerebral ischemia in rats. Effect of hypervolemic hemodilution with diaspirin cross-linked hemoglobin versus albumin on brain injury and edema. *Anesthesiology* 1993; **78:**335-342.

353. Tu YK, Heros RC, Karacostas D, et al: Isovolemic hemodilution in experimental focal cerebral ischemia. Part 2: Effects on regional cerebral blood flow and size of infarction. *J Neurosurg* 1988; **69:**82-91.

354. Koller M, Haenny P, Hess K, Weniger D, Zangger P: Adjusted hypervolemic hemodilution in acute ischemic stroke. *Stroke* 1990; **21:**1429-1434.

355. Goslinga H, Eijzenbach V, Heuvelmans JHA, et al: Cust-tailored hemodilution with albumin and crystalloids in acute ischemic stroke. *Stroke* 1992; **23:**181-188.

356. Italian Acute Stroke Study Group: Haemodilution in acute stroke: Results of the Italian hemodilution trial. *Lancet* 1988; **i:**318-321.

357. Scandinavian Stroke Study Group: Multicenter trial of hemodilution in acute ischemic stroke. I. Results in the total patient population. *Stroke* 1987; **18:**691-699.

358. The Hemodilution in Stroke Study Group: Hypervolemic hemodilution treatment of acute stroke. Results of a randomized multicenter trial using pentastarch. *Stroke* 1989; **20:**317-323.

359. Mast H, Marx P: Neurological deterioration under isovolemic hemodilution with hydroxyethyl starch in acute cerebral ischemia. *Stroke* 1991; **22:**680-683.

360. Todd MM, Wu B, Maktabi M, Hindman BJ, Warner DS: Cerebral blood flow and oxygen delivery during hypoxemia and hemodilution: The role of arterial oxygen content. *Am J Physiol* 1994; **267:**H2025-H2031.

361. Lee SH, Heros RC, Mullan JC, Korosue K: Optimum degree of hemodilution for brain protection in a canine model of focal cerebral ischemia. *J Neurosurg* 1994; **80:**469-475.

362. Reasoner DK, Ryu KH, Hindman BJ, Cutkomp J, Smith T: Marked hemodilution increases neurologic injury following focal cerebral ischemia in rabbits. *Anesth Analg* 1996; **82:**61-67.

363. Practice guidelines for blood component therapy. A report by the American Society of Anesthesiologists Task Force on blood component therapy. *Anesthesiology* 1996; **84:**732-747.

Index